Biological Control of Locusts and Grasshoppers

Proceedings of a Workshop held at the International Institute of Tropical Agriculture, Cotonou, Republic of Benin, 29 April–1 May 1991

Edited by

C.J. Lomer & C. Prior

International Institute of Biological Control

C·A·B International

in association with

International Institute of Tropical Agriculture

C·A·B International
Wallingford
Oxon OX10 8DE
UK

Tel: Wallingford (0491) 32111
Telex: 847964 (COMAGG G)
Telecom Gold/Dialcom: 84: CAU001
Fax: (0491) 33508

Published on behalf of
International Institute of Tropical Agriculture
Oyo Road
PMB 5320
Ibadan
Nigeria
Tel: (234 22) 400 300
Telex: TDS IBA NG 31417 TROPIB NG

in association with

International Institute of Biological Control
(an Institute of C·A·B International)
Silwood Park
Buckhurst Road
Ascot
Berkshire SL5 7TA
UK
Tel: 0344 872999
Telex: 9312102255 BC G
Telecom Gold/Dialcom: 84: CAU015
Fax: 0344 872901

For full details of services available from the International Institute of Biological Control please contact the Institute Director at the address given here

A catalogue entry for this title is available from the British Library

ISBN 0 85198 779 6

Typeset by Leaper & Gard Ltd, Bristol
Printed and bound in the UK by Redwood Press Ltd, Melksham

Contents

Foreword
Locust control – cause for concern ix
Lukas Brader

Preface xi

Acknowledgements xii

Welcome address 1
Representative of the Minister for National Education

Keynote address
Biological control as a potential tool for locust and grasshopper control 4
D.J. Greathead

The IIBC/IITA/DFPV collaborative research programme on the biological control of locusts and grasshoppers 8
C. Prior, C.J. Lomer, H. Herren, A. Paraïso, C. Kooyman & J.J. Smit

Section I: Organizations Concerned with Locust and Grasshopper Control, and Country Reports

APHIS; grasshopper integrated pest management in the United States – a co-operative project with emphasis on biological control 21
G.L. Cunningham

CEC; biological control of locusts with entomopathogens 26
B. Zelazny

CILSS/DFPV; the Permanent Interstate Committee for Drought Control in the Sahel, and the Department of Crop Protection Training, Niger 30
J.J. Smit

CNLA; short report on the control strategy of acridids in Morocco 1987–89 38
A. Mouhim

DLCOEA; pest control: the begging questions 41
R.A. Kitenda

GTZ; the integrated biological control of locusts and grasshoppers – a GTZ research project 44
S. Krall & O.M. Nasseh

IAPSC/OAU; communiqué from the Inter-African Scientific Secretariat of the OAU, with comments on the application of the Inter-African Plant Protection Convention 50
N. Nkouka

ICIPE; development of a biocontrol strategy for the management of the desert locust, *Schistocerca gregaria* 54
S.K. Raina

IRLCOCSA; perspectives and prospects of biological control of the red locust, *Nomadacris septemfasciata* 57
J.W. Bahana & E.K. Byaruhanga

NRI; statement of position 64
J.I. Magor

OCLALAV; biological control of migratory pests, and perspectives in Africa 70
A.B. Ndiaye

PRIFAS: notes from PRIFAS on biological control of locusts and grasshoppers 75
M.H. Launois-Luong

Country Reports

Congo; the acridid situation in the Congo 79
G. Bani

Mali; notes on the acridid problem in Mali 82
B. Maiga

Republic of Benin; the acridid situation in the Republic of Benin 86
A. Coffi

Senegal; grasshopper and locust control in Senegal 90
A. Niassy

Sudan; the situation of desert locust, tree locust and grasshoppers in the Sudan (1990–91) 97
A. Abdalla

Discussion: precis 99

Section II: Agents for Biocontrol

Natural enemies of tropical locusts and grasshoppers: their impact and potential as biological control agents 105
D.J. Greathead

Fungal agents for biocontrol 122
M.S. Goettel

Preliminary studies on the ecology of *Zonocerus variegatus* in the Republic of Benin 133
A. Paraïso, C.J. Lomer, I. Godonou & D. Kpindu

Effects of neem oil treatment on the phase status of desert locust, *Schistocerca gregaria* 142
J. Langewald & H. Schmutterer

Panel discussion: precis 155

Section III: Exploration and Characterization

Discovery and characterization of fungal pathogens for locust and grasshopper control 159
C. Prior

Mechanisms of fungal pathogenesis in insects with particular reference to locusts 181
A.K. Charnley

Molecular approaches to the study of entomopathogenic fungi 191
J.M. Clarkson

Selection and characterization of strains of *Metarhizium anisopliae* for control of soil insects in Australia 200
R.J. Milner

Exploration for locust and grasshopper pathogens 208
C. Kooyman & P. Shah

Panel discussion: precis 214

Section IV: Mass Production, Application and Formulation

Mass production, formulation and application of fungi as biocontrol agents 219
B.A. Auld

Mass production, formulation and field application of entomopathogenic fungi 230
M.S. Goettel & D.W. Roberts

Mass production, application and formulation of *Metarhizium anisopliae* for control of sugarcane froghopper, *Mahanarva posticata*, in Brazil 239
A.F. Mendonça

The principles of ultra-low volume spraying in relation to the application of microbial insecticides for locust control 245
G.A. Matthews

Controlled droplet application of mycopesticides to locusts 249
R.P. Bateman

Development of a novel field bioassay technique for assessing mycoinsecticide ULV formulations 255
R.P. Bateman, I. Godonou, D. Kpindu, C.J. Lomer & A. Paraïso

Panel discussion: precis 263

Section V: Biology, Ecology, Field Experimentation and Environmental Impact

Introduction: biology, ecology, field experimentation and environmental impact 267
D.L. Johnson

The *Beauveria–Melolontha* project: experiences with regard to locust and grasshopper control 279
S. Keller

Biological control of grasshoppers in the Cape Verde Islands 287
M.L. Lobo Lima, J.M. Brito & J.E. Henry

Field trials with the entomopathogenic fungus *Beauveria bassiana* against grasshoppers in Mali, West Africa, July, 1990 296
D.L. Johnson, M.S. Goettel, C. Bradley, H. van der Paauw & B. Maiga

Field cage trials on the effects of enriched neem oil, insect growth regulators and the pathogens *Beauveria bassiana* and *Nosema locustae* on desert locusts in the Republic of Niger 311
O.M. Nasseh, T. Freres, J. Wilps, E. Kirkilionis & S. Krall

Effects of neem oil, *Beauveria bassiana* and dieldrin on non-target tenebrionid beetles in the desert zone of the Republic of Niger 321
R. Peveling & J. Weyrich

The effect of various neem products on the survival and flight activity of adult *Schistocerca gregaria* 337
H. Wilps, O. Nasseh & S. Krall

A review of field studies of the environmental impacts of locust/grasshopper control programmes in Africa 347
P.C. Matteson

Environmental impact and safety of fungal biocontrol agents 356
M.S. Goettel & D.L. Johnson

Panel discussion: precis 362

Section VI: Closing Session

Discussion: precis 369

Acronyms and abbreviations 375

Addresses of delegates 378

Author index 387

Subject index 388

Foreword
Locust control – cause for concern

Lukas Brader

Director General, International Institute of Tropical Agriculture (IITA), Ibadan, Nigeria, former Director of the FAO Emergency Centre for Locust Operations (ECLO), Rome, Italy.

Locusts have caused problems to man's agricultural efforts and well being ever since the first historical records. During the 1930s to 1960s, a period of sustained locust attack, research by a number of institutions including the Anti-Locust Research Centre led to the development of effective control strategies. These were based on effective monitoring and forecasting and using mainly dieldrin, primarily to lay down persistent barriers to control hopper bands.

The period from 1960s to 1985 was a remarkably quiet time for locusts, the longest inter-plague period known. Regretfully, locust surveillance, control and research were allowed to run down at the same time. Also during this period, the rise of environmental concerns led to the banning of many persistent organochlorine insecticides including dieldrin. Another development of note was that legislation adopted in the USA (and later elsewhere) arising from concerns about dumping of toxic chemicals in developing countries, made it impossible for countries in receipt of US aid to carry on using dieldrin.

Thus when locust plagues did recur in 1985, not only were organizations charged with control and monitoring unprepared, they had also been deprived of their most powerful weapon for hopper control. The less persistent organophosphates, carbamates and more recently the synthetic pyrethroids used in place of dieldrin made hopper control more complicated because they had to be sprayed over the whole infested area and had to be applied much more frequently. As such, they have led to undesirable environmental effects of their own. However, for the control of adults, these new insecticides proved very useful.

The challenge is now to develop effective control measures and strategies, including biological control methods, which will have reduced environmental effects, lower costs and equal or greater effectiveness than existing methods. Problems in application will always remain; the huge extent of the locust recession areas, and their inaccessibility will make locust control always a difficult job. Models predicting outbreaks are still unreliable and despite the advances made in the use of satellite technology, we still rely on ground reports for most of our information.

The ideas presented in this volume give some indication of the new possibilities for control offered by biological means.

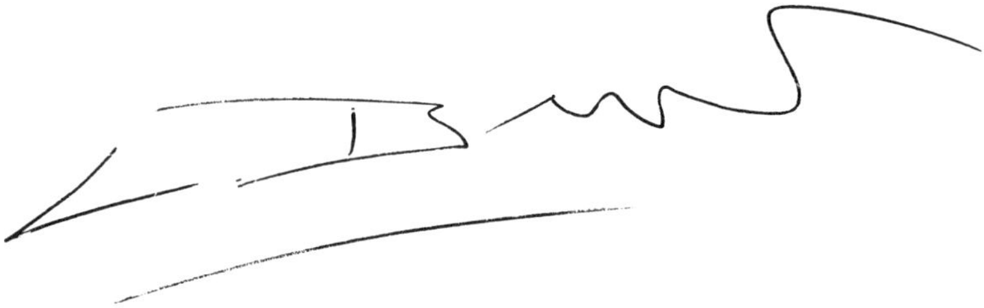

Preface

This volume contains the proceedings of a workshop on biological control of locusts and grasshoppers, held at Cotonou, Republic of Benin, from 29 April to 1 May 1991. The workshop was funded by a grant from USAID, and organized as part of the joint IIBC/IITA/DFPV collaborative research programme on the biological control of locusts and grasshoppers. Details of the programme are given in the relevant section of this book. The programme is funded by CIDA, USAID, ODA and DGIS.

The workshop was originally planned as a working forum to discuss subjects specifically relevant to the programme; however, the response to invitations sent out was so great that the concept had to be expanded to include a variety of peripheral topics. Nevertheless, useful discussion took place, some of which is summarized here.

The talks presented at the workshop have been edited, translated from French where necessary, and refereed in the case of all but the first section. The first section (I) consists of summaries of the activities of various organizations involved in locust and grasshopper control and some country reports.

The remaining sections cover technical aspects of locust and grasshopper biocontrol; (II) agents for biocontrol; (III) exploration and characterization; (IV) mass production, application and formulation; and (V) biology, ecology, field experimentation and environmental impact. An edited precis of the discussions in the closing session (VI) is also presented. We invited speakers who have had practical experience in the use of fungi for biocontrol in a variety of situations; in sugarcane in Brazil, in forests in Switzerland, in grassland in Australia. As the reader will note, there seems to be a great mood of optimism concerning the possibilities for control using fungi, and we hope that the information presented here will encourage others to try for themselves.

A French version will be produced in due course.

Acknowledgements

The conference organizers greatly appreciate the consideration and co-operation shown by the government of our host country, the Republic of Benin.

We would like to thank all the speakers who presented papers and also those who contributed from the floor to the discussions. Speakers and referees provided their written texts promptly and we thank them for enabling us to produce these proceedings with the minimum of delay.

Jacob Quaye and Samson Acheyompong (IITA-BCP) provided invaluable logistical support.

We are very grateful to Annette Greathead for meticulous copy editing, to Clare Lord, Oscar Hounvou and Carole Moudachirou for simultaneous translation during the meeting, and to Cecile Lomer who collated the manuscripts and translated the French texts.

The workshop was financed out of grant AFR-0517-G-IN-9096-00 from USAID and we are grateful to Dr W. Knausenberger of USAID (Africa Bureau) and to all our donors for their material support and encouragement.

Welcome address

Representative of the Minister for National Education

The Representative of the Minister for Rural Development and Cooperative Action, Representatives of International Organizations, Representatives of Donor Agencies, The Director of the International Institute of Biological Control, The Representative of the International Institute of Tropical Agriculture, The Director of the Biological Control Centre for Africa, Representatives of National Plant Protection Organizations, Honoured Guests and Research Scientists, Ladies and Gentlemen:

I am delighted to welcome to Cotonou scientific experts and all those partners in scientific development who have kindly come to Africa to the free territory of Benin to exchange views and experiences in the field of biological control of locusts and grasshoppers, which are major pests of crops in the tropical and Mediterranean zones of Africa and also world-wide.

Your acceptance of this invitation from IITA and IIBC demonstrates without doubt, the interest which the international community shows in the vast regions of Africa which are subject to invasions by grasshoppers. Those of you here in Cotonou, are, by your very presence, lending your support to the new biological control project run jointly by IITA and IIBC at the IITA research station at Abomey-Calavi, which is trying to curb this scourge. This is a project in which the Beninois government and people, and all African farmers have a great deal of hope.

In fact, despite strenuous financial efforts by donors, it is an inescapable fact that chemical means of control are not sufficient to give lasting respite from the pressure of locusts and grasshoppers, which jeopardise the best laid plans for ensuring adequate food supplies every year, in every affected region. Besides this, when one knows that the solution offered by chemical pesticides is compromised by the environmental effect of the chemicals entering the food chain and affecting the environment, the importance of biological control in this domain can be clearly appreciated.

Ladies and gentlemen involved in scientific research:

Let me tell you that all African farmers, people concerned with socio-economic development and the populations of both town and country await with impatience new technical packages which your work will bring to National Plant Protection programmes and to farmers. I must remind you that this workshop gives you a good opportunity to examine critically your results, your methods and the obstacles which impede the rapid development of biological control techniques for locusts and grasshoppers. This forum also gives you a chance to work out the most effective strategies for acquiring a better grasp of the pathology of these insects, production of pathogens, application and field trials, related ecological problems and regional and international co-operation.

In this respect, this workshop – the first of its kind – is only the first step in a long process, for there is still so much work to be done, the stakes are so important and the subject so interesting. Here we should thank the donors for making their funds available and for their solicitude. I am convinced that they still believe in the cause and will spare no effort to hold regular meetings of this kind where scientists from different disciplines and sectors can meet to agree upon effective action.

Now I shall address myself particularly to the representatives of National Plant Protection organizations.

In the process of developing appropriate biological control techniques against locusts and grasshoppers, it seems to me that you have a particularly heavy responsibility, since you are at the same time those who must act and those who benefit.

Your active contribution is required in the exploration phase and in the characterization of diseases of local Orthoptera, in identifying fungi and other natural pathogens of the insects and in defining optimum rearing conditions. As beneficiaries, you are under an obligation to master the techniques for *in situ* experimentation, methods of evaluating the impact of biological pesticides on the environment and the norms and methods of applying formulations in the field. You will not be able to fulfill your role without interesting the powers that be whom you must inform, and enlisting the co-operation of the populace whom you must impress and whose confidence you must gain.

The Representative of the Minister for Rural Development and Cooperative Action, Ladies and Gentlemen:

The organization of a forum at this level involves important undertakings and this is why I should like to thank all those who have been kind enough to lend their support.

I should like to mention USAID, GTZ, UNDP, USDA/APHIS.

My thanks also to IITA and IIBC who have made this workshop possible.

Once more, I thank national, international and non-governmental organizations and institutes, from far or near, who have all contributed to the present gathering, and all those research scientists who agreed to come here and take part in this meeting.

Wishing you the very best success in your work, I declare open, on this day Monday 29 April at Cotonou, the Workshop on Biological Control of Locusts and Grasshoppers.

Thank you.

Keynote address
Biological control as a potential tool for locust and grasshopper control

D.J. Greathead

International Institute of Biological Control.

In 1985, near normal rains over much of Africa for the first time after a prolonged period of dry years triggered the development of widespread infestations of grasshoppers in West Africa; principally the Senegalese grasshopper, *Oedaleus senegalensis* (Krauss) in the northern part but also several other species further south. There were also simultaneous upsurges in the populations of the four species of locusts of major importance in tropical Africa for the first time in 50 years. A year later desert locust, *Schistocerca gregaria* (Forskål), numbers had reached plague proportions and threatened countries throughout its invasion area in Africa, the most alarming development since the last major plague collapsed in 1963. Breeding conditions remained favourable through 1986–88. During this period countries from Senegal and Mauritania in the west to Iran in the east were affected by swarms and hopper bands (Brader, 1988; OTA, 1990). Also, desert locust swarms crossed the Atlantic confounding the predictions of the experts that this could not happen (Ritchie & Pedgley, 1989). However, the desert locust plague collapsed in 1989 after failure of the rains during the winter breeding season. Unfortunately, because of the unprecedentedly long recession period, national and regional locust control organizations had been allowed to run down and were short of resources and expertise to combat the plague.

Locust control had depended on ultra-low volume (ULV) application of dieldrin for many years following research during the 1949–63 plague. This technique was particularly valuable for controlling hopper bands because a grid of sprayed swaths could be laid down which persisted throughout a season and killed any bands stopping to feed as they crossed them. Dieldrin was also valuable for swarm control but had begun to be replaced by less persistent organophosphates such as malathion. However, concern about the effects of persistent pesticides on the environment and the banning of dieldrin in many countries at the end of the 1970s, including countries affected by locusts, forced the abandonment of this product. One consequence is the need to apply repeated blanket sprays over large areas to achieve the same results as formerly provided by single applications of dieldrin over a fraction of the area (Brader, 1988; OTA, 1990).

The donor community responded to the crisis by contributing some US$275 million towards locust and grasshopper control mainly in the Sahel and north-west Africa (Table 1). As a result of this donor assistance and their own resources, about 4.6 million ha of land in 10 countries received aerial or ground insecticide treatments in 1986–7 against locusts or grasshoppers, and 10 million ha were sprayed in 1988. Some 13 million l of insecticides were applied, mostly malathion and fenitrothion. The large-scale repeated application of insecticides raised concern about the possible impact on the environment as well as on human health (OTA, 1990). A pilot study on behalf of the FAO measured the impact of organophosphate insecticides and an insect growth regulator on insects, birds, aquatic invertebrates and fish. Adverse effects were recorded on all these categories of non-target organisms, including families containing natural enemies of locusts and grasshoppers, by one or more of the test chemicals (Everts, 1990).

Clearly, a reassessment of locust control methods was required and the FAO convened a desert locust research conference entitled *Defining Future Research Priorities* in October 1988. *Inter alia* the conference considered alternatives to chemical pesticides for locust control and 'expressed its great interest in the ideas' put forward by IIBC for research on the possibility of developing a biological pesticide (FAO, 1989). These ideas (Prior & Greathead, 1989) were developed into a proposal for a research programme by the International Institute of Biological Control (IIBC) of CAB International. This was eventually funded by the Canadian International Development Agency (CIDA), the Directorate General for Development Cooperation of the Netherlands (DGIS), the Overseas Development Administration of the UK (ODA) and the United States Agency

Table 1. Donor assistance to locust and grasshopper control programmes, 1986–89 in US$.

Bilateral donors	192,060,553
Multilateral donors	60,545,175
NGOs	2,455,460
Additional contributions	20,000,000
Total	**275,061,188**

From OTA (1990).

for International Development (USAID). It began in 1989 as a collaborative three year programme being undertaken by IIBC, the International Institute of Tropical Agriculture (IITA) and the Département de Formation en Protection des Végétaux (DFPV) in Niger.

This programme, entitled *Biological Control of Locusts and Grasshoppers*, has as its essential objective demonstration of the technical feasibility of killing locusts and grasshoppers using an oil-based formulation of a fungal pathogen, and involves the following components:

1. exploration for pathogens
2. evaluation of these pathogens as potential active ingredients of a biological pesticide
3. population ecology of locusts and grasshoppers in relation to the effects of pathogens
4. formulation of pathogens for ULV application
5. application of pathogens to demonstrate their efficacy as a control agent
6. development of mass production methods for pathogen spores (IIBC, 1990)

Although the programme had its origin in the concern generated by the desert locust plague and the massive application of pesticides applied to control it, the objective includes grasshoppers. The reasons for this are very important. Firstly, analysis of the desert locust plague by the US Congress Office of Technology Assessment (OTA), based partly on a questionnaire sent to individuals and organizations concerned with locust control, concludes that grasshoppers may be responsible for 5–18% of crop loss in each year (OTA, 1990) whereas locusts do not cause more than 4% loss even in peak plague years (Bullen, 1972). Thus, grasshoppers constitute a continuing and more serious threat every year than locusts during plague years only. Secondly, because of the intermittent nature of locust plagues, a product used for locust control and which cannot be stockpiled is most unlikely to continue to be produced during inter-plague periods unless it has other uses. Therefore, a product which is used to control grasshoppers will be in continuous production so that all that is needed if there is an upsurge in locust activity will be an increase in production to meet the emergency.

This address has outlined the circumstances leading to the initiation of the locust and grasshopper biological control programme and its rationale. We, the collaborating institutes, believe that we have made good progress in meeting the objectives of the programme and are proud of our achievements so far. This conference has been convened to discuss progress, obtain the views of specialists in the various disciplines involved in its execution, and most important, to inform and solicit guidance from the countries and organizations which will eventually have the opportunity to use any product which is developed. Steps are being taken on behalf of the donors to ensure, by means of protective patents, that the results will be freely available to affected countries so that they can benefit from setting up their own production plants, and as far as possible make use of cheap locally available materials to manufacture the product.

The conference has been planned in such a way as to provide an authoritative review of each main topic by a specialist, followed by a discussion led by expert panellists during which it is hoped that you will contribute. The formal reviews, contributed papers, and a summary of the discussions and conclusions will be published to provide a statement of the state of the art for biological control of locusts and grasshoppers in the tropics. I look forward to an informative and stimulating few days, and in advance would like to thank all those whose efforts have made this conference possible and hopefully a big success.

References

Brader, L. (1988) Control of grasshopper and migratory locusts. *Brighton Crop Protection Conference (Pests and Diseases)* **1988**, 283–288.

Bullen, F.T. (1972) A review of the assessment of crop losses caused by locusts and grasshoppers. In: Hemming, C.F. & Taylor, T.H.C. (eds), *Proceedings of the International Study Conference on Current and Future Problems of Acridology*, London, 6–16 July 1970. Centre for Overseas Pest Research, London, 163–169.

Everts, J.W. (Ed.) (1990) *Environmental Effects of Chemical Locust and Grasshopper Control. A Pilot Study.* Project ECLO/SEN/003/NET Project Report FAO, Rome.

FAO (Food and Agriculture Organization of the United Nations) (1989) Report of the meeting on desert locust research. 'Defining future research priorities'. 18–20 October 1988. FAO, Rome.

IIBC (1990) *Biological Control of Locusts & Grasshoppers. A Collaborative Programme.* CAB International leaflet, Wallingford.

OTA (Office of Technology Assessment) (1990) *A Plague of Locusts – Special Report OTA-F-450.* US Government Printing Office, Washington, DC.

Prior, C. & Greathead, D.J. (1989) Biological control of locusts: the potential for the exploitation of pathogens. *FAO Plant Protection Bulletin* **37**, 37–48.

Ritchie, M. & Pedgley, D. (1989) Desert locusts across the Atlantic. *Antenna* **13**, 10–12.

The IIBC/IITA/DFPV collaborative research programme on the biological control of locusts and grasshoppers

C. Prior, C.J. Lomer

International Institute of Biological Control.

H. Herren, A. Paraïso

International Institute of Tropical Agriculture.

C. Kooyman, J.J. Smit

Département de Formation en Protection des Végétaux.

Introduction

Locusts (particularly the desert locust, *Schistocerca gregaria* (Forskål)) and grasshoppers (*Oedaleus senegalensis* (Krauss), *Kraussaria angulifera* (Krauss) and many other species) are the most serious insect pests of agriculture in the Sahel (Geddes, 1990). In plague years swarms of the desert locust may attack crops from West Africa to India (Steedman, 1990). Both grasshoppers and locusts frequently require chemical control measures. The campaign against the desert locust outbreak which began in 1985 had cost US$150 million by 1988, with approximately US$70 million of this cost borne by the afflicted countries (Brader, 1988). In 1988 alone, US$100 million was spent on desert locust control (Anon., 1990). Costs for grasshopper control in 1986–87 amounted to US$62 million (Brader, 1988).

The insecticide formerly favoured for desert locust control was dieldrin, which persists for months after application. This was very effective at very low doses per hectare, but is now banned in most countries where control is required because of concern about environmental damage and the hazard to health of humans and livestock. The most recent plague was fought with a variety of less persistent pesticides, of which the most frequently used were fenitrothion and malathion. These are less effective precisely because they are less persistent, and may give inadequate control (Brader, 1988). As a result of the switch to these somewhat more environmentally acceptable pesticides, control costs have risen tenfold (Brader, 1988). The amounts of pesticide applied have also greatly increased, because several applications may now be necessary instead of only one of dieldrin.

The very high cost of these control operations and the concerns expressed about their effectiveness have led to unease among the donor community, especially in the USA which provides 20% of donor support (Anon., 1990). Brader (1988) noted that the ban on dieldrin should be an incentive to review control strategies and to carry out research on new control methods, including biological control. This approach was reviewed by Prior & Greathead (1989), who discussed the range of biological agents that may attack the desert locust and concluded that the only viable approach was to develop the entomopathogenic Deuteromycotina *Metarhizium* spp. and *Beauveria* spp. as biological insecticides. The reasons for this are reviewed below.

Biology of locusts and their natural enemies

During recession periods between plagues, desert locusts occur as very sparse populations of individuals in the solitary phase, which cause no damage. When conditions for breeding become more favourable, usually as a result of rainfall which provides more areas of soft soil for egg laying, populations increase and the insects switch to the gregarious phase. Hopper bands and adult swarms then form and the latter migrate very large distances by flying, following well-documented wind patterns. Because of the great fecundity of locusts, huge numbers may appear very rapidly when breeding conditions are favourable: a swarm may contain up to 50 million adults/km^2, and in 1988 there were swarms in Sudan covering 150 km^2 (Brader, 1988). A major invasion of swarms may weigh 100,000 tonnes and eat this much green vegetation every day.

If breeding areas were both predictable and accessible, treatment of egg fields or hopper bands would be the preferred approach to control. When dieldrin was used, swaths were laid down in the desert which persisted for many months and effectively controlled hoppers which marched into them. If hoppers are to be treated with non-persistent insecticides it is essential either to treat the whole area or to find and treat every band, but neither of these approaches is feasible. The total areas involved are too great for economic treatment and the environmental damage would also be unacceptable. Surveys for hoppers cannot normally hope to detect more than a small fraction of the bands in a given area, but >90% must be killed to give useful control (Brader, 1988). In addition many breeding areas are not accessible due to remoteness or military activity. It is therefore often necessary to adopt a 'firefighting' approach which involves detecting adult swarms and treating them before they arrive at agriculturally important areas.

If adult swarms are the target then a suitable biological agent must have certain properties to be effective against them. Prior & Greathead (1989) noted that although the arthropod predators and parasitoids of locusts had a major role in hastening the end of plagues they were unsuitable for manipulation, and migratory pests such as the desert locust were poor targets for classical biological control. Pathogens showed more promise, because some of these could be manipulated as biological pesticides. This allows the possibility of using conventional application technology, including aerial spraying, which is already highly developed for locust control.

The known pathogens of locusts and grasshoppers include entomopoxviruses of unknown host range and pathogenicity, a single record of a baculovirus in desert locust, several protozoa including the well-studied *Nosema locustae* Canning, mermithid nematodes, several opportunistic, wound-infecting bacteria such as *Serratia marcescens* Bizio and *Pseudomonas aeruginosa* (Schroeter) with a wide host range including mammals, the fungus *Entomophaga grylli* (Fresenius) Batko, sensu lato, and deuteromycete fungi in the genera *Metarhizium, Beauveria, Nomuraea, Paecilomyces* and *Verticillium* (Prior & Greathead, 1989).

To be effective as a biopesticide, the properties of a pathogen must include cheap and easy production, safety and host specificity, application using existing technology, rapid action. Only the entomopathogenic deuteromycetes, especially *Metarhizium* spp. and *Beauveria* spp., fulfil these requirements. They also have the additional advantage of penetration directly through the cuticle, whereas all other agents have to be ingested. These fungi can therefore be used as contact pesticides, and there is no need for them to persist in the harsh desert environment for the target insects to find and eat them before infection can occur. However, it will be necessary to show that they can infect successfully under conditions of high temperature and low relative humidity.

Formulation and application of fungal pathogens for locust control

In 1988/89, IIBC developed a joint proposal with the Biological Control Programme Centre of the International Institute of Tropical Agriculture (IITA) at its station in Cotonou, Republic of Benin, and the Département de Formation en Protection des Végétaux (DFPV) in Niger for the biological control of locusts and grasshoppers. The core of this proposal was research on the development of formulations of the conidia of entomopathogenic deuteromycetes which would be effective under arid conditions and suitable for application using controlled droplet application (CDA) technology at ultra-low volume (ULV) rates.

The most commonly recorded fungi in this group which attack locusts and grasshoppers are *Metarhizium anisopliae* (Metschnikoff) Sorokin, *M. flavoviride* W. Gams & J. Rozsypal and *Beauveria bassiana* (Balsamo) Vuillemin. Conidia, the natural units of dispersal, and blastospores, which are thin-walled spores produced in submerged culture, are both pathogenic but conidia are more stable. The conidia of *Metarhizium* spp. and *Beauveria* spp. are hydrophobic and difficult to disperse in water, but they are lipophilic and can be suspended easily in oils. Insect cuticles are also hydrophobic, but oils spread readily over the epicuticle which contains a high proportion of waxes. A suspension of conidia in oil therefore adheres readily to the cuticle. The oils may also have the additional advantages of protecting the conidia from desiccation, thus encouraging germination when ambient humidity is low, and spreading them to the intersegmental membranes where penetration may occur most easily. Some evidence for this was obtained by Prior *et al.* (1988), who found that the LD_{50} of conidia of *B. bassiana* for the cocoa weevil pest *Pantorhytes plutus* (Oberthür) (Coleoptera: Curculionidae) was over thirty times lower if the conidia were suspended in a vegetable oil instead of water.

There was no evidence from the work on *P. plutus* that such an effect could be demonstrated at low humidities. However, Marcandier & Khachatourians (1987) showed that when the grasshopper *Melanoplus sanguinipes* (Fabricius) was inoculated with an aqueous suspension of *Beauveria bassiana* conidia, the rate and level of mortality was unaffected by the relative humidity during subsequent incubation, and the LT_{50} was 7–8 days whether the RH was 100%, 33% or 12%.

It thus appears possible to kill grasshoppers by topical application of *B. bassiana* even at very low relative humidity, and to greatly reduce the dose of fungus required by formulating in oils instead of water. Oil formulation would have the additional advantage that conventional CDA equipment could be used, at ULV rates. CDA is a more efficient way to apply pesticides than conventional methods of atomization, but it is essential to formulate in non-volatile diluents to avoid evaporation of the very small spray droplets. Oils are frequently used for this purpose.

CDA techniques are well-adapted to ULV application rates and are essential where the formulation must be applied by air, as is often the case for *Schistocerca gregaria* (Forskål). The technology of ULV application was developed for locust control and the logistical infrastructure already exists. There are also good prospects for controlling a variety of economically important grasshoppers by ULV spraying. Unlike locusts, it would be feasible to tackle grasshoppers by ground based spraying. The technology for fungus production and application would be in place for grasshopper control at times when locusts are in recession and this would also ensure its availability for locust control in plague years.

Four international donor agencies agreed to contribute to a three year research programme to demonstrate the feasibility of this approach to locust and grasshopper control. These are the Canadian International Development Agency (CIDA), the Netherlands Directorate General for Development Cooperation (DGIS), the UK Overseas Development Administration (ODA) and the USA Agency for International Development (USAID). Work began in October 1989.

Research organization and progress October 1989–April 1991

The programme at IIBC, UK

Are suitable fungal pathogens available?

Surveys are being undertaken in West Africa, Oman and Pakistan for new isolates of suitable fungi, and existing isolates from culture collections are also being tested. An assay technique has been developed using topical application of a standard dose of 75,000 conidia/insect in oil to adult *S. gregaria.* After inoculation the insects are held unfed in plastic boxes at 30°C and mortality is measured over a 7 day period. This method discriminates satisfactorily between the majority of isolates which cause no mortality during this period, and a few which cause mortality beginning on day 4 and rising to >90% by day 6.

All isolates highly virulent to *S. gregaria* which have been tested to date are in the genus *Metarhizium* and have originated from Orthoptera. The isolate adopted as a standard and used in all assays for comparison is *M. flavoviride* IMI 330189 which originated from the grasshopper *Ornithacris cavroisi* (Finot) collected in Niger. Other isolates which are highly virulent to *S. gregaria* are: *M. flavoviride* IMI 324673 ex *Zonocerus elegans* (Thunberg), Tanzania; *M. anisopliae* IMI 168777ii ex *S. gregaria,* Ethiopia; *M. anisopliae* ARSEF 324 ex *Austracris guttulosa* (= *Patanga guttulosa* (Walker)), Australia.

No highly virulent isolates have yet been found originating in non-orthopteran hosts, although some coleopteran isolates showed moderate virulence. No isolates of *Beauveria* spp. have yet been found which are more than weakly virulent to *S. gregaria,* even those which originated from the host itself or other acridids. This may be due to the high temperature (30°C) at which the assays are conducted.

It would appear from the limited evidence to date that *Metarhizium* spp. are more likely than *Beauveria* spp. to be virulent, and isolates from Orthoptera are more likely to be virulent than those from other orders. However, many cases are known of an isolate from one order showing virulence to an insect in another order (Prior, 1990) and it would be premature to draw any conclusions yet on the most favourable sources of useful genotypes. It is clear that highly virulent isolates are available, both from *S. gregaria* and from taxonomically related hosts, even if the latter are geographically isolated from it.

Can infection occur at low humidity and high temperature using suitable diluents?

The relative humidity in the bioassay boxes is approximately 35% and it would therefore appear that these results support the claim by Marcandier & Khachatourians (1987) that infection can occur at low RH following topical application. Mortality also occurs under these conditions following inoculation with an aqueous suspension of conidia, but the mortality peak is delayed by about two days. Comparative LD_{50} determinations for oil and water have not yet been carried out, but it would appear that there is a reduction in LD_{50} with oil formulations similar to that observed by Prior *et al.* (1988).

Are the formulations stable at high temperatures and high incident levels of ultra-violet radiation?

Studies have been carried on the effect of temperature on the survival of conidia of isolate IMI 330189 suspended in various oils. In the most benign oils, such as soyabean oil and mineral kerosene, there was only a 5% loss of viability after 20 weeks at 5° and 15°C, but a similar decline occurred in 2–4 weeks at 25°C and in < 1 week at 35°C. No attempt was made in these experiments to improve stability by the use of additives or by pre-treating the conidia, although several approaches are feasible. It appears that long-term storage will require cooling. Conidia are probably sufficiently stable to allow spraying under desert conditions, but more research is required to improve temperature tolerance.

Ultra-violet radiation in the UVB range is lethal to many fungal spores. A range of compounds is available which absorb UVB and have been used to improve the stability of biological pesticides. Those which are compatible with oils have been investigated in an attempt to improve the survival of conidia of IMI 330189 on exposure to tropical sunlight. Oil suspensions of conidia with added chemical sunscreens have been exposed to the UV component of tropical sunlight using an 'Oriel' brand sunlight simulator.

Oils themselves have a considerable absorbance for UVB but conidial suspensions in oils without added sun-screens decline to approximately 25% of their initial viability after 60 min exposure and < 1% after 100 min. The addition of a single sun-screen chemical can increase survival to approximately 45% after 60 min, and a combination of two chemicals can increase it to approximately 65%. Care must be taken in selecting combinations of additives, because some combinations have a cancelling effect and the conidial survival is worse than in the unamended suspension.

Can the required lethal dose of spores be delivered to the target?

Under field conditions the biopesticide will impact on the target as very small droplets, probably approximately 75 μm VMD. The lethal dose must therefore be applied in a large number of very small droplets rather than the single large drop used in the laboratory assay. In order to study the deposition of formulated conidia under more realistic conditions, an experimental track sprayer has been built in which the target insects are passed on a conveyor belt at controlled speed through a cloud of spray droplets produced by a conventional CDA rotary atomizer. The technique can also be used to study the effects of varying the droplet size by adjusting the speed of rotation of the atomizer. The experiments are carried out at 30°C and 30–35% RH but these environmental conditions can also be varied. Mortality occurs in 5–8 days depending on dose and droplet size. This suggests that the formulation is suitable for field testing using similar rotary atomizers, which are available commercially as hand-held sprayers.

The programme at IITA, Cotonou

Work at the IITA Biological Control Centre for Africa, Republic of Benin, fits into the joint locust programme as the field site for initial testing of formulations developed in UK, and for basic ecological work on local grasshoppers. The project will also investigate methods of mass production, and initiate a training programme.

Grasshopper ecology

The first six months' data on local grasshopper ecology are summarized in the paper by Paraïso *et al.*, these proceedings. *Zonocerus variegatus* (Linnaeus) is the commonest grasshopper encountered in the humid zone in West Africa. *Z. variegatus* is generally ignored by predators, but is host to a variety of interesting pathogens and parasites, of which *Entomophaga grylli* is the most prevalent. Outbreaks are closely associated with rainfall, but epidemics are very localized, and some mini-climate studies are planned to see if we can predict *E. grylli* outbreaks, and possibly find some way of enhancing them.

Several isolates of *Beauveria bassiana* on *Z. variegatus* have been found, and the best is being developed as a mycopesticide using the same system as for locusts. Despite the controversy over the pest status of *Z. variegatus*, farmers still worry about this insect, and large amounts of insecticide are applied to control it. For these reasons, development of a mycopesticide which could be produced locally and applied by farmers is justified. So long as a pathogen and application system similar to that being developed for use in the Sahel can be shown to be effective, *Z. variegatus* provides us with an accessible model system. Preliminary results have been encouraging.

Of the other grasshoppers in south Benin (Fishpool & Popov, 1984) none are reported as major pests, but local populations can cause damage to a variety of crops. Our interest in them is primarily as a source of pathogens. Project work has focussed on assembling a reference collection of grasshoppers, so that incoming material can be given a positive identification before being dissected to look for pathogens. Some interesting nematodes have been found, and various bacteria and fungi, particularly in *Zonocerus variegatus.*

Field testing of formulations

The main thrust of the work at Cotonou is the field testing of formulations of *Metarhizium flavoviride* developed by IIBC. This work is presented in more detail in the paper by Bateman *et al.* (these proceedings). The most recent field bioassay resulted in 95% mortality in 10 days in adult *Schistocerca gregaria.* However, these insects were infected with *Malamoeba locustae* (King & Taylor) which may have predisposed them to infection. This work is at an early stage of development, and more results will be reported as they emerge.

Production

Fungus spore production is a key element in assessing the potential applicability of any mycopesticide. Fungal spores have been applied at a rate of 2×10^9 spores/ml with 2 to 3 l of formulation/ha (= 4–6 $\times 10^{12}$ spores/ha), and we must solve the problems of production if we are to apply sufficiently high doses in the field. With insecticides, it is common to apply 2.5×10^7 LD_{90}s/ha and this is the level we should aim to apply with biologicals too. So far, requirements for arena trials and laboratory bioassay have been met by producing spores in medical flats and various locally available bottles, the most suitable being square-sectioned spirits bottles. Molisch's agar is used as the medium. This method suits oil extraction of the spores very well. Other papers in these proceedings (Roberts; Mendonça) discuss mass production in developing country settings. This work has not yet been carried out in any African country; it is likely that the Brazilian methods, such as production on rice grains, would provide a better model than methods used in Czechoslovakia or China based on a slightly higher level of technology or experience with fungal fermentation for food production.

Local support

The project has been very favourably received by the plant protection authorities in the Republic of Benin. Issues which we need to face are whether farmers are likely to use mycopesticides, or whether we should think in terms of specialist plant protection teams. In assessing the applicability of proposed methods, it is essential that national programmes are involved early on in the research and development process so that African solutions can be found to African problems.

Training needs which should be addressed at this stage are both graduate specialist training in insect pathology, and training for professional entomologists who are interested in conducting work on insect pathogens. Until we are more confident of our results, we are concentrating on training for research scientists, not for practical implementation.

Environmental monitoring

Environmental monitoring will also form part of our studies. As discussed by Matteson (these proceedings) environmental impact studies are an essential prerequisite to field application. Although pathogens are inherently far more selective than chemical insecticides, and already exist in the environment, the amount of inoculum may be raised above natural levels. We need to know the effect of this on non-target organisms.

The programme at DFPV, Niamey

The DFPV in Niamey, Niger, is predominantly a training organization and provides training for crop protection at a variety of levels. The department also provides a base for exploration and networking activities carried out by the DFPV part of the locust project. DFPV is on the same site as AGRHYMET, and this link provides access to a large body of expertise on acridology.

Exploration and collection

Work started at DFPV in May 1990 with the arrival of the locust control expert. The first season's field work took place largely in Niger and established a network of collaborators who would be prepared to help collect grasshopper pathogens. This network has subsequently been expanded to all the mainland CILSS countries visited (see paper by Smit, these proceedings); collaborators have been identified in each country. Several notices have been placed in the SAS (Surveillance des Acridiens du Sahel) newsletter produced by PRIFAS. The most recent notice included the offer of cash bonuses for any useful pathogens found; exploration and collection strategies are discussed in greater detail in the paper by Kooyman & Shah (these proceedings).

Subsequent field seasons will be spent travelling throughout the countries of the Sahel and visiting desert locust breeding grounds in Niger and Mali. However, political instability is likely to circumscribe the extent of some of the visits.

Laboratory work

Cultures of *Schistocerca gregaria* and migratory locust, *Locusta migratoria* (Linnaeus), are maintained at DFPV by Mr Tahir Diop, an acridologist of long standing. *Oedaleus senegalensis* (Krauss), *Kraussaria angulifera* (Krauss), *Hieroglyphus daganensis* Krauss and several other pest species have also been brought into culture. By manipulating day-length, it has proved possible to break diapause in *O. senegalensis* enabling continuous reproduction to occur.

Facilities are in place in Niamey for the culture of fungi, and some bioassays of fungi in locusts and grasshoppers have been carried out. Recently, some large cages have been constructed which will allow us to spray locusts with fungal spore preparations under natural conditions and leave them undisturbed after spraying.

Conclusion

The results of this research programme have shown that it is possible to formulate the conidia of *M. flavoviride* in oil diluents suitable for CDA using rotary atomisers and to apply the formulations successfully in the field to kill locusts. Research will now concentrate on improving the formulation, particularly with regard to its stability at high temperatures and its resistance to ultra-violet light. Since isolates of *Metarhizium* and *Beauveria* show considerable specificity it will also be necessary to continue screening for isolates with virulence to other target acridids. The programme has established contacts throughout a vast area of West Africa to provide a source of isolates and, eventually, to participate in the field testing of fungal formulations.

References

Anon. (1990) A plague of locusts – special report, OTA-F-450. US Congress, Office of Technology Assessment, Washington, DC. US Government Printing Office, July, 1990.

Brader, L. (1988) Control of grasshoppers and migratory locusts. *Proceedings of the Brighton Crop Protection Conference – Pests and Diseases* **1988**, 283–288.

Fishpool, L.D.C. & Popov, G.B. (1984) The grasshopper faunas of the savannas of Mali, Niger, Benin and Togo. *Bulletin de l'Institut Française d'Afrique Noire* **43**, 275–410.

Geddes, A.M.W. (1990) The relative importance of crop pests in sub-Saharan Africa. *Natural Resources Institute Bulletin* **no. 36**, 69 pp.

Marcandier, S. & Khachatourians, G.G. (1987) Susceptibility of the migratory grasshopper, *Melanoplus sanguinipes* (Fab.) (Orthoptera: Acrididae) to *Beauveria bassiana* (Bals.) Vuillemin (Hyphomycete): influence of relative humidity. *Canadian Entomologist* **119**, 901–907.

Prior, C. (1990) The biological basis for regulating the release of micro-organisms, with particular reference to the use of fungi for pest control. *Aspects of Applied Biology* **24**, 231–238.

Prior, C. & Greathead, D.J. (1989) Biological control of locusts: the potential for the exploitation of pathogens. *FAO Plant Protection Bulletin* **37**, 37–48.

Prior, C., Jollands, P. & le Patourel, G. (1988) Infectivity of oil and water formulations of *Beauveria bassiana* (Deuteromycotina: Hyphomycetes) to the cocoa weevil pest *Pantorhytes plutus* (Coleoptera: Curculionidae). *Journal of Invertebrate Pathology* **52**, 66–72.

Steedman, A. (1990) *The Locust Handbook.* (3rd edn). Natural Resources Institute, Chatham, UK.

Section I

Organizations Concerned with Locust and Grasshopper Control, and Country Reports

APHIS; grasshopper integrated pest management in the United States – a co-operative project with emphasis on biological control

G.L. Cunningham

USDA, APHIS, PPQ, Grasshopper Integrated Pest Management Project.

Abstract

The Grasshopper Integrated Pest Management (GHIPM) Project was organized in 1987 in response to record-setting grasshopper infestations that blanketed millions of hectares of US rangeland in the mid-1980s. Initiated as a pilot study, the project is designed to develop and integrate grasshopper control strategies into a total system for use by managers of public and private rangelands. Two areas in Idaho and North Dakota are used as integrated pest management (IPM) demonstration sites. Management studies in these areas include population dynamics, economics, environmental consequences, bait applications, and biological controls. The GHIPM Project is a co-operative effort managed by the Animal and Plant Health Inspection Service in association with other agencies of the US Department of Agriculture and the US Department of Interior, Environmental Protection Agency, State Universities, and rancher associations.

Introduction

Combatting rangeland grasshopper infestations in the western USA is well beyond the abilities of individuals or community organizations. As a result, in 1934 Congress charged the US Department of Agriculture (USDA) with assisting in grasshopper control efforts. USDA's Animal and Plant Health Inspection Service (APHIS) provides direct supervision and leadership for grasshopper management programmes in co-operation with other federal agencies, state departments of agriculture, and private ranchers. APHIS's authority to conduct control programmes is provided by the Incipient Control of Pests Act (1937), the Organic Act of the Department of

Agriculture (1944), the Cooperation With State Agencies in the Administration and Enforcement of Certain Federal Laws Act (1962), and the Food Security Act (1985).

Co-operative control programmes for grasshoppers on rangeland occur every year and were most visible in 1985, when 22 million hectares were heavily infested. In Idaho alone, more than 2.4 million hectares were treated that year. Treatments of this magnitude, usually with aerially applied liquid insecticides in blocks of 4000 hectares or more, raised concern about the effects on nontarget organisms, environmental contamination, and other related problems. The American public and scientists jointly developed considerable interest in integrated pest management (IPM) as a result, and IPM is now the preferred alternative for federal control programmes on rangeland grasshoppers.

GHIPM Project

The Grasshopper Integrated Pest Management (GHIPM) Project was initiated in 1987 as a 5-year pilot programme. Its goal is to develop, evaluate, and implement a grasshopper management scheme that can maintain populations at noneconomic levels and that is cost effective, technically feasible, and environmentally acceptable. Plans are being made to extend the project for three more years, to September 30, 1994, to allow for technology transfer.

The GHIPM Project has its headquarters in Boise, Idaho. Field work is accomplished at two rangeland areas in McKenzie County, North Dakota, and the Shoshone Bureau of Land Management District in Idaho. These rangelands represent the major western ecosystems in which grasshopper outbreaks usually occur. Three distinct study areas are contained in each of the two sites – a no-treatment area, a standard treatment area, and the demonstration area.

No-treatment area

In no-treatment areas, neither APHIS, the GHIPM Project, nor any other co-operator funds or participates in any programme to control grasshoppers. The no-treatment alternative enables the GHIPM Project to study the impact of allowing grasshopper populations to develop without intervention. This study provides a benchmark against which the success rate of other alternatives can be gauged.

Standard treatment area

Within standard treatment areas, APHIS guidelines govern the management of grasshopper infestations. Typically, APHIS implements biological or chemical control methods when grasshopper populations exceed 8 per square yard ($8.7/m^2$). Local factors such as grasshopper life stage and species as well as range condition affect the decision to treat.

Demonstration area

The GHIPM Project tests IPM strategies at selected demonstration sites. Based on grasshopper management needs, these strategies help identify feasible control options.

Research and evaluation of IPM methods in the demonstration area include:

1. formulation of selective grasshopper bran baits
2. development of biological control agents
3. improvement of range management techniques
4. monitoring of environmental effects
5. evaluation of post-treatment effectiveness.

Most of the GHIPM Project's research is done by university cooperators funded with federal tax dollars. Studies fall into one of four categories: forecast, survey, decision making, or options.

Forecast studies are conducted to help predict the time of year when grasshopper outbreaks will occur, the age structure of grasshopper populations during outbreaks, and changes in grasshopper density. Research covers such topics as range management, grasshopper biology, and phenology.

Survey studies are conducted to improve the accuracy of field observations. Research results help establish guides to assist field personnel in identifying nymph and adult grasshoppers. The published field guides portray economically significant grasshopper species, including information on distribution, habitat, and food preferences.

Research on decision making looks at the benefits and costs of grasshopper suppression and the environmental impacts of grasshopper control. Studies cover treatment efficacy, relationships between grasshopper density and forage loss, and the effect of control programmes on threatened and endangered plant and animal species.

Options studies are designed to evaluate current control tactics and to develop new strategies that take into account environmental sensitivity. The project is studying the effectiveness of bran bait formulations for pesticide delivery and possibilities for using reduced active ingredients. Options studies also involve work on the development and application of biological control.

Biological control emphasis

The GHIPM Project emphasizes research, development, and implementation of biological control for grasshoppers (Anon. 1987, 1990). The 1990s promise to be the decade of the environment with increased public pressure for farmers to lessen their dependence on chemical pesticides. Concern about pesticide residues and ground water contamination by agrichemicals is growing. As a consequence, the use of chemicals is likely to be more restricted in the future. These concerns, coupled with increased federal and state regulations to protect threatened and endangered plant and animal species, push biological control to the forefront as a possible alternative to conventional control techniques.

Unfortunately, the need for research toward the use of biological control agents for grasshoppers has been given lower priority until now because of the availability of inexpensive and effective chemicals. Ranchers and land managers, who expect quick kill with pesticides, will have to readjust their thinking about biological control because it is relatively slow acting. Other barriers, such as economics, mass production, viable shelf life, quality control standards, and governmental regulation, pose significant hurdles to the use of natural controls.

Using combinations of parasites, predators, and pathogens, investigators in the GHIPM Project are addressing biological control on several fronts. The protozoan, *Nosema locustae* Canning is approved for use in Federal co-operative control programmes. Its utility on rangeland continues to be studied. Exotic isolates of the obligate fungal pathogen *Entomophaga grylli* (Fresenius) Batko are undergoing experiments on epizootiology and field release. Entomopox viruses have been isolated from at least eight grasshopper species and studies are ongoing to maximize production efficiency for field release. The microsporidium *Vairimorpha* sp. has been found to cause natural epizootics with mormon cricket, *Anabrus simplex* Haldeman (Orthoptera: Tettigoniidae). Accordingly, studies have been initiated to develop protocols for production of inoculum for field introduction. The fungal pathogen *Beauveria bassiana* (Balsamo) Vuillemin is being investigated to determine its effect on several species of rangeland grasshoppers. Cell culture systems for production of host cell dependent grasshopper pathogens have been initiated along with formulation additive studies for solar-irradiation protection of fungal pathogens. Foreign exploration for grasshopper biological control agents has been focused on Australia and the Soviet Union. Results to date include the collection and quarantine screening of grasshopper egg parasitoids from the genus *Scelio* (Hymenoptera: Scelionidae). Finally, impact studies of large scale grasshopper control programmes on insect parasites and pathogens continue in the IPM demonstration areas of North Dakota and Idaho.

Co-operative effort

The GHIPM Project is a co-operative effort managed by the USDA's Animal and Plant Health Inspection Service. Other USDA agencies involved include the Agricultural Research Service, Economic Research Service, Forest Service, and Extension Service. Three branches of the US Department of Interior are also co-operating: the Bureau of Land Management, Fish and Wildlife Service, and National Park Service. The US Environmental Protection Agency, 10 state universities, and the McKenzie County North Dakota Grazing Association are also directly involved in the co-operative effort.

References

Anon. (1987) *Rangeland Grasshopper Cooperative Management Program: Final Environmental Impact Statement.* USDA, APHIS, Washington, DC 221 pp.

Anon. (1990) *Cooperative Grasshopper Integrated Pest Management Project: Annual Report.* USDA, APHIS, Washington, DC 282 pp.

CEC; biological control of locusts with entomopathogens

B. Zelazny

Biologische Bundesanstalt für Land- und Forstwirtschaft, Institut für Biologischen Pflanzenschutz, Darmstadt, Germany.

Abstract

The structure of the CEC locust entomopathogen project is described. The project has only recently started and at present links five European and two African countries. The emphasis is on collection and identification of pathogens, and contact points for three groups of pathogens (bacteria/protozoa, fungi and viruses) are given.

The Commission of European Communities sponsors a project entitled 'Biological control of locusts by entomopathogens'. The project supports research on the use of insect disease agents against locusts and grasshoppers in five European and two African countries. The project has only started recently and little practical work has so far been done. It is scheduled to operate for three years until the end of 1993.

The main objectives of the project are to find diseases for the microbial control of locusts and grasshoppers, to accomplish the necessary isolations, characterizations and testing of such agents, and to develop effective formulations of these pathogens for practical use. These formulations might contain synergistic compounds like chemical insecticides in reduced concentrations or insect growth regulators.

The Institute for Biological Pest Control in Darmstadt, Germany, is the main contractor for the project. The main function of the institute in the CEC project is to co-ordinate activities. It also helps other participants to identify locust diseases and trains staff of African institutes. Its practical research on locust control falls mainly under a national GTZ-sponsored project: 'Biological and integrated locust control'. The institute is part of the Biologische Bundesanstalt für Land- und Forstwirtschaft (BBA, Federal Biological Research Centre for Agriculture and Forestry). The BBA is presently arranging four associated contracts with European institutions and two subcontracts with African organizations. The following institutes will be participating in the project under these contracts.

The INRA Research Station of Biological Control in La Minière, France, will study mainly the persistence of microbial control agents in the environment, that is how disease agents can survive under the influence of factors such as radiation, temperature or low humidity. The research is led by Dr J. Farques who has extensive experience in this field. Connected to such research will be attempts to improve the persistence of promising agents through suitable methods of formulation. The institute will also search for new pathogens of locusts and grasshoppers and in the past has studied many different types of insect diseases, particularly fungi.

The Laboratory of Comparative Pathology in Saint-Christol-Les-Alès in France is a second INRA institute participating in the project. A group under Prof. M. Bergoin will be mainly involved in the characterization and testing of promising viruses which will be hopefully discovered during the duration of the project. In this connection it should be mentioned that a virus belonging to the group of entomopoxviruses has been recently found in field populations of *Schistocerca gregaria* (Forskäl) in the Yemen, but the material has been subsequently lost.

The International Institute of Biological Control in close collaboration with the University of Bath in England is attempting to enhance the infectivity of fungi against locusts through the addition of chemical insecticides (at low concentrations) or insect growth regulators. Dr C. Prior is leading the locust group at IIBC; the work at the University of Bath is headed by Dr A.K. Charnley. If time permits it will also be investigated whether the addition of certain compounds to the food or to baits could facilitate fungal infections through the gut.

A group at the University of Crete under Dr A. Legakis is studying the ecology and control of local species of grasshoppers which are causing crop damage in Greece. The group will mainly attempt to identify diseases suitable for microbial control and to develop methods of producing, formulating and applying these.

The entomological institute of the University of Bologna in Italy has a similar type of programme. The research is conducted by Dr G. Briolini and Dr K. Deseö. The most destructive species of grasshopper is *Calliptamus italicus* (Linnaeus). The ecology of this grasshopper is being studied, especially how populations are regulated by the fungus *Entomophaga grylli* (Fresenius) Batko. The development of microbial control methods will be attempted.

The Desert Locust Control Organization for Eastern Africa (DLCOEA) is starting efforts under the project to find and develop suitable microbial control agents against the desert locust. Mr Musa of the DLCOEA will be in charge of this work. The research will be done in close collaboration with the participating institutes in Europe. Because the DLCOEA regularly conducts control campaigns in a number of East African countries, it already has a very suitable organization for conducting surveys and field trials.

At the University of Cairo Dr Said Abol-Ela leads a group which will collect locusts and grasshoppers in Egypt and study their diseases. Apart from project contributions this work is strongly supported by ORSTOM. The group and collaborating ORSTOM scientists are mainly interested in viruses. Viruses of locusts and grasshoppers will be isolated, tested and, if found promising, developed as microbial control agents.

Apart from supporting the research work described above, an important function of the project is to encourage collaboration between the participating institutes. Such collaboration was discussed recently at a meeting in Wageningen, Holland. There was a general consensus at the meeting to extend such collaborations also to workers and institutes which are not officially part of the project, if these find such an arrangement mutually beneficial. In fact the meeting was attended by a number of scientists from outside the project. The CEC project is also linked via IIBC to the IIBC/IITA/DFPV Locust and Grasshopper Biological Control Programme and the two projects are co-operating fully in the exchange of pathogens.

Initially a number of areas of collaboration were identified which will increase the overall output of the project. The most important one was mutual assistance in the identification of new diseases. A number of participating institutes are engaged in collecting locusts and grasshoppers, but each worker has only a limited knowledge in recognizing and identifying potentially useful diseases. So that valuable collected material is carefully inspected for all promising groups of insect diseases, the project participants have worked out a system of helping each other in the search for the identification of new diseases. This includes the establishment of three contact points, Saint-Christol-Les-Alès for viruses, IIBC for fungi, and BBA Darmstadt for protozoa and bacteria. Other areas of collaboration would be the exchange of disease agents and locusts for laboratory testing. Some of the disease agents will be used as standards, in order to make results from different laboratories comparable.

Contact points for the identification of insect pathogens:

1. Viruses
Dr M. Bergoin
Institut National de la Recherche Agronomique (INRA)
Station de Recherches de Pathologie Comparée
F-30380 Saint-Christol-les-Alès
France
Tel: (33) 6652 2017

2. Fungi
Dr C. Prior
International Institute of Biological Control
Silwood Park
Ascot
Berkshire
SL5 7TA
UK
Tel: (44) 0344 872999

3. Bacteria and protozoa
Dr B. Zelazny
Biologische Bundesanstalt für Land- und Forstwirtschaft
Institute for Biological Pest Control
Heinrichstrasse 243
D-6100 Darmstadt
Germany
Tel: (49) 6151 44061

CILSS/DFPV; the Permanent Interstate Committee for Drought Control in the Sahel, and the Department of Crop Protection Training, Niger

J.J. Smit

Département de Formation en Protection des Végétaux, Centre CILSS AGRHYMET

Abstract
The Permanent Interstate Committee for Drought Control in the Sahel (CILSS) was set up by nine Sahelian countries following the drought of 1968–73, and agreed in 1974 to improve crop protection services. A joint CILSS/Netherlands mission agreed in 1977 to strengthen training in crop protection with emphasis on integrated methods. The Département de Formation en Protection des Végétaux (DFPV) was set up in 1981 in Kolo, Niger and moved to its present site in Niamey in 1987. The main course lasts two years and leads to a Higher Diploma in Crop Protection. Short language training courses, specialized crop protection courses, and seminars are also held. Dissemination of information is also a very important activity. DFPV is well equipped with modern training equipment.

Following the drought years of 1968–73 six Sahelian countries, later followed by three others, created in 1973 the Permanent Interstate Committee for Drought Control in the Sahel, commonly known by the initials of its French name, Comité Permanent Inter-Etats de Lutte contre la Sécheresse dans le Sahel, CILSS.

This Committee then represented its member states in dealing with their principal donor countries on the subject of support for economic and social development.

Right from the beginning CILSS has given a very high priority to agricultural development, in order to achieve its goal of food self-sufficiency.

The member countries of CILSS are:

Burkina Faso

The Republic of the Cape Verde Islands
The Republic of the Gambia
The Republic of Guinea-Bissau
The Republic of Mali
The Islamic Republic of Mauritania
The Republic of Niger
The Republic of Senegal
The Republic of Chad.

Having experienced serious insect invasions after the drought years, the CILSS countries agreed in 1974:

1. to strengthen their crop protection services and regional institutes for the control of migrating insect pests such as locusts and grasshoppers
2. to develop research and training in crop protection.

After consultations with interested donor countries and international organizations such as FAO and the Club du Sahel, agreements were finally reached for the financial, material and expert support of the following activities:

1. strengthening of national crop protection services
2. development of a system of integrated control methods against pests and diseases of important food crops in the Sahel region
3. development of information services and training facilities in crop protection.

In 1977 a joint mission CILSS/The Netherlands agreed on the kind of training most needed to strengthen national crop protection services in the Sahel and concluded that to protect the environment an integrated control system should be developed, secondly, that there was an urgent need to adapt crop protection training to Sahelian conditions and, thirdly, that there was a most urgent need for mid-level field and laboratory staff in crop protection that could strengthen and improve the efficiency of national crop protection services.

DFPV: a centre for training and information in crop protection

The project for Training in Crop Protection was established in 1981, following a request by the member states of CILSS. It is funded by the Netherlands, following an agreement between that country and the CILSS.

Objective

To contribute to food self-sufficiency by improving the protection of crops and stored products against pests, diseases, and weeds.

The status of DFPV

In 1981, an agreement was signed between the CILSS and the Netherlands to implement a training project for Crop Protection. This project was situated at the Institute for Practical Rural Development (IPDR) in Kolo, Niger.

The urgent need for crop protection expertise, as well as for the various project activities, has been well recognized. Therefore, during the meeting of the Council of Ministers of the CILSS in Dakar, on 25 and 26 January 1986, the member states formulated Resolution No 7/21/CM/86, which conferred permanent status to the Project by creating a Department for Training in Crop Protection, within the AGRHYMET Centre. In January, 1987, the DFPV moved into its new quarters in Niamey.

Two statutory bodies define the DFPV's activities:

1. The Scientific and Pedagogical Committee (CSP)
2. The Management Committee (CG).

The Scientific and Pedagogical Committee is responsible for examining and approving all suggestions of pedagogical and scientific nature, as well as all changes in the orientation of training. The committee is composed mainly of directors of National Crop Protection Services.

The Management Committee, composed of CILSS experts as well as experts from the Netherlands and all other donor countries, approves the budget and accounts of the department as well as the financial consequences of the CSP's decisions.

These two committees meet at least once every year.

Short-term objectives of the Department of Crop Protection Training

The immediate objective of the project is to reinforce the National Crop Protection Services by training medium level personnel working directly in the field.

This is accomplished in part by the dissemination of crop protection information relating to the Sahelian countries but more importantly by the various training activities of the DFPV.

Activities of the DFPV

- A two-year Higher Diploma training course for Crop Protection Technicians (TSPV)
- A four-month French language course for English and Portuguese speaking students from The Gambia, Guinea-Bissau and the Cape Verdian Islands, prior to their two-year training course in Crop Protection mentioned above
- A four-month training course in Crop Protection, intended for the following professional categories:
  — crop protection teachers at agricultural schools
  — senior technicians and agronomists
- Specialization of agricultural technicians and agronomists in their last year of study
- The organization of workshops, covering certain specialized topics in Crop Protection
- The dissemination of information on Crop Protection in the Sahel.

The training course for crop protection technicians

Candidates recruited for the training course for Crop Protection Technicians (TSPV) must fulfill the following requirements:

1. be a national of one of the member states of the CILSS (candidates from non-Sahelian countries may be accepted under special circumstances)
2. possess a baccalaureate certificate, a secondary school certificate or an equivalent certificate in crop protection
3. have preferably two years of professional experience
4. be under 40 years old.

The instruction consists of theoretical courses, as well as practical work in the laboratory and in the field; other appropriate methods are used as needed.

In the first year basic subjects are covered, whereas more specific crop protection topics are treated in the second year. A practical training period and a research project are also part of the TSPV course.

Approximately 25 students are now being trained each year. At the end of the course, after receiving their diplomas, the students return to their duties in their home countries.

Specialization courses

The objective of this education programme is to reinforce crop protection expertise within the national structures by addressing the following professional categories:

1. crop protection teachers at agricultural schools
2. senior technicians and agronomists working in plant protection and research services.

Training workshops

The objective of these workshops is to broaden the basic understanding of topics of current concern in crop protection; other topics could be covered, as judged necessary by member states.

Crop protection training results

- To date 111 students successfully completed the two-year training course in crop protection and left for their home countries with a Higher Diploma in Crop Protection
- Five students from the Gambia were trained at the Ahmadu Bello University in Zaria, Nigeria
- Twelve students so far followed the French language training course for English and Portuguese-speaking students
- Twenty-five agricultural technicians and higher technicians were given training in crop protection
- Twelve agricultural school teachers were given crop protection training and educational materials were supplied by the project for use in their schools of work
- To date 142 trainees from crop protection services in the Sahel region took part in training workshops organized by the DFPV.

Training courses were organized on the following themes:

1986: Safe and efficient use of pesticides
1987: Phytosanitary aspects of seeds
1988: Rodent pest control
1989: Phytosanitary control
1990: Surveillance of locusts and grasshoppers
1990: Bird pest control
1991: Rodent pest control (April)
1991: Ecology and identification of immature grasshoppers and eggpods (June–August).

Information

The recently created information package is designed to complement the training. Its purpose is to disseminate crop protection information throughout the Sahel.

A database of crop protection documentation has been created at the DFPV, as an integral part of the Sahelian Documentation Network (RESADOC) of the Sahel Institute (INSAH) in Bamako.

Available are AGRIS and CAB ABSTRACTS databases and the DFPV database which will soon contain 4,000 bibliographic references.

Upon request bibliographic searches may be performed free of charge.

Publications

- Descriptive bulletins
- Technical bulletins
- Brochures, technical notes
- Workbooks and lecture notes
- Slides
- Technical documents relating to the workshops
- A newsletter to maintain contact between alumni and other persons connected with the project.

Outside experts are invited to contribute to the publications of the department.

Publications on acridology

The Netherlands Ministry of International Cooperation financially supports the publication of a series of booklets in the French language prepared by CIRAD/PRIFAS, which are being distributed by the DFPV. The series is called *Collection Acridologie Opérationelle* and contains considerable information on acridology for workers in the field.

The following titles are already published:

No 1: Les criquets du Sahel (Grasshoppers of the Sahel)
No 2: La surveillance des criquets du Sahel (The surveillance of Sahelian grasshoppers)
No 3: La lutte chimique contre les criquets du Sahel (Chemical control of grasshoppers in the Sahel)
No 4: *Oedaleus senegalensis*: sauteriau ravageur du Sahel (*Oedaleus senegalensis*: a grasshopper pest of the Sahel)
No 5: Vade-mecum des principaux criquets ravageurs du Sahel
No 6: Le criquet pèlerin au Sahel (The desert locust in the Sahel)

No 7: Les oothèques des criquets du Sahel (Eggpods of sahelian grasshoppers).

In preparation:

No 8: Les ennemis naturels des criquets du Sahel (The natural enemies of grasshoppers in the Sahel).

General equipment of the DFPV

The DFPV has available several types of audiovisual and other equipment (video, slide and transparency projectors) and photographic, printing and photocopying apparatus. The DFPV library is well stocked with publications in the field of crop protection: entomology, ecotoxicology, acridology, ornithology, phytopathology, nematology, virology, phytopharmacy, weed science, rodentology) and related fields of plant and soil science.

Every section of the department has its own systematic collection of insects, fungi, nematodes, weeds, rodents and diapositive slide collections on these important organisms and the damage they cause.

Ample laboratory research facilities for entomology, phytopharmacy, nematology, virology, and ecotoxicology are provided for at the DFPV, as they go hand in hand with practical training of students. An irrigated area of about two hectares is available for out-of-season growing for various crops and three air-conditioned greenhouses built for growing and testing crops are now near completion.

Transport facilities for teaching and research purposes consist of a fleet of three landcruisers, one pick-up, one bus for 30 persons and three smaller cars for the directorate and administration. Two class-rooms for 25 students each are available for regular teaching purposes and there is a spacious conference room for staff meetings, seminars and workshops.

Special equipment in acridology

The DFPV is well equipped for the rearing of grasshoppers in its insectary which is now exclusively used for this purpose. There is also a large mosquito-netted greenhouse which provides facilities for biopesticide tests on grasshoppers.

Rearing of grasshoppers has so far been very successful. *Locusta migratoria migratorioides* (Reiche & Fairmaire), *Schistocerca gregaria* (Forskål) and *Oedaleus senegalensis* (Krauss) are now routinely reared without interruption as we were able to solve problems of reproduction and diapause in the latter species. Rearing of *Kraussaria, Ornithacris* and *Hieroglyphus* will be started in the very near future.

Three pathogenic fungal strains are now being grown at the DFPV, *Metarhizium flavoviride* (W. Gams & J. Rozsypel), *Sorosporella* sp. and *Aspergillus flavus* Link ex Fries. Testing with the pathogenic fungi now available in pure culture will continue on several other species of grasshoppers, notably *O. senegalensis* and *Locusta migratoria* (Linnaeus).

Acridology staff

Two acridologists have been assigned at the DFPV and they co-operate in activities such as grasshopper rearing and surveillance work. They are assisted by four laboratory assistant staff and they have available two drivers for travelling within the Sahel region to visit locust areas. Funding of these activities is by the Dutch Ministry of International Cooperation (DGIS) through the DFPV, which is the home base of the grasshopper project known as the SPC, the French acronym for Surveillance des Pathogènes des Criquets.

CNLA; short report on the control strategy of acridids in Morocco 1987–89

A. Mouhim

Centre National de la Lutte Anti-Acridienne, Morocco.

Abstract

Locust monitoring is carried out by the National Centre for Acridid Control at Ait-Melloul. When action is required the Ministries of Agriculture, Agrarian Reform, Interior and of Information and also the National Defence are also mobilised. Over 2 million ha were treated in 1987–88. The principal strategy is one of destroying adult locusts outside crop zones before they can oviposit.

Introduction

Among the 206 species of locusts and grasshoppers known in Morocco, only two species of locusts cause serious damage to crops. These are the Moroccan locust, *Dociostaurus maroccanus* (Thunberg) and the desert locust, *Schistocerca gregaria* (Forskål). *D. maroccanus* is a native and univoltine species. The control of its gregarious foci has meant that the population has remained at a controllable level. On the other hand, *S. gregaria* is a visiting species which enters Morocco at the end of September to mid-October.

The resurgence of the locust pest problem was encouraged by favourable climatic conditions in the permanent habitat zones of *S. gregaria* and by the paucity of preventative control exercised in the gregarious foci. Thus several uncontrollable swarms formed and engendered an invasion from 1987 to 1989.

In the south and south-east of Morocco there was an unprecedented invasion by massive swarms of locusts coming from Algeria and other

Sahelian countries. During this time, 4,802,805 ha were treated with pesticides.

Organization of acridid control on a national scale

Strategy

The National Centre for Acridid Control (CNLA) at Ait-Melloul does extensive exploration annually in the south of the country, where swarms of *S. gregaria* might infiltrate. If there is much activity in the summer reproduction zones of *S. gregaria* then preparations for preventative control are begun in strategic zones. Usually, this will comprise between three and five aeroplanes and seven to ten 4-wheel drive vehicles with ground spraying equipment and large stocks of insecticide for use over a period of two to three months.

In Morocco, in addition to the people themselves, the Ministries of Agriculture and Agrarian Reform, the Interior and Information, and National Defence are mobilized in the fight against locusts. Co-ordination is undertaken by a Central Command Post (CCP) at Rabat and 12 Regional Command Posts (RCP) in the affected regions.

The CNLA not only contributes to control but ensures technical assistance to every RCP and is concerned with training personnel for locust control. It also ensures that every RCP obtains the pesticides and equipment which it needs.

More than 3,600 people from different ministries took part in control operations; 28% were technicians or qualified research scientists. Sprayers used were atomizers, hydraulic pressure sprayers, and exhaust nozzle sprayers mounted on vehicles. 57 aeroplanes were used of 13 different types, depending on the topography of the area and with a capacity of 200–12,000 l. In addition, there is a well established radio network with 108 radio posts, 66 mobile and 42 fixed.

The pesticides used were selected on the basis of toxicological data (rapid action against the locust, but less toxic to man, fauna and flora), the types of sprayers which were available and storage conditions. 5,981,146 l were sprayed at low dosages: 0.8–1 l/ha by air and 2–5 l/ha on the ground (Table 1).

In 1987–88, 2,813,182 ha were treated, 1,201,245 against larvae and 1,611,937 against adults. In 1988–89, acridid populations were exclusively swarms of immature locusts. 1,989,622 ha were treated, thus, the total in these two seasons was 4,802,805 ha.

During the two years 0.85 billion francs were spent on fighting acridids, 54% of which was donated from abroad, with a cost of US$12/ha.

Table 1. Volumes of insecticides and carrier used in Morocco during locust campaigns 1987/88 and 1988/89.

Product	Dose (g a.i./ha)	Amounts used (litres) 1987–88	1988–89	Total (litres)
Dichlorvos (DDVP 96%)	200	88,702	401,251	489,953
Fenitrothion (1000 ULV)	350	412,790	4,400	417,190
Fenitrothion 500 ULV	350	120,600	48,400	169,000
Malathion 96% ULV	700	781,526	661,327	1,442,853
Carbaryl 4% oil	480	42,784	–	42,784
Diazinon 90% ULV	900	8,200	–	8,200
Deltamethrin 12.5% ULV	12.5	0	56,700	56,700
Deltamethrin 25% EC	12.5	0	22,325	22,325
Lambdacyhalothrin 4% ULV	20	8,900	5,825	14,725
Organic diluent for ULV formulations (HAN)		1,900,000	1,417,416	3,317,416
Total		3,363,502	2,617,644	5,981,146

The acridid problem is not just a national one, but regional throughout the Sahel and even international. In this context a conference was held in Fes in 1988 with the idea of creating an international acridid control force. The aims of this body are to reinforce exploration and control of the desert locust and to ensure a better evaluation of the acridid situation. There are three units in Mauritania, Mali and Tchad and two others in Sudan and on the Red Sea.

Conclusion

The invasions of locusts between 1987–89 were the largest this century. The success of control measures prevented enormous damage. The efficiency of the interventions are based on the following:

1. the adoption of a new concept in acridid control, that of destroying adults outside crop zones before oviposition
2. the use of qualified and experienced personnel
3. the improvement of spraying techniques
4. the selection of more appropriate methods of control according to the size of swarm and the kind of terrain
5. the increased use of large trucks and aeroplanes.

Morocco has become one of the pilot countries in the organization of acridid control, thanks to the enriching experience undergone during the last few years.

DLCOEA; pest control: the begging questions

R.A. Kitenda

Desert Locust Control Organization for Eastern Africa.

Abstract

The possible ways in which schemes for the biological control of locusts and grasshoppers might fit in with existing modes of operation are discussed. Particular attention is paid to the problems experienced by locust control organizations in recent years with a run-down in resources.

Biological control of locusts and grasshoppers is a subject I am not at all familiar with. However, looking at the approach being made from an educated and experienced view point, I am of the opinion that a great step indeed is being made.

It is a great step considered in relation to past and present measures and means of locust control in my area of specialization which is aerial control.

The biological control programme when being developed is likely to have some teething problems and perhaps when fully evolved would have its limitations just like any other. It is however, a very welcome element in an integrated pest control approach in general. We must endeavour to reduce pollutants.

Aerial control of locusts and grasshoppers (area of specialization)

Locusts have existed for as long as man can remember. Various ways and means have been employed in every effort to try and contain the scourge since the beginning of history; some very crude and others refined as time went by. All these measures have succeeded to some extent in containing the threat. The degree of success by the means employed has, however, depended to a large extent on the size of infestation and the experience and expertise of personnel employed. This state of affairs is as true today as it was in yester years and it will remain tomorrow, whatever the methods.

Constraints

There are various bottlenecks which have and still continue to afflict effective locust and grasshopper control:

1. finance
2. trained manpower
3. effective monitoring
4. research.

The financing of control organizations remains a very big problem and in many cases a burden to participating states. This situation is not helped in any way when conservation of resources is undertaken by incompetent personnel.

The future can only be improved if the burden is carried by the international community and management handed to competent heads with sufficient expertise. The donor community must reconsider assistance strategy.

Trained manpower in the area of locust control is almost extinct. The reasons are manifold, poor remuneration, difficult working conditions, poor recruitment decision making, and again lack of funds and facilities.

Unnecessary amounts of pollutants are still being dispersed in the atmosphere because of untrained manpower incapable of equipment calibration and adjustment.

Without ways and means to effectively monitor areas of outbreak and breeding, it is impossible to cope with the demand of the job regardless of the method employed. The task of monitoring has unfortunately become increasingly difficult, given that many key geographical areas are also zones of conflict. We must therefore seek alternative ways of gaining access to breeding territory using available technology to reduce outbreaks. The question remains how to adapt and utilize such technology.

Research in locust and grasshopper control has for a long time now been dormant. The advent of biological control research is therefore very welcome.

Where there is research being conducted, it is incomplete, in that it ends in the laboratory without being extended to real field trials.

Research does not have continuity and therefore leaves unfilled gaps. In many instances researchers leave their jobs taking the records of their work with them.

The list of deficiencies in locust research is long but one of vital importance is the failure to establish the economics involved as in the final analysis everything depends upon money.

This means that the next person on the job has to start afresh or on very scanty information. Since locust outbreaks occur after lapses of time, some many years apart, the would-be researcher may never have fulfilment of knowledge gained in the laboratory under actual field conditions. We know the history of control measures, we have the present in hand, but what does the future hold in store when we consider the experience gained to-date! The future survival of locust and grasshopper control lies in a co-ordinated international effort through a recognized body with a specialized group of experts.

The biological control approach is welcome and must be pursued relentlessly as part of an integrated effort.

The programme must avoid the present pitfalls in existing programmes; namely, allowing a run-down of trained manpower, gaps and deficiency in research, employing incompetent or disinterested staff and over-extending resources; high-tech application must be seriously enhanced to help in reducing the pressure on limited resources; we know how far history has brought us today. We must therefore build a more certain future based on knowledge so far gained and the desire to reduce the threat of locusts and grasshoppers to our food supply.

GTZ; the integrated biological control of locusts and grasshoppers – a GTZ research project

S. Krall & O.M. Nasseh

GTZ-Projekt.

Abstract

The aim of the integrated biological control project of the GTZ is to develop more acceptable alternative non-chemical methods of controlling locusts and grasshoppers. The existing control measures still rely heavily on chemical pesticides which are the only method available at the present time for cases of severe infestation. The most effective pesticide, dieldrin, is banned in most countries. The substitutes are less effective, more expensive and require multiple applications. It is therefore essential to search for more acceptable, non-chemical alternatives. Preliminary tests have shown that one such alternative could be the use of pathogens and insect growth regulators. The final goal of the project is to localize and attack the problem at the earliest possible stage of development of locust upsurge. This will comprise identifying the problem in the recession areas of the desert locust (*Schistocerca gregaria* (Forskål)) and then treating the insects. In this way the impact on the environment is minimized, the required treatment area is limited, the costs of control are reduced and the potential for crop and grassland damage is negligible. An additional biological, non-chemical alternative method would support this strategy. The programme of the project has nine principal objectives:

- mapping the locust habitat by satellite
- research into gregarization pheromone, to prevent swarm formation
- locust control with insect growth regulators, especially synthetic juvenile hormone analogs
- biological control of the locust with entomopathogenic micro-organisms
- pest management with the help of pyrrolizidine alkaloids
- seed components from *Melia volkensii* and their use for locust control
- field trials with non-chemical alternatives
- research on environmental aspects of the new compounds

- loss assessment and economic studies relating to the effects of locust and grasshopper attack/damage.

Introduction

From 1985–88, after an interval of almost twenty years, outbreaks of the desert locust (*Schistocerca gregaria* (Forskål)) occurred in Africa and the Near East. Climatically favourable conditions in conjunction with the neglect of the warning services and the inaccessibility of some areas due to armed conflict contributed to this mass reproduction. The countries affected were largely unprepared and poorly equipped to cope with the plague. Moreover both donors and recipient countries discovered that since the last plague, hardly any research had been carried out into developing better and more environmentally acceptable control methods. An additional handicap was represented by the banning of the insecticide dieldrin. The advantage of this insecticide, which had been used in all previous plagues, was that, due to its persistence it needed to be applied in the breeding grounds only in widely spaced bands, at large intervals. On crossing these bands the larvae became contaminated and died. When dieldrin was banned the effects of this special method of locust control in Africa had not been analysed sufficiently. Accordingly no alternative agent or methods had been developed to replace dieldrin and in the case of the recent outbreaks, this resulted in mainly short-life insecticides being applied. This in turn resulted in much larger areas having to be treated, and in multiple applications, with all the accompanying negative effects on the environment. On the basis of this unsatisfactory situation a discussion was instigated on the promotion of research into new, biological and integrated control methods. Programmes along these lines were elaborated at international level. The Deutsche Gesellschaft für Technische Zusammenarbeit (GTZ) submitted a proposal to the Federal Ministry for Economic Cooperation (BMZ) who made almost 6 million DM available for research into integrated biological control of locusts and grasshoppers. Under the leadership of the GTZ and German research institutions in co-operation with international institutes and organizations as well as technical co-operation projects, research programmes were begun. The first phase of the project will be a three year term which will deal chiefly with practice-oriented research approaches. These approaches are outlined briefly in the following pages. It is intended that the results will be published at appropriate intervals. Field trials in the Sudan, on the Cape Verde Islands and in the Republic of Niger have already produced interim results.

Approaches for research into alternative methods of locust control

Early and remote sensing

Control measures for locust pests can be made environmentally more acceptable by identifying potential epidemics at their beginning and initiating control measures in good time. This is currently effected primarily by surveys and information from the local population, in particular from nomads. This system is efficient but it cannot always be implemented globally and will now be supported by the most modern methods of satellite photography. By evaluating satellite photos (Landsat), maps will be drawn up on a model basis for the Red Sea coast of Sudan, identifying areas which are potentially suitable for mass reproduction of locusts. Such satellite maps, in combination with normal maps, could be of great assistance to prospectors and pilots in the performance of their tasks in future. The present state of technology does not permit a direct identification of locusts by satellite, even when they appear in swarms. The programme outlined here will be implemented under the leadership of Professor Voss at the Institute for Geography of the Technical University Berlin.

Prevention of swarm formation by pheromones

Schistocerca gregaria occurs in a solitary and in a swarming (gregarious) form. In the solitary phase the locusts live in isolation, inconspicuously and as a useful element of a labile ecosystem in areas known as recession areas. Sustained favourable conditions of life lead to explosive mass reproduction. This is accompanied by a gradual change from the solitary to the swarm-forming (gregarious) phase. Adult *S. gregaria* occurring in vast aggregations are able to fly very long distances. They can thus reach areas of agricultural use and cause devastating damage. It appears that the aggregation may be induced by pheromones which influence the behaviour, the appearance, and many of the physiological properties of the locusts. So far none of these potential phase pheromones has been identified, nor is anything known about where they are formed, or their chemical nature. Under the leadership of Professor Ferenz, attempts will be made in the Department of Biology at the University of Oldenburg to identify, isolate and analyse the chemistry of the gregarization pheromone(s). Once the pheromone is synthesized it will be possible to examine the formation and the mode of action of the substance in the locusts. From the resulting knowledge of such a gregarization pheromone and the biological foundations of gregarization, possibilities for targeted intervention in the gregarization process will be developed. However, it is not yet possible to define the exact details of this intervention scheme.

Locust control with juvenile hormone analogs

Juvenile hormones are formed in the insect. They are inter alia, antagonists of the metamorphosis hormone, ecdysone. They prevent metamorphosis to the adult insect; in the case of *S. gregaria,* for instance, there are between five or six larval stages. It is only at the final moulting that the juvenile hormone titre drops so low that an imaginal moulting to the complete insect stage takes place. A synthetic increase in the juvenile hormone titre by additional administration brings about disturbances in the moulting process. The insects die since they are unable to free themselves from the old larval skin. Furthermore, juvenile hormones play an important role in the phase change of *S. gregaria,* affecting the mating behaviour of the male, the egg maturation in the female and possibly the accumulation of lipids (energy reservoirs for the long migration flights). Juvenile hormones have been biochemically analysed so that in the meantime it has been possible to synthesize more than 2,000 analogs. Under the leadership of Professor Dorn of the Institute of Zoology at the University of Mainz, juvenile hormone analogs from as many different chemical groups as possible will be screened for effective interference with the above processes. Tests to investigate the active mechanisms will also be conducted. This concerns both the role of the endogenous juvenile hormone in disturbing physiological processes, and the effects achieved by the analogs. Alongside the juvenile hormones, the so-called anti-juvenile hormones which have not yet been the subject of much research will be examined.

Locust control with entomopathogenic microorganisms

Locusts are attacked by viruses, bacteria, fungi and protozoa. It is the task of the Institute for Biological Pest Control at the Federal Biological Institute for Agriculture and Forestry in Darmstadt (Biologische Bundesanstalt für Land- und Forstwirtschaft) to conduct surveys of the occurrence of microbial antagonists of various types of locust and grasshopper, of their isolation, characterization and behaviour in response to environmental factors, and to test their effectiveness under laboratory conditions (Zelazny, these proceedings). To this end, specimens of dead or suspected diseased locusts and soil samples from various regions of Africa are collected and screened. Both new and previously recognized pathogens are tested in the laboratory for their effectiveness and their environmental behaviour. The aim is to elaborate formulations which can then be used in the field.

Pest management on the basis of pharmacophagous reactions to pyrrolizidine alkaloids

Pyrrolizidine alkaloids are secondary plant substances which occur in many plant species and serve primarily as protection against being eaten. Professor Boppré of the Institute of Forestry Zoology at the University of Freiburg is heading research into the relations between a specific locust species (*Zonocerus variegatus* (Linnaeus)) and one of its host plants which contains pyrrolizidine alkaloids (*Chromolaena odorata*). The alkaloids are taken up by the locusts and exercise the same function as in the plants – protection against being eaten. They do not serve nutritional purposes. For this reason such behaviour is termed pharmacophagy. The plants exert a strong attraction on the insects. Whether the alkaloids have additional influence on *Z. variegatus* is a subject for research. It is known that certain butterflies use pyrrolizidine alkaloids as precursors in the synthesis of sexual pheromones. The goal of the research is to use the alkaloids for the production of bait-like substances, and thus lure the locusts so as to tackle them selectively in small areas. Field trials are being conducted in the Republic of Benin (West Africa). The extent to which this insect-plant relation exists in *S. gregaria* also is to be investigated in preliminary laboratory tests.

Plant components as locust control agents

As in *Azadirachta indica* (neem), compounds suitable for insect control also occur in *Melia volkensii.* Under the leadership of Professor Rembold, the Max-Planck Institute in Martinsried will investigate this component. Seeds of the plant are to be collected and treated in co-operation with an international institute in Kenya. The active agents will be isolated and analysed. Laboratory tests will be conducted with crude extracts in order to test the development-inhibiting impact on locusts. By clarifying the structure of the active agents it may be possible to provide initiatives for the synthesis of new control agents.

Test of new products under practical conditions

There are already new kinds of product on the market or at the checking stage, which might represent promising alternatives to the synthetic insecticides employed so far. These include in particular the development of moulting inhibitors. They act in a manner similar to that of the juvenile hormone analogs already described. Pathogenic micro-organisms which have been formulated as control preparations also exist. These and the other preparations derived from the previously described research approaches must be tested under field conditions. Only in this way will it be possible to assess their potential for subsequent large-scale application. Testing of these agents will be conducted under the leadership of the GTZ in various African countries. The microsporidian *Nosema locustae* Canning (as bait formulation) has so far been tested on the Cape Verde Islands against *Oedaleus senegalensis* (Krauss) and *Diabolocatantops axillaris* (Thunberg). In 1991 series of trials were conducted in Niger. In field cage trials, beside the pathogenic effects of *Beauveria bassiana* (Balsamo) Vuillemin and *Nosema locustae*, the impact of neem and teflubenzuron were tested on *S. gregaria.*

Parallel ecotoxicological tests

Since the new kinds of products are not necessarily environmentally benign, even though they possess a lower degree of toxicity for warm-blooded animals than conventional insecticides, a continuous ecotoxological back-up programme will be implemented. Professor Müller from the Institute for Biogeography of the University of the Saarland heads a team which is backing up all practical trials with tests for possible side-effects of the agents employed. This has already been implemented for the Sudan, the Cape Verde Islands and Niger. In addition, preliminary tests with new active agents will be conducted in the laboratory.

Studies on economic aspects and loss assessment

Our present knowledge concerning the potential and actual damage caused by locusts to food crops and pasture plants is extremely meagre. Under the direct leadership of the GTZ losses on millet will be investigated and economic calculation models will be set up. Model field tests are being conducted in Niger in co-operation with the GTZ plant protection project. Papers on losses due to grasshopper and locust damage and on loss assessment on millet in Niger are available.

Prospects

The initial term of the project is three years. For this reason approaches have been selected which may reasonably be expected to produce results within this period. These approaches include testing the latest generation of preparations, research on pathogenic micro-organisms, or production of bait based on pyrrolizidine alkaloids. Other components, such as research into pheromones, must be considered as more long-term programmes. Should this first phase of the project be successful and further research appear necessary and promising, an extension could follow.

IAPSC/OAU; communiqué from the Inter-African Scientific Secretariat of the OAU, with comments on the application of the Inter-African Plant Protection Convention

N. Nkouka

Organization of African Unity.

Abstract

The Organization of African Unity approved a Phytosanitary Convention for Africa in 1967 and resolved to make member states apply it. The implementation of quarantine precautions varies among states, and breaches of quarantine which have occurred in other parts of the world serve as examples for the need for vigilance in maintaining quarantine standards at the national level. However, the convention allows member states to import small quantities of prohibited material for research purposes provided they observe precautions recommended by the OAU.

Your Excellency the Minister, Representatives of International Organizations, Honourable Delegates, Ladies and Gentlemen.

In the name of His Excellency, Dr Salim Ahmed Salim, Secretary General of the OAU, I should like to thank IITA for associating itself with our organization in participating in this workshop on the biological control of locusts and grasshoppers. In fact, the felicitous convergence of IITA projects dealing with plant protection in Africa and of the OAU's Interafrican Phytosanitary Council, demonstrates, if indeed it were necessary, the concerns of our countries.

The fact that we are here today to work in Cotonou in the Republic of Benin, proves again how officials of State and the people of Benin have remained true to the great African qualities of hospitality, availability, dialogue. We thank them gratefully for this.

We have taken this opportunity of reminding you in this message from the OAU, which I have the honour to bring to this workshop, and as a base-line from which to work, of the guide-lines given in Resolution 119

(IX) of the OAU Council of Ministers held at Kinshasa in September 1967. This adopted resolution states, and I quote:

'The Council of Ministers of the Organisation of African Unity, assembled in its ninth ordinary session at Kinshasa from the 4th to 10th September 1967.
— Having examined the proposal to establish a continent-wide phytosanitary convention for Africa, to protect plant health;
— noting that the scientific council for Africa, which held its second session at Addis-Abeba, Ethiopia from 8 to 12 April 1967, recommended that this convention should be accepted;
— noting, moreover, that the OAU charter advocates the coordination, harmonisation and intensification of the activities in such areas as these; we are convinced that if properly applied, this convention would allow us better to control the pests and plant diseases which rage in Africa and in this way to increase production and economic yields.

It is decided:

a. To approve the Phytosanitary Convention for Africa:
b. To make the member states of the OAU apply it.'

These provisions give quite precise directives to member states on taking proper quarantine precautions, control and inspection measures and in general any measures judged necessary by the OAU, concerning organisms living off plants, parts of plants, seeds, land, manure or packing materials, including containers and all articles which the OAU declares dangerous to agriculture throughout Africa.

No provision in the Articles of the Convention prevents any member state from importing small quantities of plant or other prohibited material, whilst observing precautions recommended by the OAU, in order to do basic or applied research. It is understood however, that such imports of prohibited material will only be made if absolutely necessary. The specific member states will inform the OAU of all such imports which are normally prohibited and the OAU in turn will inform other member States.

Constraints to the application of the Inter-African Plant Protection Convention

Despite the adoption by Ministers of the OAU of the Inter-African Phytosanitary Convention, it must be stated that its application by the member states and partners does not seem satisfactory. We cannot doubt the political will of the authorities since the legal framework exists.

During this workshop on biological control of locusts and grasshoppers there are at least two issues which we should address, since there may well be imports of live organisms to the continent for this kind of work. These two issues are at different levels:

1. the existence of national legal documentation concerning plant protection regulations
2. the implementation of these laws on plant protection legislation in our countries.

It should be noted that the situation varies considerably from country to country. In fact, Ivory Coast, Senegal and Cameroun already have quite solid legal barriers concerning plant protection.

It should be remembered that all member states of the OAU have ratified the Inter-African Phytosanitary Convention. Another question which could be asked, is why the adoption of national plant protection regulations runs into difficulties. Here, I ask for action from the Directors of National Plant Protection Services who are, in point of fact, technical advisers in this domain to their governments.

Scientific and popular knowledge seem, in the final analysis, to be two of the determining factors in decision making and in the perfection of the responses necessary when faced with the problems of plant protection regulation.

These issues are in everyone's interest. We scientists know what happened, in Europe, for example, concerning the pests of potato and grape vines. African countries can and must take these catastrophes as warnings.

Prevention depends on what responses are possible. These responses can be translated into documentation, attitudes, particularly when people travel, and in migrations. People should be aware that taking a plant or an insect in a handbag across borders, can create danger for a whole country.

Economic crises and agricultural production particularly require rapid solutions and in these conditions practising research scientists will, from time to time, have to convince our decision makers on the necessity for introducing such and such an organism in order to fight a specific pest; thus, in the name of the Inter-African Phytosanitary Council of the OAU, for whom you are the prime movers chosen for and privileged by your active participation in the creation of coordinated phytosanitary regulation in each country, take every care in order to avoid wrong decisions being made as the result of contradictory interpretations.

Today, we are engaged in biological control of locusts and grasshoppers in the same way as yesterday we fought against *Rastrococcus invadens* Williams and *Phenacoccus manihoti* Matile-Ferrero (Homoptera; Pseudococcidae). It seems that here we have two examples which may help us better to ascertain possible constraints for future projects.

In passing, I should like to mention that a consultative scientific report initiated by the Phytosanitary Council on *Zonocerus variegatus* (Linnaeus) is available at our offices in Yaoundé, Cameroun and we would like to make effective use of this study through a network of researchers in collaboration with IITA and other institutions.

Whilst reminding you of the legal framework for introducing live organisms to our continent, we have an opportunity for the OAU to lend its support to federal biological control programmes which are carried out by various international organizations.

Perhaps you already know that the OAU wishes in the near future, to redefine itself as an Economic Commission for Africa and the agro-food dimension will be seriously considered in all its aspects, including that of research.

Your contribution to the work in progress will be faithfully relayed to the Secretariat General of the OAU.

I wish you every success for this workshop and thank you for your kind attention.

ICIPE; development of a biocontrol strategy for the management of the desert locust, *Schistocerca gregaria*

S.K. Raina

International Centre of Insect Physiology and Ecology.

Abstract

Intervention for prevention of locust swarms may be contemplated either by disrupting gregarisation or manipulating solitarious populations to keep numbers low. The former could be achieved by manipulating pheromones and the latter by the augmentation of indigenous natural enemies. Protozoan and viral pathogens may have potential for use in arid conditions because the protein coats render them resistant to extremes of temperature. They also show host specificity and transovarial transmission. ICIPE has initiated a programme to select and evaluate these agents for introduction into pregregarious populations, with emphasis initially on the protozoan *Malamoeba locustae* and entomopoxvirus.

The desert locust, *Schistocerca gregaria* (Forskål), has a vast invasion area of around 29 million km^2 in which farming communities from 57 countries in the continents of Africa and Asia are affected. The devastating outbreaks of locusts in Africa which have plagued the mid-1980s, reflect a long-lasting problem with chemical control. The current method of control is mainly based on application of toxic chemicals which are detrimental to the flora and fauna of the treated areas and can result in the development of new pests because of the disruption of the natural enemy complex. Moreover, the present control strategies become operative only when locusts reach outbreak status. In ICIPE's view, prevention of locust outbreaks would be a more attractive management strategy than attempts to control populations that have already reached swarm levels. Conceptually, at least two levels of intervention, which may pre-empt or prevent the formation of swarms are possible:

1. the first involves the disruption of the process of gregarization
2. the second involves the manipulation of the population equilibrium of the solitary locust, to levels less likely to develop into swarms.

Successful research and development leading to viable interventions at these levels through the induction of chronic diseases, could virtually contain the locust menace and minimize the present reliance on large-scale use of environmentally detrimental insecticides.

Some research groups working on biocontrol of locusts have been engaged in developing biocides for direct hit on desert locust swarms. This is basically different from our approach at ICIPE, which focuses on colonization of selected pathogens, augmentation of indigenous inoculum to induce an epizootic, and conservation of inoculum following enzootics or epizootics within pre-gregarious locust populations.

Due to the severe conditions prevailing in the desert locust recession and breeding zones, candidate pathogens which require high humidity, such as fungi, and those which cannot perpetuate in the desert environment (bacteria and nematodes) are considered unsuitable components of a sustainable locust management package. However, some protozoans and insect viruses, if appropriately formulated, could tolerate the extremes of temperature and humidity because of their protein coverings. Both groups can perpetuate through transovarial transmission and are known to be specific to their target hosts (Henry, 1971; Summers *et al.*, 1975; Menapace *et al.*, 1978; Kurstak *et al.*, 1978; Canning *et al.*, 1985; Henry, 1985; Raina *et al.*, 1987, 1990).

In view of the envisaged potential of microbial control, ICIPE has initiated a biocontrol research programme, based on the above concept, which is to be executed in two phases:

1. to evaluate, isolate and characterize virulent protozoan and entomopoxviruses likely to be associated with desert locusts in their recession and breeding areas

2. **(a)** to develop methods for colonization and augmentation of the effective micro-organisms in selected pregregarious populations
(b) to devise production and formulation technology for field release.

Investigations in phase 1 have started using initially the known protozoan candidate (*Malamoeba locustae* (King & Taylor)). Other protozoans and viruses are also being considered. The biochemical characterization, pathogenicity evaluation through bioassay techniques, virulence improvement by selection procedures and extensive biosafety tests, would make it possible to establish the potential of these protozoans and viruses as biocontrol agents for sustainable management of the pregregarious population of the desert locust. A thorough study of the population dynamics of pregregarious desert locust in recession areas would help develop the proper methodology for dispersal of these microorganisms in the field after proper formulations. This is expected to be part of a comprehensive strategy, integrating biocontrol agents with selected semiochemicals (pheromones and kairomones).

References

Canning, E.U., Barker, R.J., Page, A.M. & Nicholas, J.P. (1985) Transmission of Microsporidia (Canning 1960) especially *Orthosoma operophterae* between generations of winter moth *Operophtera brumata* (L.) (Lepidoptera: Geometridae). *Parasitology* **90**, 11–19.

Henry, J.E. (1971) Experimental application of *Nosema locustae* for control of grasshoppers. *Journal of Invertebrate Pathology* **18**, 389–394.

Kurstak, E., Tijssen, P. & Maramorosch, K. (1978) In: Kurstak, E. & Maramorosch, K. (eds), *Viruses and Environment*, Academic Press, New York, pp. 571–592.

Menapace, D.M., Sackett, R.R. & Wilson, W.T. (1978) Adult honey-bees are not susceptible to infection by *Nosema locustae. Journal of Economic Entomology* **71**, 304–306.

Raina, S.K., Rai, M.M. & Khurad, A.M. (1987) Grasshopper and locust control using microsporidian insecticides. In: Maramorosch, K. (ed.), *Biotechnology in Invertebrate Pathology and Cell Culture.* Academic Press, New York, pp. 345–365.

Raina, S.K., Khurad, A.M., Rai, M.M. & Pandharipande, T.N. (1990) *Final Technical Report (Phase II) Biological Pest Management Project (IDRC Canada).* Nagpur University CSBR publication. 125 pp.

Summers, M., Engler, R., Falcon, L.A. & Vail, P. (eds) (1975) *Baculoviruses for Insect Pest Control: Safety Considerations.* American Society for Microbiology, Washington, DC.

IRLCOCSA; perspectives and prospects of biological control of the red locust, *Nomadacris septemfasciata*

J.W. Bahana & E.K. Byaruhanga

International Red Locust Control Organisation for Central and South Africa.

Abstract

The increasing awareness of environmental safety in recent years has brought to the forefront the dangers posed by chemical pollution from insect pest control. Although advances have been made in the search for alternative strategies to chemical pest control, the successes of such methods have been limited to a few insect pests.

Locusts pose formidable problems and their control has so far been possible only through intensive chemical spraying. Hitherto, other methods have not had any significant impact on prevention of locust outbreaks. On the other hand, the success of chemical control appears to have masked the development of alternative control methods.

The red locust, *Nomadacris septemfasciata* (Serville), is no exception to the locust story, but this locust has peculiarities in its ecosystem that allow alternative control strategies. This paper reviews areas in which such strategies could be developed and proposes that the red locust can be a model in the development of biological control for locusts in general.

Introduction

The red locust, *Nomadacris septemfasciata* (Serville), has been responsible for four major plagues in Africa south of the Sahara in the past 150 years but little is known of the first two. Records show that there were plagues about the periods 1847 to 1854, 1892 to 1910, 1913 to 1919, and 1930 to 1944. However, most of the information on red locust plague dynamics and progression is available only for the 1930 to 1944 plague when extensive studies were carried out to try and find a solution to the locust menace.

Evidence from the studies revealed that *N. septemfasciata* plagues originated from definite source areas where simultaneous and widespread breeding was initiated. Consequently, there were swarm escapes and further breeding both inside and outside the source areas. After a period which varied with each plague, there was collapse of locust populations. Later, breeding was limited to the source areas, and at very low levels.

Control methods employed during the first three plagues were rudimentary and ineffective. Although chemical pesticides, particularly arsenic compounds, were applied in an attempt to control locust upsurges, their use was not widespread but was restricted to the source areas. It can hardly be claimed, therefore, that pesticides were effective in ending the red locust plague. Moreover, the more effective acridicides that were introduced, such as dieldrin, came on the scene only much later, after the plague had dissipated. So, what triggers population upsurges that initiate plagues, and what is responsible for the population collapse? What role did ecological factors play in bringing about the collapse of *N. septemfasicata* populations, four times in the last 150 years? Was there a significant role by biocontrol agents in these wild fluctuations?

The ecology of *N. septemfasciata* and its outbreak areas

During the last plague of 1930–44, swarms of the red locust covered virtually all the areas south of the equator, and even as far north as Sudan and Somalia (Steadman, 1990). Studies, in part triggered by the effects of the recurring plagues, were initiated in the 1930s to try and find the origin of plagues, with a view to stopping them at source. The search for outbreak areas was based on the theory of the great acridian scientist Sir Boris Uvarov, who postulated that plagues were initiated from a few special ecosystems, later to be referred to as 'outbreak areas'.

Field investigations and subsequent analysis of reports of locust occurrence led to the conclusion that swarms which had apparently started the plague had initially formed in the grass plains of Mweru-wa-Ntipa in northern Zambia. It appeared that another source area was the Rukwa Valley in Tanzania, but there is no concrete evidence to support this (Symmons, 1978). Areas which were later found either to have produced migrating swarms, or to be capable of producing one if not controlled, were designated recognized outbreak areas (Symmons, 1978). Since 1944, these outbreak areas (Fig. 1) have at one time or another produced swarming populations (Table 1).

The outbreak areas of *N. septemfasciata* have a number of common ecological features which have been described by Gunn (1955, 1956,

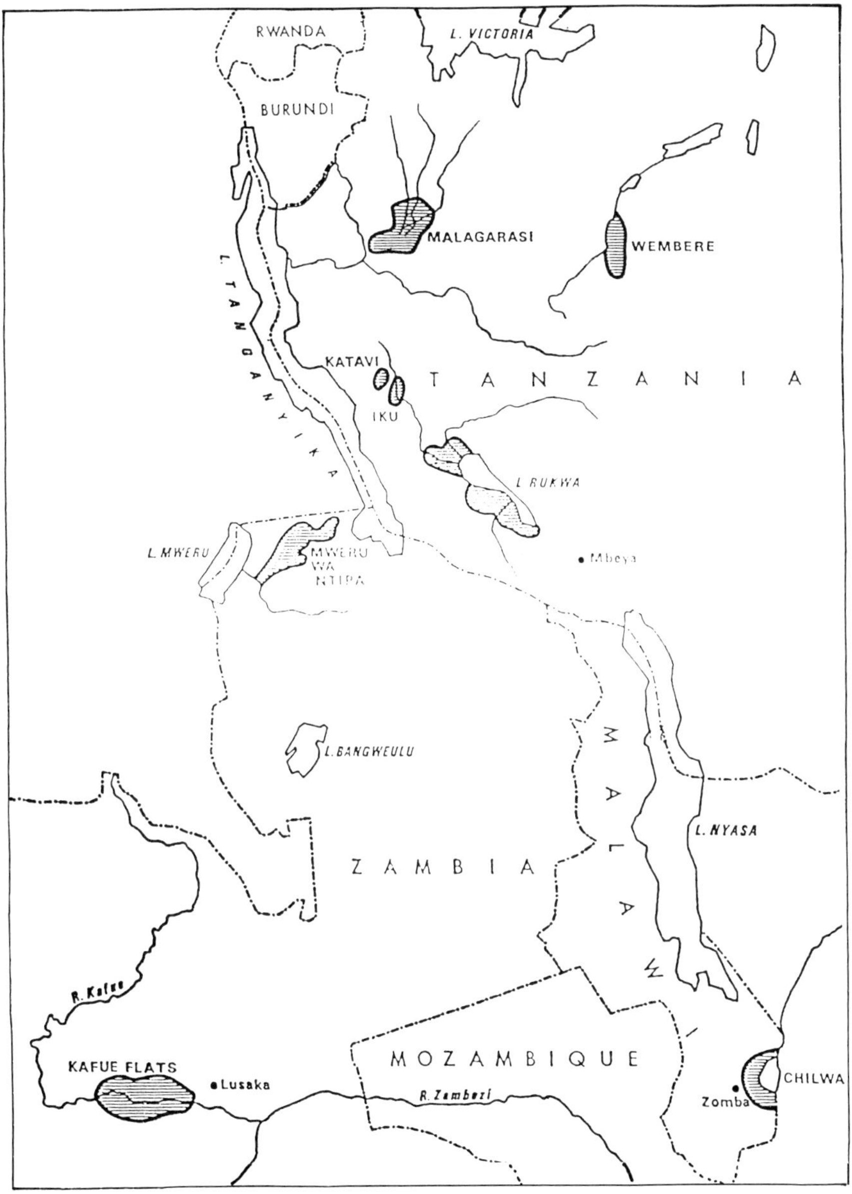

Figure 1. The recognized outbreak areas of the red locust. Shaded areas are those actually or potentially capable of producing swarms. (From Stortenbeker, 1967).

Table 1. Frequency of recorded and probable swarm formation and escape from the recognized outbreak areas of the red locust between 1945 and 1987.

	Number of years			
Area	Swarm escaped	Swarms within outbreak area only	Swarm formation possible without control	Total
Wembere	8	4	5	17
Rukwa	5	7	4	16
Malagarasi	3	3	4	10
Iku/Katavi	2	5	3	10
Buzi/Gorongosa	5	2	0	7
Kafue Flats	0	6	0	6
Mweru-wa-Ntipa	2	1	2	5
Chilwa	0	1	0	1

1960), Symmons (1978) and Materu (1984). Briefly, they are areas of extensive and open grasslands with impeded or closed drainage, consequently, they are subject to prolonged flooding during the rainy season, whereas during the latter part of the dry season, conditions can be extremely hot and dry. Generally, they are well defined areas, and it is here that red locust numbers fluctuate widely from scattered populations to swarm density, even during recession.

Vesey-Fitzgerald (1964) and Materu (1984) reviewed the ecological niches of different stages of *N. septemfasciata* in outbreak areas and reiterated an earlier view (Clark, 1947) that the ecological niche essentially consists of food-shelter and oviposition habitats. Materu (1984) then went on to suggest that it is these two habitat factors which influence the size of the population and, consequently, swarm formation. However, no definite studies have been conducted to determine the extent of this influence. Nonetheless, it is not clear if these are the only factors that influence the numbers of *N. septemfasciata*, and the role of natural enemies in the population fluctuations is not known.

Life cycle

In central and southern Africa *N. septemfasciata* lives in a region with one dry season per year. The wet season begins around November and lasts until May; oviposition coincides with the beginning of the wet season and the eggs hatch about 30–40 days later. The emerging hoppers pass through

6–7 instars, and become adult around February or March. The adults live through the dry season in immature state until the beginning of the rains when maturation is initiated. Mating and oviposition then follow.

Population dynamics

There have been few investigations on the population dynamics of *N. septemfasciata*, particularly in the field. Robertson (1954, 1958) investigated reproduction of the red locust in an outbreak area and Albrecht (1959) and Norris (1959) independently studied the dynamics of laboratory populations, but their investigations have not been corroborated by field studies.

Symmons (1959) and Symmons & Carnegie (1959) studied the effect of climate and weather on *N. septemfasciata* populations, as well as factors that affect breeding. In his studies on influence of climate and weather, Symmons (1959) demonstrated that fluctuations in numbers from one generation to the next are inversely correlated with the rainfall total in the last but one rainy season. In these studies, no mention was made of the influence of biotic factors on population numbers.

More comprehensive work in the field, however, was the study by Stortenbeker (1967) who investigated population dynamics of *N. septemfasciata* in an outbreak area. In addition to corroborating Symmons' (1959) work, Stortenbeker (1967) also showed that reductions of the parent numbers and the fledging process in the filial populations were correlated with rainfall. Stortenbeker (1967) went on to make a number of conclusions on various factors affecting population fluctuations. Significantly, again none of these were biotic factors.

Although it was not the main part of his study, Stortenbeker (1967) made a number of observations on biotic agents that were causing mortality to *N. septemfasciata.* He observed, for example, that Odonata (dragonflies and damsel flies) population numbers appeared to be correlated with the previous year's rainfall and suggested that species of Odonata were probably the most important agents causing fluctuations in the breeding success of the red locust.

Prospects of biological control – a review of natural control agents

Several investigations and reviews of population dynamics of *N. septemfasciata* (e.g. Dean, 1964; Stortenbeker, 1967; Materu, 1984) have reported a number of natural enemies in its outbreak areas. Thus, Materu (1984) listed the multimammate rat (*Mastomys natalensis*) and mites (Acarina) as egg predators. The hymenopteran *Scelio howardi* Crawford was also found parasitizing the eggs. Predators of hoppers he listed were *Alcimus* sp., *Ommatius variabilis* Engel and *Philodicus nigrescens* Ricardo (as *P. nigripes*) (all Diptera: Asilidae), *Anisoptera* spp. (Odonata) and larvae of Tabanidae (Diptera). Other workers (e.g. Chapman, 1962; Stortenbeker, 1967) have also observed a number of natural enemies of adult locusts. These included parasitic nematodes, a tachnid, *Metacemyia calleti* (Seguy), as *Ceracia nomadacris*), birds, and the fungus *Beauveria* sp.

There are thus, a large number of biocontrol agents causing mortality of different stages of *N. septemfasciata* in its outbreak areas. Unfortunately, even with such a long list of natural enemies, an impact assessment of their influence on populations has never been done. Moreover, insecticides have regularly been sprayed to suppress locust upsurges in outbreak areas and yet the effect of these pesticides on the populations of the biocontrol agents in these areas is also not known. There is, therefore, a challenge for biological control scientists to exploit the special ecosystem of *N. septemfasciata* in their quest to provide a solution to the locust menace.

Acknowledgements

The authors wish to acknowledge the expert typing of the manuscript by C. Musonda.

References

Albrecht, F.O. (1959) Facteurs internes et fluctuations des effectifs chez *Nomadacris septemfasciata* (Serv.) *Bulletin Biologique de la France et de la Belgique* **4**, 414–461.

Chapman, R.F. (1962) *Ceracia nomadacris* Van Emden (Diptera: Tachinidae) parasitising *Nomadacris septemfasciata* (Serville) (Orthoptera: Acrididae). *Proceedings of the Royal Entomological Society of London* (A) **37**, 69–71.

Clark, L.R. (1947) An ecological study of the Australian plague locust, *Chortoicetes terminifera* Walk in the Bogan-Macquaire outbreak area, N.S. Wales *CSIRO Bulletin* **226**, 71 pp.

Dean, G.J.W. (1964) Stork and egret as predators of the red locust in the Rukwa Valley outbreak areas. *Ostrich* **35**, 95–100.

Gunn, D.L. (1955) Mweru wa Ntipa and the red locust. *Northern Rhodesia Journal* **2**, 3–15.

Gunn, D.L. (1956) A history of Lake Rukwa and the red locust. *Tanganyika Notes* **42**, 1–18.

Gunn, D.L. (1960) Nomad encompassed. *Journal of the Entomological Society of South Africa* **23**, 65–125.

Materu, M.E.A. (1984) The ecology and control of the red locust (*Nomadacris septemfasciata* Serv.) *Insect Science and its Application* **5**, 79–82.

Norris, M.J. (1959) The reproduction of the red locust (*Nomadacris septemfasciata* Serville) in the laboratory. *Anti-Locust Bulletin* **36**, 46 pp.

Robertson, I.A.D. (1954) The numbers of eggs in pods, of the red locust *Nomadacris septemfasciata* (Orthoptera, Acrididae), Serville. *Entomologists Monthly Magazine* **90**, 254–255.

Robertson, I.A.D. (1958) The reproduction of the red locust, *Nomadacris septemfasciata* Serville (Orthoptera: Acrididae), in an outbreak area. *Bulletin of Entomological Research* **49**, 475–496.

Steedman, A. (1990) *Locust handbook*, 3rd edn. Natural Resources Institute, Chatham.

Stortenbeker, C.W. (1967) Observations on the population dynamics of the red locust *Nomadacris septemfasciata* Serville in its outbreak areas. *Instituut voor Toegepast Biologisch Ondorzoek in de Natuur Mededeling* **No 84**, 118 pp.

Symmons, P.M. (1959) The effect of climate and weather on the numbers of the red locust in the Rukwa Valley outbreak area. *Bulletin of Entomological Research* **50**, 507-521.

Symmons, P.M. (1978) The prevention of plagues of the red locust *Nomadacris septemfasciata* Serv. *Acrida* **7**, 55–78.

Symmons P.M. & Carnegie A.J.M. (1959) Some factors affecting breeding and oviposition of the red locust, *Nomadacris septemfasciata* (Serv). *Bulletin of Entomological Research* **50**, 333–353.

Vesey-Fitzgerald, D.F. (1964) Ecology of the red locust. *Monographiae Biologicae* **24**, 255–268.

NRI; statement of position

J.I. Magor

Natural Resources Institute, UK.

Abstract

The Natural Resources Institute (NRI) has a long history of multi-disciplinary research on problems in tropical agricultural development and is an integral part of the British Government's overseas aid programme. NRI generates income from commissions with the Overseas Development Administration (ODA) as well as from other donor agencies. It has three operational divisions, of which one, Pest Management, contains the Windborne Pest Programme, in which locust and grasshopper research falls. Current research includes pesticide bioassays, grasshopper taxonomy, outbreak forecasting and egg diapause in *Oedaleus senegalensis* (Krauss). The extensive library facilities are particularly strong on locust and grasshopper literature.

Introduction

The Natural Resources Institute (NRI) was established as an Executive Agency in April 1990. It is the scientific arm of Britain's Overseas Development Administration (ODA) within the Foreign and Commonwealth Office.

NRI has a tradition of multi-disciplinary problem solving, research and development which goes back through the Tropical Products Institute, the Land Resources Development Centre, the Centre for Overseas Pest Research, and others including the Anti-Locust Research Centre to the Imperial Institute founded in the late nineteenth century.

The institute forms an integral part of the British Government's overseas aid programme. Its principal aim is to alleviate poverty and hardship in developing countries by increasing the productivity of their renewable natural resources.

NRI's main fields of expertise are:

1. resource assessment and farming systems
2. integrated pest management
3. food science and crop utilization.

It carries out research and surveys; develops pilot-scale plant, machinery and processes; identifies, prepares, manages and executes projects; provides advice and training; and publishes scientific and development material.

This paper first outlines the structure of British Aid and its interface with NRI, then summarizes the organization of work within NRI, and finally, describes facilities for visitors and NRI's current work on locusts and grasshoppers.

British aid programme

The ODA is responsible for Britain's aid programme to developing countries which in 1990/91 amounted to over £1,600 million. It has development projects and programmes in more than 120 countries. ODA works through its five Development Divisions and with British Embassies and High Commissions overseas to manage the aid programme.

ODA staff have professional advisers dealing with economic and social development, agriculture and renewable resources, engineering, health and population, education and the environment.

Resources are allocated between bilateral aid provided on a country by country basis and multilateral aid, which is Britain's contribution to International Organizations and Institutions.

Research & development in NRI

NRI as an Agency has to cover its full costs with income. This is generated through commissions with ODA's Natural Resources and Environment Department, Geographical Desks and Development Divisions as well as through other donor agencies.

The pattern for Natural Resources Division expenditure is based on a Research Strategy for Renewable Natural Resources. Nine priority areas were identified and are managed at UK Institutes for ODA. The strategy Areas are Resource Assessment and Farming Systems, Agricultural

Engineering, Integrated Pest Management, Food Science and Crop Utilization, Animal Health, Forestry and Agroforestry, and Fisheries.

The three operational divisions at NRI Resource Assessment and Farming Systems, Pest Management and Food Science and Crop Utilization each manages a strategy area within which work is grouped into programmes containing problem areas. The emphasis within these strategy areas is for multi-disciplinary studies and the Institute's 400 professional staff cover a wide range of disciplines, notably anthropology, biochemistry, chemistry, economics, entomology, engineering, food technology, geography, information technology, land use, livestock nutrition, meteorology, physics.

Each problem area covers the whole spectrum of research from generating new knowledge, converting it into new technologies and finally adapting and transferring them for use in developing countries.

Locust and grasshopper research

Work on locusts and grasshoppers comes under the umbrella of the Integrated Pest Management (IPM) Strategy Area in the Windborne Pest Programme. The Strategy Area contains five Programmes aimed at developing IPM systems for controlling pests and diseases of annual, perennial and industrial crops in intensive and subsistence agriculture.

Migrant insects and disease vectors are important epidemic pests and the ability to quantify and forecast their dispersal is a critical factor in limiting crop damage and in developing appropriate control strategies and early warning systems.

Control and forecasting are based on a knowledge of the physiology and behaviour of the pest and their interaction with weather, climate, topography and agriculture. These facts together with a study of historical analogues predict pest incidence and severity in space and time.

The programme uses a wide group of specialists at NRI and in other UK and overseas institutes to investigate the population dynamics, epidemiology, migration, host-plant interactions, pheromones and control of rice pests and vectors, the African armyworm, locusts, grasshoppers and disease agents.

Results are used in other NRI programmes, international institutes, the IRRI rice IPM network and in regional locust organizations and are disseminated in publications and at conferences and workshops. Overseas scientists train with us and come to NRI as visiting experts.

Current locust and grasshopper research

Work on locusts and grasshoppers expanded in response to needs identified during recent outbreaks which matched NRI areas of expertise. Taxonomic revisions of East African grasshoppers are preceding the preparation of an *Identification Handbook.* Insecticides bioassays are in progress and staff have taken part in pesticide and application equipment trials. Information on the recent desert locust plague (1985–89) is being analysed so that the causes of its onset, spread and rapid decline are made available to forecasters. Finally, an examination has started of diapause in the Senegalese grasshopper *Oedaleus senegalensis* (Krauss) as part of a larger project looking at millet production and protection in Mali.

This programme does not address the biocontrol aspects of this workshop but facilities at NRI will be of interest, and an understanding of the art of forecasting grasshopper and locust outbreaks is necessary to those who wish to implement biological control.

NRI facilities

Locust archives

NRI links with locust survey and control go back fifty years to the anti-locust unit selected to hold and analyse reports collected to determine the causes of intermittent plagues. The main body of reports has been microfilmed. It starts in 1929 and ends in 1973 when FAO assumed the responsibility for maintaining the forecasting and central collection of reports. References to locusts from literature before 1929 are also in the archives.

Maps of locust outbreaks which were used in forecasting and other studies are lodged in the archives; *Locusta migratoria migratorioides* (Reiche & Fairmaire) (1928–41) red locust (*Nomadacris septemfasciata* (Serville)) (1925–41) and desert locust (*Schistocerca gregaria* (Forskål)) (1926–73). Temperature, relative humidity and rainfall maps of the desert locust area are available from 1925–37 and there are synoptic weather charts and rainfall maps of this area for 1961–73. Less detailed maps are also available for *Anacridium melanorhodon* (Walker), *Patanga succincta* (Linnaeus), the brown locust (*Locustana pardalina* (Walker)), and *Schistocerca cancellata* (Serville) in Argentina.

NRI library and information services

Resources

NRI library specialises in the literature of tropical agriculture and is recognized as a major world resource in this field. It incorporates the library of its antecedents including the Anti-Locust Research Centre (ALRC), Centre for Overseas Pest Research (COPR) and the Tropical Development Research Institute (TDRI).

The library stock includes journals, books, pamphlets, reprints, theses, annual reports and technical reports in series. Over 2,000 current journal titles are received, many through exchange arrangements.

TRAIS (Tropical Agriculture Information Service) is the name given to the library's in-house computerized bibliographic database. Bibliographic records for literature published from 1980 onwards are held on the computer database. About 11,500 new records are added each year. For earlier literature manual catalogues and indexes have been retained.

The library has on-line access to commercially available external databases, and holds CD-ROM copies of certain databases including Agricola (USDA), AGRIS (FAO) and CAB Abstracts (CABI).

Locust and grasshopper literature was collected comprehensively until about 1980. For this period there are two keys to the literature: a card index arranged by subject and by species which is available for consultation in the NRI library, and Acridological Abstracts, the published abstracts of literature on locusts and grasshoppers which are available from NRI Publications Distribution Officer.

For the period since 1980 the locust and grasshopper collection is less complete. However, it does contain most of the specialist publications and report literature on locusts and grasshoppers of economic importance, but only selected journal articles.

Services available to external users

Visitors – NRI library is open by appointment to visiting readers, for reference purposes only, from 09.00 h to 16.30 h Monday to Friday (excluding public holidays).

Enquiries – library and information services staff are available to answer bibliographic enquiries from external UK and overseas enquiries by letter, telephone or in person. Enquirers should define the subject of their enquiry as precisely as possible. Literature searches can be made for enquirers using the in-house computerized database and manual indexes. In addition the external databases which NRI library holds on CD-ROM can also be searched, but the library does not normally undertake on-line searches on external databases on behalf of external enquirers.

Photocopying – the library can only supply limited numbers of photocopies of articles. Enquirers should first try the library resources within their own country and only ask NRI library to supply what is not available locally. Copies are charged at 10 pence per page (plus VAT) but are free to organizations in developing countries eligible for British aid. Photocopying of copyright material is undertaken strictly within the UK copyright regulations (only one article from a journal or up to 10% of a book).

Remote sensing and GIS

Satellite observations of cloud duration and temperature when suitably calibrated against point surface rainfall measurements can give rapid estimates of rainfall. The TAMSAT system of Primary Data User Systems with micro computers developed in the UK by Bradford University Research Ltd, TAMSAT Research, and the Department of Meteorology at Reading University offer a cheap and robust system for monitoring rainfall using data from METEOSAT.

This system is in operational use by the meteorological services of Morocco (Casablanca); Algeria (Algiers, Tamanrasset); Tunisia (Tunis); Sudan (Khartoum); Jordan (Amman); Ethiopia (Addis Abeba); Somalia (Mogadiscio); Botswana (Gaberone) and by the Desert Locust Control Organization for Eastern Africa (DLCO-EA) in Nairobi. Cost to buy and install, with training is about £20,000.

Another exciting development by this group with Silsoe and NRI is a system to receive NOAA AVHRR data which in the absence of clouds allows vegetation changes to be monitored and from which Normalized Difference Vegetation Indices NDVIs, the greennesss maps used by locust units, are calculated. NOAA is a polar orbitting satellite, and the AVHRR sensor has a swathe width of 1500 km which enables it to complete global coverage every 12 h.

The dish on the receiver has to be steered to the point in the sky at the time the satellite is passing. A manual system has been fully tested and an automatically steered dish is under test. Software for improved geographical correction is scheduled for June. Cost with training is estimated as £25,000 to 30,000.

Publications and training

Results are published and distributed to scientists and plant protection services overseas and training is given.

OCLALAV; biological control of migratory pests, and perspectives in Africa

A.B. Ndiaye

OCLALAV, Dakar, Senegal.

Abstract

The present structure of OCLALAV is outlined, and a description of biological control as it might be applied to migratory pests is described. Work to date on biological control of locusts and grasshoppers is reviewed.

Introduction

OCLALAV, with its headquarters in Dakar, Senegal, is a regional organization for acridid control, begun in 1965 at N'Djamena (Chad) by amalgamating the Communal Organisation for Control of Acridids (Organisation Commune de Lutte Anti-Acridienne – OCLA) and the Organisation for Control of Bird Pests (Organisation Commune de Lutte Anti-Aviaire – OCLAV). The organization's mandate is to undertake control measures against locusts and grain-eating birds. Member countries are: Republic of Benin, Burkina Faso, Cameroun, Côte d'Ivoire, Gambia, Mali, Mauritania, Niger, Senegal and Chad. In 1986, the administrators of OCLALAV decided to restructure the organization, considerably reducing the number of employees.

Biological control

At the end of the Second World War, chemical control was considered as the ultimate weapon for mankind to defend itself against all ills, particularly crop pests. After a decade of spraying, and following the appearance of resistant species and the first signs of a negative impact on man and the environment, people began to consider other pest control techniques. Rather than banning the use of pesticides outright, it proved necessary to forbid the use of first generation (organochlorine) products and to opt for moderate use of second generation pesticides (organophosphates). In almost all countries DDT, HCH and dieldrin were prohibited.

There are many definitions of biological control, the most relevant of which states that biological control 'consists in putting together all appropriate means and methods which can be used by man to make changes in a biological equilibrium in a way which benefits man in a given environment'.

There are many difficulties in applying biological control methods to migratory pests as the pests may be more mobile than their control agent. We will quickly review the few biological control trials carried out in Africa for the control of migratory pests.

Biological control of locusts and grasshoppers

Bacteria

Bacillus thuringiensis Berliner was one of the first bacteria used against insects, but no strains virulent against Orthoptera have yet been found. Some early laboratory work using different bacterial species has been carried out (Stephens, 1959; Stevenson, 1959).

Other infections

Other infective organisms have been tried with variable results. In 1989, a microsporidian called *Nosema locustae* Canning was used in Mali. This protozoan was discovered on *Locusta migratoria migratorioides* (Reiche & Fairmaire) and has already been used in acridid control in North America. Trials have been carried out in the Cape Verde Islands (Lobo-Lima *et al.*, these proceedings) and in Mali but the results have been disappointing to date.

Chemical attractants

Experiments have been done taking into account the well-developed olfactory sense in insects, in order to concentrate and destroy pest species. Until now, very few viable results have been obtained in Africa.

Use of hormones or pheromones

Hormones, especially those which control growth and moulting in insects, have been used in experiments to disturb moulting patterns or growth of young larvae. It has proved possible to cause atypical moulting or to maintain individuals in the larval state. Pheromones were used because of their attractant powers on mature adults in particular. Hormones and pheromones are specific to arthropods, therefore risks to human health and to the environment are very small.

Unappetizing substances in plants

Trials using sprays made from fruits and leaves of neem, *Azadirachta indica*, have given encouraging results for certain sedentary species of grasshopper and this led to the isolation of azadirachtin, the active ingredient of fruits and leaves of neem. The use of this plant as a reforestation tree shows that its use on a large scale could be envisaged. Since neem is so abundant, it is readily available to all farmers at little or no cost. It has a repellent effect on grasshoppers; other studies on neem seem to show an effect as a growth regulator (see Langewald, these proceedings).

Cultural control

Agricultural control measures (digging up egg-pods and desiccation of embryos) could be achieved, especially with those species of grasshopper such as *Zonocerus variegatus* (Linnaeus), which lay their eggs in groups. The development of such procedures should occur in the framework of an integrated pest management programme.

However, for the time being, the use of chemical pesticides is the only efficient means of grasshopper control.

Other control possibilities

There are a great number of insectivorous vertebrates, such as rodents many species of birds and reptiles. The impact of these vertebrates as auxiliaries in the reduction of insect populations is important naturally, but they cannot be manipulated at will.

Control measures for small vertebrates (grain eating birds)

Bacteria

The impact of bacteria on birds and rodents has been investigated, but no proposals for their use as control agents have been made because of the health risk.

The contribution of predators

Destruction of nests and small dormitories by flights of migrating raptors such as kites, sparrow-hawks and eagles has been observed.

Advantages of biological control and the future for its use in Africa

Biological control has the following advantages:

1. it may be relatively cheap
2. it does not cause resistance as in use of pesticides
3. it can be used where chemical control is unacceptable.

Use of biological control in Africa

Difficulties in using biological control methods should not lead to discouragement, on the contrary, it is sufficient to weigh the advantages against the disadvantages to be immediately aware of the benefit of these methods. Africa is rich in human resources, but it does not have the financial resources to undertake the research which will lead to the perfecting of appropriate technology and to organizing training sessions.

Constraints for biological control in Africa

For the efficient use of these procedures a minimum level of scientific knowledge is necessary. It is also necessary to:

1. know the environment in which one is working
2. study the biology and behaviour of the pest in depth
3. understand the biology and behaviour of host populations
4. carry out much research and training at all levels.

Conclusion

In 1986, 1987 and 1988 unprecedented quantities of pesticides were sprayed in the fight against acridids. Biological control could help to reduce the amounts of pesticide applied and thus conserve the sahelian ecosystem.

We know that when we have mastered the use of biological control this formidable tool will open up the prospect of a great victory over enemies of crops in Africa.

References

Stephens, J.M. (1959) Note on the effects of feeding grasshoppers two pathogenic species of bacteria simultaneously. *Canadian Journal of Microbiology* **5**, 313–315.

Stevenson, J.P. (1959) Epizootiology of a disease of the desert locust *Schistocerca gregaria* (Forskål) caused by a non-chromogenic strain of *Serratia marescens* Bizio. *Journal of Insect Pathology* **1**, 232–244.

PRIFAS; notes from PRIFAS on biological control of locusts and grasshoppers

M.H. Launois-Luong

CIRAD-PRIFAS, Département GERDAT.

Abstract
PRIFAS has not so far been involved in work on biological control of locusts and grasshoppers. However, PRIFAS scientists have extensive experience in detailed ecological work on acridids which would be of great value in implementing any biological control programme.

Apart from observations on natural enemies carried out during studies of acridid population dynamics, PRIFAS has not yet undertaken specific research into biological control. Nevertheless, it may be able to contribute some ideas towards consolidating research aims using a global bioecological approach, through simultaneous studies on all aspects of the ecology of individual acridids, of acridid communities and of their natural enemies.

The reduction in numbers of acridids by biological agents occurs in natural conditions through the action of predators, scavengers, parasites and/or pathogens (fungi, viruses, bacteria). The list is very long and particularly concerns major acridid pests where there is potential for a population explosion. To these can be added indirect methods, such as the use of pheromones which encourage individuals to group together, thus making interventions easier, or insect growth regulators, which aim specifically at larvae by inhibiting feeding.

Before control of an organism is undertaken, in-depth knowledge of its ecological behaviour should be available. It is crucial to be able to decode the multi-factorial system which creates situations favourable to population explosions. Knowing when to intervene is the main problem. The answer is not always clear, since so little is known about the bioecology of the pest and its natural enemies. According to what criteria should the threshold of vulnerability of a given taxon be defined? Should we wait for economic evidence or act at periods of maximum vulnerability, when the organism is already in difficulties due to eco-meteorological problems, for example? Whether to intervene or not, must depend on the ecological characteristics of each species.

Specific situations occur when the organism is at the limit of its natural distribution. The prognosis for the species could be favourable or unfavourable, depending on its ecological flexibility and its capacity for survival under adverse conditions. Once removed from its centre of ecological stability, the organism may become more vulnerable. This is the case with the migratory locust *Locusta migratoria* (Linnaeus) in its gregarious phase, when it overflows from the humid tropical zone. Alternatively, the species may develop a new survival strategy as migratory locusts have done, by becoming sedentary in artificial oases (in Sarir in Libya), in an area far to the north of its normal area of distribution.

Voltinism also influences the chances of success of a control measure. Univoltine taxa such as *Zonocerus variegatus* (Linnaeus) or *Kraussaria angulifera* (Krauss) are targets for which control has longer lasting effects than for plurivoltine species such as *Schistocerca gregaria* (Forskål) or *Oedaleus senegalensis* (Krauss), especially if populations of adults are very mobile and capable of dispersing over very long distances.

There are as many intervention strategies as there are species and one cannot be limited to only two strategies, for example one for locusts and one for grasshoppers.

The synecological framework defines communities of species which colonize the same habitats. Time and space variants are the indices of stability or instability in a particular ecological zone. The specificity of actions of natural enemies is an important point to establish, since control efforts should be targeted towards economically important species which are already in population imbalance. Many observations have been made and studies carried out on the biology and ecology of certain natural enemies. It is to be hoped that taxonomic inventories complemented by already existing bio-ecological data, continue to be updated and made accessible.

Biocoenotic studies define the host ecological niche, by describing vegetation groupings which are true ecological indicators of the environment, and integrating them with static and dynamic components of local or regional ecometeorological events. These will show the likelihood of proliferation, the degree of aggressiveness or simply the possibilities of survival of an external pathogen in its new habitat.

The biogeography of acridids is an important indicator to ascertain the importance and the type of ecological zones where control measures could take place. The type of habitat indicates the likely success of a biological control measure. Thus, the harshness of the climate of desert regions, where most of the gregarious foci of migratory locusts in Africa are situated (apart from those around the Red Sea), is in itself a major difficulty for the survival and proliferation of a pathogen.

On islands such as the Cape Verde Islands there is a closed system which is favourable for biological control, as long as safety of the agent for non-target organisms is assured. An imbalance introduced into a biocoenosis can last for a long time, due to slow exchanges with the continent and other islands, and will lead eventually to a new equilibrium of the organism. Exploration carried out in different islands revealed a significant population of acridids parasitized by Diptera larvae at the end of the rainy season which leads to speculation about the impact which this natural limiting factor could have on the population. At the same time, trials with *Nosema locustae* on *Oedaleus senegalensis* have not been conclusive, probably because of the great mobility of the adults, which prevented good contamination of the population.

An oasis effect created on a continent by deforestation does not generate such an impervious environment as an island, and exchanges are more difficult to control.

This global approach, ecological, synecological, biocoenotic, biogeographic, of the host and its aggressor, allows us to define the outlines of their respective ecological niches. The cross-checking of their ecology with behaviour will provide the spatial and temporal framework for the optimum moments of vulnerability of the acridid at the same time as those of the optimum harmfulness of its natural enemy. Many questions could be partially answered:

1. what are the encounter strategies of the natural enemies with their hosts? Do they show active identification, interception or attack modes, or are they passive modes using proliferation of the inoculum to increase the chances of encounter?
2. what are the modes of action and eco-meteorological conditions necessary for an optimum expression of their harmfulness?
3. how long will the pathogen remain active or alive, what is the likelihood of proliferation and survival?
4. what are the alternative hosts or the forms of survival if the host is absent?
5. what guarantee is there that they have a specific action and that they are innocuous to the environment?

PRIFAS is ready to invest in this kind of approach, alone or in collaboration, as long as there are visible sources of funding. It is probable that the species of acridids most likely to become the object of biological control, apart from *Zonocerus variegatus*, which is already being studied, are *Kraussaria angulifera*, *Cataloipus cymbiferus* (Krauss), *Hieroglyphus daganensis* Krauss, *Kraussella amabile* (Krauss), species which are having an increasing economic impact on the Sahel.

Field trials could be complemented by studies in the laboratory in Africa or at Montpellier and in the latter case, in the framework of the proposed Inter-Organism Centre (CIO). This is a specialist research structure which would regroup INRA, CIRAD, ORSTOM, CNRS, ENSAM, USTL, in the context of the international biological control complex of AGROPOLIS, CILBA which includes Australian partners (CSIRO) and Americans (USDA), and which represents the emergence of an accumulation of knowledge and skills in operational biological control.

COUNTRY REPORTS

Congo; the acridid situation in the Congo

G. Bani

Direction Générale de la Recherche Scientifique, Brazzaville.

Introduction

The Congo, with a surface area of 342,000 km^2 of forest and savanna, has a humid tropical climate with an average temperature of 26°C, 85% relative humidity and rainfall of 2,000 mm. The wet season is from October to May and the dry season from June to September. There are approximately 2,000,000 inhabitants in the Congo, whose basic staple is cassava, not only the tubers, but the leaves also, form an important part of the diet.

There are many crop pests and diseases in the Congo. Crop pests identified include acridid species such as the variegated grasshopper, *Zonocerus variegatus* (Linnaeus) which is, at the moment, the only species to have attained the status of economic pest.

Distribution and habitat

Z. variegatus can be found in all regions of the Congo, on the edges of paths, close to villages, vegetable growing areas and cassava agro-ecosystems. It is not found in uncultivated forests and savanna.

Damage

The importance of the damage caused by *Z. variegatus* varies according to ecological zones and crops; in the forest zone of Mayombe, it is the single most important pest of cassava (*Manihot esculenta*). Damage occurs in the first month after the cutting is planted and usually it is completely destroyed. Farmers may replant two or three times but only cuttings planted later on manage to avoid the ravages of early attack. Nevertheless, next year's attacks are also important, since defoliation by grasshoppers affects farmers who themselves consume the leaves and can also sell them for a high price.

In vegetable growing zones, *Z. variegatus* is a permanent menace to green leafy vegetable production, since it diminishes the commercial value of the product by the damage it causes.

Biological cycle

Research carried out shows that the biological cycle of *Z. variegatus* is univoltine and variable. Hatching can occur from May to August, depending on the location. Oviposition occurs from December to January or a little later. Some hatching has been observed in January/February in certain areas but this is not a bivoltine cycle, since there are two univoltine populations present reproducing at different times of the year. This case is being studied.

Control

Until recently, chemical methods have been used to control populations of *Z. variegatus* around cash crop plantations, coffee (*Coffea* spp.), cocoa (*Theobroma cacao*), citrus (*Citrus* spp.). In cassava plantations man simply harvested what the undesirable visitor left for him. However, we have been able to institute a strategy which allows us to reduce or avoid early attacks on cassava. This consists of staggering the times when cuttings are taken, depending on hatching times. This practice has already been adopted by a few forward-thinking farmers. It is only applicable to cassava and only in the first months of planting.

Suggestions

Control of *Z. variegatus* in the Congo is a real need and, recognizing the limits of chemical control, we think that everything possible should be done to institute a system of control which does not damage the environment and is economically viable. In order to do this, it is necessary to understand all the biotic factors for population regulation so that we can reinforce the action still further. Thus, specific attention should be given to the parasitoid complex of *Z. variegatus.* We are in favour of all endeavours in this direction and we firmly uphold any initiatives for co-operation in research for biological control agents of *Z. variegatus.*

COUNTRY REPORTS

Mali; notes on the acridid problem in Mali

B. Maiga

Service de la Protection des Végétaux, Mali.

Introduction

Mali has a varied collection of pests: locusts and grasshoppers, birds, rodents, beetles (leaf miners and leaf beetles) which cause considerable damage to crops and crop yields every year. Since they appear so regularly, locusts and grasshoppers are by far the most important of these pests. In fact, since the droughts began in 1970, there have been problems with grasshoppers every year, and this necessitates the deployment of great financial, material and human resources; Mali finds itself obliged to request financial aid in order to finance its plant protection campaigns.

Strategy and control methods used against acridids

In Mali, the Plant Protection Service (PPS) uses the following strategies and methods:

1. Locusts. Preventative control consisting of intensive observation of gregarious foci, with the aim of stopping locusts becoming gregarious and so preventing swarms from spreading and reaching crop zones.
2. Grasshoppers. Since acridids are a semi-permanent scourge throughout the Sudano-sahelian belt, the accent is more and more on preventative control. First, mobilizing farmers to dig up egg-pods in their fields and the immediate surroundings during the dry season and secondly treating larvae at the beginning of the rainy season.

In keeping with its resources, the PPS opted for grass-roots protection of crops, with the farmer as a key element in protecting his own crops and the officers of the PPS taking charge of remote areas, pasture and uninhabited areas. Farmers are organized into plant protection brigades, trained and equipped to protect village crops. Digging up egg-pods and early control of larvae gives a significant reduction in the use of pesticides. Further control measures are only used if necessary.

The main species of economic importance are:

1. *Hieroglyphus daganensis* Krauss
2. *Kraussaria angulifera* (Krauss)
3. *Oedaleus senegalensis* (Krauss)
4. *Cataloipus fuscocoeruleipes* Sjöstedt
5. *Cataloipus cymbiferus* (Krauss)
6. *Kraussella amabile* (Krauss)
7. *Aiolopus simulatrix* (Walker)
8. *Diabolocatantops axillaris* (Thunberg)
9. *Cryptocatantops haemorrhoidalis* (Krauss)
10. *Ornithacris turbida cavroisi* (Finot)
11. *Pyrgomorpha cognata* Krauss

These species can co-exist at high densities and can cause serious damage.

Area covered by exploration

Observation

All the Sahelian and Saharo-sahelian region is under direct observation by teams of plant protection explorers, these comprise at least 15 exploration teams deployed throughout the region.

Areas treated with chemicals against different pests

During the last five years an average of 516,000 ha per year has been treated in Mali (Table 1). Although acridids are the main targets of treatments, the chemicals affect all pests in treated areas.

Cost of plant protection campaigns over the past five years

The PPS has received funds from the Department of Agriculture, the National Budget, foreign governments and international organizations.

Table 1. Area treated with chemicals 1987–91.

Campaign	Area treated	Area infested
1986–87	595,337 ha	1,000,000 ha
1987–88	330,597 ha	800,000 ha
1988–89	502,098 ha	1,200,000 ha
1989–90	722,492 ha	1,500,000 ha
1990–91	459,471 ha	525,000 ha

National budget

1986–87	121,622,000 CFA Fr
1987–88	150,000,000 CFA Fr
1988–89	250,000,000 CFA Fr
1989–90	310,000,000 CFA Fr
1990–91	297,000,000 CFA Fr

International Organizations – Emergency funds

1986–87	268,453,000 CFA Fr
1987–88	1,102,515,000 CFA Fr
1988–89	1,575,779,000 CFA Fr
1989–90	1,032,685,000 CFA Fr
1990–91	297,000,000 CFA Fr

Conclusion

In Mali, there are a variety of crop pests but acridids are the most important and every year enormous resources are deployed to control their increase. These resources are often greater than the country has at its disposal, hence the plea for urgent help from the international community. To combat these difficulties, the PPS in Mali has opted for a grass-roots approach which means that the farmer must assume responsibility for the protection of his own fields and immediate surroundings. However, enormous quantities of chemical pesticides (more than 200,000 l of liquid chemical and 500 t of powder each year) are still being used with all the risks that this entails for man and his environment. The PPS recognises the dangers, which is why it is turning towards research into and application of alternative methods, digging up egg-pods, end of season cultivation, proper field and border sanitation, trials of biological products, harvest and trial rearing of egg-pod parasites, etc. This research is aimed at the reduction of the use of chemcial pesticides and is carried out in collaboration with partners such as FAO, USAID, Ciba-Geigy, etc.

COUNTRY REPORTS

Republic of Benin: the acridid situation in the Republic of Benin

A. Coffi

Service Protection des Végétaux, Benin.

Introduction

For the past ten years Benin has undergone wide-ranging attacks by grasshoppers in the north (near the border with Niger), on crops such as maize (*Zea mays*), sorghum (*Sorghum* sp.) rice (*Oryza sativa*) and cassava (*Manihot esculenta*). *Zonocerus variegatus* (Linnaeus) has become a pest of some importance in the south since 1985. It has become necessary to formulate a national strategy against grasshoppers.

1982 saw an unprecedented proliferation of grasshoppers. The FAO collaborated with the government of Benin to spray an area of 20,000 ha in the north from the air. Since then, Benin has treated an average of 6,000 ha of crops and fallow annually.

Organization

Training of extension workers and farmers

There are approximately 20 especially recruited extension officers, who have helped farmers and involved them in control measures.

Exploration

We have found about 15 very common species of grasshopper (Acrididae) of which six are of economic importance:

1. *Hieroglyphus daganensis* Krauss
2. *Kraussaria angulifera* (Krauss)

3. *Oedaleus senegalensis* (Krauss)
4. *Oedaleus nigeriensis* Uvarov
5. *Cataloipus fuscocoeruleipes* (Sjöstedt)
6. *Zonocerus variegatus* (Linnaeus)

Population density during infestations is from 50 to 230 larvae/m^2, counting all species. Pressure from grasshoppers was intense until 1988, when due to exceptionally heavy rains grasshoppers drowned and crops were lost.

In 1989, there was calm, but in 1990 a resurgence took place from those areas which had not been flooded, and from external populations borne in on the winds.

Treatment

Spraying takes place from June to September or October, during the rainy season. The primary target is the population of young larvae in fallow, and in crops damaging growing tips, and for this we use powder formulations (propoxur, carbaryl, fenitrothion, Table 1).

From August to September there follows an intensive treatment

Table 1. Anti-grasshopper activities in Benin.

Year	Insecticides used	Quantity	North Area treated ha	South Area treated ha
1986	propoxur	4.0 t	2,980	6,666
	HCH	1.9 t		
	fenitrothion	3390.0 l		
	dieldrin			
1987	propoxur	2.0 t	6,578	7,964
	γ-HCH	0.5 t		
	fenitrothion	60.0 t		
1988	fenitrothion	25.7 t	6,758	4,712
	propoxur	6.7 t		
	malathion	5400.0 l		
1989	propoxur	13.5 t	6,285	
	carbaryl	11.6 t		
	fenitrothion	0.8 t		
	malathion	1310.0 l		
1990	propoxur	15.3 t	4,614	
	carbaryl	0.5 t		

against advanced larvae and adults with ULV formulations (malathion, fenitrothion, Table 1).

Evaluation of treatments takes place to see how effective they have been and whether isolated pockets need to be treated again.

Future aims

- Organization of farmers into farmer brigades
- Providing brigades with means of treatment
- Reviving observation posts in the north
- Training

Zonocerus variegatus – the variegated grasshopper

This grasshopper lives in the southern part of the country and attacks maize, cotton (*Gossypium* spp.), cassava and teak (*Tectona grandis*), especially in the long dry season, causing defoliation and bark-stripping on cassava. The longer the dry season, the worse the threat. From 1986–89 there were three control campaigns over 20,000 ha and due to this successful treatment the situation is calm at the moment.

There is still much work to be done (real damage, effect of attacks on tubers), since although *Z. variegatus* is not a problem now, there are still ecological zones favourable to grasshopper proliferation in areas of natural forest surrounded by planted forest, as in the Lama forest.

Complementary to these activities research work has been done in the laboratory and in the field.

Laboratory

The influence of neem oil on different stages of *Zonocerus variegatus* larvae was investigated, at 5 l/ha and 10 l/ha.

Results: neem oil inhibits moulting and affects the antennae.

In the field

Z. variegatus damage was simulated on cassava.

Results: the damage made no significant difference in yield.

Conclusion

In Benin, we have used only chemical insecticides against locusts and grasshoppers, which may well present great risks for the environment, man and other animals.

The insecticides used only limit the damage done to crops, without any respect for non-target species.

Although the use of insecticides is in response to a pressing need for the elimination of insects in crops, when possible long- and short-term harmful effects are taken into account, it becomes imperative to identify other approaches which can take the protection of nature into account.

COUNTRY REPORTS

Senegal; grasshopper and locust control in Senegal

A. Niassy

Directorate of Plant Protection, Dakar, Senegal.

Abstract

In Senegal, grasshopper control represents 80% of pest control activities organized by the Directorate for Plant Protection (DPP) in collaboration with OCLALAV and FAO amongst others. Until now, mainly chemicals have been used for control purposes, but now different ideas are being developed, more extension workers are receiving training and more farmers closely monitored. Thus, from large-scale spraying by helicopter, the trend is towards small scale interventions, even by the farmer himself. This new outlook means that we will soon be in a position to introduce biological control methods in an experimental form.

Locust control strategies

Basic findings

In order to define the strategy for the next year, we have to examine population dynamics from preceding campaigns in conjunction with climatic conditions and the results of exploration for egg pods during the previous season.

There are two main groups in locust and grasshopper populations.

Migratory grasshoppers

These move in relation to the intertropical convergence zone (ITCZ). *Oedaleus senegalensis* (Krauss), for example, often causes major damage to cereal crops in the north of Senegal. The behaviour of this species is well known since it has been extensively studied by researchers from PRIFAS. Control begins by observing the ITCZ and studying vegetation maps to predict or locate outbreaks. If the results of this method seem positive, the model will become the main tool in observation of the species. The Pest Forecasting Bureau at the Crop Protection Service started to use the PRIFAS biomodel in 1990.

Sedentary species

These can be divided into two main groups:

1. Wet season grasshoppers; univoltine with embryonic diapause (*Kraussaria angulifera* (Krauss), *Cataloipus cymbiferus* (Krauss), *Hieroglyphus daganensis* Krauss, *Acorypha* spp., etc.). These insects hatch in July/ August and become adult by mid-September. Diapausal eggs are laid at the end of September/ beginning of October. Density and damage can be quite substantial depending on the area. During the 1990–91 campaign 261,601 ha were treated (Table 1).

2. Dry season grasshoppers; univoltine with either adult diapause (*Ornithacris turbida* Walker, *Diabolocatantops axillaris* (Thunberg), or egg diapause (*Zonocerus variegatus* (Linnaeus)), or bivoltine with adult diapause (*Aiolopus simulatrix* (Walker), *Acanthacris ruficornis* (Fabricius)). These attack vegetable and fruit crops. *O. turbida* and *A. ruficornis* have become endemic in the Nioro area and they cause significant damage to cashew tree (*Anacardium occidentale*) plantations; sometimes the whole crop can be lost. Spraying with insecticides is effective but does not solve the whole problem.

Table 1. Summary of the results of treatments in the 1990–91 campaign.

	Area treated (ha)			Proportion of area with acridids (%)
Type of intervention	Acridids	Others	Total	
1. Ground-based applications				
Village committees	30,519	16,309	46,828	65
DPP	198,938	34,248	233,186	85
Total terrestrial	229,457	50,557	280,014	82
2. Aerial applications				
ECOFORCE (French Cooperation Project)	32,144	–	32,144	100
Total aerial	32,144	–	32,144	100
Overall total	261,601	50,557	312,158	84

Source: Anon. (1991b)

Strategies

Chemical control of wet season grasshoppers

The main methods of control are:

1. early intervention (farmers' level) in small areas concentrating on groups of larvae in fields using powder and emulsifiable concentrates
2. intervention on the ground over larger areas on fallow land and in forests; control of adults is done using ULV sprayers and emulsifiable concentrates
3. aerial intervention when the infestation is general and cannot be treated on the ground.

The type of control strategy used depends on the following points:

1. the importance of the crop to be protected
2. the nature and developmental stage of the pest
3. surface area infested and location
4. resources available.

Thanks to the efforts of the state in conjunction with the European Community, the Directorate has large human and logistical resources at its disposal.

Human resources

At Directorate level there are 273 personnel. In addition, there are village pest control committees, extension officers and experts from the international community (computer specialists, aeroplane mechanics and pilots). Local labour may be employed as necessary.

Material resources

201 vehicles for application, liaison, exploration and maintenance, 31 of them with proper equipment. 900 pairs of boots, 900 goggles, 900 masks and 99 pairs of gloves are available at the ten regional Plant Protection Inspectorates.

During extensive infestations in certain regions close to Dakar, the French Cooperation Project (ECOFORCE) allocated a helicopter to Senegal for 90 flying hours.

Ground spraying

This was done by motorized units from the DPP and anti-locust village committees. The surface area treated was 229,457 ha, with 198,938 ha by the DPP and 30,519 by village committees. There was about 90% mortality in 48 hours.

Aerial spraying

This was carried out by helicopter on areas of massive infestation of five species of grasshoppers over a total of 32,144 ha in different regions. Using fenitrothion there was 81.8% mortality after 24 hours and 90.4% after 48 hours.

A total of 312,158 ha was treated. Treatments affected grasshoppers and other pests (hairy caterpillars, scale insects and cantharid beetles) and birds.

The total of chemicals used was as follows:

393 t of powder
14,469 l of emulsifiable concentrate
169,390 l of ULV formulations

The pesticides were fenitrothion, carbaryl, chlorpyriphos, malathion and lambdacyhalothrin (Table 2).

It is obvious from these figures, which reflect a fairly calm period of activity, how expensive locust and grasshopper control can be. Chemical control needs vast financial and material resources and risks polluting the environment. Therefore, other methods of control should be considered, especially now that environmental protection has become so important world-wide.

Control using poisoned baits

This has certain advantages for grasshopper control if well thought out. The surface area treated can be considerably smaller and can affect winged adults and larvae in the dry season or at the beginning of the wet season, using a base (bran) provided by the farmer himself. This method involves the farmer in the monitoring and protection of his own farm. In Senegal, control with insecticide baits using millet bran with carbaryl and certain feeding stimulants has been effective (82% mortality) against *Ornithacris turbida.* It may be worth using against *Zonocerus variegatus* and *Aiolopus simulatrix* which threaten crops in southern and northern areas of the country respectively.

Trials are in progress to assess the effectiveness and economic impact

Table 2. Summary of nationally approved chemical insecticides.

Product	Application kg (wp) or L (ec and ULV)			National total
	DPP	Village committees	Aerial	
Wettable powders				
Fenitrothion 3%	13,997	339,794	–	
Propoxur 2%	–	7,690	–	
Propoxur 1%	–	800	–	
Carbaryl 5%	–	9,100	–	
Chlorpyriphos 5%	9,395	12,655	–	
Total wp	23,392	370,039	–	393,431
Emulsifiable concentrates				
Fenitrothion 50	7,151	2,502	–	
'Sumicombi 30'*	1,726	3,089	–	
Total ec	8,877	5,591	–	14,468
ULV formulations				
Fenitrothion 500	44,086	284	–	
Fenitrothion 250	26,565	–	29,930	
Malathion 95%	15,808	–	–	
Chlorpyriphos**	23,031	–	–	
Lambdacyhalothrin 1%	3,200	–	16,792	
Chlorpyriphos 24	9,695	–	–	
Total ULV	122,385	284	46,722	169,391

*50:1 mixture of fenitrothion and fenvalerate
**Concentration not specified

of this method. We will try to use these baits containing pathogens, as well as chemical insecticides, more often in future.

Biological control

This method may be useful against sedentary species (see above) since they develop in relatively small areas and it should be possible for natural enemies and pathogens to maintain high enough levels to control pest populations. Studies on the impact of natural enemies on egg pods of *Cataloipus cymbiferus* (Anon., 1991a; Niassy, in press) have shown that the level of attack can be as high as 60% on egg pods. On *Kraussaria angulifera* and *Hieroglyphus daganensis* 11% were affected three months after the start of the rainy season.

Predators of egg pods include tenebrionids such as *Pimelia senegalensis* Olivier, *Vieta senegalensis* (Klug) and carabids such as *Styphlo-*

merus sp. etc. *P. senegalensis* larvae are often seen on *K. angulifera* egg cases. Comprehensive studies on insect enemies have been done by Greathead (1963), Popov (1980), Van der Valk (1990) and Popov *et al.* (1990). Van der Valk's study, carried out in Senegal, stressed the abundance of certain locust enemies and their susceptibility to chemical insecticides.

Work has also been done on pathogens. Prior & Greathead (1989) discussed the possibilities in this area. In Senegal, investigations on the use of pathogens such as *Nosema locustae* Canning have been done at DPP with the help of USAID. These trials included different species of grasshopper including *Zonocerus variegatus* and *Oedaleus senegalensis* (Fishpool, 1982).

Growth regulators have also been used against locusts and the results were interesting, but methods are still experimental. However, the pilot project (Niassy, 1990) showed that they can compete with chemical insecticides such as fenitrothion and chlorpyriphos.

Two new projects are about to start. The first will deal with biological control using entomopathogens and is financed by the governments of the Netherlands, USA, Canada and UK. It will concern itself with Sahelian countries and is based at IIBC (UK), IITA (Benin) and DFPV in Niger (see paper by Prior *et al.*, these proceedings). Senegal will participate in this project.

The second project is a study of the impact of pesticides on the environment, with a sub-programme dealing with useful entomofauna. It will be based in Senegal and is financed by the Netherlands and co-ordinated by FAO and the National Plant Protection Service.

Senegal is ready to lend every effort towards developing biological control.

References

Anon. (1991a) Direction de la Protection des Végétaux. 1991 Rapport des missions de prospection d'oothèques dans les zones Nord et Centre du Sénégal. Période du 26.12.90 au 19.01.91. DPV, B.P. 20 054 Thiaroye, Dakar, Senegal.

Anon. (1991b) Direction de la Protection des Végétaux. 1991 Bilan des activités de la campagne phytosanitaire 1990/1991. DPV, BP 20 054, Thiaroye, Dakar, Senegal.

Fishpool, L.D.C. (1982) *Control of Grasshoppers in West Africa using* Nosema locustae. *A Report of the 1982 Field Trial.* COPR, London.

Greathead, D.J. (1963) A review of the insect enemies of Acridoidea (Orthoptera). *Transactions of the Royal Entomological Society of London* **114**, 437–517.

Niassy, A. (1990) The grasshopper complex. In: Everts, J.W. (ed.), *Environmental Effects of Chemical and Grasshopper Control: a Pilot Study.* FAO, Rome. Report on Project ECLO/SEN/003/NET, pp. 126–139.

Niassy, A. (in press) Etude de l'impact des traitements antiacridiens: au fénitrothion, chlorypyriphos et diflubenzuron sur la prédation et le parasitisme des oothèques des populations acridiennes résiduelles. Cas de *Cataloipus cymbiferus* Krauss (1877) Acrididae Eyprepocnemidinae.

Popov, G.B. (1980) *Studies on Oviposition, Egg Development and Mortality in* Oedaleus senegalensis *(Krauss) Orthoptera, Acridoidea) in the Sahel.* COPR report no. 53. COPR, London.

Popov, G.B., Launois-Luong, M.H. & Van der Weel, J.J. (1990) *Les Oothèques des Criquets du Sahel. Collection Acridologie Opérationelle.* Ministère des Affaires Etrangères des Pays-Bas et CIRAD/PRIFAS, France.

Prior, C. & Greathead, D.J. (1989) Biological control of locusts: the potential for the exploitation of pathogens. *FAO Plant Protection Bulletin* **37**, 37–47.

Van der Valk, H.C.H.G. (1990) Beneficial arthropods. In: Everts J.W. (ed.), *Environmental Effects of Chemical Locust and Grasshopper Control: a Pilot Study.* FAO, Rome, Report on Project ECLO/SEN/003/NET, pp. 171–224.

COUNTRY REPORTS

Sudan; the situation of desert locust, tree locust and grasshoppers in the Sudan (1990–91)

A. Abdalla

Locust and Grasshopper Control Unit, Plant Protection Directorate, Sudan.

Abstract

The status of the two main locust species, *Schistocerca gregaria* (Forskål) and *Anacridium melanorhodon* (Walker), and of grasshoppers in the Sudan in 1990 and 1991 is briefly reviewed.

Introduction

During 1990 in the Sudan, rainfall was generally below average and this meant that breeding conditions for locusts and grasshoppers were not favourable. In fact, survey operations in summer breeding zones between latitudes 12°N–18°N, showed that no locusts were present.

Desert locust, *Schistocerca gregaria* (Forskål)

During the summer campaign, all areas were calm and only a few scattered individuals were found in three localities in the Central region of Sudan during August, at a density of one locust/km^2. Both ground and aerial surveys produced the same conclusions. The main crops in the surveyed areas were vegetables, millet, and sorghum, and no damage was reported.

Tree locust, *Anacridium melanorhodon* (Walker)

The same survey teams were used for tree locust as for desert locust and here too the local population reflected the low rainfall with tree locusts concentrated in relatively high rainfall areas. In June, ground surveys in Central region indicated some threat by tree locusts to orchard crops. In July, in Darfur the total infested area was about 1,700 ha with a medium density of locusts and in north Kordufan the infested area was 100,000 ha, but most swarms dispersed since low rainfall made conditions unsuitable for egg laying. In September in Kadugli, more rain encouraged egg-laying which resulted in a high density presence at 60–70 individuals per tree, of 2nd–5th instar. The area infested from August to October 1990 was 28,660 ha, with less than half affected by adults.

During this period, 3,000 ha were sprayed aerially and 17,000 ha on the ground using propoxur dust 1%, diazinon EC 60% and fenitrothion 96%.

Grasshoppers

After some rainfall in July, grasshoppers (1–5 individuals/m^2) were seen in Darfur and Eastern region. In August, after more rain, there were outbreaks in Darfur of several species of grasshopper, attacking mainly millet. In one area of about 4,000 ha, up to 80% damage to millet and sorghum was noted with a grasshopper density of 20–70 individuals/m^2. Propoxur was sprayed.

1990–91

During the winter breeding season the desert locust situation was generally calm. The Tokar Delta is the most ecologically suitable habitat for the desert locust to breed, since it is flooded annually. The area cultivated here is usually about 30,000 ha and can be as large as 80,000 ha, but this year was exceptionally small with only about 85 ha flooded – a completely new phenomenon.

In November, some scattered individuals were found in the Tokar Delta over an area of 200 ha at a density of one individual/ha. The crops cultivated here are sorghum and millet. All other areas were found free from locusts. The vegetation varied from very dry to green, and included some favourable ecological breeding conditions. During December and January there was still no problem and up until March no gregarious activity was reported, so it seems likely that the calm situation regarding the desert locust will persist throughout 1991, despite the likely presence of scattered adults in the traditional breeding grounds of the Sudan.

Discussion: precis

Dr Johnson congratulated Dr Ndiaye on his talk, but asked why, in Dr Ndiaye's opinion, the *Nosema* trial in Mali in 1989 did not work, since it was not a temperature problem as he had been present when frozen spores arrived from Evans Biocontrol. Dr Ndiaye and Dr Knausenberger were agreed that it was a logistic problem.

Dr Bateman commented to Captain Kitenda that his comments on the involvement of farmers and other practical realities were taken very seriously. Could Captain Kitenda help make laboratory studies more realistic by suggesting what might be typical temperatures during spray operations? Captain Kitenda replied that temperatures vary between 10°C and 20°C in the mornings, and that between 07.00 and 10.00 h they may be as low as 8–12°C in some areas.

Dr Niassy commented to Mr Mouhim that a figure of six million litres of chemicals used during the campaign against locusts seemed huge when one considers the risks and the means necessary to put this into practice. Could Mr Mouhim give some information about the logistic framework and equipment necessary on the one hand and on farmer participation on the other. Mr Mouhim responded that the fight against locusts used land based resources, but the greater part of the intervention was from the air. The application was at a dosage of between 0.8 l and 1 l of ULV product/ha. Farmers were especially valuable in warning us and this is what they have mostly been trained to do. Concerning the environment, Dr Ndiaye spoke of the ECOTOX project in Senegal which is concerned about the effects on the environment of chemicals used in the fight against locusts.

Dr Oomen commented to Dr Zelazny that the number of activities described which are aimed at finding and developing biological control agents is impressive. Many questions to be studied are, however, easily comparable in the different research institutes involved, (e.g. surveying, isolating, bio-assay, formulation, application). In order to obtain results efficiently, considerable co-ordination and co-operation are very desirable. How does the EC provide for and assure such co-operation? Dr Zelazny responded that the co-ordination of research activities is a very important aspect of the CEC project. At the moment, such co-ordination involves mainly identification, processing of collected material and exchange of pathogens to establish standards during testing. The main aim at this stage is to search for and find new and promising disease agents. If the work in the future concentrates more on application and formulation, such co-ordination will have to be intensified.

Dr Ba-Diallo asked Dr Zelazny whether he would welcome collaboration with the newer research institutes from the Sahelian region. Dr Zelazny replied that GTZ has offered fellowships to four people, but it is difficult to find people to go to Germany and funds were very tight.

Mr Shah asked Dr Raina what microbial agents should be used in the pre-gregarization phase of desert locust and how could they be used in the field given that they would need to be easily applicable, persistent and cover an extensive area. Dr Raina responded that biological agents which can perpetuate in the harsh environment of the desert locust through transovarial transmission and which are sustainable with proper formulations in the field are the most preferred. Mr Shah further asked Dr Raina what steps had been taken to ensure that desert locust in culture at ICIPE are solitarious as claimed. Dr Raina responded that morphometric measurements such as femur size, body length, elytra size, etc., had been used, and that biochemical markers using SDS PAGE of haemolymph proteins is under investigation. Dr Johnson asked Dr Raina whether the data on host specificity and host range changes in *Nosema* referred to in his talk had been published; Dr Raina replied that the work was not published, but that a draft article was available for those interested. Dr Johnson commented that enormous quantities of inoculum would be required to treat all recession areas, and that baits would need to remain palatable for many years.

Panel discussion

Dr Cunningham began the discussion, saying that most farmers and the general public are familiar with chemical pesticides and how they work but not with biological control agents. He was of the opinion that 98% of the general public want biological control and that we need training for both farmers and the public, but that we should be careful not to oversell the capabilities of biological control. There should be co-ordination to implement the research which has already been developed. Many technical reports have been produced and implementation teams set up to use and implement the technologies.

What about field implementation? Dr Goettel urged that caution was needed not to push the research too much before it was ready, because of the danger of raising expectations unduly.

Dr Magor discussed a donor's point of view. Donors want results because they see so much research work published. We have a problem now and we need to do something about it now. Maybe we would get better results later on when much more research has been done, but in the meantime we need to go forward with what we have.

Dr Krall felt it was important to involve the farmers wherever possible and collaborate with them in the form of farmer brigades and with the plant protection services. Some basic research still needs to be done in laboratories. Where there are no farmers as such in the recession areas, monitoring and control will have to be done in collaboration with plant protection services. Various people stressed the need to demonstrate safety in the laboratory and efficiency in the field. We should not at this stage promise viable biological control agents to the farmers.

Section II

Agents for Biocontrol

Natural enemies of tropical locusts and grasshoppers: their impact and potential as biological control agents

D.J. Greathead

International Institute of Biological Control.

Abstract

There are numerous records of natural enemies of Acridoidea but few in-depth studies on natural mortality of tropical species. These chiefly relate to the desert locust, *Schistocerca gregaria* (Forskål), African grasshoppers, *Zonocerus variegatus* (Linnaeus) and *Oedaleus senegalensis* Krauss), and the Australian plague locust, *Chortoicetes terminifera* (Walker). The principal groups of natural enemies - vertebrate and invertebrate predators, insect parasitoids, parasitic nematodes and pathogens - are reviewed with emphasis on their importance as mortality factors and potential for manipulation as biological control agents. The conclusions of population dynamic studies on the impact of natural enemies are summarized and it is shown that there is a consensus that natural enemies are unable to prevent locust outbreaks but can provide a useful constraint on the rate of population increase and may hasten the collapse of plagues. The possibilities for biological control are discussed and it is concluded that there is little prospect for classical biological control of mobile locusts but that there may be some opportunities for introduction of insect predators for suppressing static grasshopper populations. Augmentative release programmes are not considered feasible. However, the most promising approach to biological control appears to be the development of pathogens, particularly those fungi which can be cultured *in vitro*, as biological pesticides.

Introduction

There are numerous records of natural enemies of locusts and grasshoppers beginning with the monumental study of Künkel D'Herculais (1893–1905) in Algeria. The natural enemies which have been recorded include predators, parasitoids and pathogens. Many of those recorded are rare or incidental but there remains a formidable list of potentially important mortality factors to be evaluated.

Insect natural enemies were reviewed and catalogued by Greathead (1963). Information on arthropod and nematode natural enemies in America north of Mexico was summarized by Rees (1973) and lists of natural enemies of tropical species are included in *The locust and grasshopper manual* (COPR, 1973). Knowledge on the pathogens of grasshoppers has been reviewed recently by Streett & McGuire (1990), and Prior & Greathead (1989) have provided an evaluation of the various groups as potential biological control agents for tropical locusts and grasshoppers. There are also some important studies on particular species of natural enemies which are cited below in discussions on these species.

Less information is available on the impact of natural enemies on populations of Acridoidea, especially in the tropics. Studies on populations of the desert locust, *Schistocerca gregaria* (Forskål), were carried out during the 1950–62 plague by scientists of the Anti-Locust Research Centre and the Desert Locust Survey (e.g. Stower *et al.*, 1958; Ashall & Ellis, 1962; Stower & Greathead, 1969). This and other work was summarized by Greathead (1966a) who showed that although the impact of natural enemies is considerable (Tables 1–3) and may reduce the population growth rate of gregarious populations from 11 per generation to 6–8.5 (Table 4), natural enemies are incapable of preventing outbreaks although they may contribute to the collapse of plagues.

The only other relevant studies in Africa are those of Chapman & Page (1979) on *Zonocerus variegatus* (Linnaeus) and by Cheke *et al.* (1980) and Popov (1980) on egg mortality of *Oedaleus senegalensis* (Krauss) (Table 5). Studies have also been made in Australia on the population dynamics of *Chortoicetes terminifera* (Walker) (Farrow, 1977, 1982a, 1982b; Table 6).

Table 1. Estimates of egg mortality of gregarious desert locusts in north-eastern Africa and the Red Sea basin.

Cause	Mortality
Stomorhina lunata (Calliphoridae)	<90%
Systoechus spp. (Bombyliidae)	<30%
Trox procerus (Trogidae)	<10% (75%)*
Fungi, etc.	<30%
Inviability	c. 10%
Hatching failure	c. 4%

*On Saudi Arabian coast only.

Table 2. Estimates of parasitism of nymphs and adults of the desert locust in north-eastern Africa.

Cause		Mortality
Trichopsidea costata (Nemestrinidae)		<30%
Blaesoxipha spp. (Sarcophagidae)	in *gregaria*	<5% – <45%
	in *transiens*	<40%

Table 3. Examples of bird predation on desert locusts in north-eastern Africa.

Bird	Population type	Daily loss
Marabou	swarms	650,000
White stork	swarms	200,000
Eagles	swarms	25,000
Raven	hopper bands	168,000
Hornbill	hopper bands	140,000
Wheatear, etc.	*transiens*	1,200
Kestrel	*transiens*	1,000

Table 4. Desert locust multiplication rates in north-eastern Africa.

Rates of increase	*solitaria*	*transiens*	*gregaria*
Potential rate of increase	65+		50
Actual rate of increase:			
a. without natural enemies	16.5		11
b. with natural enemies			
i. Somali Peninsula	–		6–8.5
ii. Red Sea coast	–	0.03	

Data from Greathead (1966)

This review discusses the important groups of natural enemies in relation to their value as mortality factors and their potential as biological control agents with particular reference to tropical Asia and Africa.

Principal groups of natural enemies

Different suites of natural enemies attack the egg and post-embryonic stages, but there is no useful distinction between those of the nymphs and adults, thus they are best treated as two categories.

Table 5. Mortality of Senegalese grasshopper eggs.

Cause	Niger[a]	Oman[b]
Systoechus sp. (Bombyliidae)	11%	–
Xeramoeba oophaga (Bombyliidae)	4%	2%
Mylabris sp. (Meloidae)	3%	0.5%
Pimelia sp. (Tenebrionidae)	40%	–
Tenebrionid	–	11%
Unidentified	–	27.5%

Data from Popov (1980)
a. means of 104 samples.
b. single sample.

Table 6. Mortality rates for the Australian plague locust during 1971–4.

Cause	Rate (range)	Remarks
Unrealized natality	33.5 (7–57)	minor influence of gregarines
Egg mortality	27.2 (7–60)	83% due to *Scelio*, ants, etc.
Hopper mortality	30.4 (12–58)	mostly rainfall, some predation
Dispersal	6.8	net loss/gain over all generations
Adult mortality	1.5 (<1–11)	parasitoids and mermithids
	—	
	99.4	

Data from Farrow (1982a) means of 17 generations.

Natural enemies of the egg stage

All locusts and grasshoppers, except a few specialized species, oviposit in the ground and deposit a batch of eggs which are protected by secretions from the accessory glands – referred to as an 'egg pod'. The secretions form a 'froth plug' which blocks the hole above the eggs and provides both protection from predators and an escape route for the hatching nymphs. In those species with diapausing eggs the secretions may also form a hard capsule of cemented soil around the pod and even occasionally a cap at the soil surface which provide further protection from predators.

Egg predators

Many of the insect natural enemies of eggs consume all or part of the eggs in an egg pod and remain in it throughout their larval life. Thus, they behave more like parasitoids than predators and so are treated as a separate category from conventional predators which move from egg pod to egg pod.

Diptera: Bombyliidae

Bee-flies of the genera *Systoechus* and *Anastoechus* are usually associated with egg pods in North America, Africa and Eurasia. Other genera also contain species specialized as egg predators, e.g. *Xeramoeba oophaga* (Zhakvatkin) on *O. senegalensis*, or sometimes in limited geographical areas, e.g. *Cytherea* spp. in the Mediterranean Basin and Central Asia. They are frequently the most important cause of egg mortality. They are not host specific but individual species attack either non-diapausing egg pods (without hardened walls) or diapausing egg pods which have hardened walls (Greathead, 1963).

The eggs are minute, thin-walled and sticky and are coated with sand in a special chamber formed by the invagination of the posterior abdominal segments which is filled prior to oviposition. The sand covered eggs are ejected onto the ground or into irregularities in the soil surface and the tiny triungulin-like first instar larvae wander in search of their prey. After completing feeding the larvae become dormant until pupation is triggered by a weather event. In the arid parts of Africa this is a rain storm which wets the soil (Hynes, 1947), thus synchronizing emergence with the appearance of a flush of flowers on which the adults feed. Mating requires a large space for courtship flights. This and the fragility of the adults makes breeding of bee-flies in captivity extremely difficult and this has only been achieved rarely and only on an experimental basis (Du Merle & Delpech, 1973).

Diptera: Calliphoridae

Stomorhina lunata (Fabricius) is an unique egg predator within the family Calliphoridae. It is widespread in Africa (except West Africa) and its distribution extends northwards into the Mediterranean Basin and eastwards to the Indus River. Although it is a major predator on egg pods of gregarious desert locusts, it has not been recovered from the egg pods of solitary locusts and grasshoppers so that its alternative hosts in the absence of locusts remain a mystery.

Oviposition takes place into the froth plug and the larvae move down into the egg mass to feed, movement within the egg mass causes extensive damage and ensures infection by fungi and bacteria so that a single larva may cause the destruction of an entire pod. There is no diapause and adult predators emerge shortly after the nymphs from undamaged egg pods. The adult flies feed on flowers, consuming both nectar and pollen, which is essential for maturation. Flies congregate in large numbers around ovipositing swarms and there is circumstantial evidence that the adults migrate and are thus brought into areas where locust breeding is likely.

Breeding has been carried out on an experimental scale on hen's egg yolk without difficulty (Greathead, 1962).

Coleoptera: Trogidae

Beetles of the genus *Trox* are usually considered to be scavengers but two species have been identified as egg predators, one in southern South America (*T. suberosus* Fabricius) and one in Africa-Arabia (*T. procerus* Harold). On the Red Sea coasts the latter is often an important egg-predator of gregarious desert locusts. Adults burrow in the ground to oviposit near egg pods and the larvae feed indiscriminantly on the eggs. Adults are attracted to ovipositing locusts and feed on cadavers (Roffey, 1958).

Coleoptera: Meloidae

Larvae of *Mylabris* spp. (Africa and Eurasia) and *Epicauta* spp. (North America) prey on eggs of locusts and grasshoppers in most regions but usually their numbers are low and they do not appear to have a significant impact. The numbers of adults may be greater than seems reasonable to account for the number of larvae observed in egg pods, suggesting that there may be other undetected hosts. The life cycle is complex and exhibits hypermetamorphosis. The adults lay large numbers of minute eggs (like the Bombyliidae) which hatch into triungulin larvae. These seek egg pods in which they feed and pass through three instars, as a 'caraboid' and then two 'scarabaeoid' larvae, before moulting into a resting stage, the 'coarctate' larva. In the arid tropics further development seems to require rain. Then there is a further moult, into a 'scolytoid' larva, before pupation. The adults feed on flowers and some species are important pests of crops, especially beans.

Miscellaneous

Egg pods are also attacked by generalist insect predators living in the soil. The most important of these are larvae of Asilidae (Diptera), and Carabidae and Tenebrionidae (Coleoptera). These predators may cause important mortality and can be present consistently at oviposition sites of particular species or at particular localities. However, none of them seems to be dependent on locust and grasshopper eggs for their survival.

Egg parasitiods

Hymenoptera: Scelionidae

The only true parasitoids of the eggs of Acridoidea belong to the genus *Scelio sensu lato*, excepting a few records of chalcidoids from some very specialized grasshoppers which oviposit above ground, e.g. *Oxya* spp. which lay between the leaves of rice plants above the water level.

The African species of *Scelio* were revised by Nixon (1958). Adults penetrate the froth plug to reach the eggs in which they lay their own eggs. The developing stages remain within the chorion until the emerging adult cuts its way out.

There does not seem to be any host specificity but there is a tendency for particular species to be reared from particular hosts (Irshad *et al.*, 1978), possibly egg size and habitat are the chief determinants of host selection. Although *Scelio* spp. can be abundant in grasshopper eggs they are rare or absent from the egg-fields of gregarious locusts in Africa and Asia. However, in Australia *S. fulgidus* Crawford can achieve very heavy mortality (over 90%) of eggs of *Chortoicetes terminifera* in declining populations (Farrow, 1977). Some authors claim to have detected a tendency to density dependence in levels of parasitism but there is often extreme patchiness of attack.

Some species exhibit phoresy and Farrow (1981) has presented evidence that *S. fulgidus* migrates on air currents in such a way that it will be transported to the same areas as migrating *C. terminifera.*

These parasitoids are easily cultured on grasshopper eggs and *S. pembertoni* Timberlake is, so far, the only insect parasitoid to have been successfully introduced as a biological control agent of a grasshopper – against *Oxya chinensis* (Thunberg) in Hawaii (Clausen, 1978).

Pathogens

Investigators studying egg mortality frequently report significant losses due to 'mould' but there have not been any studies which have identified the causal agents. The record of *Cunninghamella* sp. as a pathogen by Daguerre (1937, cited in Roffey, 1968) is dubious since this is a common genus of saprophytes in soil. However, a true pathogen, *Paecilomyces lilacinus* (Thom) Samson, has been isolated from eggs of *Segestidea* sp. (Tettigoniidae) in Papua New Guinea (Prior & Greathead, 1989).

Natural enemies of the post-embryonic stages

Predators

Nymphal and adult Acridoidea are preyed on by a large number of vertebrate and invertebrate predators most of which are generalists. Gregarious locust populations are particularly attractive concentrations of food, and both swarms and hopper bands are often followed by predators, notably migrant birds and sphecid wasps. The only quantitative studies are to be found in the papers cited above but there are also some useful observations scattered in the literature which are cited below in discussing the contribution of particular groups of predators.

Terrestrial vertebrates
Mammals (small carnivores, insectivores and rodents) and reptiles (particularly lizards) are frequently reported as predators but there are no quantitative assessments in the tropics except the study of a *transiens* population of desert locusts in Ethiopia (Stower & Greathead, 1969) and on that occasion they were of negligible importance.

Birds
Predation by birds can be significant (Table 3) and there are reports of birds congregating on small hopper bands and remaining with them until the population has been completely eliminated. This behaviour has been reported both for resident species (passerines, hornbills, rollers, etc.) attacking early instars (Huddleston, 1958, and references therein) and also for storks, especially migrant populations of European and Abdim's storks, attacking bands of older instars and swarms (Smith & Popov, 1953). Raptors have also been credited with causing substantial mortality (e.g. Smith & Popov, 1953) many of these are also migrant.

Migrant birds from the Palaearctic Region, including many of the important predators cited above, arrive in the winter breeding areas of the desert locust and remain there throughout the season (Moreau, 1972) and are thus able to exploit locusts and grasshoppers breeding at this time, but are absent during the summer breeding period and thus insects breeding at this time probably suffer much less bird predation, e.g. those in the Sahel.

Invertebrates
Scorpions and insects, such as ground beetles, have been reported as predators but there is no evidence that they cause significant mortality.

Hymenoptera: Sphecidae
Some sphecid wasps are specialist predators using Acridoidea to provision their nests. In Africa the best known is *Sphex aegyptiacus* Lepeletier which has been observed to accompany swarms (Haskell, 1955).

Parasitoids

The nymphs and adults of Acridoidea are unusual in that they do not have hymenopterous parasitoids, but they do have an unusually rich assemblage of dipterous parasitoids which can cause substantial mortality.

Diptera: Nemestrinidae

Several genera of nemestrinids parasitize Acridoidea, the most important of these in the Old World is *Trichopsidea. T. costata* Loew has a remarkably wide distribution and is present throughout Africa and the Mediterranean Basin parasitizing a wide range of species, possibly because it is dispersed as larvae within parasitized hosts. The adults lay large numbers of minute eggs in holes in wood, irregularities in the ground and other similar sites. The tiny triungulin-like hatchling larvae seek and enter their acridoid hosts where they feed attached to a respiratory tube growing from the entry point. Death of the host usually follows the exit of the fully fed third instar larva which burrows into the ground. Pupation is delayed until triggered by rain, as with bombyliid egg predators. Although adults of some genera have fully formed mouthparts and are able to feed, those of *Trichopsidea* spp. are vestigial (Greathead, 1958).

Diptera: Sarcophagidae

A large number of species of sarcophagid flies has been reared from Acridoidea, but many of them are saprophages (e.g. *Sarcophaga* spp.) or facultative parasitoids of newly moulted or moribund individuals (e.g. *Wohlfahrtia* spp.) so records need careful evaluation. Most true parasitoids belong to the genus *Blaesoxipha.* These flies are larviparous and place their larvae on the host which is entered through an intersegmental membrane. The species are not host specific but the host range is determined by the behaviour of the ovipositing female; thus, of the two most common African species, *B. filipjevi* Rohdendorf is attracted to crawling hosts and so is reared from nymphs and adults of a wide range of species but *B. lineata* (Fallén) attacks flying hosts and so is usually only reared from adults.

The number of larvae developing in a host is limited only by host size. Fully fed larvae leave the host, which usually dies rapidly from desiccation, and pupate immediately in the ground. There is no diapause in tropical species (Greathead, 1966b). They are easily cultured by teasing larvae from the ruptured bodies of gravid females and placing them on the open stump of an amputated leg.

Diptera: Tachinidae

Several genera of Tachinidae have been reported as parasitoids of Acridoidea, those most frequently encountered are *Acemyia* and *Ceracia.* They appear to be rare in Africa but Chapman (1962) reported up to 13%

parasitism of female *Nomadacris septemfasciata* (Serville) by *Ceracia nomadacris* van Emden in its outbreak area, the Rukwa Valley in Tanzania. Like *Blaesoxipha* spp. the tachinids are not host specific but tend to have favoured hosts, suggesting that they too select hosts in particular situations. They are viviparous or lay macrotype eggs on the host. The larva penetrates the host and feeds attached to the cuticle by a breathing tube. More than one larva may develop in each host.

Tachinids are usually less abundant than sarcophagids and have seldom been reported as important mortality factors. In fact there are no records of substantial parasitism of the larger pest species and no authenticated records from the desert locust.

Diptera: Muscidae

Muscid parasitoids have not been reared in the tropics but *Acridomyia* spp. are important parasitoids in North America and Eurasia. They are gregarious with up to one hundred larvae developing in a single host (e.g. Rees, 1973).

Parasites

Nematodes

Mermithid worms are frequently reported and have been studied extensively in North America. Although high levels of parasitism have been recorded in favourable habitats, they require moisture for maturation and oviposition and so are rare except in humid environments where grasshoppers are not usually a serious problem. See Rees (1973) for references and a discussion.

Pathogens

A wide range of pathogens have been isolated from Acridoidea but there are few quantitative assessments indicating their importance as mortality factors. Only the more important ones will be discussed.

Protozoa

Acridoid digestive tracts are frequently infected with protozoan parasites, e.g. *Malamoeba locustae* (King & Taylor) (Henry, 1968) and Eugregarina (Canning, 1956), which are often a problem in laboratory cultures but these parasites seem to be of little significance in field populations.

A more serious infection is caused by *Nosema locustae* Canning, which was first isolated from an insectary colony of *Locusta migratoria* (Linnaeus) in the UK (Canning, 1953). It causes a debilitating disease which reduces the life-span and fecundity of infected insects. *N. locustae* is now known to be widespread in field populations of locusts and grasshoppers and has been the subject of intensive research as a potential biological control agent (Brooks, 1988).

Bacteria

Bacterial infections recorded to date have all been due to non-specific agents which are potential human pathogens and so have been discounted as possible control agents. The most notorious of these was the disease reputedly caused by '*Coccobacillus acridiorum* d'Herelle' and used in abortive field trials as a potential biological pesticide until it was found that it was in fact a strain of a coliform bacterium, *Aerobacter aerogenes* (Kruse) (Steinhaus, 1949). Another bacterial disease isolated from a laboratory colony of desert locusts, due to a nonchromogenic strain of *Serratia marcescens* Bizio, was investigated by Stevenson (1959) who carried out a field trial with a bran bait inoculated with the bacteria but with equivocal results.

Spore forming bacteria, most notably *Bacillus thuringiensis* Berliner, have not been isolated from Orthoptera. The low pH of the gut would prevent the toxic crystal of most known strains from dissolving (Prior & Greathead, 1989).

Viruses

There are few records of virus infections from Acridoidea and most of these have only been reported once. The best known are entomopox viruses which have now been isolated from specimens collected in North America, Africa and Arabia (see table of records in Streett & McGuire, 1990). These large DNA viruses resemble vertebrate pox viruses superficially and therefore have been treated with caution; however, they are now known to have no close biochemical similarity and do not infect vertebrates (Streett & McGuire, 1990). Isolates from North American grasshoppers have been obtained and are being studied as potential control agents. However, entomopox viruses are not highly virulent and debilitate, rather than kill, the host. Furthermore, being obligate intra-cellular parasites they cannot be cultured *in vitro*.

The only other naturally occurring virus of Acridoidea, of possible interest as a control agent, is the crystalline array virus (CAV) isolated from grasshoppers in the USA. However, CAV was found to resemble picornaviruses of vertebrates and so studies on it were abandoned.

Nuclear polyhedrosis viruses are not known from Acridoidea in nature but there is an interesting report of the oral transmission of *Spodoptera littoralis* NPV to both *Schistocerca gregaria* and *Locusta migratoria* which causes visible symptoms termed 'dark cheeks disease' (Bensimon *et al.*, 1987).

Fungi
Fungi are among the most frequently reported pathogens affecting Acridoidea and records have been tabulated by Prior & Greathead (1989).

The best known fungal infections of insects are those caused by *Entomophaga* (*Entomophthora*) spp., known as the 'summit disease' because dying insects climb to the tops of stems where they die clasping the stem. Thus the dead insects are conspicuous and this may account for the frequency of reports of this disease compared with others which do not induce this behaviour. Epidemics in locusts and grasshoppers, usually identified as *E. grylli* Fresenius, have been reported from all regions where pest species have been studied, e.g. Skaife (1925) in South Africa, Chapman & Page (1979) in Nigeria, Pickford & Riegert (1964) in Canada, Roffey (1968) in Thailand and Milner (1978) in Australia (see also table in Streett & McGuire, 1990). Accounts note that prolonged periods of rain or warm humid weather are necessary to initiate and sustain epidemics and that although some acridoid species may be decimated others escape or are hardly affected. This variability in susceptibility has led to the recognition of many strains and some are now described as separate species. These fungi are obligate parasites and so cannot, at present, be cultured *in vitro*, furthermore, the resting spores have so far proved impossible to germinate artificially (Carruthers *et al.*, 1991).

Epidemics caused by Deuteromycotina, usually by *Beauveria* spp. and *Metarhizium* spp., have also been reported under similar circumstances to those reported for *E. grylli.* For example, Balfour-Browne (1960) provides a detailed description of the almost complete destruction of a swarm of desert locusts by *M. anisopliae* (Metschnikoff) Sorokin in Eritrea (Ethiopia) during unusually humid conditions.

Strains of these fungi do not always exhibit host specificity in laboratory tests but there are marked differences in pathogenicity to a range of test insect species which do not necessarily conform with the taxonomic affinity of the insects. The biosystematics and ecology of these associations are poorly understood and are the subject of current research. These fungi can be cultured readily *in vitro* on simple media and are already being exploited as biopesticides for froghoppers (Cercopidae) and other pests (McCoy *et al.*, 1988).

Impact of natural enemies on locust and grasshopper populations

There have been few rigorous studies on the population dynamics of Acridoidea which attempted to measure the role of natural enemies in population regulation. Quantitative studies over several years on essentially static populations in temperate regions include those of Richards & Waloff (1954) on grasshoppers in England; Dempster (1957) on the Moroccan locust (*Dociostaurus maroccanus* (Thunberg)) in Cyprus and Smith (1965) on grasshoppers in Ontario. These studies indicate that natural enemies can cause important mortality but present no conclusive evidence that natural enemies are able to prevent outbreaks.

Zonocerus variegatus is the only tropical grasshopper on which quantitative population studies have been made. Chapman & Page (1979) found a surprising absence of egg parasitiods and predators but substantial mortality due to *Entomophaga grylli*, *Blaesoxipha filipjevi* and mermithid nematodes. However, the key factor in population regulation appeared to be fungal infection following rain.

The investigations on the desert locust mentioned in the introduction, and summarized by Greathead (1966a), point to the importance of natural enemies in contributing to the collapse of plagues but question their ability to prevent them.

The most comprehensive quantitative studies have been those on *Chortoicetes terminifera* by Farrow (1977, 1982a, 1982b) on populations in experimental plots. He concludes that natural enemies are only able to attain high mortality when generations overlap or when the population remains static. Key factor analysis identified migration as the factor determining population size. Natural enemy impact decreased during upsurges and increased during population decline, hastening the collapse of outbreaks.

Farrow & Longstaff (1986) modelled information on population dynamics of four tropical locusts: *L. migratoria*, *S. gregaria*, *Nomadacris septemfasciata* and *C. terminifera*. They concluded that in each instance weather and emigration were the key factors and that emigration prevented populations exceeding the carrying capacity and stopping natural enemies exerting any regulating influence. This result confirms beliefs of the authors cited above that natural enemies have little influence in plague dynamics.

Thus, natural enemies may on occasion provide a useful constraint on the rate of population increase, although they cannot prevent plagues, but probably have their greatest impact on declining populations. As such they merit conservation.

Potential of locust and grasshopper natural enemies for biological control

Classical biological control with insect natural enemies has been attempted on a number of occasions (Prior & Greathead, 1989) but with no success, and only two of nine introductions resulted in establishment. The possibilities for classical biological control of static grasshopper populations merit further consideration. Some insect natural enemies can be eliminated from consideration because they are not amenable to handling in captivity, e.g. the egg predators (Bombyliidae, Meloidae) and nemestrinid parasitoids. *Stomorhina lunata* can be reared but there are questions to be answered about its biology before it can be recommended: viz. where does it breed in the absence of gregarious hosts, why is it absent from West Africa when it is present in the rest of the continent? The muscoid parasitoids are easy to multiply but introductions into North America and Hawaii have failed, suggesting that more careful selection of species for introduction is necessary before embarking on an introduction programme. Finally the scelionid egg parasitoids appear to merit further consideration. They are easy to rear but more information is required about host selection before recommendations can be made. There is currently renewed interest in the USA where species from Australia are being imported for trial (Dysart, 1991).

Multiplication of insect natural enemies for augmentative release is not considered feasible because of the large numbers required, problems of timing production in relation to phenology in areas of uncertain rainfall and the logistics of delivery. Pathogens are more promising for this purpose and *Nosema locustae* has been commercialized as a bait (Brooks, 1988). Although some promising results have been reported on the North American prairies overall the results have been equivocal and trials in the tropics have failed. Entomopox viruses are currently being investigated in the USA but the problem of economic production in living tissue is likely to restrict their use severely in the near future.

For swarming populations and also static populations the most promising approach to biological control appears to be the development of pathogens as biological pesticides. Here for the reasons already given those fungi which can be cultured *in vitro* are considered the most promising and are the subject of the current programme.

Since natural enemies have been shown to have an impact on acridoid populations they merit conservation and other control measures which have an adverse impact on them should be avoided or actions should be taken to minimize the damage. In particular it is necessary to monitor the environmental impact of chemical pesticides since a recent pilot study (Everts, 1990) has shown that fenitrothion and chlorpyriphos, now being applied for locust and grasshopper control in Africa following the banning of dieldrin, have an adverse effect on non-target organisms, including entomophagous arthropods and predatory birds which are natural enemies of Orthoptera.

References

Ashall, C. & Ellis, P.E. (1962) Studies on numbers and mortality in field populations of the desert locust (*Schistocerca gregaria* Forskål). *Anti-Locust Bulletin* **no. 38**, 59 pp.

Balfour-Browne, F.L. (1960) The green muscardine disease of insects, with special reference to an epidemic in a swarm of locusts in Eritrea. *Proceedings of the Royal Entomological Society of London* (A) **35**, 65–74.

Bensimon, A.S., Zinger, E., Gerasi, A., Hauschner, I. & Sela, I. (1987) 'Dark cheeks', a lethal disease of locusts provoked by a lepidopterous baculovirus. *Journal of Invertebrate Pathology* **50**, 254–260.

Brooks, W.M. (1988) Entomogenous Protozoa. In: Ignoffo, C.M. & Bushan Mandava, N. (eds), *Handbook of Natural Pesticides. Vol. 5. Microbial Pesticides. Part A. Entomogenous Fungi and Protozoa.* CRC Press, Florida, pp. 1–149.

Canning, E.U. (1953) A new microsporidian, *Nosema locustae* n. sp., from the fat body of the African migratory locust, *Locusta migratoria migratorioides* R. & F. *Parasitology* **43**, 287–290.

Canning, E.U. (1956) A new eugregarine of locusts, *Gregarina garnhami* n. sp., parasitic in *Schistocerca gregaria* Forsk. *Journal of Protozoology* **3**, 50–62.

Carruthers, R.I., Humber, R.A. & Ramos, M.E. (1991) Development of *Entomophaga grylli* as a biological control agent of grasshoppers. In: *Cooperative Grasshopper Integrated Pest Management Project. 1990 Annual Report.* USDA, Boise, Idaho, pp. 220–226.

Chapman, R.F. (1962) *Ceracia nomadacris* van Emden (Diptera: Tachinidae) parasitising *Nomadacris septemfasciata* (Serville) (Orthoptera: Acrididae). *Proceedings of the Royal Entomological Society of London* (A) **37**, 69–71.

Chapman, R.F. & Page, W.W. (1979) Factors affecting the mortality of the grasshopper, *Zonocerus variegatus*, in southern Nigeria. *Journal of Animal Ecology* **48**, 271–288.

Cheke, R.A., Fishpool, L.D.C. & Ritchie, J.M. (1980) An ecological study of the egg-pods of *Oedaleus senegalensis* (Krauss) (Orthoptera: Acrididae). *Journal of Natural History* **14**, 363–371.

Clausen, C.P. (1978) Introduced parasites and predators of arthropod pests and weeds: a world review. *US Department of Agriculture Agriculture Handbook* **no. 480**, 545 pp.

COPR (Centre for Overseas Pest Research) (1982) *The Locust and Grasshopper Agricultural Manual.* Centre for Overseas Pest Research, London.

Dempster, J.P. (1957) The population dynamics of the Moroccan locust (*Dociostaurus maroccanus* Thunberg) in Cyprus. *Anti-Locust Bulletin* **no. 27**, 60 pp.

Du Merle, P. & Delpech, M. (1973) Dispositifs de terrain destines à l'étude de la biologie et du rôle limitif de *Villa brunnea* (Dipt., Bombyliidae) vis-à-vis de *Thaumetopoea pityocampa* (Lep., Thaumetopoeidae). *Annales de la Societé Entomologique de France* INS) **9**, 471–482.

Dysart, R. (1991) Australian egg parasites for grasshopper biocontrol. In: *Cooperative Grasshopper Integrated Pest Management Project. 1990 Annual Report.* USDA, Boise, Idaho, pp. 279–280.

Everts, J.W. (ed) (1990) *Environmental Effects of Chemical Locust and Grasshopper Control. A Pilot Study.* FAO, Rome Project ECLO/SEN/003/NET. 277 pp.

Farrow, R.A. (1977) Origin and decline of the 1973 plague locust outbreak in central western New South Wales. *Australian Journal of Zoology* **25**, 455–489.

Farrow, R.A. (1981) Aerial dispersal of *Scelio fulgidus* (Hym.: Scelionidae), parasite of eggs of locusts and grasshoppers (Ort.: Acrididae). *Entomophaga* **26**, 349–355.

Farrow, R.A. (1982a) Population dynamics of the Australian plague locust, *Chortoicetes terminifera* (Walker) in central western New South South Wales III. Analysis of population processes. *Australian Journal of Zoology* **30**, 569–579.

Farrow, R.A. & Longstaff, B.C. (1986) Comparison of the annual rates of increase of locusts in relation to the incidence of plagues. *Oikos* **46**, 207–222.

Greathead, D.J. (1958) Notes on the life history of *Symmictus flavopilosus* Bigot (Diptera: Nemestrinidae) as a parasite of *Schistocerca gregaria* (Forskål) (Orthoptera: Acrididae). *Proceedings of the Royal Entomological Society of London* (A) **33**, 107–119.

Greathead, D.J. (1962) The biology of *Stomorhina lunata* (Fabricius) (Dipt., Calliphoridae), predator of the eggs of Acrididae. *Proceedings of the Zoological Society of London* **138**, 139–180.

Greathead, D.J. (1963) A review of the insect enemies of Acridoidea (Orthoptera). *Transactions of the Royal Entomological Society of London* **114**, 437–517.

Greathead, D.J. (1966a) A brief survey of the effects of biotic factors on populations of the desert locust. *Journal of Applied Ecology* **3**, 239–250.

Greathead, D.J. (1966b) Notes on *Blaesoxipha* spp., (Dipt. Calliphoridae) parasitising Acridoidea in eastern Africa. *Commonwealth Institute of Biological Control Technical Bulletin* **no. 7**, 91–100.

Haskell, P.T. (1955) Further observations on the occurrence of *Sphex aegyptius* Lep. (Hym., Sphecidae) with swarms of the desert locust. *Entomologist's Monthly Magazine* **91**, 284–285.

Henry, J.E. (1968) *Malamoeba locustae* and its antibiotic control in grasshopper cultures. *Journal of Invertebrate Pathology* **11**, 224–233.

Huddleston, J.A. (1958) Some notes on the effects of bird predators on hopper bands of the desert locust (*Schistocerca gregaria* Forskål). *Entomologist's Monthly Magazine* **94**, 210–214.

Hynes, H.B.N. (1947) Observations on *Systoechus somali* Oldroyd (Diptera: Bombyliidae) attacking the eggs of the desert locust, *Schistocerca gregaria* (Forskål) in Somalia. *Proceedings of the Royal Entomological Society of London* (A) **223**, 79–85.

Irshad, M., Ahmad, M., Ghani, M.A. & Ali, R. (1978) Parasites of grasshopper (Acridoidea: Orthoptera) eggs: distribution and life history of *Scelio* spp. (Hymenoptera: Scelionidae) in Pakistan. *Canadian Entomologist* **110**, 449–454.

Künkel D'Herculais, J. (1893–1905) *Invasions des Acridiens, Vulgo Sauterelles, en Algérie.* Algiers.

McCoy, C.W., Samson, R.A. & Boucias, D.R. (1988) Entomogenous Fungi. In: Ignoffo, C.M. & Bushan Mandava, N. (eds), *Handbook of Natural Pesticides. Vol. 5. Microbial Pesticides. Part A. Entomogenous Fungi and Protozoa.* CRC Press, Florida, pp. 151–236.

Milner, R.J. (1978) On the occurrence of *Entomophthora grylli*, a fungal pathogen of grasshoppers in Australia. *Journal of the Australian Entomological Society* **17**, 293–296.

Moreau, R.E. (1972) *The Palearctic-African Bird Migration Systems.* Academic Press, London.

Nixon, G.E.J. (1958) A synopsis of the African species of *Scelio* Latreille

(Hymenoptera: Proctotrupoidea, Scelionidae). *Transactions of the Royal Entomological Society of London* **110**, 303–318.

Pickford, R. & Riegert, P.W. (1964) The fungous disease caused by *Entomophthora grylli* Fres., and its effects on grasshopper populations in Saskatchewan 1963. *Canadian Entomologist* **96**, 1158–1166.

Popov, G.B. (1980) Studies on oviposition, egg development and mortality on *Oedaleus senegalensis* (Krauss), (Orthoptera, Acridoidea) in the Sahel. *Centre for Overseas Pest Research Miscellaneous Report* **no. 53**, 48 pp.

Prior, C. & Greathead, D.J. (1989) Biological control of locusts: the potential for the exploitation of pathogens. *FAO Plant Protection Bulletin* **37**, 37–48.

Rees, N.A. (1973) Arthropod and nematode parasites, parasitoids, and predators of Acrididae in America north of Mexico. *USDA, ARS, Technical Bulletin* **no. 1460**, 288 pp.

Richards, O.W. & Waloff, N. (1954) Studies on the biology and population dynamics of British grasshoppers. *Anti-Locust Bulletin* **no. 17**, 182 pp.

Roffey, J. (968) The occurrence of the fungus *Entomophthora grylli* Fresenius on locusts and grasshoppers in Thailand. *Journal of Insect Pathology* **11**, 237–241.

Skaife, S.H. (1925) The locust fungus, *Empusa grylli*, and its effects on its host. *South African Journal of Science* **22**, 298–308.

Smith, K.D. & Popov, G.B. (1953) On birds attacking desert locust swarms in Eritrea. *Entomologist* **86**, 3–7.

Smith, R.W. (1965) A field population of *Melanoplus sanguinipes* (Fab.) (Orthoptera: Acrididae) and its parasites. *Canadian Journal of Zoology* **43**, 179–201.

Steinhaus, E.A. (1949) *Principles of Insect Pathology*. McGraw-Hill, New York.

Stevenson, J.P. (1959) Epizootology of a disease of the desert locust, *Schistocerca gregaria* (Forskål), caused by nonchromogenic strains of *Serratia marcescens* Bizio. *Journal of Insect Pathology* **1**, 232–244.

Stower, W.J. & Greathead, D.J. (1969) Numerical changes in a population of the desert locust, with special reference to factors responsible for mortality. *Journal of Applied Ecology* **6**, 203–235.

Stower, W.J., Popov, G.B. & Greathead, D.J. (1958) Oviposition behaviour and egg mortality of the desert locust (*Schistocerca gregaria* Forskål) on the coast of Eritrea. *Anti-Locust Bulletin* **no. 30**, 33 pp.

Streett, D.A. & McGuire, M.R. (1990) Pathogenic diseases of grasshoppers. In: Chapman, R.F. & Joern, A. (eds), *Biology of Grasshoppers*. John Wiley & Sons, New York, pp. 484–516.

Fungal agents for biocontrol

M.S. Goettel

Agriculture Canada Research Station, Lethbridge, Alberta.

Abstract

Fungi have much potential to play a key role in the microbial control of grasshoppers. Successful development of a microbial insecticide will require careful selection of the best species and isolates. A brief review of the attributes and limitations of fungi as potential microbial control agents and of the several species of fungi commonly associated with grasshoppers are presented. Unlike most other insect pathogens which must be ingested in order to invade their host, fungi generally invade via the external cuticle. As with other biological control agents, fungi are limited by an array of biotic and abiotic factors. Although more than 700 species of entomopathogenic fungi are known to occur world-wide, only a handful are known to affect grasshoppers; among the most common are *Beauveria bassiana* (Balsamo) Vuillemin, *Metarhizium anisopliae* (Metschnikoff) Sorokin and *Entomophaga grylli* (Fresenius) Batko. It is concluded that there is presently an urgent need for a concerted effort to search for and isolate fungal pathogens world-wide.

Introduction

The first step in the development of a microbial control agent is the identification of those pathogens which infect the pest in nature. Among the different types of pathogens affecting grasshoppers are fungi. Fungal diseases in insects are common and widespread and often decimate insect populations in spectacular epizootics. This phenomenon illustrates the promising potential of fungi and has resulted in a considerable research effort in an attempt to exploit these organisms as insect control agents; however, much more research is required and many problems must be solved before these organisms can be utilized on a larger scale for insect control. Recent reviews on the development of entomopathogenic fungi as microbial control agents are those of Hall & Papierok (1982), Lisansky & Hall (1982), Ferron (1985), Wraight & Roberts (1987), McCoy *et al.* (1988), Samson *et al.* (1988) and McCoy (1990).

Pathogenesis

Unlike most other insect pathogens which must be ingested in order to invade their host, entomopathogenic fungi usually invade via the external cuticle (Charnley, 1984; St Leger, in press). The infective propagule, usually a spore, attaches itself onto the integument surface, germinates, and penetrates the host cuticle. In some instances, fungi may also enter the host via the digestive tract or spiracles. Once the fungus has entered the body cavity, it spreads and colonizes the host's haemocoel. Some species produce a toxin within the host, and in such cases, host death may be rapid (Roberts, 1981). In species or strains that do not produce a toxin, host death is usually delayed and is generally thought to be the result of depletion of nutrients. After host death, the fungus emerges from the cadaver and, in the presence of high relative humidity, produces more infective propagules on the surface.

A full understanding of the factors affecting the ability of a fungus to enter and kill its host is paramount in the development of fungi as control agents. Factors that interfere in any of the critical steps could render the pathogen less efficient if not useless. Only recently have we begun to unravel the complex interactions between the host integument and fungal pathogen (St Leger, in press). Factors affecting these interactions include moulting, host defence mechanisms, fungal strain, presence of nutrients on host integument, and humidity, to name a few. Further details are given in the paper by Charnley (these proceedings).

Host range, specificity and virulence

Fungi have one of the widest host ranges among entomopathogens and, consequently, have the potential for use against most pest insects. Reports on wide host ranges of entomopathogenic species, however, are based on fungal species as a whole whereas laboratory studies demonstrate that different isolates of the same species may have varying degrees of specificity;

isolates are generally more virulent to the host from which they were first isolated (Goettel *et al.*, 1990a). Furthermore, fungi may even be more specific under field conditions and especially during epizootics.

Enhancement of virulence in entomopathogenic fungi has been a particularly neglected area of research. It has been demonstrated that, in general, virulence increases following successive passage through a host and decreases following repeated subculturing on artificial media (Aizawa, 1971; Roberts & Yendol, 1971; Daoust & Roberts, 1982). Such changes were thought to be due to gradual selection of genotypes; however, recently it was demonstrated that levels of cuticle-degrading enzymes were higher in conidia from infected tobacco hornworm larvae than those harvested from artificial culture, indicating that environmental conditions in which spores develop can pre-adapt them for the pathogenic mode (St Leger *et al.*, 1991).

Host specificity and virulence optimization need further investigation from the point of view of the range of insects infected, the virulence towards the target host, and the biotic and abiotic factors responsible for the extension or restriction of that virulence. Such information would enhance the development or choice of strains with optimal potential as control agents for specific pests or pest complexes and with minimal adverse effects on non-target organisms.

Biotic and abiotic limitations

As with other biological control agents, fungi are limited by an array of biotic and abiotic factors. The former limitations are still poorly understood. They include microbial antagonists on the host integument, leaf surface or in the soil; host feeding behaviour, physiological condition and age; and fungal strain. Abiotic factors include inactivation by sunlight, desiccation, presence of insecticides or fungicides, and temperature and humidity thresholds for germination and growth. Traditionally, because of a germination requirement for free water or a relative humidity of over 90%, relative macrohumidity has been considered as the most serious constraint on the use of fungi for insect control. However, recent studies indicate that fungal infections can occur at relatively low macro-humidities (Marcandier & Khachatourians, 1987). Indications are that the micro-humidities at the surface of the host integument or on the foliage may be sufficient for spore germination and host penetration (St Leger, in press); fungal spores formulated in oil have been shown to kill locusts at ambient humidities of 35% R.H. (Prior *et al.*, these proceedings).

As our knowledge of the biology, pathogenesis, and epizootiology of entomopathogenic fungi increases, novel strategies are being applied to overcome some of the many limitations. Through strategies such as selection of strains or recombinant DNA technology and proper formulation, many limitations may be overcome. The recent transformation of *Metarhizium anisopliae* (Metschnikoff) Sorokin to benomyl resistance through the introduction of a benomyl resistance gene from a non-entomopathogenic fungus, *Aspergillus nidulans* (Eidam) Vuillemin is the first example of the use of DNA recombinant technology in an entomopathogenic fungus (Goettel *et al.*, 1990b).

Fungal pathogens of grasshoppers

More than 700 species of entomopathogenic fungi are known to occur world-wide, but only a handful are known to affect grasshoppers (Table 1; see also Prior & Greathead (1989) for a list of species recorded from Orthoptera). Furthermore, most records are based on single occurrences. There is presently a need for a world-wide concerted efffort to identify and isolate fungal pathogens of grasshoppers.

Some promising candidates

Beauveria bassiana (Balsamo) Vuillemin

This fungus has been developed recently as a control agent of pest insects. It is being used in the USSR for control of the Colorado potato beetle

Table 1. Host records of fungal pathogens in grasshoppers.

Class/Species	Relative abundance[1]	Geographical area
Hyphomycetes		
Aspergillus sp.	rare	Spain
Beauveria bassiana	frequent	Africa, Australia, Brazil, North America
Metarhizium anisopliae	frequent	Africa, Australia, South-east Asia, South America
Metarhizium flavoviride	rare[2]	Ecuador, Africa
Sorosporella sp.	rare	USA, Africa
Entomophthorales		
Entomophaga sp.	rare	Indonesia
Entomophaga grylli (species complex)	frequent	Africa, Australia, Europe, North America, South-east Asia

[1]Abundance based on numbers of host records from various sources.
[2]This assessment may need to be changed in the light of recent discoveries in Africa.

(*Leptinotarsa decemlineata* (Say) (Coleoptera: Chrysomelidae)) and in the People's Republic of China for control of the pine caterpillar (*Dendrolimus punctata* (Walker) (Lepidoptera: Lasiocampidae)). Other isolates are being investigated as potential control agents of other pest insects, including *L. decemlineata*, fire ants (*Solenopsis* spp. (Hymenoptera: Formicidae)), black vine weevils (*Otiorhynchus sulcatus* (Fabricius) (Coleoptera: Curculionidae), and citrus root weevils (*Diaprepes* spp. (Coleoptera: Curculionidae)) (McCoy, 1990). Although this fungus has a very wide host range, with over 700 insect species being susceptible, recent research indicates that certain strains of the fungus are much more host specific (Goettel *et al.*, 1990a).

There are several records of *B. bassiana* infecting grasshoppers (Table 1; Dresner, 1949; MacLeod, 1954; Humber & Soper, 1986; Li, 1987; Moore & Erlandson, 1988) and it has been documented as the cause of an epizootic in a swarm of red locusts (*Nomadacris septemfasciata* (Serville)) in South Africa (Schaefer 1936). Some recent experimental studies have also demonstrated its pathogenicity to grasshoppers under laboratory conditions (Marcandier & Khachatourians, 1987; Moore & Erlandson, 1988). Other recent research has shown that grasshoppers are highly susceptible to a strain of *B. bassiana* isolated from a dead grasshopper in Montana (Johnson *et al.*, 1988). Grasshoppers that were fed wheat leaves treated with spores produced from a Mycotech isolate died within 10 days. In subsequent laboratory dose-mortality tests, spores of *B. bassiana* sprayed in water or applied on lettuce disks were found to infect and kill grasshoppers of other species and ages at economically reasonable levels of application. Experiments in which third-instar grasshoppers were fed lettuce disks treated with droplets of spores indicated mortality of over 60% at one million spores per hopper (Goettel & D.L. Johnson, unpublished data).

Although *B. bassiana* may infect insects via the respiratory system (Clark *et al.*, 1968) and alimentary tract (Gabriel, 1959; Bao & Yendol, 1971; Broome *et al.*, 1976; Yanagita, 1987), penetration through the external integument is the most common route of invasion (Vey & Fargues, 1977; Pekrul & Grula, 1979; Atuahener & Doppelreiter, 1982; Allee *et al.*, 1990). The route of invasion in grasshoppers is unknown; however, histopathological studies are under way in Lethbridge to determine the mode and site of infection in grasshoppers. Such information may greatly aid in the selection of the most effective methods for host targeting, product formulation and field application.

The development of methods for the mass production of this strain by Mycotech Corporation, Butte, MT, (see Goettel & Roberts, these proceedings) has allowed preliminary field trials to be conducted against grasshoppers in Alberta, Montana, Saskatchewan (C. Bradley, M.A. Erlandson, Goettel and D.L. Johnson, unpublished data), and Mali (see Johnson *et al.*, these proceedings). These applications included treatment of caged grass and crop, and also treatment of whole fields, using bran bait and oil-based spray formulations. Economic analysis by Mycotech has indicated that, if successful, an application rate of 10^{13} conidia/ha can be competitive in price with chemicals currently used for grasshopper control in the United States.

Metarhizium anisopliae and *M. flavoviride* W. Gams & J. Rozsypal

M. anisopliae is presently used on a wide scale in Brazil to control the sugarcane spittle bug (*Mahanarva posticata* (Stål)) (Roberts *et al.*, 1991; Mendonca, these proceedings); *M. flavoviride* has been successfully field-tested against the rice brown planthopper (*Nilaparvata lugens* (Stål) in the Philippines (Rombach *et al.*, 1986). There are numerous records of *M. anisopliae* from grasshoppers world-wide (Table 1; Balfour-Browne, 1960; Veen, 1968a; Humber & Soper, 1986) and it has been documented as causing an epizootic in a swarm of desert locusts in Ethiopia (Balfour-Browne, 1960). *M. flavoviride* was isolated from a grasshopper in the Galapagos Islands (Evans & Samson, 1982). Although this fungus has not been observed causing an epizootic in grasshoppers, recent laboratory studies have demonstrated that it is highly virulent against locusts (see Prior *et al.*, these proceedings).

There have not been any field tests to evaluate the potential of *M. anisopliae* or *M. flavoviride* against grasshoppers. However, such tests are warranted. *M. anisopliae* can be cultured using the solid-state fermentation technology developed by Mycotech (C. Bradley, pers. comm; Goettel & Roberts, these proceedings), or by low-tech methods discussed by Mendonça (these proceedings). Laboratory studies have demonstrated that *M. anisopliae* conidia ingested by desert locusts are killed by antifungal toxins produced by the gut bacteria; axenic locusts which were starved post-inoculation succumbed to the disease (Dillon & Charnley, 1986). Therefore, an innovative strategy for formulation of *M. anisopliae* would be to incorporate both an antimicrobial and stomach poison which would allow the fungus to penetrate via the gut.

Entomophaga grylli (Fresenius) Batko complex

E. grylli is an obligate grasshopper pathogen responsible for numerous epizootics in grasshoppers world-wide (Table 1; Skaife, 1925; Pickford & Riegert, 1964; Roffey, 1968; Milner, 1978; Chapman & Page, 1979; Erlandson *et al.*, 1988). It is regarded as the key factor regulating many grasshopper populations, often reducing populations to below economic thresholds. For instance, an epizootic in the clear-winged grasshopper

(*Camnula pellucida* (Scudder)) in the 1960s resulted in an 80% reduction in the required insecticide control costs of previous years saving farmers $30 million (D.L. Johnson, pers. comm.). It is generally believed that such epizootics require relatively humid environments with frequent dew formation; however, epizootics sustained in very dry environments have been recorded (R.S. Soper, R.A. Humber & B. Martinell, unpublished data as cited by Soper *et al.*, 1983). Several years of data from grasshopper populations in isolated mountain valleys of Arizona suggest that a combination of host and pathogen density-dependent relationships, spatial dynamics, and varying environmental conditions regulate disease prevalence (R.S. Soper, unpublished data as cited by Carruthers & Soper, 1987). More research is needed to fully elucidate the epizootiology of this fungus. (See also Paräso *et al.*, these proceedings).

Grasshoppers succumbing to *E. grylli* climb to the top of vegetation and die in the late afternoon with their heads pointing upwards (Skaife, 1925; MacLeod, 1963). Cadavers remain on the vegetation until they are either blown away by the wind or are washed off by rain. Soon after death, if the humidity is very high, fungal mycelia emerge through the intersegmental membranes and gradually encompass the cadaver. This mycelium produces numerous conidiophores which give rise to conidia which are forcibly discharged, showering many of the grasshoppers in the area. Conidia germinate on the host cuticle and penetrate into the grasshopper. Some cadavers killed by the fungus produce resting spores which develop within the host body. These are long-lived and initiate the disease cycle in another season.

Although presently recognized as a single species, *E. grylli* is actually a complex of pathotypes or possible species. These pathotypes may be recognized by host specificity and isozyme patterns (Soper *et al.*, 1983; Ramoska *et al.*, 1988). The existence of such great genetic variability throughout this taxon offers the potential for its use for classical biological control; recent work by Carruthers *et al.* (1991) is aimed at the importation of a particularly virulent pathotype of *E. grylli* from Australia for release in the USA.

Although *E. grylli* can be grown *in vitro* as protoplasts (MacLeod *et al.*, 1980), it produces infective stages only *in vivo*. Therefore, until an *in vitro* method for spore production can be developed, use of this fungus as a microbial insecticide would require mass production *in vivo* (see Goettel & Roberts, these proceedings). It may be possible to use *E. grylli* in the inoculative approach in order to initiate epizootics.

Conclusions

Fungi have the potential to play a key role in the microbial control of grasshoppers. However, our understanding of the epizootiology of fungal diseases is rudimentary; much research is needed before we can successfully use a fungus such as *E. grylli* to cause epizootics in grasshopper populations. Furthermore, very few fungal isolates from grasshoppers are available. Successful development of a microbial insecticide will require careful selection of the best isolates. There is presently an urgent need for a concerted effort to search and isolate fungal pathogens from grasshoppers world-wide – and the joint IIBC/IITA/DFPV programme provides an excellent opportunity to do this.

References

Aizawa, K. (1971) Strain improvement and preservation of virulence of pathogens. In: Burges, H.D. & Hussey, N.W. (eds), *Microbial Control of Insects and Mites.* Academic Press, New York, pp. 655–699.

Allee, L.L., Goettel, M.S., Gol'berg, A., Whitney, H.S. & Roberts, D.W. (1990) Infection by *Beauveria bassiana* of *Leptinotarsa decemlineata* larvae as a consequence of fecal contamination of the integument following per os inoculation. *Mycopathologia* **111**, 17–24.

Atuahene, S.K.N. & Doppelreiter, H. (1982) Histopathological observations on *Beauveria bassiana* in larvae of *Lamprosema lateritialis* (Lepid., Pyralidae). *Zeitschrift für Angwandte Entomologie* **93**, 456–463.

Balfour-Browne, F.L. (1960) The green muscardine disease of insects, with special reference to an epidemic in a swarm of locusts in Eritrea. *Proceedings of the Royal Entomological Society of London* (A) **35**, 65–74.

Bao, L. & Yendol, W.G. (1971) Infection of the eastern subterranean termite, *Reticulitermes flavipes* (Kollar) with the fungus *Beauveria bassiana* (Balsamo) Vuill. *Entomophaga* **16**, 343–352.

Broome, J.R., Sikorowski, P.P. & Norment, B.R. (1976) A mechanism of pathogenicity of *Beauveria bassiana* on the larvae of the imported fire ant, *Solenopsis richteri. Journal of Invertebrate Pathology* **28**, 87–91.

Carruthers, R.I. & Soper, R.S. (1987) Fungal diseases. In: Fuxa, J.R. & Tanada, Y. (eds), *Epizootiology of Insect Diseases.* Wiley, Chichester, UK, pp. 357–416.

Carruthers, R.I., Humber, R.A. & Ramos, M.E. (1991) Development of *Entomophaga grylli* as a biological agent of grasshoppers. In: *Cooperative Grasshopper Integrated Pest Management Project 1990 Annual Report.* USDA, APHIS TPQ-Boise Idaho, Boise, Idaho, pp. 220–231.

Chapman, R.F. & Page, W.W. (1979) Factors affecting the mortality of the grasshopper, *Zonocerus variegatus,* in southern Nigeria. *Journal of Animal Ecology* **48**, 271–288.

Charnley, A.K. (1984) Physiological aspects of destructive pathogenesis in insects by fungi: a speculative review. In: Anderson, J.M., Rayner, A.D.M. & Walton, D.W.H. (eds), *Invertebrate-Microbial Interactions, British Mycological Society Symposium.* Cambridge University Press, Cambridge, pp. 229–270.

Clark, T.B., Kellen, W.R. Fukuda, T. & Lindegren, J.E. (1968) Field and laboratory studies of the pathogenicity of the fungus *Beauveria bassiana* to three genera of mosquitoes. *Journal of Invertebrate Pathology* **11**, 1–7.

Daoust, R.A. & Roberts, D.W. (1982) Virulence of natural and insect-passaged strains of *Metarhizium anisopliae* to mosquito larvae. *Journal of Invertebrate Pathology* **40**, 107–117.

Dillon, R.J. & Charnley, A.K. (1986) Invasion of the pathogenic fungus *Metarhizium anisopliae* through the guts of germ-free desert locusts, *Schistocerca gregaria. Mycopathologia* **96**, 59–66.

Dresner, E. (1949) Culture and use of entomogenous fungi for the control of insect pests. *Contributions. Boyce Thompson Institute for Plant Research* **15**, 319–335.

Erlandson, M.A., Johnson, D.L. & Olfert, O.O. (1988) *Entomophaga grylli* (Fresenius) infections in grasshopper (Orthoptera: Acrididae) populations in Saskatchewan and Alberta, 1985–1986. *Canadian Entomologist* **120**, 205–209.

Evans, H.C. & Samson, R.A. (1982) Entomogenous fungi from the Galapagos Islands. *Canadian Journal of Botany* **60**, 2325–2333.

Ferron, P. (1985) Fungal control. In: Kerkut, G.A. & Gilbert, L.I. (eds), *Comprehensive Insect Physiology, Biochemistry and Pharmacology.* Pergamon Press, Oxford, New York, pp. 314–338.

Gabriel, B.P. (1959) Fungus infection of insects via the alimentary tract. *Journal of Insect Pathology* **1**, 319–330.

Goettel, M.S., Poprawski, T.J., Vandenberg, J.D., Li, Z. & Roberts, D.W. (1990a) Safety to nontarget invertebrates of fungal biocontrol agents. In: Laird, M., Lacey, L.A. & Davidson, E.W. (eds), *Safety of Microbial Insecticides.* CRC Press, Boca Raton, pp. 209–231.

Goettel, M.S., St Leger, R.J., Bhairi, S., Jung, K., Oakley, B.R., Roberts, D.W. & Staples, R.C. (1990b) Pathogenicity and growth of *Metarhizium anisopliae* stably transformed to benomyl resistance. *Current Genetics* **17**, 129–132.

Hall, R.A. & Papierok, B. (1982) Fungi as biological control agents of arthropods of agricultural and medical importance. *Parasitology* **84**, 205–240.

Humber, R.A. & Soper, R.S. (1986) USDA-ARS collection of entomopathogenic fungal cultures. Catalog of strains. USDA, Ithaca, New York, 56 pp.

Johnson, D.L., Pavlik, E. & Bradley, C. (1988) Activity of *Beauveria bassiana* sprayed onto wheat against grasshoppers. Expert Committee on Pesticide Use in Agriculture, Pesticide Research Report. Ottawa, Agriculture Canada.

Li, Z. (1987) A list of the insect hosts of *Beauveria bassiana.* In: *First National Symposium on Entomogenous Fungi,* Gongzhuling, Jilin, People's Republic of China.

Lisansky, S.G. & Hall, R.A. (1982) Fungal control of insects. In: Smith, J.E., Berry, P.R. & Kristonson, B. (eds), *The Filamentous Fungi.* Edward Arnold, London, pp. 127–345.

McCoy, C.W. (1990) Entomogenous fungi as microbial pesticides. In: *New Directions in Biological Control: Alternatives for Suppressing Agricultural Pests and Diseases.* Alan R. Liss, Inc., New York, pp. 139–159.

McCoy, C.W., Samson, R.A. & Boucias, D.G. (1988) Entomogenous fungi. In: Ignoffo, C.M. & Bushan Mandava, N. (eds), *CRC Handbook of Natural Pesticides, Vol V: Microbial Insecticides: Part A Entomogenous Protozoa and Fungi.* CRC Press, Boca Raton, pp. 151–236.

MacLeod, D.M. (1954) Investigations on the genera *Beauveria* Vuill. and *Tritirachium* Limber. *Canadian Journal of Botany* **32**, 818–890.

MacLeod, D.M. (1963) Entomophthorales infections. In: Steinhaus, E.A. (ed.),

Insect Pathology: An Advanced Treatise. Academic Press, New York, pp. 189–231.

MacLeod, D.M., Tyrrell, D. & Welton, M.A. (1980) Isolation and growth of the grasshopper pathogen, *Entomophthora grylli. Journal of Invertebrate Pathology* **36**, 85–89.

Marcandier, S. & Kachatourians, G.G. (1987) Susceptibility of the migratory grasshopper, *Melanoplus sanguinipes* to *Beauveria bassiana*: influence of relative humidity. *Canadian Entomologist* **119**, 901–907.

Milner, R.J. (1978) On the occurrence of *Entomophthora grylli*, a fungal pathogen of grasshoppers in Australia. *Journal of the Australian Entomological Society* **17**, 293–296.

Moore, K.C. & Erlandson, M.A. (1988) Isolation of *Aspergillus parasiticus* Speare and *Beauveria bassiana* (Bals.) Vuillemin from melanopline grasshoppers. (Orthoptera: Acrididae) and demonstration of their pathogenicity in *Melanoplus sanguinipes* Fabricius *Canadian Entomologist* **120**, 989–991.

Pekrul, S. & Grula, E.A. (1979) Mode of infection of the corn earworm (*Heliothis zea*) by *Beauveria bassiana* as revealed by scanning electron microscopy. *Journal of Invertebrate Pathology* **34**, 238–247.

Pickford, R. & Riegert, P.W. (1964) The fungous disease caused by *Entomophthora grylli* Fres., and its effects on grasshopper populations in Saskatchewan in 1963. *Canadian Entomologist* **96**, 1158–1166.

Prior, C. & Greathead, D.J. (1989) Biological control of locusts: the potential for the exploitation of pathogens. *FAO Plant Protection Bulletin* **37**, 37–48.

Ramoska, W.A., Hajek, A.E. Ramos, M.E. & Soper, R.S. (1988) Infection of grasshoppers (Orthoptera: Acrididae) by members of the *Entomophaga grylli* species complex (Zygomycetes: Entomophthorales). *Journal of Invertebrate Pathology* **52**, 309–313.

Roberts, D.W. (1981) Toxins of entomopathogenic fungi. In: Burges, H.D. (ed), *Microbial Control of Pests and Plant Diseases 1970–1980.* Academic Press, London, pp. 441–464.

Roberts, D.W., Fuxa, J.R., Gaugler, R., Goettel, M., Jaques, R. & Maddox, J. (1991) Use of pathogens in insect control. In: Pimentel, D. (ed.), *CRC Handbook of Pest Management in Agriculture.* CRC Press, Boca Raton, pp. 243–278.

Roberts, D.W. & Yendol, W.G. (1971) Use of fungi for microbial control of insects. In: Burges, H.D. & Hussey, N.W. (eds), *Microbial Control of Insects and Mites.* Academic Press, New York, pp. 125–149.

Roffey, J. (1968) The occurrence of the fungus *Entomophthora grylli* Fres. on locusts and grasshoppers in Thailand. *Journal of Invertebrate Pathology* **11**, 237.

Rombach, M.C., Aguda, R.M. Shepard, B.M. & Roberts, D.W. (1986) Infection of the rice brown planthopper, *Nilaparvata lugens* (Homoptera: Delphacidae), by field application of entomopathogenic Hyphomycetes (Deuteromycotina). *Environmental Entomology* **15**, 1070–1073.

St Leger, R.J. (in press) The integument as a barrier to microbial infections. In: Retnakaran, A. & Binnington, K. (eds), *The Physiology of Insect Epidermis.* Inkata Press, Victoria.

St Leger, R.J., Goettel, M., Roberts, D.W. & Staples, R.C. (1991) Pre-penetration events during infection of host cuticle by *Metarhizium anisopliae. Journal of Invertebrate Pathology* **58**, 168–179.

Samson, R.A., Evans, H.C. & Latgé, J.P. (1988) *Atlas of Entomopathogenic Fungi.* Springer-Verlag, New York.

Schaefer, E.E. (1936) The white fungus disease (*Beauveria bassiana*) among red locusts in South Africa, and some observations on the grey fungus disease (*Empusa grylli*). *Science Bulletin Department of Agriculture & Forestry Union of South Africa* **160**, 28 pp.

Skaife, S.H. (1925) The locust fungus *Empusa grylli* and its effect on its host. *South African Journal of Science* **22**, 298–308.

Soper, R.S., May, B. & Martinell, B. (1983) *Entomophaga grylli* enzyme polymorphism as a technique for pathotype identification. *Environmental Entomology* **12**, 720–723.

Veen, K.H. (1968) Liste d'hôtes. *Mededelingen Landbouwhogeschool Wageningen* **68**, 19–24.

Vey, A. & Fargues, J. (1977) Histological and ultrastructural studies of *Beauveria bassiana* infection in *Leptinotarsa decemlineata* larvae during ecdysis. *Journal of Invertebrate Pathology* **30**, 207–215.

Wraight, S. & Roberts, D.W. (1987) Insect control efforts with fungi. *Journal of Industrial Microbiology* **28**, 77–87.

Yanagita, T. (1987) Studies on oral infection of the silkworm, *Bombyx mori*, with *Beauveria bassiana. Journal of Sericulture Japan* **56**, 279–284.

Preliminary studies on the ecology of *Zonocerus variegatus* in the Republic of Benin

A. Paraïso[1], C.J. Lomer[2], I. Godonou[1] & D. Kpindu[1]

[1]*International Institute of Tropical Agriculture, Benin:*
[2]*International Institute of Biological Control.*

Abstract
Zonocerus variegatus (Linnaeus) is a very prevalent grasshopper species in Benin and forms a major focus of present ecological studies on grasshoppers. Parasites found so far include mites (Trombidiidae), the calliphorid fly *Blaesoxipha filipjevi* (Rohdendorf) and mermithid nematodes. The nematodes also attacked *Eyprepocnemis plorans ornatipes* (Walker). Quantitative studies on *B. filipjevi* are reported. Fungal infestation by *Entomophaga grylli* (Fresenius) Batko on *Z. variegatus* was observed in four regions. Several isolates of *Beauveria bassiana* (Balsamo) Vuillemin have been obtained from *Z. variegatus.* Some preliminary observations on other species of grasshoppers have been made. *Z. variegatus, Oedaleus nigeriensis* Uvarov, *E. plorans ornatipes* and several species of locusts and grasshoppers are being bred for pathology studies.

Introduction

Locusts and grasshoppers pose a continuing threat to food production in several African countries. An average swarm of locusts contains, in each square kilometre, 20–50 million insects weighing 40–100 t which can consume 40–100 t of vegetation per day. During a plague of locusts a swarm may cover a total area of several thousand square kilometres (Courshee, 1990). However, locust plagues occur sporadically while grasshoppers are more consistent in their occurrence in several countries, including Benin.

Zonocerus variegatus (Linnaeus) is the most important grasshopper pest in Benin. The most heavily infested areas, covering the four southern provinces, are about 150,000 ha (Anon., 1986); but the insect occurs throughout the country, particularly in riverine habitats.

Other grasshoppers affect crops in northern Benin along the banks of the Niger river (Coffi, these proceedings). To date, the only means of controlling these pests has been to use insecticides (e.g. propoxur and fenitrothion) which are toxic to non-target organisms. With an increasing awareness of environmental problems associated with the use of chemical insecticides, it is important to consider non-chemical alternatives.

Numerous efforts were made to control locusts and grasshoppers with microbial agents, during the end of 19th century and the first half of the 20th century (Streett & McGuire, 1990). Several pathogens have been isolated from grasshoppers by different authors; microsporidians (Canning, 1953; Henry, 1967, 1971); viruses (Henry & Jutila, 1966; Henry *et al.*, 1969); bacteria (Stevenson, 1959); fungi (Chapman & Page, 1979); and nematodes (Denner, 1976).

Ecological studies on *Z. variegatus* and its natural enemies were made in West Africa by Chapman & Page (1979); work by other authors has been reviewed by Chiffaud & Mestre (1990). No studies on the ecology of *Z. variegatus* in Benin have been reported previously. The present study concentrates on the effects of parasites and pathogens.

Other species of grasshoppers have been little studied in Benin, although Fishpool & Popov (1984) provided an annotated species list.

Materials and methods

Surveys took place every month in the four provinces of southern Benin; Atlantique, Mono, Zou and Ouemé. Densities of *Z. variegatus* and other grasshoppers were recorded per square meter (Lecoq & Mestre, 1988). Information on host vegetation and damage was recorded. Collected *Z. variegatus* and other grasshoppers were brought to the laboratory and placed in cages to check for mites, parasitoids, nematodes and pathogens (Oma *et al.*, 1990). Samples of grasshoppers were dissected to evaluate the parasitism by flies and nematodes (Taylor, 1964). Diseased and dead grasshoppers were dried and incubated in moist petri dishes to look for fungi; tissues from dead and moribund grasshoppers were examined microscopically for other pathogens. Where disease symptoms were evident in the field (e.g. of *Entomophaga grylli*), counts were made of the number of diseased insects/m^2 to obtain approximate estimates of percentage mortality.

Results

Maps of the areas infested by *Z. variegatus* at high ($>20/m^2$) and medium density ($5–20/m^2$) are shown in Fig. 1. *Oedaleus nigeriensis* Uvarov was discovered in high densities of up to 5–7 adults/m^2 and 3–4 larvae/m^2 in some areas. *Eypreprocnemis plorans ornatipes* was the second most commonly encountered grasshopper in southern Benin after *Z. variegatus*, although it was never present at high densities.

In the Lama forest, Zou Province, the density of *Z. variegatus* was 275 larvae/m^2 in October before the start of the survey, but decreased in November (Fig. 2). After November the density increased again due to recruitment of newly hatched larvae. Parasitism by mites reached 30% by December and 55% in March. In March up to 45 mites were counted on one grasshopper. This period coincided with the oviposition period when most of the adult *Z. variegatus* are crawling on the soil. By 15 April, the next generation of newly hatched larvae was present. Parasitism by *Blaesoxipha filipjevi* (Rohdendorf) (Diptera: Calliphoridae) was first noticed at the end of January and reached 15% by February, and 50% by mid-April (Fig. 3). In the Lama region, fungal infection by *Entomophaga grylli* (Fresenius) Batko was not observed during our surveys. However, in Covè region, epizootics of *E. grylli* occurred and led to 90 to 95% mortality of the population of *Z. variegatus*. The density of the dead grasshoppers reached $10/m^2$.

In Mono province, high densities of *Z. variegatus* occurred in Lalo, Aplahoue, Athieme and Djakotomey. In Aplahoue the density was 380 larvae/m^2 in November, this decreased to 40 in January, coinciding with an increase in parasitism by mites and flies (Fig. 3). No fungal infection was recorded, and parasitism by nematodes in this region was very low. We also observed very low level of parasitism by the mites which increased in January, and in March reached 15%. Parasitism by *B. filipjevi* also began in January with 10% and increased to 22% by March (Fig. 3).

The second region in which a high level of infestation of *Z. variegatus* by *E. grylli* was observed was Ouemé. Here the level of parasitism by *B. filipjevi* increased from 0% in December 1990 to 50% in March 1991 (Fig. 4). At the end of this generation the complex of parasites and pathogens decreased as the *Z. variegatus* density fell below $10/m^2$. In this region, mites parasitized 10% of *Z. variegatus* in January, increasing to 20% by March. The fungus *E. grylli* killed up to 80% of the *Z. variegatus* population in Sakete region decreasing the population density to $7/m^2$.

In Atlantique province, one of the most infested regions is Niaouli, where the population density was more than 275 per m^2 in November. The level of parasitism due to mites was 3% in November and rose to 30% in March. In this region *E. grylli* killed 95% of the population of

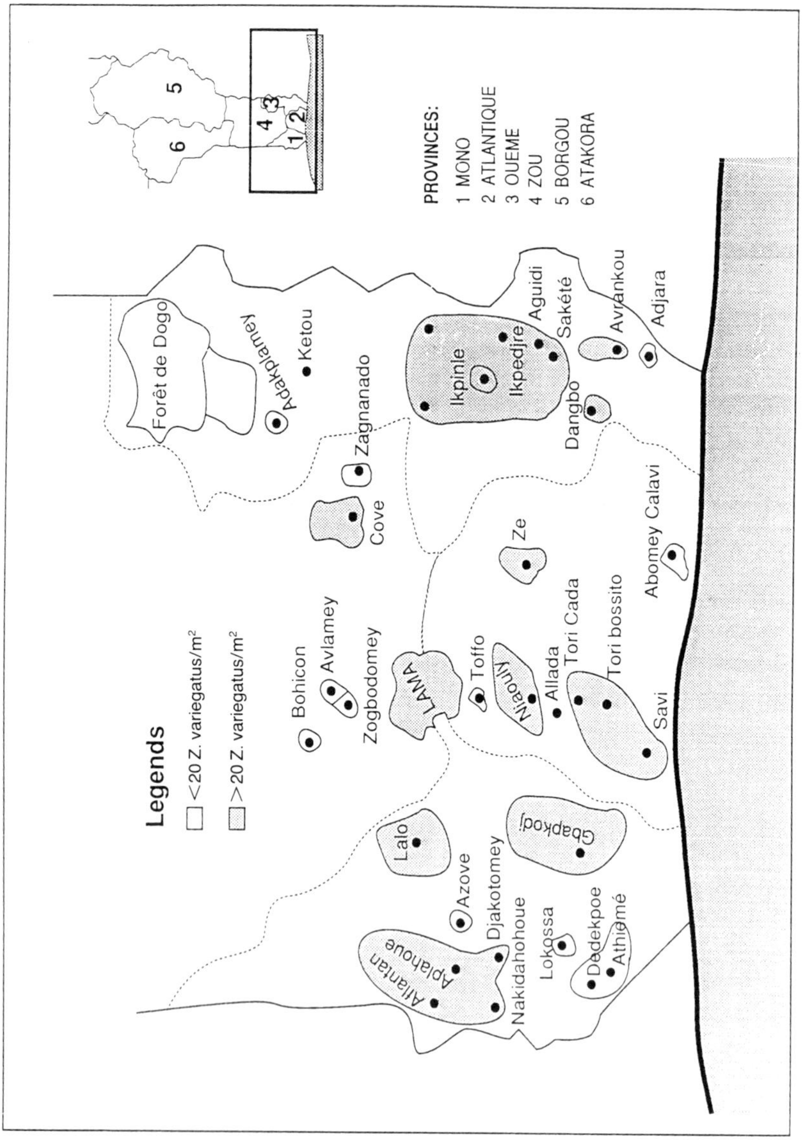

Figure 1. Map of areas infested by *Zonocerus variegatus* in southern part of Benin.

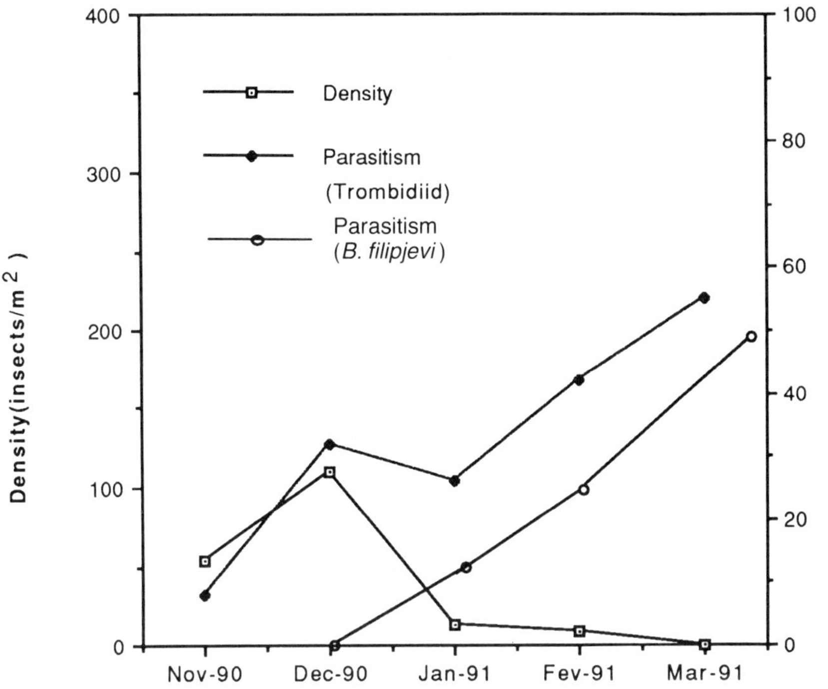

Figure 2. Density and level of parasitism of *Z. variegatus* in Lama, (ZOU Province).

Z. variegatus during February. Two isolates of *Beauveria bassiana* have been found in this region. The high density observed in November decreased in March to less than one *Z. variegatus*/m^2. Also in Atlantique, in Zê region, we observed an epizootic of *E. grylli* leading to the suppression of 90% of the *Z. variegatus* population; this was observed in both January and March. *B. filipjevi* parasitized 16% of the population in the same area in January and 60% by March (Fig. 5). In Zê, the level of parasitism due to mites was 30% in January. A third *B. bassiana* isolate was found about 50 km from Niaouli.

In all the regions we visited, oviposition sites of *Z. variegatus* were identified. Soil samples were taken from these different regions.

Pathogens

So far, three isolates of *Beauveria bassiana* (Balsamo) Vuillemin have been recovered from dead insects in the field; one was found on fifth instar larvae and the others on adults. The regions in which they were discovered

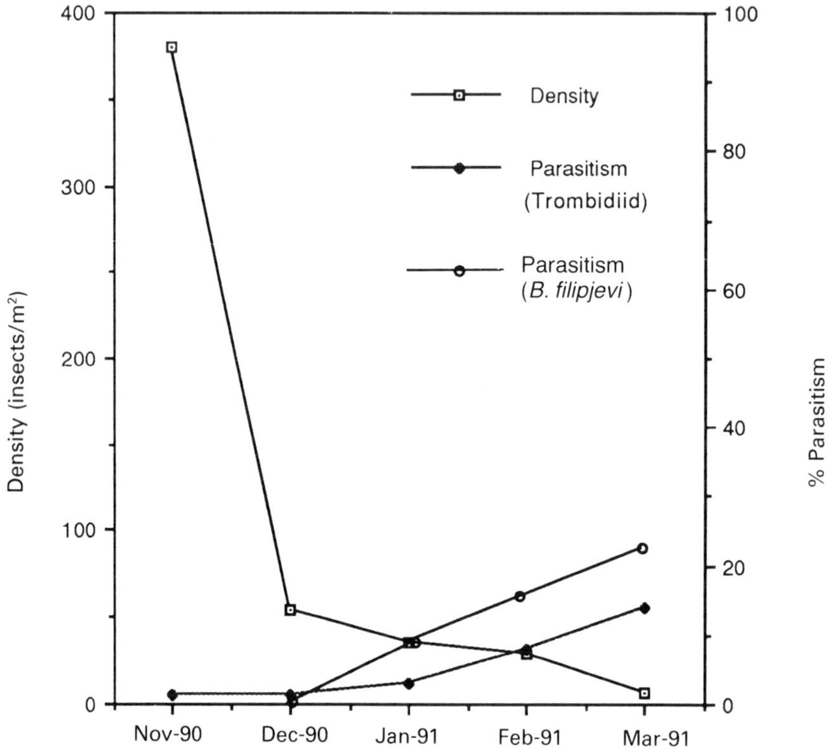

Figure 3. Density and level of parasitism of *Z. variegatus* in Aplahoué, (MONO Province).

are characterized by high levels of infestation of *E. grylli.* Unlike the *E. grylli* epizootics, which seemed to have a significant effect on the *Z. variegatus* populations, no epizootics of *B. bassiana* were observed in the field. We isolated *Fusarium* sp. from *Z. variegatus*, but it did not prove to be pathogenic on reinoculation. Laboratory tests have begun with the three isolates of *B. bassiana.*

Discussion

Oedaleus nigeriensis has not previously been reported in southern Benin. The zone in which it was found is characterized by the presence of young millet and wild Gramineae. However, severe damage by this grasshopper was not observed and the high density was very local.

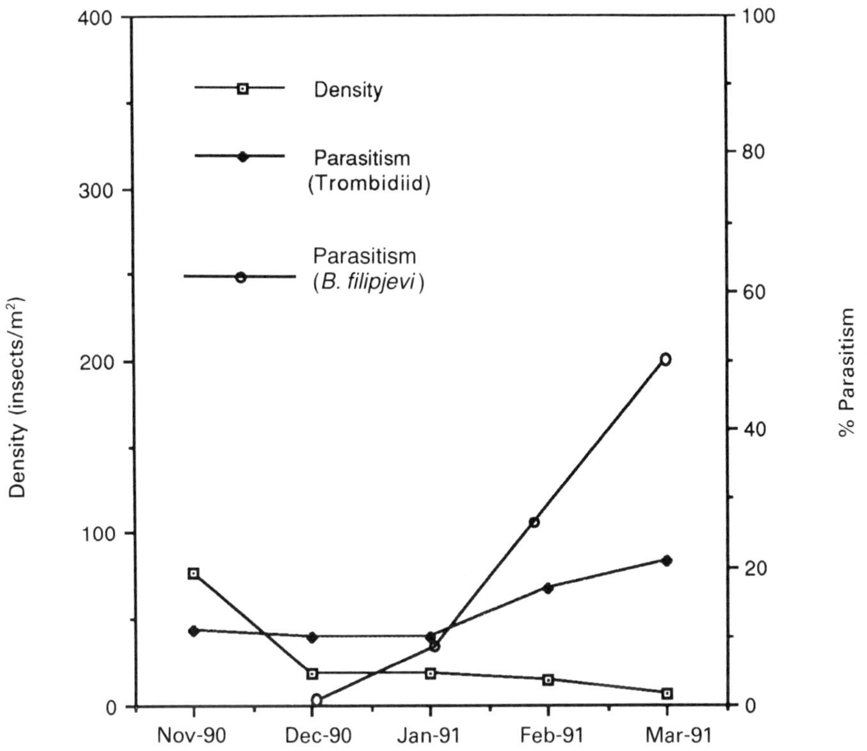

Figure 4. Density and level of parasitism of *Z. variegatus* in Avrankou, (OUEME Province).

Eyprepocnemis plorans ornatipes (Walker) is the second most often encountered grasshopper in southern Benin after *Z. variegatus.* Despite its density, little damage to crops was observed during current surveys in different localities in southern Benin.

A wide range of natural enemies is known to attack grasshoppers (see Greathead, these proceedings). Studies on *Z. variegatus* in Nigeria undertaken by Taylor (1964) and by Chapman & Page (1979) showed that *Blaesoxipha filipjevi* is the most prevalent parasitoid, with up to 60% of adults attacked. Similar levels were observed in the present study, e.g. 50% in Ouemé and 60% in Atlantique in March.

Chiffaud & Mestre (1990) in a review of the literature concluded that parasitized females would be unable to lay eggs and that levels of parasitism were sufficient to regulate *Z. variegatus* populations; however, critical studies to confirm a regulatory effect are lacking.

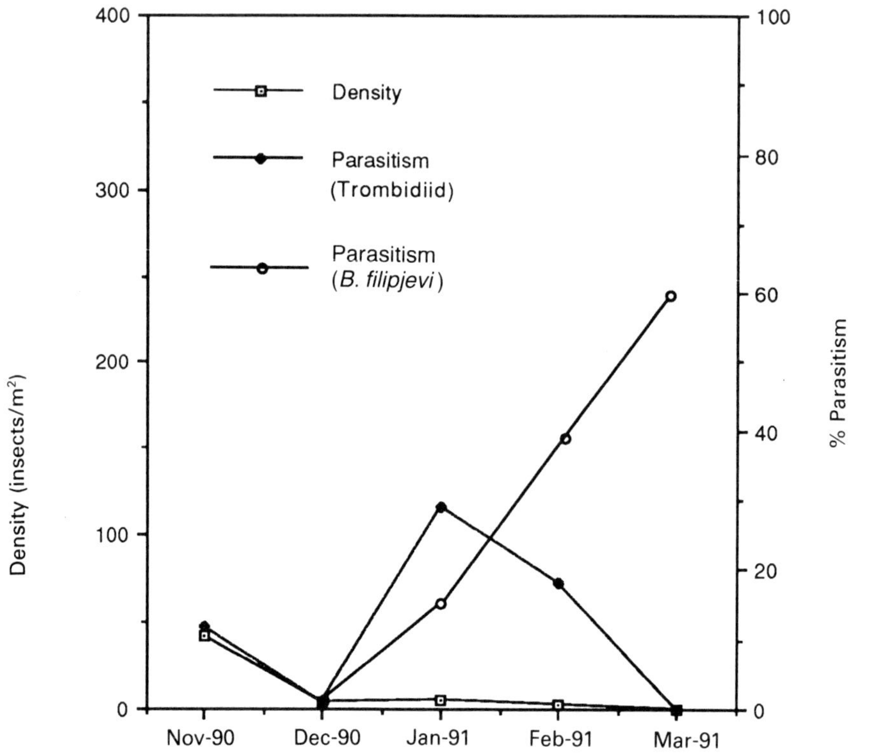

Figure 5. Density and level of parasitism of *Z. variegatus* in Zê, (Atlantique Province).

Studies on fungal pathogens showed that epizootics of *E. grylli* often led to 80% (Chapman & Page, 1979) or 99% infestation (Coulibaly *et al.*, 1988). In Benin, epizootics of *E. grylli* were observed in four regions leading to the suppression of 80% to 90% of the population of *Z. variegatus*.

Our isolates of *Beauveria bassiana* from *Z. variegatus* are the first reported. Preliminary laboratory tests with the three isolates indicated good virulence in *Z. variegatus*, and will be the subject of our next publication.

The high level of parasitism by trombidiid mites seemed not to affect *Z. variegatus*, despite the high numbers occasionally observed on grasshoppers at the time of oviposition.

Parasitism by nematodes was very low, less than 1%, and in many places they did not appear at all. They seemed not to be specific to *Z. variegatus*.

References

Anon. (1986) Annual report. Crop protection service of Benin.

Canning, E.U. (1953) A new microsporidian, *Nosema locustae* sp. n., from the fat body of the African migratory locust, *Locusta migratoria migratorioides* R. and F. *Parasitology* **43**, 287–290.

Chapman, R.F. & Page, W.W. (1979) Factors affecting the mortality of the grasshopper, *Zonocerus variegatus* in southern Nigeria. *Journal of Animal Ecology* **48**, 271–288.

Chiffaud, J. & Mestre, J. (1990) Le criquet puant, *Zonocerus variegatus* (Linné, 1758). CIRAD-PRIFAS. Department GERDAT.

Coulibaly, N., Decasy, B. & Duverger, B. (1988) *Lutte Contre le Criquet Puant,* **1980–April 1988**. Institut de Recherches du Café et du Cacao. CIRAD, Montpellier.

Courshee, R.J. (1990) Desert locust and their control. *International Pest Control* **32**, 16–18.

Denner, M.W. (1976) Preliminary studies on the pathology caused by *Mermis nigrescens* in Orthoptera. *Proceedings of the Indiana Academy of Science* **85**, 258–261.

Fishpool, L.D.C. & Popov, G.B. (1984) The grasshopper faunas of Mali, Niger, Benin and Togo savannas. *Bulletin de l'Institut Française d'Afrique Noire* **43** A, 275–410.

Henry, J.E. (1967) *Nosema acridophagus* sp. n, a microsporidian isolated from grasshopper. *Journal of Invertebrate Pathology* **9**, 331–341.

Henry, J.E. & Jutila, J.W. (1966) The isolation of a polyhedrosis virus from a grasshopper. *Journal of Invertebrate Pathology* **8**, 417–418.

Henry, J.E. (1971) *Nosema cuneatum* sp. n. (Microsporida: Nosematidae) in grasshoppers (Orthoptera: Acrididae). *Journal of Invertebrate Pathology* **17**, 164–171.

Henry, J.E., Nelson, B.P. & Jutila, J.W. (1969) Pathology and development of the grasshopper inclusion virus in *Melanoplus sanguinipes. Journal of Virology* **3**, 605–610.

Lecoq, M. & Mestre, J. (1988) *La Surveillance des Sauteriaux du Sahel. Collection Acridologie Opérationnelle* no. 2. CIRAD-PRIFAS, Montpellier.

Omar, E.A., Streett, D.A. & Henry, J.E. (1990) Establishment of a nondiapause *Melanoplus differentialis* (Thomas) Orthoptera: Acrididae colony. *Canadian Entomologist* **122**, 583–584.

Stevenson, J.P. (1959) Epizootiology of disease of the desert locust *Schistocerca gregaria* (Forskål) caused by a non-chromogenic strain of *Serratia marescens* Bizio. *Journal of Insect Pathology* **1**, 232–244.

Streett, D.A. & McGuire, M.R. (1990) Pathogenic diseases of grasshoppers. In: Chapman, R.F. & Joern, A. (eds), *Biology of Grasshoppers.* John Wiley & Sons, New York, 483–516.

Taylor, T.A. (1964) *Blaesoxipha filipjevi* Rohd. (Diptera: Sarcophagidae) parasitizing *Zonocerus variegatus* (Linné) (Orthoptera: Acridoidea) in Nigeria. *Bulletin of Entomological Research* **55**, 83–86.

Effects of neem oil treatment on the phase status of desert locust, *Schistocerca gregaria*

J. Langewald[1] & H. Schmutterer[2]

[1]*International Institute of Tropical Agriculture:* [2]*Institut für Phytopathologie Universität Giessen.*

Abstract

Gregarious desert locust (*Schistocerca gregaria* Forskål) hoppers were treated with neem oil formulations containing different concentrations of azadirachtin in laboratory and field trials. Effects on the colour, morphology, and behaviour of the hoppers were examined.

First and second instar locusts were treated with neem oil at a concentration of 10 l/ha. Their aggregation behaviour was tested in small arenas after each moult following the treatment. The capability of the treated adults to aggregate, especially in larger groups, was significantly reduced compared to the untreated control.

For cage trials in the field, two neem oil formulations containing 0.2% and 0.4% azadirachtin, respectively, were each sprayed on 600 third instar hoppers which were then separated in four cages containing 150 hoppers each. An untreated control was also replicated in four cages. Each surviving locust was observed daily for damage to antennae and legs and for colour change. The results clearly show differences in the proportions of damage to antennae in the fifth instar and the adults. In the fourth instar, proportions of yellow hoppers were higher in the treatments compared with the control. In the fifth instar green coloured hoppers were found in higher proportions than in the controls. Positive correlations between the green (solitary phase) colour and antennae damage were observed in the fourth instar in the treatments and the control. In the fifth instar strong positive correlations could be found between the green colour and damaged antennae or legs in the treatments and the control.

Introduction

The neem tree (*Azadirachta indica*), indigenous to Burma and India, is now very common in Africa, especially in the sahelian region. The properties of this fast-growing tree are various. In India, neem products are commonly used for medicinal purposes and soap production. The timber is termite resistant and because of its drought resistance, grows well in arid zones. With regard to plant protection the secondary compound azadirachtin, a triterpenoid, is most interesting. Azadirachtin affects insects in different ways (Schmutterer, 1990).

Compared to other insect species, *Schistocerca gregaria* (Forskål) seems to be extremely sensitive to azadirachtin (Nicol, 1991).

Material and methods

Formulation

In the laboratory trials pure neem oil with an azadirachtin content less than 0.05% was used to avoid high mortality and therefore allow a range of sub-lethal effects to be studied. In the field, oil enriched with methanolic extracts from neem cake (residue of the oil pressing) was sprayed at azadirachtin concentrations of 0.2% and 0.4%.

Experiments

Behaviour trials

In the laboratory on a small scale, a design airbrush was used as a sprayer. 100 first and 100 second instar hoppers in the gregarious phase were placed in a 25 × 25 × 40 cm glass tray in the middle of one square meter of ground. The area was sprayed with one ml neem oil. After each moult the aggregation behaviour was tested. A method similar to Gillet (1973) was used in this trial. The groups 'treated as first instar' and 'treated as second instar' were studied separately. After each subsequent moult ten treated and ten untreated hoppers were placed in a round arena 30 cm (for the second to the fourth instar) or 45 cm in diameter (for the fifth and the adult instar). The observations were made under natural light conditions in a greenhouse at a temperature of 28°C. The locusts were crowded together and 30 min later when they had settled down, a photograph was taken and they were crowded again. Further pictures were taken in the same way after 60 and 90 min. The pictures were analysed in two ways. First, the aggregation behaviour in general was evaluated by counting locusts sitting together at a distance, less than one body length. Secondly, their capability to aggregate in larger groups was evaluated by counting locusts sitting together in groups of more than three individuals. The counts for the three replicates (30, 60, 90 min) were added. Each trial was repeated ten times.

Semi-field trials

The aim of these trials was to analyse effects of neem oil treatments under small scale field conditions and to test the above mentioned enriched neem oil formulations. For this purpose small mosquito screen cages with 1.5×1.5 m ground surface and 1 m height were installed in a cassava field. Two cassava plants in each cage provided shelter. Because of the high cyanide content of the cassava these plants were not eaten. Two neem oil formulations containing 0.2% and 0.4% azadirachtin were tested on late second and third instar hoppers.

For oil application, a Micro-Ulva sprayer with a red restrictor loaded with five batteries, providing a flow rate of approximately 20 ml/min and a droplet size of 80–100 μm was used. For each treatment 600 third instar hoppers were sprayed in a 25 m^2 arena using a dosage of 10 l/ha. After the treatment, the hoppers were separated in groups of 150 individuals and placed in the cages. Four cages with untreated controls were also installed. Then the instar, colour (black-brown, green, yellow) and morphological damage (antennae, legs) to each surviving locust were recorded daily during a 33 day period until all locusts were adult.

Results

Behaviour trials

The results for both groups 'treated as first instar' and 'treated as second instar' were very similar. During the larval instars there were no significant differences in aggregation behaviour, while for the adults the number of locusts was significantly ($P < 0.05$, Wilcoxon Signed-Rank Test) lower in a distance closer than one body length (Figs 1 and 2) and the number of locusts in groups of more than three individuals was highly significantly lower ($P < 0.01$, Wilcoxon Signed-Rank Test) (Figs 3 and 4) than in the controls. The medians of the ten replicates are shown in Figs 1–4.

Semi-field trials

The first effects on treated locusts could be expected in the fourth instar, i.e., after the first moult following the treatment. Since adult locusts have

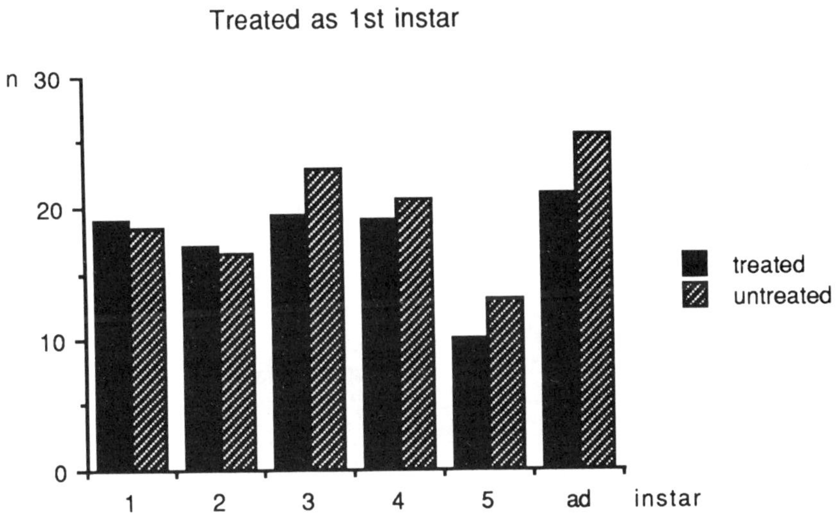

Figure 1. Number of grouped locusts in each instar.

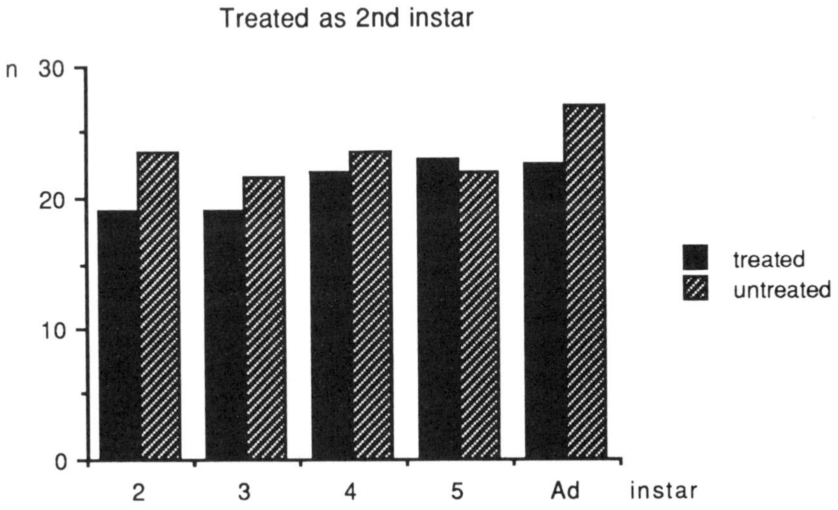

Figure 2. Number of grouped locusts in each instar after treatment.

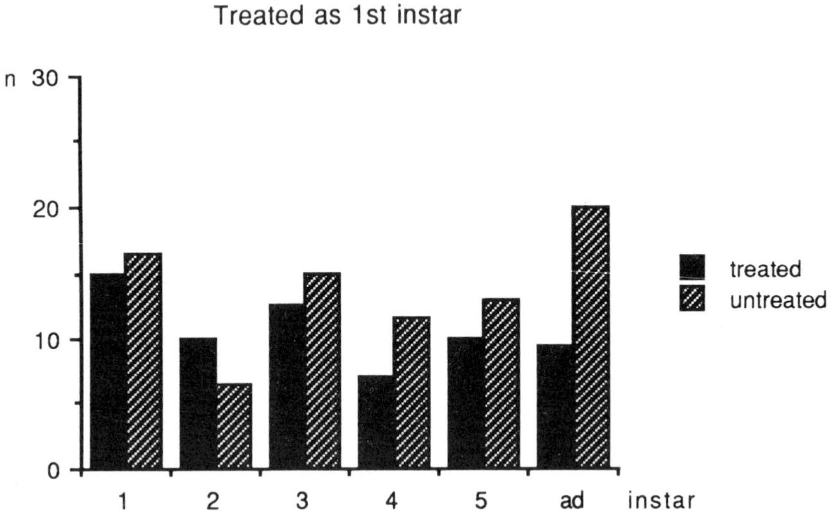

Figure 3. Number of locusts in groups composed of more than three specimens in each instar.

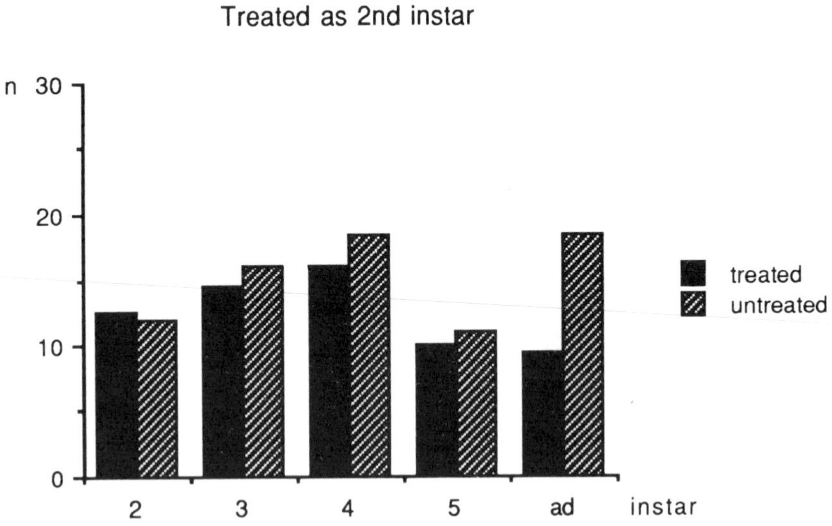

Figure 4. Number of locusts in groups composed of more than three specimens in each instar after treatment.

different colour characterisics from nymphs, the colours were not evaluated. For the presentation of results, the three day moving averages of proportions of damaged and differently coloured locusts are shown in Figs 5 to 8. To avoid misinterpretation, only those values from the period when >50% of the population was in that instar (indicated in each case by the dotted lines) should be examined. Outside of these values proportions could result from low numbers of locusts. The values of the replicates, for the days representing 50% of the population maximum were utilized in a one factor analysis of variance (Scheffe F-test and Dunnett t-test).

Morphological damage

Fourth instar
There was no significant difference between the treatments.

Fifth instar
On the 14th day the damage to antennae in the 0.4% treatment was significantly higher ($P < 0.05\%$) than in the 0.2% treatment and the control. The damage to antennae in the 0.2% treatment was also significantly higher than in the control of ($P < 0.05$).

On the 25th day the 0.4% treatment and the 0.2% treatment differed significantly from the control ($P < 0.05$) (Fig. 5).

There were no significant differences in the damage to legs.

Adults
On the 25th day damage to antennae was significantly higher in the 0.4% and 0.2% treatments compared to the control ($P < 0.05$) (Fig. 6). Damage to legs differed only significantly between the 0.4% treatment and the control on the 25th day in the fifth instar ($P < 0.05$) (Fig. 6).

Colours

Fourth instar
On the 14th day the proportion of yellow coloured locusts in the 0.2% treatment was significantly higher than in the control ($P < 0.05$) (Fig. 7).

Fifth instar
On the 14th day the proportion of yellow coloured locusts in the 0.4% treatment was significantly higher than in the control ($P < 0.05$) (Fig. 8).

On the 25th day the proportion of green coloured locusts in the 0.2% treatment and the control ($P < 0.05$), and the 0.4% treatment and the control differed significantly (Fig. 8).

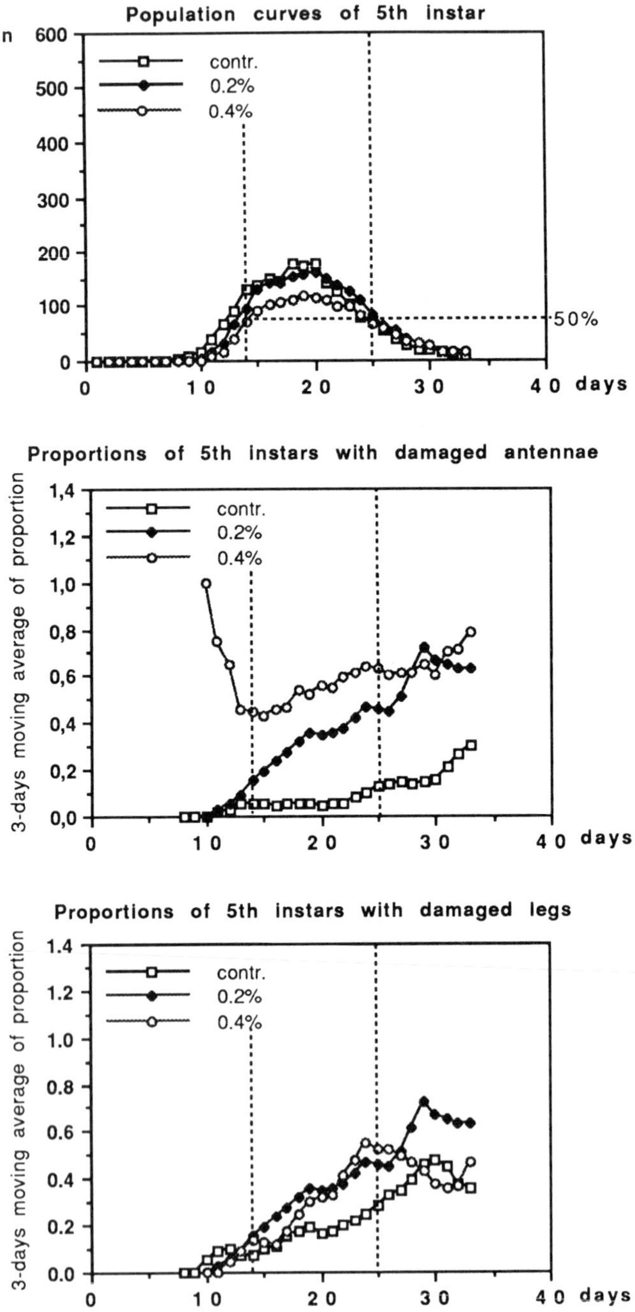

Figure 5. Proportions of damaged 5th instars during the experimentation period.

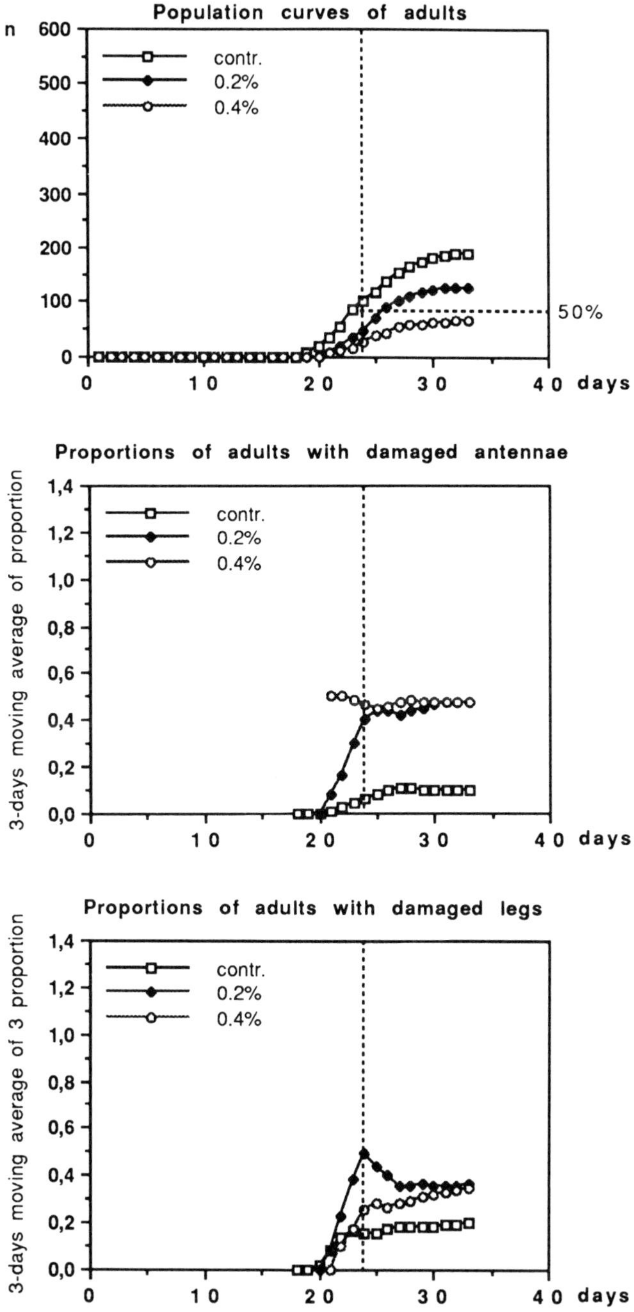

Figure 6. Proportions of damaged adults during the experimentation period.

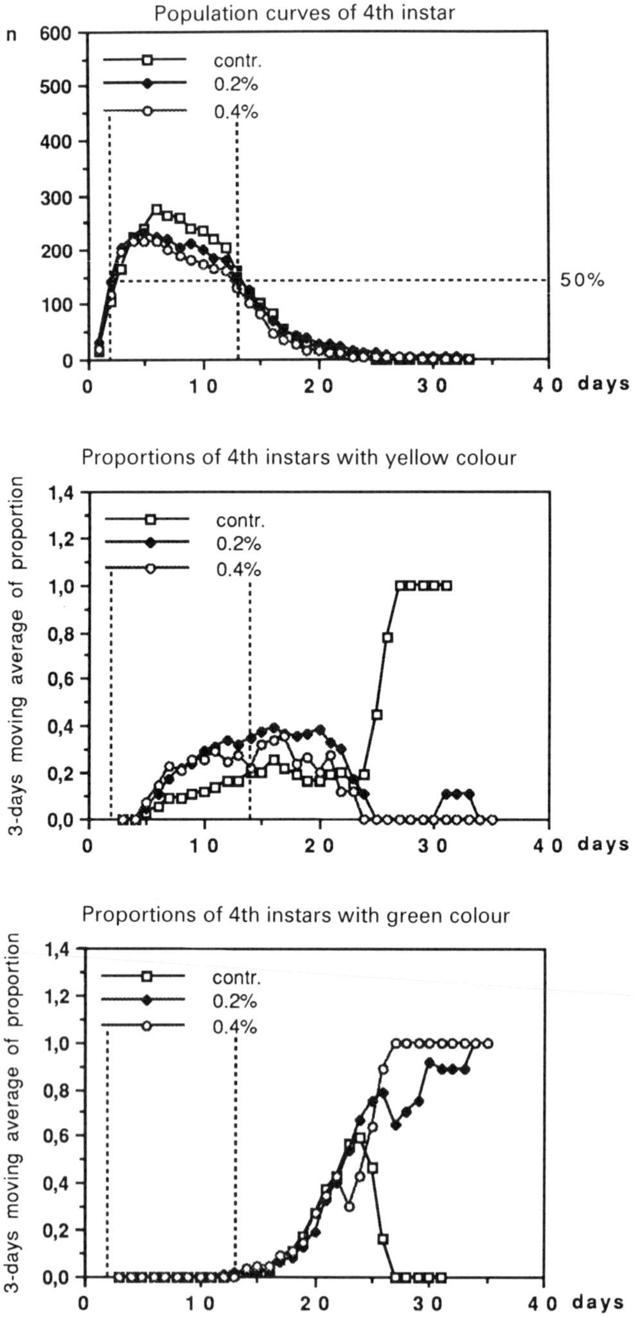

Figure 7. Proportions of 4th instars with yellow and green colour during the experimentation period.

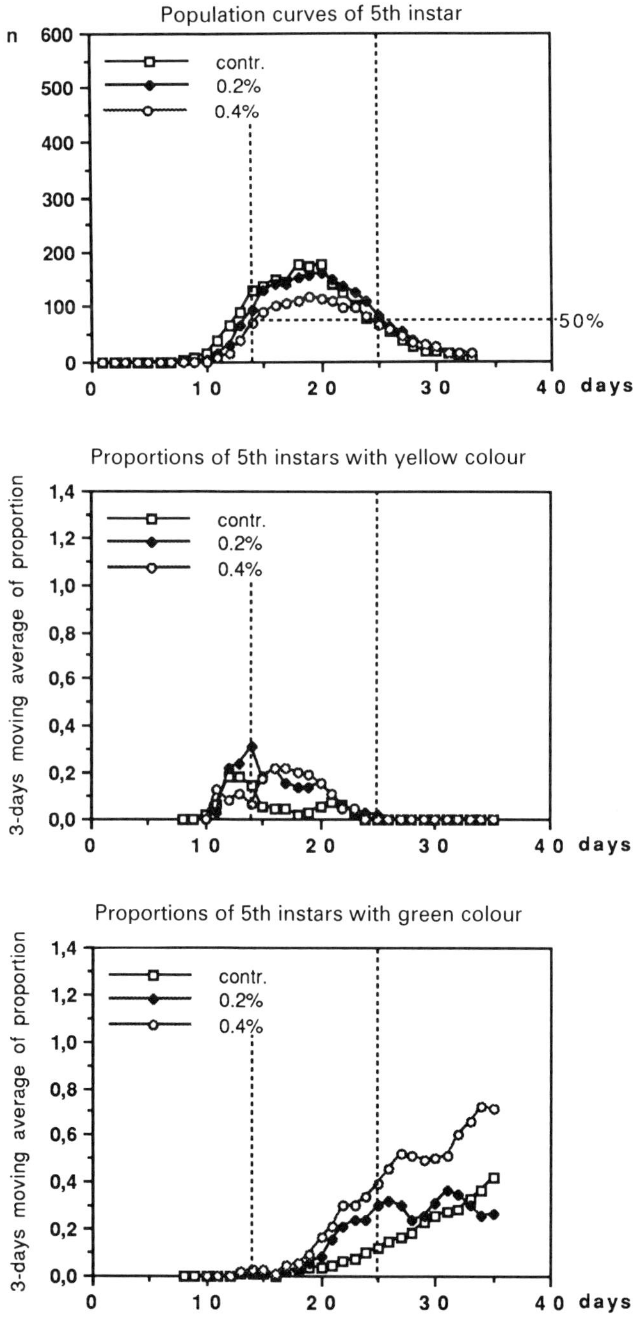

Figure 8. Proportions of 5th instars with yellow and green colour during the experimentation period.

Correlations

When the proportions of different coloured locusts are plotted against the proportions of locusts with damaged antennae and the proportions of locusts with damaged legs, in each treatment, clear correlations can be seen only for the fifth instar (see Table 1).

Fourth instar
In the fourth instar significant positive correlations between the proportions of green coloured locusts and the proportions of locusts with damaged antennae was found in the control (r=0.7; P=0.01) and the 0.4% (r=0.78; ($P < 0.01$) treatment.

Table 1. Correlations between proportions of different coloured locusts and proportions of locusts with damaged antennae or with damaged legs in each treatment, in the 5th instar.

		Correlations	
		r	*P*
Proportion damaged antennae			
Control	yellow	−0.55	0.04
	green	0.84	<0.01
	brown/black	−0.29	0.15
0.20%	yellow	−0.86	<0.01
	green	0.81	0.01
	brown/black	−0.19	0.47
0.40%	yellow	−0.71	0.01
	green	0.82	0.01
	brown/black	−0.52	0.13
Proportion damaged legs			
Control	yellow	−0.55	0.04
	green	0.84	<0.01
	brown/black	−0.29	0.15
0.20%	yellow	−0.86	<0.01
	green	0.81	0.01
	brown/black	−0.19	0.47
0.40%	yellow	−0.71	0.01
	green	0.82	0.01
	brown/black	−0.52	0.13

A significant correlation was found between the proportions of the yellow coloured and the proportions of the locusts with antennae damages in the control ($r=0.7$; $P=0.02$).

No significant correlation between leg damage and colour was observed.

Fifth instar
In the fifth instar the results were more obvious. It is clear that proportions of green locusts have a significant positive correlation, while the proportions of the yellow coloured locusts have a significant negative correlation, with the proportions of locusts with damaged antennae in all three treatments.

Exactly the same is true for the correlations between the proportions of green and yellow (except yellow in the control) coloured locusts and the proportions of locusts with damaged legs (see Table 1).

Discussion

The experiments show that damage to extremities, caused by neem, leads to a change of colour in locust hoppers towards green, the colour of solitary nymphs. It was observed that this solitarizing effect also influences the aggregation behaviour. It is known from the literature (Mordue, 1977) that locusts at a certain population density may produce a gregarization pheromone which may be perceived by the antennae. If the neem oil treatment causes damage to the antennae, the affected locusts are no longer able to receive this pheromonal input and show a tendency towards solitarization. Since the change of colours in locusts treated with neem oil is much more intensive than in locusts with amputated antennae, damage to antennae cannot be the only explanation for solitarization (Schmutterer & Freres, 1990). The decline of juvenile hormone titres in treated locusts may also contribute to this phenomenon (Rembold, 1986). For practical locust control, a solitarizing effect as found after neem oil application could play an important role.

Acknowledgements

These studies were conducted at the International Institute of Tropical Agriculture, Biological Control Program, Cotonou, Benin, in collaboration with the University of Giessen, Germany and the Deutsch Gesellschaft für Technische Zusammenarbeit in Eschborn, Germany.

References

Gillet, S.D. (1973) Social determinants of aggregation behavior in adults of the desert locust. *Animal Behaviour* **21**, 599–606.

Mordue, A.J. (1977) Some effects of amputation of the antennae on pigmentation growth and development in the locust *Schistocerca gregaria. Physiological Entomology* **2**, 293–300.

Nicol, C.M.Y. (1991) Contact effects of seed from the neem tree, *Azadirachta indica* (A. Juss.), on nymphs of the gregarious phase of the desert locust, *Schistocerca gregaria* (Forsk.). *Journal of Applied Entomology* **111**, 197–205.

Rembold, H. (1986) Effect of azadirachtin A on hormone titers during the gonadotrophic cycle of *Locusta migratoria. Proceedings of the Third International Neem Conference* Nairobi, 81–93.

Schmutterer, H. (1990) Properties and potential of natural pesticides from the neem tree *Azadirachta indica. Annual Review of Entomology* **35**, 271–297.

Schmutterer, H. & Freres, T. (1990) Influence of neem-seed oil on metamorphosis, colour and behaviour of the desert locust, *Schistocerca gregaria* (Forsk.), and of the African migratory locust, *Locusta migratoria migratorioides* (R.&F.). *Journal of Plant Diseases and Protection* **97**, 431–438.

Panel discussion: precis

Mr Niassy asked about egg parasites, the possibilities of fungal epizootics in the desert and the cost of formulations of fungal pathogens. Dr Greathead replied that there was little possibility of manipulating egg parasitoids as control agents. Concerning epizootics in the desert, Dr Goettel mentioned the possibility of conditions of high humidity following rain. Dr Prior added that formulating fungal spores in oil would reduce the requirement for high humidity; the cost of additions to the formulation, such as stabilizers, would be minimal.

Mr Adam commented that in Togo, *Verronia* sp. was found to act as a trap plant for *Zonocerus variegatus.* Dr Paraïso replied that this had not been tried in Benin. Mr Saizonou (Benin) commented that parasitism of *Zonocerus variegatus* builds up towards the end of the season. It is not clear whether the parasitic fly *Blaesoxipha filipjevi* has an effect on the population or not.

Captain Kitenda asked about the time to kill, and the survival of microbial control agents in the field. Dr Henry replied that while fungi could cause mortality in a few days, agents such as *Nosema* took several weeks. Activity of the microbes is reduced after 4 to 6 days; *Nosema* spores can persist for one year in the field, but cause insignificant mortality by that time.

Section III

Exploration and Characterization

Discovery and characterization of fungal pathogens for locust and grasshopper control

C. Prior

International Institute of Biological Control.

Abstract

An effective biopesticide must be based on a pathogen isolate with high virulence to the target pest, an acceptable host range and proven safety. Isolates of *Metarhizium* spp. with virulence to the desert locust, *Schistocerca gregaria* (Forskål), have been obtained both from within its known distribution and also outside it. All isolates with high virulence have been obtained from Orthoptera, but not necessarily from acridids. However, in other studies highly virulent isolates have been obtained from insects taxonomically unrelated to the target. Although such 'new encounter' isolates may be found they may be difficult to use because of quarantine concerns about their release in a new environment and their impact on non-target organisms. All isolates used as biopesticides for pest control must be proven harmless to the environment, and this will require the use of biochemical and genetic 'fingerprinting' in field tests to distinguish them from indigenous isolates already present. Concern may also be expressed over the stability of isolate genotypes which survive after application. Instability in *Metarhizium* spp. may arise either from mutation or from recombination via the parasexual cycle, but evidence suggests this may be rare under field conditions and restricted by incompatibility mechanisms. The known facts concerning the nature, geographical range and stability of genotypes in *Metarhizium* spp. do not support restriction on the distribution or use of these fungi for pest control.

Introduction

Locusts, especially the desert locust, *Schistocerca gregaria* (Forskål), and grasshoppers, including *Oedaleus senegalensis* (Krauss), *Hieroglyphus* spp. and *Kraussaria angulifera* (Krauss), are major pests in the Sahel and during plague years the desert locust may also cause damage to the more humid zones of Africa and Asia (Brader, 1988; Steedman, 1990). Pyrgormorphids, especially *Zonocerus variegatus* (Linnaeus), may also be targets for control. Grasshopper control costs in 1986–87 amounted to US$62 million (Brader, 1988). International donor contributions to desert locust control during the last plague 1985–89 were US$275 million (Anon., 1990). The scale of the problem is immense and the volume of chemical pesticides used in control has caused great concern to donors and the afflicted countries (Anon., 1990).

The collaborative research programme for biological control of locusts and grasshoppers being carried out by IIBC, IITA and DFPV seeks to develop pathogens as biological pesticides which may be integrated into the existing control infrastructure and thereby lessen the dependence on chemical control. The pathogens which have the most potential are members of the entomopathogenic Deuteromycotina, because these organisms are readily produced on simple culture media, have a proven safety record and are formulable as biological pesticides suitable for spraying using controlled droplet application technology at ultra low volume (ULV) rates of 1–2 (< 5) l/ha (Prior & Greathead, 1989). They have been used in commercial pest control operations in USSR and Brazil for many years.

Species in the two Deuteromycete genera *Metarhizium* and *Beauveria* have been recorded from a very wide range of host arthropods and there are several records from Orthoptera (Prior & Greathead, 1989). Other entomopathogenic Deuteromycete genera which have been recorded occasionally from Orthoptera include *Paecilomyces* and *Verticillium*, but the former includes some species pathogenic to mammals, and the latter are slime-spored and difficult to formulate in non-aqueous diluents for application at ULV rates. The joint programme is therefore concentrating on *Metarhizium* spp., which have proved more pathogenic than *Beauveria* spp. in assays to date.

The range of target species within the Orthoptera is wide. Although locusts and grasshoppers are taxonomically related, there are substantial differences in their ecology which affect control strategies. There is much evidence from studies on other insect pest groups that isolates of *Metarhizium* spp. and *Beauveria* spp. show considerable host specificity and will even show differential virulence to taxonomically related target pests. Both these factors indicate a need for careful selection of isolates with high virulence to the specific target pest under field conditions. Since it is not clear from the currently available information whether the best isolate for controlling a particular pest will originate from that pest, or even from one related to it (Prior, 1990), it is possible that a desirable isolate may originate from a country or even a biogeographical zone different from the one in which it must be used. If the chosen isolate is exotic to the country where it must be used, it will be prudent to obtain quarantine clearance prior to import (Greathead & Prior, 1990).

In many countries, pathogens are subject to requirements for registration before they can be used in the same way as pesticides. The requirements include both mammalian safety testing, and environmental safety. The latter involves assessment of the impact on non-target organisms and of environmental contamination. An essential part of any work to meet the registration requirements will be adequate techniques to monitor the impact of the fungus after use. Since the species of *Metarhizium* and *Beauveria* are ubiquitous, a test is required to distinguish the test genotype from those already present in the test ecosystem. This requires characterization of the isolate using methods other than classical morphology because morphological criteria are insufficient to separate genotypes at the sub-specific level.

There are thus three questions to be answered with respect to selection of the best isolates for development:

1. where is the best place to seek the required virulent isolate?
2. if it is exotic in the country where it must be used, how can it be characterized so that its environmental impact, if any, can be monitored?
3. if it is exotic what are the risks, if any, involved in its use?

This paper discusses these questions, both in a general context and in the specific context of the discovery, development and characterization of isolates of *Metarhizium* spp. and *Beauveria* spp. for locust and grasshopper control.

Discovery – where to search?

What characteristics?

In order to develop fungal pathogens for controlling insects it is necessary to select genotypes which combine the best possible characters for killing the target pest under field conditions. It is obvious that the very best can never be achieved because the number of genotypes available is effectively limitless. It is therefore necessary to decide how to sample them adequately with the limited resources that are usually available. The characteristics that are desirable in an entomopathogenic fungal genotype can be divided into good production features, such as high sporulation, optimum utilization of available substrate and genetic stability, and good field performance, which can be summarized as high virulence to the target coupled with suitable host range.

Good production characteristics can be determined adequately in the laboratory. They have been reviewed frequently (McCoy *et al.*, 1988; Bartlett & Jaronski, 1988). A high rate of conidial production per unit of substrate is very important. Conidiation in submerged culture would be most advantageous and is known for a few isolates of *Hirsutella thompsonii* Fisher (van Winkelhoff & McCoy, 1984) and *Beauveria bassiana* (Balsamo) Vuillemin (Thomas *et al.*, 1987), but not *Metarhizium* spp. Stability in storage is important and *Metarhizium* spp., in particular, are prone to lose the ability to sporulate if maintained on rich media or if subcultured frequently: storage in liquid nitrogen is recommended to avoid these changes. The main requirement for selecting optimum production characters is a wide range of genetic diversity to choose from, but criteria for identifying these characters in the field are difficult to define.

Virulence under field conditions is determined by a complex of characteristics, not all of which can be quantified under laboratory conditions. The terms virulence and pathogenicity are often used interchangeably and it is worth noting that there are clearly defined differences, at least in plant pathology (Talboys *et al.*, 1973):

- **pathogenicity** is the ability to cause disease and is used as a qualitative description of a genus or species. For example, *M. anisopliae* (Metschnikoff) Sorokin is pathogenic to a wide range of arthropods
- **virulence** is a quantitative measure of the capacity of an individual pathogen genotype to cause infection. Thus one may have an avirulent isolate (genotype) of a pathogenic species with respect to an individual host: many of the isolates tested against *Schistocerca gregaria* in the current programme have had little or no virulence to that host, but are none the less pathogenic because they are virulent to other hosts

When selecting for virulence in isolates for mycopesticide development, not all determinants may be relevant. Adhesion may play an important role in the natural infection process. However, the mechanical requirement for adhesion is circumvented in a contact biopesticide formulation by applying the conidia directly to the cuticle in a diluent. Similarly, the ability to produce conidia under dry conditions would be advantageous in the field because this would extend the time period in which natural spread would occur. The use of the fungus as a biopesticide also circumvents this requirement, since the conidial inoculum is produced artificially.

In the current programme for locust and grasshopper control, considerable effort has been made to search for new isolates in the breeding grounds of the desert locust and the main grasshopper species. A major reason for this is the existence of evidence for differences in temperature optima among isolates. McCoy *et al.* (1988) noted that entomogenous fungi are mesophiles, with temperature optima in the 20–30°C range. However, Milner (1989) noted the existence of a high-temperature isolate of *M. anisopliae* attacking termites from northern Australia which had an optimum of 30°C and could sporulate at 37°C. Rath *et al.* (1990) reported a 'cold-active' isolate DAT F-001 of *M. anisopliae* which is under development for control of the pasture pest *Adoryphorus couloni* (Burmeister) (Coleoptera: Scarabaeidae) in Tasmania. Thus genotypes discovered in hot dry climates are more likely to be adapted to those climates.

A very high temperature optimum would however be undesirable because the risk of mammalian infection would cause great concern. Most isolates of *Metarhizium* spp. and *Beauveria* spp. show reduced or no growth at 37°C. It is not clear whether the hot- and cold-tolerant isolates obtained by Milner and Rath are stable for the temperature tolerance characteristic. This has been examined in other fungi and Burnett (1983) discussed warm-environmental and cool-environmental 'races' of *Helminthosporium maydis* (Nisikado), the cause of southern corn blight in the USA. These were not stable and adapted to the alternate regime if exposed for 6–7 generations. There is thus a distinction to be noted here between selecting an existing isolate with an ecological adaptation to the higher or lower end of the mesophile range (as in *H. maydis*) and an attempt to extend that range beyond its limits by culturing and selecting at very high temperatures. It is not clear if the latter is possible and Milner's high temperature isolate may represent the limits of what is available.

Isolates of *Metarhizium* spp. or *Beauveria* spp. with tolerance of low humidity do not seem to have been detected, but Drummond *et al.* (1987) detected ability to grow at unusually low humidities in an isolate of *Verticillium lecanii* (Zimmermann) Viégas from aphids, suggesting that this trait would be worth seeking in other entompathogens.

'New encounter' or 'old association'?

The successful use of natural enemies for biological control was pioneered by entomologists and initially concentrated on the use of parasitoids or phytophages from the centre of origin of an insect pest or weed to control the pest in an outbreak area from which the natural enemies were absent. This 'classical' approach has been extended recently to the use of pathogens, particularly rust fungi, for weed control but has very rarely been attempted with pathogens for insects – the baculovirus of *Oryctes* is an exception. In the 1980s there has been considerable debate about the relative merits of old association versus new encounter agents for classical biocontrol (Hokkanen & Pimentel, 1984; Waage, 1990). The old association agents are those that have co-evolved with the target. They thus tend to have a high specificity, but some have suggested that they also have a lower impact because they have reached an evolutionary equilibrium with the host. By contrast, new encounter agents may have a devastating impact but by their nature cannot be specific, because they must occur on at least one other host, the one on which they existed before the new encounter host arrived. There are not yet sufficient data to decide which of these two alternatives will provide the 'best' pathogen for development as a mycopesticide, but there are important implications in seeking a new encounter isolate.

The current research programme is concentrating on searches in the major breeding grounds of the desert locust, on the assumption that the most likely place to find isolates which combine virulence with host specificity is where the host is most constantly present. In the case of the desert locust the difference between old and new encounter pathogens is obscured by the locust's migratory habit, and it is likely that isolates might be obtained from anywhere within the plague area where breeding occurs. However, the greatest likelihood of finding locust-adapted isolates must still be in the areas where locusts occur most frequently.

There are acridid species in all hot, dry climates similar to the environments where the desert locust occurs, and in the New World there are many other species of *Schistocerca.* Since the range of hosts to which isolates of *Metarhizium* show virulence is usually wider than a single species, and often wider than a genus, it would be predictable that isolates with virulence to *S. gregaria* would be found both among New World *Schistocerca* spp. and among related orthopterans. While it is too early to draw conclusions, it is notable that all isolates of *Metarhizium* spp. which have shown high virulence to *S. gregaria* during the current work have originated from Orthoptera. These are listed in Table 1. It is also notable that not all isolates from orthopterans are virulent: a *M. anisopliae* isolate from an acridid in Pakistan and a *B. bassiana* isolate from *Zonocerus variegatus* in Benin were not virulent to *S. gregaria* using the standard bioassay.

To date, no examples have been found of non-orthopteran isolates of *Beauveria* spp. or *Metarhizium* spp. with high virulence to *S. gregaria.* However, Prior (1990) noted many examples from the literature where this was the case for other target insects (Table 2). Of particular interest is the routine use at the University of Bath of *M. anisopliae* isolate ME1 for studies on infection processes in several insects including *S. gregaria*: this isolate originated from the pecan weevil *Curculio caryae* (Horn) (Coleoptera: Curculionidae) in the USA (Dillon & Charnley, 1986), neither a host nor a country ever encountered by *S. gregaria.* This and other virulent isolates from non-hosts will be included in the current assays.

It would appear that a search among isolates from the target host and its relatives will reliably yield examples with high levels of virulence. The detection of high virulence in ARSEF 324 from *Patanga guttulosa* (Walker) is an example of a new encounter, albeit from a related host. The possibility that isolates from non-related hosts such as pecan weevil may

Table 1. Isolates of *Metarhizium* spp. tested against *Schistocerca gregaria.*

Isolate	Species*	Host	Country	% Mortality 5d	6d
ARSEF 324	*M. a.*	*Patanga guttulosa* (Walker) (as *Austracris guttulosa*) (Orthoptera: Acrididae)	Australia	88	88
IMI 330189	*M.f.*	*Ornithacris cavroisi* (Finot) (Orthoptera: Acrididae)	Niger	76	90
IMI 330189**	*M. f.*	*Ornithacris cavroisi*	Niger	81	96
IMI 324673	*M. f.*	*Zonocerus elegans* (Linnaeus) (Orthoptera: Pyrgomorphidae)	Tanzania	56	60
IMI 324673**	*M. f.*	*Zonocerus elegans*	Tanzania	32	72
IMI 168777ii	*M. a.*	*Schistocerca gregaria* (Forskål) (Othopera: Acrididae)	Ethiopia	48	56
IMI 152222	*M. a.*	*Myllocerus discolor* Boheman (Coleoptera: Curculionidae)	India	16	40
ARSEF 2023	*M. f.*	Unidentified acridid	Galapagos Is	8	40
IMI 298059	*M. a.*	*Scapanes australis* Boisduval (Coleoptera: Scarabaeidae)	Papua New Guinea		20
IMI 047038	*M. a.*	*Aeneolamia varia* (Fabricius) (as *A.* (*Tomaspis*) *saccharina* (Homoptera: Cercopidae)	Venezuela	0	4
IMI 298061	*M. a.*	*Brontispa longissima* (Gestro) (Coleoptera: Chrysomelidae)	Papua New Guinea	0	0
IIBC I90–574	*M. a.*	*Acrotylus humbertianus* Saussure (Orthoptera: Acrididae)	Pakistan	0	0

**M. a.* = *Metarhizium anisopliae* (Metschnikoff) Sorokin; *M. f.* = *M. flavoviride* W. Gams & J. Rozsypal.
**Single conidium isolates from original mass conidial cultures. ARSEF = Agricultural Research Service Entomopathogenic Fungus collection; IMI = International Mycological Institute;
IIBC = International Institute of Biological Control.

also be virulent indicates that the geographical and biological distribution of virulence is wider than the host and its near relatives.

There have been suggestions that virulence is associated with high levels of protease, particularly chymoelastase, produced by the appressorium during cuticle penetration and ME1 produces high levels of this enzyme (St Leger, 1990). This might mean that there are general virulence determinants as well as the currently unknown specific determinants of

Table 2. Some examples of virulence in isolates of *Metarhizium* spp. and *Beauveria* spp. from taxonomically, ecologically or geographically isolated hosts.*

Fungus	Target/location	Source/location of most pathogenic isolate
Beauveria bassiana (Balsamo) Vuillemin	*Hypothenemus hampei* (Ferrari) (Coleoptera: Scolytidae) **Colombia**	*Cossus cossus* (Linnaeus) (Lepidoptera: Cossidae) **Italy**
Beauveria bassiana	*Chalcodermus bimaculatus* Fiedler (Coleoptera: Curculionidae) **Brazil**	unidentified vespid (Hymenoptera: Vestpidae) **Brazil**
Beauveria bassiana	*Diuraphis noxia* (Mordvilko) (Homoptera: Aphididae) **USA** (introduced)	*Schizaphis graminum* (Rondani) (Homoptera: Aphididae) **USA** *'Boverin'* (unidentified source host) **USSR**
Metarhizium anisopliae (Metschnikoff) Sorokin	*Nasutitermes exitiosus* (Hill) (Isoptera: Termitidae) **Australia**	*Aeneolamia* sp. (Homoptera: Cercopidae) **Mexico**
M. anisopliae	*Diatraea saccharalis* (Fabricius) (Lepidoptera: Pyralidae) **Brazil**	*Zulia entreriana* (Berg) (Homoptera: Cercopidae) **Brazil**
M. anisopliae	*Culex pipiens* Linnaeus (Diptera: Culicidae)	many virulent isolates from Coleoptera, Lepidoptera and Homoptera hosts: none from target host
M. anisopliae	*Patanga guttulosa* (Walker) (as *Austracris guttulosa*) (Orthoptera: Acrididae) **Australia**	*Schistocerca gregaria* (Forskål) (Orthoptera: Acrididae) **Africa and Middle East**

*Examples drawn from published literature and the current IIBC/IITA/DFPV joint research programme. I am grateful to Dr J. Jimenez for permission to quote the unpublished example from *H. hampei.*

host range. There have been many attempts to correlate virulence with production of particular enzymes, especially those that assist cuticular penetration, and the results are well summarized by Heale *et al.* (1989): '... only a limited value can be assigned to any one cuticle-degrading enzyme trait amongst the many others which interact and summate in the expression of pathogenicity'. However, it would not be contradictory to claim that high production of an enzyme such as chymoelastase is a general virulence determinant (Charnley, these proceedings).

If this is eventually proved, a balance will then have to be struck between selecting strains which have good general pathogenicity determinants but are thereby relatively non host-specific, and strains which have very specific determinants and are thereby perhaps less virulent or attack too few hosts. At present, there is still insufficient evidence to use enzyme characteristics for isolate selection.

What is the true habitat of *Metarhizium* and *Beauveria* spp.?

Metarhizium spp. have been isolated from soil world-wide; *Beauveria* spp. have a similar very wide distribution, but are more frequently associated with insect remains (Domsch *et al.*, 1980). *B. bassiana* forms extensive rhizomorphs in unsterile soil in New Zealand (T.R. Glare, pers. comm.) and Germany (Keller & Zimmermann, 1989) and *M. anisopliae* does so in Australia (D. Holdom, pers. comm.); however, these would appear to be unusual cases. It is therefore not clear if these fungi genuinely flourish in soil, or whether they survive there in a dormant state awaiting a susceptible host.

Brady (1979) noted that *M. anisopliae* formed chlamydospores (asexual resting spores) but there are few references to their role in survival. The 'chlamydospores' of *M. anisopliae* from infected elaterid larvae illustrated by Zacharuk (1973) more closely resemble hyphal bodies (H.C. Evans, pers. comm.). Many experiments have been carried out on the survival of conidia in soil, and physical and chemical soil characteristics have a major influence. Conidia of *M. anisopliae* can survive at least two years in some soils (Keller & Zimmerman, 1989). *Metarhizium* spp. and *Beauveria* spp. can both be recovered from the soil either by direct plating on selective media or by baiting (Zimmermann, 1986). At present it is not clear whether what is being recovered are conidia, chlamydospores, mycelia surviving on fragments of chitin, or mycelia living on non-insect substrates.

Zimmermann (1986) used *Galleria mellonella* (Linnaeus) (Lepidoptera: Pyralidae) larvae to bait from moist soil. This insect is very susceptible to pathogens, probably because of its unusually sheltered normal habitat in beehives where fungal pathogens such as *Metarhizium* spp. do not develop. However, this may mean that isolates obtained on *G. mellonella* from soil have a low virulence to other insects. It may be more appropriate to use acridids to bait entompathogenic fungi from soil. There are no published protocols for this technique, but it is under test at present.

There is no specific information available on the relative virulence of isolates of fungi such as *Metarhizium* spp. from soil and from insects. The great majority of isolates available and used in assays are from insects, but this mainly reflects the interests of collectors. A similar situation occurs with *Bacillus thuringiensis* Berliner: this too is widely distributed in the soil but rare on insects, and many soil isolates are non-pathogenic. It may be that there are two diverse sets of selection pressures on the common entomopathogenic fungi such as *Metarhizium* spp. and *Beauveria* spp., one for optimum characteristics for soil survival and another for virulence to insects. If so, it is unlikely that the same characteristics will be optimum for both habitats.

Characterization – how much must be known?

The need for characterization at the sub-specific level

The search for superior genotypes for exploitation as biological pesticides will be a continuing process, but development can usually proceed meanwhile using the best that are available. As soon as a formulation is shown to be effective under laboratory conditions, field testing will be required. Field tests are essential to demonstrate efficacy, and also to show that the formulation is not harmful to the environment. In order to monitor the effect of a biopesticide treatment on the environment, methods must be available to detect and recover the pathogen after the treatment is applied. In the case of *Metarhizium* spp., this is complicated by the fact that, since *Metarhizium* spp. are distributed world-wide, the species will be native to the environment where the test is carried out and the test isolate must therefore be distinguished from the resident population before its effects can be clarified. There is therefore a need for methods which can distinguish genotypes at the sub-specific level. The safety and quarantine aspects of field testing of exotic isolates are dealt with in the following section.

The terms for defining variation in fungi below the species level are confusing, largely because some terms describe physiological or other phenotypic variants, and others describe the underlying differences in the genotype. Brasier & Rayner (1987) listed five disciplines, morphology, genetics, taxonomy, ecology and pathology, in which more than forty terms for variation within a species are used. The terms that commonly occur in insect pathology are variety, strain, isolate, race and pathotype.

Varieties are the only sub-specific groups that are distinguishable on morphological grounds and they may also have a distinctive host range. There are two varieties of *Metarhizium anisopliae*, *M. a.* var. *majus* (Johnston) Tulloch (conidia (9.0) 10.0–14.0 (18.0) μm long) which is confined mainly to scarabaeids, and *M. a.* var. *anisopliae* Tulloch (conidia (3.5) 5.0–8.0 (9.0) μm long with a wide host range (Tulloch, 1976). There is strong evidence that var. *majus* is diploid (Heale, 1988). *M. flavoviride* exists as *M. f.* var. *flavoviride* W. Gams & J. Rozsypal (conidia (7.0) 8.0–9.0 (11.0) μm long and *M. f.* var. *minus* Rombach, Humber & Roberts (conidia (4.0) 4.5–5.5 (6.5) μm long (Rombach *et al.*, 1986).

The term 'strain' is used by morphologists, geneticists, ecologists and pathologists, in each case with different implications (Brasier & Rayner, 1987). A strain is derived from an isolate and should be distinguishable from other strains on morphological, biochemical or pathological criteria.

Strain is a confusing term because it is defined in several ways based on different criteria for this separation and it has not been used in this paper. If attempts have been made to ensure genetic homogeneity of a culture by deriving it from a single uninucleate spore then it will normally be referred to as a strain, but in the context of insect pathology, at least for fungal pathogens, it seems safest to refer to individual fungal cultures as isolates and this is the only valid definition for initial isolations of mixed genotypes.

The feature of a pathogen that most interests insect pathologists is the possession of a unique genotype that controls virulence to a unique range of hosts. This is expressed phenotypically as a specific host range, and defines the pathotype. If there is a differential reaction between a pathotype and defined genotypes of a single host, the pathotype is the equivalent of a race in plant pathology. Unfortunately, to define a pathotype or a race rigorously requires sufficient host challenges to establish their uniqueness from all other pathotypes or races, and this is usually impractical. There is therefore much interest in the biochemical and physiological reactions of an isolate which might correlate with its host range, so that a pathotype might be defined without the need to carry out inoculations on a wide range of hosts.

In environmental studies it may be necessary to distinguish one isolate of a variety, such as *M. anisopliae* var. *anisopliae*, from other isolates of the same variety indigenous to the test area, and this cannot be done by morphology. In order to 'fingerprint' an isolate below the variety level, biochemical, physiological and genetic methods must be used.

Biochemical methods and DNA analysis for characterization

There have been several studies on variation within the species *Beauveria bassiana* using isoenzyme analysis and physiological tests, and the genus *Beauveria* was examined using similar tests to supplement differential morphological characteristics (Mugnai *et al.*, 1989). By comparing variation in isoenzyme profiles, reactions to the APIZYM test system and reactions to a wide range of nutritional and dye-based tests, a profile for each isolate can be built up. Esterases are one of the most useful isoenzymes for this purpose. Mugnai *et al.* (1989) found that *B. bassiana* was an extremely heterogeneous species but that more homogeneous groups of isolates occurred, including both those from one geographical area and those from one insect order. Bridge *et al.* (1990) examined 16 isolates of this species from a single host, the coffee berry borer *Hypothenemus hampei* (Ferrari) (Coleoptera; Scolytidae), with a pan-tropical distribution and found that there was much less variation in characteristics such as esterase bands than in the species as a whole.

By contrast, a population of 23 isolates of *B. bassiana* from the mirid *Adelphocoris lineolatus* (Goeze) in northern Italy was much more variable with respect to esterase bands, and more variable than a population of 8 French isolates examined in the same study (Riba *et al.*, 1986b). Variability in α-esterases was also used by Poprawski *et al.* (1988) to show that isolates of *B. bassiana* from the weevils *Sitona* spp. (Coleoptera: Curculionidae) were much more heterogeneous in populations from southern France than from northern France and England. Since only esterase bands were compared in these studies, it is not known if the more esterase-variable populations were also more variable in other characteristics.

A study on 96 isolates of *M. anisopliae* var. *anisopliae* and var. *majus* by Riba *et al.* (1986a) showed very similar results to that by Mugnai *et al.* (1989) on *B. bassiana.* The var. *majus* isolates were homogeneous for isoenzyme profiles but the var. *anisopliae* isolates were very heterogeneous, with more homogeneous groupings of isolates from single geographical areas or related insect hosts.

Recently DNA analysis has been used to examine genotype variability in *M. anisopliae*; Milner (1990) has shown that three native isolates of *M. anisopliae* with virulence to larvae of three scarabaeid pests of sugarcane in Australia are genetically distinct and Pipe & Heale (1990) have developed an rDNA probe from *Saccharomyces cerevisiae* Meyer ex Hansen that can detect polymorphisms in nuclear DNA of *M. anisopliae.*

Evidence for and against sub-specific populations in *Metarhizium* and *Beauveria*

There is thus evidence that within the highly heterogeneous species *M. anisopliae* and *B. bassiana* there exist groups of distinct genotypes, indistinguishable morphologically, which have narrower host range and narrower dispersal than the species as a whole. This is borne out by a large number of studies on virulence of isolates, where it has been shown many times that individual isolates have a much narrower host range than the species as a whole. To give only one example, Samuels *et al.* (1989) tested a range of isolates of *Metarhizium anisopliae* against the rice delphacid *Nilaparvata lugens* (Stål) and found that the LT_{50} ranged from five to fourteen days and that isolates from *N. lugens* itself showed an LT_{50} range of 5–11 days.

However, as already mentioned above, there are many examples where a virulent isolate originated from a host other than the target, and sometimes in a geographical area where the target does not occur (Table 2). The data of Samuels *et al.* (1989) also show that the issue of genetic adaptation is very complex, because the most virulent isolate from a host other than *N. lugens* was more virulent than the least virulent isolate from *N. lugens* itself. While the evidence certainly suggests that host-adapted genotypes and geographically distinct populations exist in *Metarhizium* spp. and *Beauveria* spp., it is also possible for new encounter genotypes to show a high degree of virulence (Prior, 1990).

Release – what are the risks?

Political and biological divisions within the environment

If the isolate used for field testing and ultimately for control is exotic to the country concerned, the quarantine authorities may wish to approve its use. It would clearly be ridiculous in biological terms to restrict the entry of an isolate of *M. anisopliae* into a country purely on the grounds that it originated in a neighbouring country if there are no ecological barriers between the two, because political boundaries defining countries are often of very recent origin and have no biological significance. The Sahel ecological zone, for example, extends unbroken across northern Africa and encompasses parts of Senegal, Mauritania, Mali, Burkina Faso, Niger, Chad, Sudan and Ethiopia. Desert locusts and many other organisms are distributed throughout this zone. When the isolate originates from outside the ecological zone in which release is contemplated however, quarantine requires more careful consideration.

The scientific basis for evaluation of the risks of release of exotic isolates

Prior (1990) discussed the scientific basis for regulating the release of naturally occurring (as opposed to recombinant) exotic isolates of entomopathogenic fungi, and noted that they posed three possible hazards: toxicity, allergenicity and direct infection of non-target organisms. The first two hazards are not unique to micro-organisms and are already covered by existing safety legislation, but infection of non-target organisms was a special issue because of the unique self-reproducing properties of biological as opposed to chemical pesticides. Prior (1990) noted that there were three questions to be answered concerning the potential hazard to non-target organisms:

1. Does the isolate show specificity at normal inoculum levels?
There is no information on the spore dose which insects receive during natural infection in the field. Under non-epizootic conditions insects would

usually be challenged by very low doses of conidia, but the dose may increase by several orders of magnitude during an epizootic in a dense insect population when conditions are suitable for sporulation. The concern is about specificity of an introduced isolate at normal inoculum levels; although the 'normal' level is difficult to define it must be assumed to be equivalent to the levels of native isolates. Therefore the issue is whether the introduced isolate poses a hazard not already posed by the native ones. Prior (1990) noted that the genes for pathogenicity (equivalent to virulence) are not closely associated with specific genes in the target pest, as is the case of gene-for-gene relationships in some plant pathogens, but seem to be widely distributed and may even occur outside the geographical or ecological range of the host itself. If this is so there cannot therefore be any additional risk in releasing what is already present. The exact extent of genotype range and diversity can only be determined by biochemical and DNA analysis on a comprehensive sample of isolates.

2. Is specificity retained at high levels of inoculum?
The concern here is that the natural specificity of the isolate may be lost when very high levels of inoculum are applied as a biopesticide for pest control. There is little evidence on this subject, but in one study on the field application of *Beauveria brongniartii* (Saccardo) Petch to control the European cockchafer *Melolontha melolontha* (Linnaeus) (Coleoptera: Scarabaeidae), Baltensweiler & Cerutti (1986) found no infection in non-target arthropods.

3. Is specificity a stable trait after release?
This is the most complex question. Stability implies that the isolate genotype will not change after release and therefore its host range and physiological requirements will remain constant. The principal fear is that if an exotic genotype did change after release it could thereby pose a threat to non-target organisms. There are only two ways that this could happen: mutation, or genetic recombination. The first can be dismissed very simply on two grounds: firstly, most mutations are deleterious and do not survive, and secondly there is no basis for assuming that a mutation is any more likely to arise in an introduced genotype than in the native genotypes which are vastly more abundant. However, the issue of recombination requires more careful examination.

Sexual reproduction has never been observed in *Metarhizium* spp. and *Beauveria* spp. and they are therefore classified in the Deuteromycotina. However, recombination without meiosis can occur in fungi through the parasexual cycle and this has been recorded several times for *M. anisopliae* (Heale, 1988) and recently for *B. bassiana* (Paccola-Meirelles & Azevedo, 1991). Thus the frequency with which parasexual recombination in these fungi may occur in nature is very important in determining their stability.

In the parasexual cycle, the monokaryotic mycelia of two different genotypes fuse and the nuclei are exchanged so that the mycelium becomes dikaryotic. The dissimilar nuclei then fuse to give a diploid nucleus. Exchange of genes between the two genotypes occurs in the diploid nucleus to give chromosomes with new gene combinations. This is followed by a process of haploidization in which there is a progressive loss of chromosomes so that the haploid number is restored, but the genotype has changed (Heale, 1988; Clarkson, these proceedings).

In *M. anisopliae* (Riba *et al.*, 1985) parasexual recombinants were forced in the laboratory between var. *majus* and var. *anisopliae*, and between two auxotrophic mutants derived from a single isolate of var. *anisopliae* virulent to *Ostrinia nubilalis* (Hübner) (Lepidoptera: Pyralidae). The segregants from the cross between the two varieties were non-virulent; some of the segregants from the cross between the two mutants showed reduced virulence and some were as virulent as the parent.

These crosses made by Riba *et al.* (1985) were forced between two mutants derived from a single parent, that is, a single genotype. If a cross is to occur between two different genotypes then these must be compatible. There is in fact much evidence that incompatibility mechanisms exist in many fungi to prevent crossing. Some isolates of *B. bassiana* studied by Paccola-Meirelles & Azevedo (1991) would not form heterokaryons, possibly because of incompatibility mechanisms. These are widespread in several intensively studied fungi and one, *Aspergillus flavus* Link ex Fries, is of particular interest because it is both a plant and insect pathogen. Numerous vegetative incompatibility groups occur in *A. flavus* and these prevent the exchange of genes. In discussing this phenomenon, Wicklow (1990) notes that: 'Asexual genetic exchange under field conditions has not been reported for *A. flavus*, or any other fungus, but is probably limited to members of the same incompatibility group.'

At present there does not seem to be any information about the existence of incompatibility groups in *Metarhizium* spp., but it would be surprising if they did not occur.

Caten (1987) had previously used similar arguments to Wicklow's (1990) to suggest that variation in fungi is not as widespread or as important for survival and evolutionary success as previously thought, and the role of the parasexual cycle in nature may have been overemphasized. Evans (1988) argued that entomopathogenic fungi such as *Metarhizium* spp. had sacrificed their teleomorphs (sexual state), and the chance of variation by sexual recombination, for the advantage of rapid and massive asexual conidial production. They did this in order to exploit ephemeral energy sources, especially the periodic population explosions of insects occurring in disturbed habitats. While parasexuality would provide the major mechanism for instability in asexual fungi, there appear to be good reasons for thinking that it is unlikely to lead to new and undesirable genetic combinations under field conditions.

The apparent absence of the teleomorph in *Metarhizium* spp. and *Beauveria* spp. deserves comment. Teleomorphs have never been detected during more than a hundred years of study in a wide range of environments. However, new teleomorph-anamorph connections are continually being established, even in fungi that are even more familiar than the common entomopathogenic deuteromycetes. The discovery of *Didymella fabae* (Jellis & Punithalingam), the teleomorph of *Ascochyta fabae* Spegazzini, which causes leaf and stem blight of faba beans, was only announced this year (Jellis & Punithalingam, 1991): this is one of the most studied of temperate pathogens of a major crop. It is often the case that fungal teleomorphs are produced in the natural environment under the influence of specific environmental and nutritional conditions, and they may therefore be transient, or rare. Such conditions are not met in artificial culture which is where the great majority of studies are carried out. Despite the continuing absence of teleomorphs for *Metarhizium* spp. and *Beauveria* spp., the possibility of their existence should not be totally discounted. It should be noted that although the teleomorph of *B. bassiana* is not known, Booth (1961) described a *Beauveria* anamorph of the Pyrenomycete *Pseudeurotium bakeri* C. Booth; in the published description it differs from *B. bassiana* principally in having conidia which are twice as large (4 µm d.).

Discussion

The alternative options for seeking microbial control agents were summarized succinctly by Pusey (1990) in the context of microbial antagonists for plant disease control. The search should always begin with the resident antagonists because these will be adapted to survive in the environment where control must be achieved. However, micro-organisms from other environments may also have good potential activity, but may be prevented from operating because of environmental constraints. These constraints may be overcome by formulation.

In the search for the best isolates for locust and grasshopper control, it may also be the case that potentially valuable isolates occur outside the environment where control must be achieved. Thus, following Pusey's (1990) guidelines, a comprehensive search should seek virulent isolates from the target, other isolates from the target which lack virulence but which may be improved by formulation, and, in addition, isolates from other hosts and regions. This includes almost all isolates that might be found, but the possibility of overlooking isolates which could be improved by formulation may be excluded by carrying out the screening using the formulation itself. Even so, the range of potentially valuable material from target and non-target hosts that remains to be screened is enormous. The policy that is being followed in the current programme is therefore to screen as wide a range of isolates as possible, but with particular emphasis on two categories: those from orthopteran hosts and those from hot, dry environments to obtain isolates with tolerance for high temperatures.

A principle that is often advocated in the search for microbial antagonists for plant pathogens is to search in areas where the problem would be expected to be serious, but is not. This is particularly clear in the case of 'suppressive' or 'pernicious' soils where plant diseases, insect pests or nematodes do not develop. The cause of the suppression is often antagonistic micro-organisms which gradually increase to high population levels if the host organism is present over several years. Thus suppression occurs either in undisturbed soils such as pastures, or in fields where the same crop is repeatedly cultivated. A case of suppression of insects was recorded by Ko *et al.* (1982) where the 'perniciousness' of an Hawaiian soil to termites was associated with the presence of two entomopathogenic fungi. It is more difficult to identify examples of soils which might be pernicious to locusts and grasshoppers because of their high mobility. However, the soil is likely to be the primary source of inoculum for occasional epizootics of *Metarhizium* spp. such as that recorded on desert locusts by Balfour-Browne (1960) and the regular outbreaks of *Entomophaga grylli* (Fresenius) Batko on *Zonocerus variegatus* noted by Chapman & Page (1979). Screening of soils from habitats frequented by target species would therefore probably be worthwhile.

Characteristics that are desirable in the chosen isolates include high virulence expressed as rapid kill and/or cessation of feeding, thermotolerance, high sporulation capacity and compatibility with the chosen spray diluent. It would also be useful to search for additional characteristics such as tolerance to ultra-violet light and efficient substrate utilization. Many of these desired characteristics are automatically selected during the assays. These are carried out at low humidity, high temperature and in the chosen formulation, in order to reproduce closely the field environment, and the isolate selected for development has performed successfully in preliminary field trials.

Pusey (1990) noted that it may be unrealistic to search for a single 'magic bullet' isolate. The range of desirable characteristics is very wide and very unlikely to occur in a single isolate. There may be some advantage in combining several different virulent isolates in a single formulation, thus widening the range of virulence determinants available to challenge the host. Synergy between isolates would be advantageous both in increasing virulence and in broadening the host range when several pest species must be controlled.

Host specificity is clearly a complex issue. Adhesion may play a role but in the case of the current work on bioassays, the mechanical aspects of adhesion are at least partly overcome by applying the conidia directly in the formulation, in which they adhere closely to the cuticle. None the less, the assays clearly demonstrate large differences in virulence, with the majority of isolates tested showing no virulence to *S. gregaria.*

The genotypes for virulence would in fact appear to be widely dispersed. It is also possible that virulence is controlled by two types of genes, those for host specificity, which restrict virulence to certain hosts, and those for general virulence which control the overall level of virulence within the whole host range. The protease *pr1* gene in *M. anisopliae* currently under study in several laboratories may be an example of one such general virulence determinant. Evidence for the existence of genes for general virulence also comes from the studies by Riba *et al.* (1982) which showed that certain isolates of *B. bassiana* were more virulent to all 'races' of *Bombyx mori* (Linnaeus) (Lepidoptera: Bombycidae) than others; presumably these isolates may have had more active genes for general virulence. Probably only extensive DNA 'fingerprinting' studies on natural populations will clarify the distribution of genotypes.

The genetic control of virulence is not yet sufficiently understood to state whether the genes for virulence are universally distributed or whether they have a more limited geographical distribution. The widespread presence of new encounter isolates would suggest the former. The hazards that might arise from movement of isolates into new areas are already identified (Prior, 1990) and are discussed further here. It would appear, from the relative ease with which new encounter virulence can be demonstrated, that genes for virulence to any specific host are already dispersed beyond the current range of that host. There does not therefore appear to be any scientific basis for restrictions on movement of genotypes from one biogeographical region to another. A satisfactory quarantine protocol for pathogen acceptance can only be based on the known biological facts and these do not suggest any reason for concern over the movement of isolates of *Metarhizium* spp. and *Beauveria* spp.

The use of pathogens for pest control could remove many of the major problems associated with chemical pesticide use, especially environmental pollution and toxicity to non-target organisms. Despite this, there exists a barrier to acceptance of pathogens that was defined by Freeman (1981) as 'pathophobia'. This irrational fear still exists and fuels ever-increasing demands for host range and safety tests (Evans & Ellison, 1990). The fear of pathogens is due largely to ignorance of their biology. Much remains to be done in convincing administrators and environmental pressure groups that the use of pathogens for pest control provides a safe alternative to chemicals. This can only be achieved by presenting a case based on an adequate basis of facts. The current research programme on locust and grasshopper control provides an excellent opportunity to gather those facts.

References

Anon. (1990) *Special Report: a Plague of Locusts.* Congress of the United States Office of Technology Assessment, Washington DC, USA, 129 pp.

Balfour-Browne, F.L. (1960) The green muscardine disease of insects, with special reference to an epidemic in a swarm of locusts in Eritrea. *Proceedings of the Royal Entomological Society of London* (A) **35**, 656–674.

Baltensweiler, W. & Cerutti, F. (1986) Bericht über die Nebenwirkungen einer Bekämpfung des Maikäfers (*Melolontha melolontha* L.) mit dem Pilz *Beauveria brongniartii* (Sacc.) Petch auf die Arthropodenfauna des Waldrandes. *Mitteilungen der Schweizerischen Entomologischen Gesellschaft* **59**, 267–274.

Bartlett, M.C. & Jaronski, S.T. (1988) Mass production of entomogenous fungi for biological control of insects. In: Burge, M.N. (ed.), *Fungi in Biological Control Systems.* Manchester University Press, Manchester, pp. 61–85.

Booth, C. (1961) Studies of Pyrenomycetes: VI. *Mycological Papers,* **83**, 15 pp.

Brader, L. (1988) Control of grasshoppers and migratory locusts. *Brighton Crop Protection Conference: Pests and Diseases* **1988**, pp. 283–288.

Brady, B.L.K. (1979) *Metarhizium anisopliae.* IMI descriptions of pathogenic fungi and bacteria no. 609. CAB, Farnham Royal, U.K.

Brasier, C.M. & Rayner, A.D.M. (1987) Whither terminology below the species level in fungi? In: Rayner, A.D.M., Brasier, C.M. & Moore, D. (eds), *Evolutionary Biology of the Fungi.* Cambridge University Press, Cambridge, pp. 379–388.

Bridge, P.D., Abraham, Y.J., Cornish, M.C., Prior, C. & Moore, D. (1990) The chemotaxonomy of *Beauveria bassiana* (Deuteromycotina: Hyphomycetes) isolates from the coffee berry borer *Hypothenemus hampei* (Coleoptera: Scolytidae). *Mycopathologia* **111**, 85–90.

Caten, C.E. (1987) Genetic integration of fungal life styles. In: Rayner, A.D.M., Brasier, C.M. & Moore, D. (eds), *Evolutionary Biology of the Fungi.* Cambridge University Press, pp. 215–229.

Chapman, R.F. & Page, W.W. (1979) Factors affecting the mortality of the grasshopper, *Zonocerus variegatus,* in southern Nigeria. *Journal of Animal Ecology* **48**, 271–288.

Dillon, R.J. & Charnley, A.K. (1986) Inhibition of *Metarhizium anisopliae* by the gut bacterial flora of the desert locust *Schistocerca gregaria*: evidence for an anti-fungal toxin. *Journal of Invertebrate Pathology* **47**, 350–360.

Domsch, K.H., Gams, W. & Anderson, T-H. (1980) *Compendium of Soil Fungi Vol. 1.* Academic Press, London, 859 pp.

Drummond, J., Heale, J.B. & Gillespie, A.T. (1987) Germination and the effect of reduced humidity on the expression of pathogenicity in *Verticillium lecanii* against the glasshouse whitefly *Trialeurodes vaporariorium. Annals of Applied Biology* **111**, 193–201.

Evans, H.C. (1988) Coevolution of entomogenous fungi and their insect hosts. In: Pirozynski, K.A. & Hawksworth, D.L. (eds), *Coevolution of Fungi with Plants and Animals.* Academic Press, London, pp. 149–171.

Evans, H.C. & Ellison, C.A. (1990) Classical biological control of weeds with micro-organisms: past, present, prospects. *Aspects of Applied Biology* **24**, 39–49.

Freeman, T.E. (1981) Use of conidial fungi in biological control. In: Cole, G.T. &

Kendrick, B. (eds), *Biology of Conidial Fungi vol. 2.* Academic Press, Inc., London, pp. 143–165.

Greathead, D.J. & Prior, C. (1990) The regulation of pathogens for biological control, with special reference to locust control. In: Somme, L. and Bie, S.W. (eds) *Proceedings of the Workshop on Health and Environmental Impact of Alternative Control Agents for Desert Locust Control. Oslo, 14–17 January, 1990. NORAGRIC Occasional Paper Series C: Development and the Environment,* **no. 5**, 67–80.

Heale, J.B. (1988) The potential impact of fungal genetics and molecular biology on biological control, with particular reference to entomopathogens. In: Burge, M.N. (ed.), *Fungi in Biological Control Systems.* Manchester University Press, Manchester, pp. 211–234.

Heale, J.B., Isaac, J.E. and Chandler, D. (1989) Prospects for strain improvement in entomopathogenic fungi. *Pesticide Science* **26**, 79–92.

Hokkanen, H. & Pimentel, D. (1984) New approach for selecting biological control agents. *Canadian Entomologist* **116**, 1109–1121.

Jellis, G.J. & Punithalingam, E. (1991) Discovery of *Didymella fabae* sp. nov., the teleomorph of *Asochyta fabae,* on faba bean straw. *Plant Pathology* **40**, 150–157.

Keller, S. & Zimmerman, G. (1989) Mycopathogens of soil insects. In: Wilding, N., Collins, N.M., Hammond, P.M. & Webber, J.F. (eds), *Insect-Fungus Interactions.* Academic Press, London, pp. 239–270.

Ko. W.J., Fuji, J.K. & Kanegawa, K.M. (1982) The nature of soil pernicious to *Coptotermes formosanus. Journal of Invertebrate Pathology* **39**, 38–40.

McCoy, C.W., Samson, R.A. & Boucias, D.G. (1988) Entomogenous fungi. In: Ignoffo, C.M. & Bhushan Mandava, N. (eds), *Handbook of Natural Pesticides Vol. 5: Microbial Insecticides Part A, Entomogenous Protozoa and Fungi.* CRC Press, USA, pp. 151–236.

Milner, R.J. (1989) Recent progress with *Metarhizium anisopliae* for pest control in Australia. In: *Proceedings of the First Asia/Pacific Conference on Entomology,* Chiang Mai November 1989.

Milner, R.J. (1990) The selection of strains of *Metarhizium anisopliae* for control of Australian sugar cane white grubs. In: *Proceedings and Abstracts of the Fifth International Colloquium on Invertebrate Pathology and Microbial Control,* Adelaide 20–24 August, 1990, p. 333.

Mugnai, L., Bridge, P.D. & Evans, H.C. (1989) A chemotaxonomic evaluation of the genus *Beauveria. Mycological Research* **92**, 199–209.

Paccola-Meirelles, L.D. & Azevedo, J.L. (1991) Parasexuality in *Beauveria bassiana. Journal of Invertebrate Pathology* **57**, 172–176.

Pipe, N.D. & Heale, J.B. (1990) DNA RFLP (restriction fragment length polymorphism) analysis and strain improvement of the entomopathogen *Metarhizium anisopliae.* In: *Proceedings and Abstracts of the Fifth International Colloquium on Invertebrate Pathology and Microbial Control,* Adelaide 20–24 August 1990, p. 471.

Poprawksi, T.J., Riba, G., Jones, H.A. & Aioun, A. (1988) Variations in isoesterase profiles of geographical populations of *Beauveria bassiana* (Deuteromycotina: Hyphomycetes) isolated from sitona weevils (Coleoptera: Curculionidae). *Environmental Entomology* **17**, 275–279.

Prior, C. (1990) The biological basis for regulating the release of micro-organisms, with particular reference to the use of fungi for pest control. *Aspects of Applied Biology* **24**, 231–238.

Prior, C. & Greathead, D.J. (1989) Biological control of locusts: the potential for the exploitation of pathogens. *FAO Plant Protection Bulletin* **37**, 37–48.

Pusey, P.L. (1990) Control of pathogens on aerial plant surfaces with antagonistic microorganisms. *Biological and Cultural Tests* **5**, v–vii.

Rath, A.C., Koen, T.B., Worladge, D. & Anderson, G.C. (1990) Control of the subterranean pasture pest *Adoryphorus couloni* (Coleoptera: Scarabaeidae) with *Metarhizium anisopliae* isolate DAT F-001. Abstract in: *Proceedings and Abstracts of the Fifth International Colloquium on Invertebrate Pathology and Microbial Control*, Adelaide, 20–24 August 1990, p. 335.

Riba, G., Katagiri, K. & Kawakami, K. (1982) Preliminary studies on the susceptibility of the silk-worm *Bombyx mori* (Lepidoptera: Bombycidae) to some entomogenous hyphomycetes. *Applied Entomology and Zoology* **17**, 238–243.

Riba, G., Azevedo, J.L., Messias, C., Dias da Silveira, W. & Tuveson, R. (1985) Studies of the inheritance of virulence in the entomopathogenic fungus *Metarhizium anisopliae. Journal of Invertebrate Pathology* **46**, 20–25.

Riba, G., Bouvier-Fourcade, I & Caudal, A. (1986a) Isoenzyme polymorphism in *Metarhizium anisopliae* (Deuteromycotina: Hyphomycetes) entomogenous fungi. *Mycopathologia* **96**, 161–169.

Riba, G., Poprawski, T.J. & Maniania, J. (1986b) Isoesterase variability among geographical populations of *Beauveria bassiana* (Fungi Imperfecti) isolated from Miridae. In: Samson, R.A., Vlak, J.M. & Peters, D. (eds), *Fundamental and Applied Aspects of Invertebrate Pathology.* Foundation of the Fourth International Colloquium of Invertebrate Pathology 1986, Wageningen, The Netherlands, pp. 205–209.

Rombach, M.C., Humber, R.A. & Roberts, D.W. (1986) *Metarhizium flavoviride* var. *minus*, var. nov., a pathogen of plant and leaf hoppers on rice in the Philippines and Solomon Islands. *Mycotaxon* **27**, 87–92.

Samuels, K.D.Z., Heale, J.B. & Llewellyn, M. (1989) Characteristics relating to the pathogenicity of *Metarhizium anisopliae* to *Nilaparvata lugens. Journal of Invertebrate Pathology* **53**, 25–31.

St Leger, R.J. (1990) The role of cuticle-degrading enzymes in fungal pathogenesis of insects. In: *Proceedings and Abstracts of the Fifth International Colloquium on Invertebrate Pathology and Microbial Control*, Adelaide, 20–24 August 1990, pp. 308–312.

Steedman, A. (1990) *The Locust Handbook.* Natural Resources Institute, Chatham, UK.

Talboys, P.W., Garrett, C.M.E., Ainsworth, G.C., Pegg, G.F. & Wallace, E.R. (1973) A guide to the use of terms in plant pathology. *Phytopathological Papers* **no. 17**, 55 pp.

Thomas, K.C., Khachatourians, G.G. & Ingledew, W.M. (1987) Production and properties of *Beauveria bassiana* conidia in submerged culture. *Canadian Journal of Microbiology* **33**, 12–20.

Tulloch, M. (1976) The genus *Metarhizium. Transactions of the British Mycological Society* **66**, 407–411.

van Winkelhoff, A.J. & McCoy, C.W. (1984) Conidiation of *Hirsutella thompsonii* var. *synnematosa* in submerged culture. *Journal of Invertebrate Pathology* **43**, 59–68.

Waage, J. (1990) Ecological theory and the selection of biological control agents. In: Mackauer, M., Ehler, L.E. & Roland, J. (eds), *Critical Issues in Biological Control.* Intercept Ltd, UK, pp. 135–157.

Wicklow, D.T. (1990) Adaptation in *Aspergillus flavus. Transactions of the Mycological Society of Japan* **31**, 511–523.

Zacharuk, R.Y. (1973). Electron-microscope studies of the histopathology of fungal infections by *Metarhizium anisopliae. Miscellaneous Publications of the Entomological Society of America* **9**, 112–119.

Zimmermann, G. (1986). The 'Galleria bait method' for detection of entompathogenic fungi in soil. *Journal of Applied Entomology* **102**, 213–215.

Mechanisms of fungal pathogenesis in insects with particular reference to locusts

A.K. Charnley

School of Biological Sciences, University of Bath.

Abstract

Control of appressorium formation may be related to host specificity among isolates of *Metarhizium anisopliae* (Metschnikoff) Sorokin. The cuticle-degrading endoprotease PR1 has an important role in host invasion. Variation in enzyme charge, and thus ability to bind to and degrade different insect cuticles, may influence isolate virulence. When fungal chitinase is slow to appear, cuticle-chitin may present a significant barrier to host penetration. Thus acylurea insecticides, which act by interfering with chitin synthesis in insects, can act synergistically with insect fungal pathogens. Antifungal phenols contribute to the gut barrier to infection in the desert locust and possibly other Orthoptera. Formulation of fungal conidia to reduce the effectiveness of the phenols may promote infection through the gut. The blood-borne cellular defences of an insect are often ineffective against virulent fungal pathogens. Secondary metabolites like the cyclic peptide destruxins produced by *M. anisopliae* may be responsible in part. Causes of death are probably complex and have not been defined adequately for any mycosis. Secondary metabolites, like destruxins, are clearly implicated in some cases. Timing and titre of production of such compounds may be amenable to selection and/or manipulation.

Introduction

It is clear from other papers in this volume that fungal pathogens of locusts and grasshoppers hold out particular promise as alternatives to chemical insecticides. Strain selection and improvement, based on a knowledge of the mechanisms of fungal pathogenesis, will be necessary to optimize the killing power of such mycoinsecticides (see Clarkson, these proceedings). The physiological and biochemical interactions between locusts and their fungal pathogens have not been studied in detail. However, because of their large size desert locusts, *Schistocerca gregaria* (Forskål), have been used in a number of model studies on insect–fungus relationships. In this brief review I will bring together what we know about the processes of invasion, host response and cause of death for deuteromycete infections in insects and, where possible, highlight *Metarhizium anisopliae* (Metschnikoff) Sorokin/*S. gregaria* interactions.

Invasion

Fungi alone among insect pathogens actively invade through the exoskeleton (cuticle). In most, but not all, cases conidia of mycopathogens attach indiscriminately to host and nonhost cuticle (Boucias & Pendland, 1991). However, for successful invasion subsequent prepenetration behaviour must be adapted to the nature of the cuticle surface. For example cuticle hardness and nutrient availability appear to govern the differentiation of infection structures (appressoria) by *M. anisopliae.* St Leger *et al.* (in press) found that strains of *M. anisopliae* isolated from Homoptera, whose cuticle surface is contaminated with high levels of sugars derived from honey dew (excreta), produce appressoria under high nutrient regimes. Conversely Coleoptera-derived isolates were adapted to a low nutrient environment, such as probably pertains on the surface of the hard, thick cuticle of their hosts. Not enough acridid isolates have been examined in this regard, however, to draw any conclusions about adapted host recognition mechanisms.

Variations in pathogenicity can be a function of a pathogen's ability to penetrate host cuticle (Vey *et al.*, 1982). The chemical complexity and resilience of the outer region of the cuticle (the epicuticle) may make it of particular importance in deterring non-pathogenic fungi; it is not known how invading fungi breach the epicuticle. Ultrastructural evidence suggests that both enzymic hydrolysis and mechanical deformation are involved. Lipoprotein lipases secreted in culture by *Metarhizium anisopliae* could perhaps combine with endoprotease PR1 (see later) to aid penetration of the inner region of the epicuticle (polymerized lipoprotein) (Charnley, 1989).

The main body of the cuticle, the procuticle, comprises primarily chitin fibrils embedded in a protein matrix, together with lipids and quinones. The mechanical properties of the different cuticles depend on the proportions of the two main constituents, the nature and extent of hydration of the proteins, and the degree of sclerotization (cross-linking of the proteins by quinones) (Hillerton, 1984). The last-named appears to have a particularly strong influence on penetrability. In the main, insects with heavily sclerotized body segments are invaded *via* intersegmental and arthrodial membranes or spiracles. Resistance to compressive force by sclerotized cuticle (exocuticle) suggests that it presents a stronger barrier than non-sclerotized endo- and mesocuticles. Since water extrusion accompanies sclerotization, water availability in addition to phenolic cross-links may be a factor limiting penetration in exocuticle. Although exocuticle from the desert locust supports growth and the production of cuticle-degrading enzyme activity by *M. anisopliae in vitro,* the cuticle remains intact (St Leger *et al.*, 1986a). Limited histolysis of the cuticle, therefore, during invasion *in vivo,* would provide sufficient nutrition to enable largely mechanical passage through the exocuticle. An ultrastructural study has shown that *M. anisopliae* can invade *via* segmental cuticle in the desert locust (E. Seyoum & Charnley, unpublished data).

Enzymatic degradation of procuticle is suggested by changes in the staining reactions of cuticles around penetrant hyphae. But in most cases absence of obvious zones of histolysis in regions where mechanical damage is reduced or non-existent suggests that fungal enzymes are active but limited to the vicinity of the fungal structure (Charnley, 1989).

In vitro studies on deuteromycete fungi grown on pulverized locust cuticle have revealed a range of extracellular cuticle-degrading enzymes that could potentially contribute to host penetration (St Leger *et al.*, 1986b). These enzymes correspond to the main components of cuticle, viz. protein, chitin and lipid. They appear sequentially. Esterase and proteolytic (endoprotease, aminopeptidase and carboxypeptidase) were produced first (< 24 h) followed by N-acetylglucosaminidase. Chitinase and lipase were produced 3–5 d later. Since chitinase from strain ME1 of *M. anisopliae* is an inducible enzyme and cuticular chitin is masked by protein, the late appearance of chitinase is presumably a result of induction, as chitin eventually becomes available after degradation of encasing cuticle proteins. The late detection of lipase appears to be due to the fact that the enzyme is largely cell-bound in young cultures.

Testing purified enzymes against locust cuticle *in vitro* showed that pretreatment or combined treatment with endoprotease (PR1, see later) was necessary for high chitinase activity. When locust exuviae (nondigested remains of old cuticle shed at ecdysis; exocuticle only) were used as substrate for purified pathogen enzymes instead of cuticle from larval sclerites (exo- and endocuticle), comparatively little hydrolysis occurred (St Leger *et al.*, 1986a). Similarly, while unsclerotized cuticle from fledgling locusts was rapidly degraded by fungal proteases, the crosslinking of cuticle proteins with gluteraldehyde (as a model for sclerotization) substantially reduced their susceptibility to proteolytic attack.

Extracellular endoprotease activity in culture filtrates of *M. anisopliae* (strain ME1) grown on locust cuticle can be resolved into three main components, a chymoelastase (PR1), a trypsin (PR2) (St Leger *et al.*, 1987a) and a cysteine protease (PR4) (S. Cole, R.M. Cooper & Charnley, unpublished data). PR1 degrades locust endocuticle very efficiently; binding of this basic enzyme to negative charges on the cuticle is necessary for activity, and solubilized peptides are further degraded until a chain length of about 5 is obtained. In contrast to PR1, PR2 and PR4 have only minor cuticle degrading activity and may be involved with cellular control mechanisms, catalysing inactivation and activation processes.

Two classes of aminopeptidases have been isolated from locust-cuticle grown cultures of *M. anisopliae* and classified as an aminopeptidase of broad specificity, but with particular activity against alanyl residues, and a post proline dipeptidyl amino peptidase 1V. Neither peptidase alone hydrolysed intact locust cuticle. However, when combined with PR1 they effected enhanced release of amino acids (R.J. St Leger, Charnley & R.M. Cooper, unpublished data). This is not surprising since the primary structure of locust cuticular proteins repeatedly contains the motif ala-ala-pro-ala/val (Hojrup *et al.*, 1986a). These exohydrolases presumably function *in situ* to break down PR1-derived peptides and thus provide nutrition for the fungus.

PR1 is produced constitutively, in the absence of repression by low molecular weight compounds containing carbon and nitrogen. Thus rapid synthesis of PR1 is only possible when the concentration of readily metabolizable compounds is low (St Leger *et al.*, 1988a). This is the case with locust cuticle as the components are largely insoluble until released by cuticle-degrading enzymes.

PR1 appears to be a pathogenicity determinant by virtue of its considerable ability to degrade cuticle (St Leger *et al.*, 1987a) and its production at high levels by the pathogen *in situ* during infection (St Leger *et al.*, 1987b; 1989; Goettel *et al.*, 1989). Simultaneous application of turkey egg white inhibitor and conidia significantly delayed mortality of *Manduca sexta* (Johannsen) (Lepidoptera: Sphingidae) larvae compared with larvae inoculated with conidia, supporting the importance of PR1 in penetration (St Leger *et al.*, 1988b). This kind of study has yet to be carried out with locusts.

Endochitinase and exochitinase (acetylglucosaminidase) have been purified from culture filtrates of *Metarhizium anisopliae* grown on chitin (St Leger *et al.*, 1991). However, there is no evidence for the production or activity of endochitinase during the first critical 40 h after inoculation of *Calliphora vomitoria* (Linnaeus) (Diptera: Calliphoridae) wings or abdominal body wall cuticle of *Manduca sexta*. The slow appearance of endochitinase *in vivo* is consistent with *in vitro* results (see earlier). It seems likely in *M. sexta–Metarhizium anisopliae* interactions that chitinase functions largely to provide nutrients during the saprophytic phase of fungal growth in cuticle of moribund insect hosts (St Leger *et al.*, 1987b). This may not be so in locusts where the thick partially sclerotized body wall cuticle could delay penetration sufficiently to allow induction and activity of endochitinase.

The importance of chitin as a barrier to penetration and as a stabilizer of the cuticular protein matrix, in the absence of fungal chitinase, is evident from a study using the insecticide diflubenzuron (= Dimilin[R]) a specific inhibitor of chitin synthesis in insects. Dual applications of diflubenzuron and *M. anisopliae* had a synergistic effect against larvae of *Manduca sexta.* Ultrastructural observations demonstrated that fungal penetration through diflubenzuron-treated cuticle was dramatically enhanced. Post-ecdysial diflubenzuron-treated cuticle (without chitin) was almost completely destroyed in contrast to pre-ecydsial cuticle (laid down prior to insecticide treatment) where hydrolysis was apparently selective (protein-only) and restricted to the vicinity of the fungal hyphae (Hassan & Charnley, 1989). Consistent with these ultrastructural observations, pharate fifth-instar *M. sexta* cuticle, produced during treatment with diflubenzuron and thus completely disrupted by the insecticide, was considerably more susceptible to Pr1 than the control cuticle. This study suggests that dual treatments of acylurea insecticides like diflubenzuron with entomopathogenic fungi could afford a useful strategy against locusts; particularly as second generation acylureas like teflubenzuron (= Nomoult[R]) have more *in vivo* persistence and significant activity against the desert locust.

Lipase(s) are produced by *Metarhizium anisopliae* in culture on locust cuticle (St Leger *et al.*, 1986b). However, a true lipase (with activity against olive oil) was not extracted from cuticles of *Manduca sexta* and *C. vomitoria* infected with *Metarhizium anisopliae* (St Leger *et al.*, 1987b). In addition, potential substrates for a lipase, viz. triacylglycerols and wax esters, appear to be comparatively minor components at least of the 'extractable' lipids of locust as of other insect cuticle. Thus it is not clear what role, if any, lipase plays in cuticular penetration (Charnley & St Leger, 1991).

If virulence among fungal isolates were correlated (at least in part) with cuticle-degrading enzyme activity then an initial target for strain selection and improvement would have been identified. However, this link is difficult to prove. Comparisons between isolates for pathogenicity and production of enzymes may only reveal the great variability within a species for numerous factors, many of which may influence, but be unrelated to, cuticle-degrading enzyme activity. From what is known about the properties and occurrence of cuticle-degrading enzymes in fungal infections in insects at the present time, endoproteases appear to be particularly important to the penetration process. However, PR1- and PR2-like endoproteases are produced in quantity by all isolates of *M. anisopliae* and other deuteromycetes looked at (Charnley & St Leger, 1991). Cuticle-degrading PR1 enzymes from *M. anisopliae, Beauveria bassiana* (Balsamo) Vuillemin, *Verticillium lecanii* (Zimmermann) Viégas, *Nomuraea rileyi* (Farlow) Samson and *Aschersonia aleyrodis* Webber differed only in charge. This has potential significance for their specificity as binding to cuticle is a prerequisite for activity. Cuticle from the migratory locust *Locusta migratoria* (Linnaeus) has a non-uniform distribution of charge, with negatively charged and positively charged groups predominating in flexible cuticle (e.g. arthrodial membranes) and rigid body-wall cuticle, respectively (Hojrup *et al.*, 1986b). What is known about the composition of desert locust cuticle suggests that it is similar to that from the migratory locust (Anderson, 1988). Thus it is possible that regions of the cuticle may be favourable or unfavourable to binding (and thus degradation) by individual enzymes, with consequences for the parts of the body which can be invaded by enzymatic action. This may influence speed of penetration and thus virulence.

Host defence

Insect alimentary canals are generally inhospitable to fungi. As a consequence, invasion rarely occurs from there despite the fact that both foregut and hindgut are lined with cuticle, which is largely unsclerotized and thus more susceptible than sclerite cuticle to pathogen enzymes. It is generally thought that anaerobiosis, digestive enzymes, adverse pH, speed of food throughput, and protection from the peritrophic membrane are primarily responsible for the gut barrier to fungi. In the case of the desert locust, however, antifungal phenols produced by the gut bacterial flora in the hindgut, make a significant contribution to host defence during periods of starvation when physical defences, such as gut movement and food throughput, prominent in fed insects, are less apparent. Fungitoxic phenols have also been found in the gut fluids of other related Orthoptera. The phenols are adsorbed by polyvinyl pyrolidone (PVP), thus formulation of conidia with PVP or other suitable material may reduce the effectiveness of the toxins and promote infection through the gut (Dillon & Charnley, 1991).

The appearance of host-produced brown or black pigments in insect cuticle in the vicinity of penetrant fungal hyphae is a common early sign of mycosis. Although the antimicrobial properties of oxidized phenols are well established, in insect cuticles melanization appears to be primarily a defence against weak or slow growing pathogens. Protease inhibitors within the cuticle may serve to restrict pathogen enzyme activity and hinder invasion (Charnley, 1989).

Once the cuticle and epidermis have been breached, the invading fungus is faced with the defence systems of the haemolymph. In the desert locust the presence of *M. anisopliae* within the cuticle elicits an inflammatory response, some 12 h before the fungus enters the haemocoel, on the basement membrane of the epidermal cells beneath the infection site. The haemocytes also invade the basement membrane and enter the epidermis. Finally, melanization occurs, starting with the endocuticle close to the epidermis and developing backwards through the capsule. Despite this intense activity on the part of the host, the fungus is not prevented from invading the haemocoel (Gunnarsson, 1988).

Within the haemocoel the main defence against an invading fungus appears to be the entrapment of small elements of the fungus in a mass of sticky blood cells (haemocytes) (nodule formation) and the encapsulation of hyphal fragments by layers of blood cells. Central to these events is the recognition of non-self, and activation of the prophenoloxidase system (ppo) may be the key (Charnley, 1989). For *M. anisopliae* (strain RS549) in the desert locust, however, the cellular response to the fungus in the haemocoel is very poor and few blood cells adhere to penetrant hyphae (Gunnarsson, 1988). A similar situation has been reported for other insect–fungus combinations. Most entomopathogenic fungi are dimorphic, existing as yeast-like hyphal bodies in the host haemolymph during the pathogenic phase and converting to a mycelial form post-mortem prior to sporulation on the cadaver. The avoidance of host defence may relate to this change in growth form. Perhaps altered cell wall composition or the production of an antihaemocyte chemical, consequent upon this change in morphology, is responsible for the failure of the cellular defence. Certainly, evidence is consistent with interference of the immune system of the desert locust by the cyclic depsipeptide toxins, the destruxins (DTX), produced by *M. anisopliae* (Huxham *et al.*, 1989).

Endogenous protease inhibitors have been reported in insect haemolymph as well as cuticle (see above). These may be involved in blood borne defence against entomopathogens. Sixth instar *Anticarsia gemmatalis* (Hübner) (Lepidoptera: Noctuidae) larvae, which are resistant to infection by *N. rileyi*, contain high levels of serum protease inhibitor (Boucias & Pendland, 1987). Susceptibility of young *A. gemmatalis* larvae and larvae of all ages of *Trichoplusia ni* (Hübner) (Lepidoptera: Nocutidae) correlates with low titre or absence of protease inhibitor, respectively. Interestingly, haemolymph of the desert locust contains a potent serum protease inhibitor with activity against the cuticle-degrading protease PR1 (M. Hoppé & Charnley, unpublished data).

Host death

Death of an insect from an entomopathogenic fungus has been variously ascribed to toxicosis, starvation (either by competition between host and fungus for nutrients, or as a result of cessation of feeding by the insect), invasion of host tissues by the fungus, asphyxiating of the insect by fungal growth within the tracheae and/or interference with host physiology. However, it is impossible to ascribe a cause of death to a mycosis with any certainty. It seems likely that several factors will be involved. From the point of view of enhancing the killing power of a biocontrol agent, the involvement of a powerful toxin in host death is more amenable to selection and/or manipulation.

Destruxins may play a significant part in host death. Fifteen related compounds in the DTX series have been isolated from culture filtrates of *M. anisopliae*, although DTX A and B tend to predominate and DTX E is generally the most insecticidal. Low doses of DTX A cause tetanic and flaccid paralysis and death in Lepidoptera and adult Diptera, by causing depolarization of muscle membranes (Samuels *et al.*, 1988a). Evidence to date is consistent with DTX A causing depolarization by opening calcium channels in the membrane. Among strains of *M. anisopliae* pathogenic for *Manduca sexta* DTXs may act as virulence determinants by virtue of their effects on muscles. Strain ME1, which produces DTX *in vitro* and *in vivo*, grows sparsely in infected larvae and causes paralysis prior to host death. However, isolates RS549 and RS1094, which were less virulent than ME1 and took longer to kill *M. sexta* larvae, grew profusely in the haemolymph, did not induce paralysis in their hosts and produced considerably less DTX in culture than ME1. In addition, no DTX was found in the haemolymph of insects infected with RS549 and RS1094 (Samuels *et al.*, 1988b).

Understanding the role of DTX in pathogenesis is complicated by the restricted susceptibility to DTX of muscles from different insect orders in comparison with the wide host range of *Metarhizium anisopliae.* Only Lepidoptera and adult Diptera respond to low doses of DTX by paralysis and death (Samuels *et al.*, 1988b). As much as 100 μg/g insect DTX did not cause paralysis upon injection into adult desert locusts, and this low *in vivo* toxicity correlated with *in vitro* insensitivity of the muscles. However, DTX does interfere with function and cause ultrastructural changes in a number of tissues (particularly Malpighian tubules and haemocytes) in a variety of insects, including locusts. It is not yet clear whether the effects of DTX on different tissues may be attributed to a common mode of action. Nor is it clear how the various cytotoxic effects (other than on lepidopteran muscle) relate to symptoms and progress of disease caused by *M. anisopliae.* A two-tier system for the involvement of destruxin in pathogenesis has been proposed (Samuels *et al.*, 1988b). On the one hand in Lepidoptera and adult Diptera DTX may have a pathogenic role *via* action on the muscles. On the other hand it may have an aggressive role in those insects such as locusts whose muscles are not susceptible to DTX, and in Lepidoptera and adult Diptera infected with low DTX producing strains. In this case DTX may assist the pathogen to establish or extend its infection. In support of this, virulence of *M. anisopliae* isolates (as measured by LT_{50}) against the vine weevil *Otiorhynchus sulcatus* (Fabricius) (Coleoptera: Curculionidae) correlated with *in vitro* DTX production (E. Moorhouse, R. Kershaw, A. Gillespie, S.E. Reynolds & Charnley, unpublished data).

DTX is possibly just one of a number of secondary metabolites that *M. anisopliae* produces to promote its parasitic existence in insects. However, it seems likely that DTX has a significant role in pathogenesis.

References

Anderson, S.O. (1988) Comparison between cuticular proteins from two locust species, *Locusta migratoria* and *Schistocerca gregaria. Insect Biochemistry* **18**, 751–760.

Boucias, D.G. & Pendland, J.C. (1987) Detection of protease inhibitors in the haemolymph of resistant *Anticarsia gemmatalis* which are inhibitory to the entompathogenic fungus *Nomuraea rileyi. Experientia* **43**, 336–339.

Boucias, D.G. & Pendland, J.C. (1991) Attachment of mycopathogens to cuticle: the initial event of mycoses in arthropod hosts. In: Cole, G.T. & Hoch, H.C. (eds), *The Fungal Spore and Disease Initiation in Plants and Animals.* Plenum Press, New York, pp. 101–129.

Charnley, A.K. (1989) Mechanisms of fungal pathogenesis in insects. In: Whipps, J.M. & Lumsden, R.D. (eds), *Biotechnology of Fungi for Improving Plant Growth.* Cambridge University Press, Cambridge, pp. 85–127.

Charnley, A.K. & St Leger, R.J. (1991) The role of cuticle degrading enzymes in fungal pathogenesis in insects. In: Cole, G.T. & Hoch, H.C. (eds), *The Fungal Spore and Disease Initiation in Plants and Animals.* Plenum Press, New York, pp. 267–287.

Dillon, R.J. & Charnley, A.K. (1991) The fate of fungal spores in the insect gut. In: Cole, G.T. and Hoch, H.C. (eds), *The Fungal Spore and Disease Initiation in Plants and Animals.* Plenum Press, New York, pp. 129–157.

Goettel, M.S., St Leger, R.J., Rizzo, N.W., Staples, R.C. & Roberts, D.W. (1989) Ultrastructural localization of a cuticle-degrading protease produced by the entomopathogenic fungus *Metarhizium anisopliae* during penetration of host cuticle. *Journal of General Microbiology* **135**, 2233–2239.

Gunnarsson, S. (1988) Infection of *Schistocerca gregaria* by the fungus *Metarhizium anisopliae,* cellular reactions in the integument studied by scanning electron and light microscopy. *Journal of Invertebrate Pathology* **52**, 9–17.

Hassan, A.E.M. & Charnley, A.K. (1989) Ultrastructural study of the penetration by *Metarhizium anisopliae* through Dimilin-affected cuticle of *Manduca sexta. Journal of Invertebrate Pathology* **54**, 117–124.

Hillerton, J.E. (1984) Cuticle: mechanical properties. In: Bereite-Hahn, J, Matoksy, A.G. & Richards, K.S. (eds), *Biology of the Integument: I. Invertebrates.* Springer-Verlag, Berlin, pp. 626–637.

Hojrup, P., Anderson, S.O. & Roepstorff, P. (1986a) Primary structure of a structural protein from the cuticle of the migratory locust *Locusta migratoria. Biochemical Journal* **236**, 713–720.

Hojrup, P., Anderson, S.O. & Roepstorff P. (1986b) Isolation, characterisation and N-terminal sequence studies of cuticular proteins from the migratory locust, *Locusta migratoria. European Journal of Biochemistry* **154**, 153–159.

Huxham, I.M., Lackie, A.M. & McCorkindale, N.J. (1989) Inhibitory effects of cyclodepsipeptides, destruxins, from the fungus *Metarhizium anisopliae*, on cellular immunity in insects. *Journal of Insect Physiology* **35**, 97–107.

St Leger, R.J., Cooper, R.M. & Charnley, A.K. (1986a) Cuticle-degrading enzymes of entomopathogenic fungi: cuticle degradation *in vitro* by enzymes from entomopathogens. *Journal of Invertebrate Pathology* **47**, 167–177.

St Leger, R.J., Charnley A.K. & Cooper R.M. (1986b) Cuticle-degrading enzymes of entomopathogenic fungi: synthesis in culture on cuticle. *Journal of Invertebrate Pathology* **48** 85–95.

St Leger, R.J., Charnley A.K. & Cooper R.M. (1987a) Characterization of cuticle-degrading proteases produced by the entomopathogen *Metarhizium anisopliae. Archives of Biochemistry and Biophysics* **253**, 221–232.

St Leger, R.J., Cooper, R.M. & Charnley, A.K. (1987b) Production of cuticle-degrading enzymes by the entomopathogen *Metarhizium anosopliae* during infection of cuticles from *Calliphora vomitoria* and *Manduca sexta. Journal of General Microbiology* **133**, 1371–1382.

St Leger, R.J., Durrands, P.K., Charnley, A.K. & Cooper, R.M. (1988a) Regulation of production of proteolytic enzymes by the entomopathogen *Metharizium anisopliae. Archives of Microbiology* **150**, 413–416.

St Leger, R.J., Durrands, P.K., Charnley, A.K. & Cooper, R.M. (1988b) The role of extracellular chymoelastase in the virulence of *Metarhizium anisopliae* for *Manduca sexta. Journal of Invertebrate Pathology* **52**, 285–294.

St Leger, R.J., Butt, T.M., Roberts, D.W. & Staples, R.C. (1989) Synthesis of proteins including a cuticle-degrading protease during differentiation of the entomopathogenic fungus *Metarhizium anisopliae. Experimental Mycology* **13**, 253–262.

St Leger, R.J., Cooper, R.M. & Charnley, A.K. (1991) Characterization of chitinase and chitobiase produced by the entomopathogen *Metarhizium anisopliae. Journal of Invertebrate Pathology* **58**, 415–426.

St Leger, R.J., May, B., Allee, L.L., Frank, D.C. & Roberts, D.W. (in press) Genetic differences in allozymes and in formation of infection structures among isolates of the entomopathogenic fungus *Metarhizium anisopliae. Journal of Invertebrate Pathology*

Samuels, R.I., Reynolds, S.E. & Charnley, A.K. (1988a) Calcium channel activation of insect muscle by destruxins, insecticidal compounds produced by the entomopathogenic fungus *Metarhizium anisopliae. Comparative Biochemistry and Physiology* **90C**, 403–412.

Samuels, R.I., Charnley, A.K. & Reynolds, S.E. (1988b) The role of destruxins in the pathogenicity of 3 strains of *Metarhizium anisopliae* for the tobacco hornworm, *Manduca sexta. Mycopathologia* **104**, 51–58.

Vey, A., Fargues, J. & Robert, P. (1982) Histological and ultrastructural studies of factors determining the specificity of pathotypes of the fungus *Metarhizium anisopliae* for scarabaeid larvae. *Entomophaga* **24**, 387–397.

Molecular approaches to the study of entomopathogenic fungi

J.M. Clarkson

School of Biological Sciences, University of Bath.

Abstract

Many molecular techniques developed for other fungi are appropriate for use with entomopathogenic species. Genetic transformation of *Metarhizium anisopliae* (Metschnikoff) Sorokin has been achieved using cloned genes from *Neurospora crassa* Sheare & Dodge and *Aspergillus nidulans* (Eidam) Vuillemin. The *pr1* gene from *M. anisopliae* which encodes a cuticle degrading protease, has been cloned recently. Improvement of strains of *Metarhizium* spp. and *Beauveria* spp. by traditional genetic methods has relied on exploitation of parasexual recombination since they lack a sexual cycle, but gene cloning methods now offer an alternative for improvement, if legislation will allow the use of laboratory produced recombinants. Molecular markers have been used to characterize the genotypes of individual fungal strains by examining gene products, but recent development of RFLP and PCR techniques allows direct examination of variability at the DNA level. Pulsed field gel electrophoresis (PFGE) is a technique which has been used to study karyotype variation in other fungi, and which could be used advantageously with entomopathogens.

Introduction

The recent development of molecular techniques for genetic engineering of filamentous fungi provides new opportunities for the study of entomopathogenic fungi. Cloning of genes encoding pathogenicity or virulence determinants will allow a rigorous testing of their role in insect pathogenesis and may provide the rationale for strain improvement by direct genetic manipulation. The identification of molecular markers for characterizing fungal genomes makes it possible to study genetic variation directly at the DNA level. These new approaches are being applied to a wide range of fungi and will give new insights into the population structure of entomopathogens. The aim of this paper is to describe some of these molecular techniques and discuss how they might be applied to entomopathogenic fungi. Deuteromycete fungi, and in particular *Metarhizium* spp. and *Beaveria* spp., show the most promise as biological control agents of locusts and grasshoppers and will form the focus of this paper.

Molecular analysis of insect pathogenesis

An essential prerequisite for the molecular analysis of pathogenesis is the development of a method for the stable introduction of exogenous DNA. DNA-mediated transformation procedures for filamentous fungi are usually based on the addition of DNA to protoplasts in the presence of Ca^{++} followed by the addition of polyethylene glycol (Fincham, 1989; Timberlake & Marshall, 1989). Transformants usually arise at low frequency (0.1–10 transformants/μg vector DNA) through the stable incorporation of DNA into the fungal chromosomes, although there are now several reports of autonomous replication of transforming DNA (Tsukuda *et al.*, 1988; Powell & Kistler, 1990). Importantly, the identification of DNA sequences that promote autonomous replication also results in high frequency (100–10,000 transformants/μg vector DNA) transformation. A variety of selectable markers has been used for fungal transformation. Initially, transformation of the genetically well characterized 'laboratory' fungi *Aspergillus nidulans* (Eidam) Vuillemin (Ballance *et al.*, 1983) and *Neurospora crassa* Sheare & Dodge (Case *et al.*, 1979) utilized genes encoding catabolic or biosynthetic enzymes to complement appropriate mutants. Subsequently, dominant selectable markers such as hygromycin, bleomycin or benomyl resistance have been used, as these can be used to transform wild type strains of a genetically uncharacterized fungus.

Bernier *et al.* (1989) demonstrated recently that *Metarhizium anisopliae* (Metschnikoff) Sorokin could be transformed to benomyl resistance using a cloned β-tubulin gene from a benomyl resistant strain of *N. crassa* (Vollmer & Yanofsky, 1986). Transformants were stable under non-selective conditions and retained pathogenicity to *Manduca sexta* (Johannson) (Lepidoptera: Sphingidae). Southern hybridization indicated that the majority of transformants arose through the random integration into the chromosomes of tandemly repeated vector sequences. Benomyl resistant transformants of *Metarhizium anisopliae* have also been selected by Goettel *et al.*, (1990) using a plasmid containing the *benA3* allele from *A. nidulans.* In both cases transformants were identified at low frequency. In *Beauveria bassiana* (Balsamo) Vuillemin resistance to chlorate has been used as a positive selection for mutants lacking nitrate reductase activity. The nitrate reductase (nia D) gene of *A. nidulans* was then used to transform a nitrate reductase mutant (Daboussi *et al.*, 1989).

Although in filamentous fungi, transformants arise mainly through the random integration of DNA, homologous integration can occur in a proportion of the transforming events (Fincham, 1989). This has been exploited to produce directed mutations by gene disruption or replacement with altered copies of cloned genes, thereby allowing a definite analysis of the role of that gene product. This strategy has been used recently to demonstrate that the cell wall-degrading enzyme polygalacturonase is not required for pathogenicity of the fungus *Cochliobolus carbonum* Nelson on its host plant maize (*Zea mays*) (Scott-Craig *et al.*, 1990). This powerful technique could also be used to investigate the role of putative pathogenicity or virulence determinants of entomopathogenic fungi.

Two areas that are already receiving attention are the production of cuticle degrading enzymes and insecticidal toxins (Charnley, these proceedings). Infection of the insect host occurs by direct penetration of the cuticle and *M. anisopliae* produces a range of enzymes capable of degrading components of the cuticle. Prominent amongst these is a protease (PR1) with chymoelastase specificity (St Leger *et al.*, 1987a). Several lines of evidence strongly implicate this enzyme as a determinant of pathogenicity. PR1 is the first of a sequence of cuticle degrading enzymes produced *in vitro* on host cuticle and is capable of extensively degrading cuticular protein (St Leger *et al.*, 1986, 1987a). It is produced in high levels by the fungus during host penetration (St Leger *et al.*, 1987b) and specific inhibition of PR1 delays disease symptoms and mortality on *Manduca sexta* (St Leger *et al.*, 1988). We have recently cloned the *pr1* gene (I. Paterson & Clarkson, unpublished data) and the production of a specific Pr1 deficient mutant of *Metarhizium anisopliae* by recombinant DNA technology should provide a definitive answer to the role of this enzyme in pathogenesis. Work on cloning the *pr1* gene is also in progress at the Boyce Thompson Institute, USA.

Insecticidal cyclic peptide toxins, destruxins, produced by *M. anisopliae* may play an important role in pathogenesis (Charnley, 1989). It is likely that destruxins are assembled extraribosomally using the thiotemplate mechanism now well established for the majority of other cyclic peptide antibiotics. The cloning of genes involved in the biosynthesis of destruxins would enable the construction of mutant strains defective for a specific biosynthetic enzyme and presumably disrupt toxin biosynthesis. Isogenic toxin-producing and toxin-less mutant strains could then be compared against a variety of insect hosts.

Strain improvement

M. anisopliae and *B. bassiana* have no known sexual stages although genetic recombination through the parasexual cycle has been demonstrated for both (Messias & Azevedo, 1980; Al-Aidroos, 1980; Paccola-Meirelles & Azevedo, 1991). The essential features of the parasexual cycle are the formation of at least a transient heterokaryon by hyphal anastomosis or protoplast fusion, rare fusions between dissimilar nuclei to produce a heterozygous diploid, and haploidization, presumably by a process of mitotic non-disjunction. Genetic recombination can occur by mitotic crossing-over between homologous chromosomes and by the random segregation of chromosomes during haploidization.

Parasexual recombination has been considered as a possible method of genetic manipulation for strain improvement in *M. anisopliae.* Heale *et al.* (1989) reported a parasexual cross between the auxotrophic mutants derived from pathogenic wild type strains, differing in sporulation rate and pathogenicity towards *Nilaparvata lugens* (Stål) (Hemiptera: Delphacidae). Two of the haploid recombinants selected from this cross combined high pathogenicity and sporulation rates. This is in contrast to parasexual crosses between isolates of *Verticillium lecanii* (Zimmermann) Viégas (Drummond & Heale, 1988) and the plant pathogenic species *V. albo-atrum* Reinke & Berthold and *V. dahliae* Klebahn (Clarkson & Heale, 1985; O'Garro & Clarkson, in press) where recombinants were generally of low pathogenicity. A possible explanation is that parasexual recombination between isolates that are normally reproductively isolated, disrupts adapted complexes of pathogenicity genes resulting in weakly pathogenic haploid recombinants.

Genetic engineering offers an exciting alternative approach to strain improvement. The cloning of genes from entomopathogenic fungi whose products are essential for pathogenicity or which contribute quantitatively to virulence may provide the basis for rational strain improvement. Increasing gene copy number and location are consequences of genetic transformation (Bernier *et al.*, 1989) which may result in over-expression of a pathogenicity gene. Gene expression could also be modified by transformation with gene constructs containing the coding region of a pathogenicity gene fused to a strong promoter. Genetic transformation will also provide a tool for moving genes from one entomopathogenic species to another. What is unclear at this stage is how legislation governing the release of genetically manipulated organisms will develop.

Molecular markers for the characterization of entomopathogenic fungi

The genetic characterization of wild-type strains of entomopathogenic fungi can provide information about variation and population structure. It may also be possible to identify individual isolates by a unique set of genetic characteristics, although this could not be done where isolates were actually clones of the same genotype, as may occur particularly in epizootics. Two types of naturally occurring genetic markers which have been used extensively for plant pathogenic fungi are mating type and specific virulence, but these are not generally applicable to entomopathogens. Molecular markers have several advantages, including co-dominance, selective neutrality, and abundance (Michelmore & Hulbert, 1987). Variations in soluble protein patterns and isozyme polymorphisms detected by electrophoresis have proved useful in a range of fungi. De Conti *et al.* (1980) examined the electrophoretic variation in esterases and phosphatases in 11 wild type isolates of *M. anisopliae* from Brazil and were able to distinguish 5 patterns for esterase. In a study of both *M. anisopliae* var. *anisopliae* Tulloch and the large spored *M. anisopliae* var. *majus* (Johnston) Tulloch, Riba *et al.* (1986) demonstrated that var. *majus* isolates were relatively homogeneous for isozyme profiles but that var. *anisopliae* isolates were highly polymorphic. Isozyme polymorphisms have also been studied in *B. bassiana* (Mugnai *et al.*, 1989).

Techniques which directly investigate genetic variation at the DNA level are rapidly gaining acceptance as the most appropriate tools for studying fungal populations. Several of these will be discussed.

Restriction fragment length polymorphisms (RFLPs) of nuclear and mitochondrial DNA

RFLPs may be detected following digestion with an appropriate type II restriction endonuclease and separation of the DNA fragments by agarose electrophoresis. Differences between isolates in DNA sequence may alter the restriction sites for endonucleases resulting in DNA fragments of varying lengths. For fungal mitochondrial genomes which are usually small (19–121 kb) and exist in relatively high copy number (Grossman & Hudspeth, 1985) RFLPs are usually easy to detect. Total DNA of the fungus is extracted and then the mitochondrial DNA separated from nuclear DNA by centrifugation in CsCl gradients containing bis-benzimide (Garber & Yoder, 1985). The small size of mitochondrial genomes results in a simple banding pattern when cut with restriction endonucleases. Mitochondrial RFLP markers have been used in a number of plant pathogenic fungi although the extent of variation differs considerably.

Although variation may sometimes be detected between strains in ethidium bromide stained gels of restriction endonuclease digests of total genomic DNA (e.g. Coddington *et al.*, 1987), labelled DNA probes are normally required. Total genomic DNA is extracted and digested with a restriction endonuclease. The complex array of DNA fragments are then size fractionated by agarose gel electrophoresis and transferred to a nylon or nitrocellulose filter (Southern blotting). The filter is then probed with a radioactive or non-radioactive labelled DNA probe and visualized by autoradiography or development of the filter, respectively. The number of bands observed depends on the copy number of DNA sequences homologous to the probe and the number of restriction sites within the sequence.

Various types of DNA probe have been used to detect RFLPs, e.g. random genomic clones containing single copy (Hulbert *et al.*, 1988) or repetitive sequences (Kistler *et al.*, 1991), rDNA (Garber *et al.*, 1988) and oligonucleotide probes (Mayer *et al.*, 1991). A. Jessop, I. Paterson & Clarkson (unpublished data) have recently used random genomic clones in the lambda vector EMBL3 to detect RFLPs in *M. anisopliae.*

Polymerase chain reaction (PCR) methods

The polymerase chain reaction (PCR) is an *in vitro* method for amplifying DNA sequences using very small amounts of target DNA (White *et al.*, 1989). The double strand target DNA is denatured by heating briefly at high temperature (ca. 95°C) and the oligonucleotide primers are allowed to anneal to their complementary sequences at low temperature (dependent on probe length and composition). DNA extension from the annealed primers proceeds using dNTPs and a thermostable polymerase, e.g. Taq polymerase, at 72°C. Repeated cycles of denaturation, annealing and extension lead to the rapid amplification of target DNA sequences which can usually be resolved by conventional agarose or polyacrylamide gel electrophoresis.

It has been demonstrated recently that PCR can be used to identify DNA sequence polymorphisms by the amplification of random DNA segments with single oligonucleotide primers, of arbitrary sequence (Williams *et al.*, 1990; Welsh & McClelland, 1990). This randomly amplified polymorphic DNA (RAPD) can be visualized on ethidium bromide stained agarose gels as discrete bands which may provide a unique genetic ‘fingerprint’ for a particular genotype. This technique is being applied to a wide range of organisms, including *Metarhizium* spp. (R. Milner, pers. comm.).

Electrophoretic karyotyping

Pulsed field gel electrophoresis (PFGE) is capable of separating DNA molecules ranging from about 20 kb to 12,000 kb (Mills & McCluskey, 1990). Schwartz & Cantor (1984) first applied this technique to the separation of the chromosomes of *Saccharomyces cerevisiae* Meyer ex Hansen. In conventional gel electrophoresis DNA molecules migrate in a single electric field. The migration rate of molecules less than approximately 20 kb is proportional to their size because they are sieved. Larger molecules are not sieved effectively and consequently migrate at similar rates. PFGE utilizes alternating electric fields which force the DNA molecules to change direction. The time required for a DNA molecule to change direction is size dependent with larger molecules requiring more time to re-orientate. The duration of each alternating electric field (or pulse) determines the resolution. Total run times may last several days.

The resolution of PFGE has been improved by modification to the original apparatus and protocol. One commonly used method is contour-clamped homogeneous electric field (CHEF) gel electrophoresis where a hexagonal array of electrodes produces a uniform electric field across the gel resulting in straight running lanes and good resolution. DNA is usually prepared from fungi by embedding protoplasts in blocks of low melting point agarose. These are mixed with a detergent (e.g. SDS), EDTA and proteinase K. The agarose blocks containing 0.5–20 μg DNA are then inserted into a well of the agarose gel and sealed with agarose.

PFGE has not been reported for entomopathogenic fungi although it has been used to study the molecular karyotypes of a wide range of plant pathogens and other fungi of commercial importance. Studies with field isolates of plant pathogenic fungi have revealed a surprising degree of variation in both chromosome number and length (e.g. Kinscherf & Leong, 1988; Mills & McCluskey, 1990) suggesting that the electrophoretic karyotypes may prove to be valuable molecular markers for entomopathogenic fungi.

References

Al-Aidroos, K. (1980) Demonstration of a parasexual cycle in the entomopathogenic fungus *Metarhizium anisopliae. Canadian Journal of Genetics and Cytology* **22**, 309–314.

Ballance, D.J., Buxton, F.P. & Turner, G. (1983) Transformation of *Aspergillus nidulans* by the orotidine-5′-phosphate decarboxylase gene of *Neurospora crassa. Biochemical and Biophysical Research Communications* **112**, 284.

Bernier, L., Cooper, R.M., Charnley, A.K. & Clarkson, J.M. (1989) Transformation of the entomopathogenic fungus *Metarhizium anisopliae* to benomyl resistance. *FEMS Microbiology Letters* **60**, 261–266.

Case, M.E., Schweizer, M., Kushner, S.R. & Giles, N.H. (1979) Efficient transformation of *Neurospora crassa* by utilizing hybrid plasmid DNA. *Proceedings of the National Academy of Sciences* **76**, 5259.

Charnley, A.K. (1989) Mechanisms of fungal pathogenesis in insects. In: Whipps, J. & Lumsden, R. (eds), *Biotechnology of Fungi for Improving Plant Growth.* Cambridge University Press, Cambridge, pp. 85–127.

Clarkson, J.M. & Heale, J.B. (1985) A preliminary investigation of the genetics of pathogenicity in hop wilt isolates of *Verticillium albo-atrum. Transactions of the British Mycological Society* **83**, 345–350.

Coddington, A., Matthews, P.M., Cullis, C. & Smith, K.H. (1987) Restriction digest patterns of total DNA from different races of *Fusarium oxysporum* f.sp. *pisi* – an improved method for race classification. *Journal of Phytopathology* **118**, 9–20.

Daboussi, M.J., Djeballi, A., Gerlinger, C., Blaiseau, P.L., Bouvier, I., Carson, M., Lebrun, M., Parisot, D. & Brygoo, Y. (1989) Transformation of seven species of filamentous fungus using the nitrate reductase gene of *Aspergillus nidulans. Current Genetics* **15**, 453–456.

De Conti, E., Messias, C., Myrina, H., De Souza, L. & Azevedo, J.L. (1980) Electrophoretic variation in esterases and phosphatases in eleven wild-type strains of *Metarhizium anisopliae. Experientia* **36**, 293–294.

Drummond, J. & Heale, J.B. (1988) Genetic studies on the inheritance of pathogenicity in *Verticillium lecanii* against *Trialeurodes vaporariorum. Journal of Invertebrate Pathology* **52**, 57–65.

Fincham, J.R.S. (1989) Transformation in fungi. *Microbiological Reviews* **53**, 143–170.

Garber, R. & Yoder, O.C. (1985) Mitochondrial DNA of the filamentous ascomycete *Cochliobolus heterostrophus. Current Genetics* **8**, 621–628.

Garber, R., Turgeon, B.G., Selker, E.U. & Yoder, O.C. (1988) Organization of ribosomal RNA genes in the fungus *Cochliobolus heterostrophus. Current Genetics* **14**, 573–582.

Goettel, M., St Leger, R., Bhairi, S., Jung, M., Oakley, B., Roberts, D. & Staples, R.C. (1990) Pathogenicity and growth of *Metarhizium anisopliae* stably transformed to benomyl resistance. *Current Genetics* **17**, 129–132.

Grossman, L. & Hudspeth, M. (1985) Fungal mitochondrial genomes. In: Bennett, J.W. & Lasure, L. (eds), *Gene Manipulation in Fungi.* Academic Press, Orlando, Fla, pp. 65–103.

Heale, J.B., Isaac, J. & Chandler, D. (1989) Prospects for strain improvement in entomopathogenic fungi. *Pesticide Science* **26**, 79–92.

Hulbert, S.J., Ilott, T.W., Legg, E.J., Lincoln, S.E., Lander, E.S. & Michelmore, R.W. (1988) Genetic analysis of the fungus *Bremia lactucae*, using restriction fragment length polymorphisms. *Genetics* **120**, 947–958.

Kinscherf, T. & Leong, S.A. (1988) Molecular analysis of the karyotype of *Ustilago maydis. Chromosoma* **96**, 427–433.

Kistler, H.C., Momol, E.A. & Benny, U. (1991) Repetitive genomic sequences for determining relatedness among strains of *Fusarium oxysporum. Phytopathology* **81**, 331–336.

Messias, C. & Azevedo, J. (1980) Parasexuality in the deuteromycete *Metarhizium anisopliae. Transactions of the British Mycological Society* **75**, 473–477.

Meyer, W., Koch, A., Niemann, C., Beyermann, B., Epplen, J.T. & Borner, T. (1991) Differentiation of species and strains among filamentous fungi by DNA fingerprinting. *Current Genetics* **19**, 239–242.

Michelmore, R.W. & Hulbert, S.H. (1987) Molecular markers for genetic analysis of phytopathogenic fungi. *Annual Review of Phytopathology* **25**, 383–404.

Mills, D. & McCluskey, K. (1990) Electrophoretic karyotypes of fungi. The new cytology. *Molecular Plant-Microbe Interactions* **3**, 351–357.

Mugnai, L., Bridge, P.D. & Evans, H.C. (1989) A chemotaxonomic evaluation of the genus *Beauveria. Mycological Research* **92**, 199–209.

O'Garro, L.W. & Clarkson, J.M. (in press) Variation in pathogenicity on tomato among parasexual recombinants of *Verticillium dahliae. Plant Pathology.*

Paccola-Meirelles, L. & Azevedo, J. (1991) Parasexuality in *Beauveria bassiana. Journal of Invertebrate Pathology* **57**, 172–176.

Powell, W.A. & Kistler, H.C. (1990) In vivo rearrangement of foreign DNA by *Fusarium oxysporum* produces linear self-replicating plasmids. *Journal of Bacteriology* **172**, 3163–3171.

Riba, G., Bouvier-Fourcade, I. & Caudal, A. (1986) Isoenzyme polymorphism in *Metarhizium anisopliae* (Deuteromycotina: Hyphomycetes) entomogenous fungi. *Mycopathologia* **96**, 161–169.

Schwartz, D.C. & Cantor, C.R. (1984) Separation of yeast chromosome-sized DNAs by pulsed-field gradient gel electrophoresis. *Cell* **37**, 67–75.

Scott-Craig, J.S., Panaccione, D., Cervone, F. & Walton, J.D. (1990) Endo-polygalacturonase is not required for pathogenicity of *Cochliobolus carbonum* on maize. *Plant Cell* **2**, 1191–1200.

St Leger, R., Charnley, A.K. & Cooper, R.M. (1986) Cuticle-degrading enzymes of entomopathogenic fungi: synthesis in culture on cuticle. *Journal of Invertebrate Pathology* **48**, 85–95.

St Leger, R., Charnley, A.K. & Cooper, R.M. (1987a) Characterization of cuticle-degrading proteases produced by the entomopathogen *Metarhizium anisopliae. Archives of Biochemistry and Biophysics* **253**, 221–232.

St Leger, R., Cooper, R.M. & Charnley, A.K. (1987b) Production of cuticle-degrading enzymes by the entomopathogen *Metarhizium anisopliae* during infection of cuticles from *Calliphora vomitora* and *Manduca sexta. Journal of General Microbiology* **133**, 1371–1382.

St Leger, R., Durrands, P., Charnley, A.K. & Cooper, R.M. (1988) Role of extra-cellular chymoelastase in the virulence of *Metarhizium anisopliae* for *Manduca sexta. Journal of Invertebrate Pathology* **52**, 285–293.

Timberlake, W.E. & Marshall, M.A. (1989) Genetic engineering of filamentous fungi. *Science* **244**, 1313–1317.

Tsukuda, T., Carleton, S., Fotheringham, S. & Holloman, W.K. (1988) Isolation and characterization of an autonomously replicating sequence from *Ustilago maydis. Molecular and Cellular Biology* **8**, 3703–3709.

Vollmer, S.J. & Yanofsky, C. (1986) Efficient cloning of genes of *Neurospora crassa. Proceedings of the National Academy of Sciences* **83**, 4869–4873.

Welsh, J.E. & McClelland, M. (1990) Fingerprinting genomes using PCR with arbitrary primers. *Nucleic Acids Research* **24**, 7213–7218.

White, T.J., Arnheim, N. & Erlich, H.A. (1989) The polymerase chain reaction. *Trends in Genetics* **5**, 185–189.

Williams, J., Kubelik, A., Lirak, K., Rafalski, J. & Tingey, S. (1990) DNA polymorphisms, amplified by arbitrary primers are useful as genetic markers. *Nucleic Acids Research* **18**, 6531–6535.

Selection and characterization of strains of *Metarhizium anisopliae* for control of soil insects in Australia

R.J. Milner

CSIRO, Division of Entomology.

Abstract

The most successful microbial pesticides are based on the bacterium, *Bacillus thuringiensis* (Berliner), with sales of over US$40M. This success has been slow to come and in part has been due to the screening of large numbers of isolates to find the most pathogenic. Recent extensions of the host range have come from searches of habitats of particular pest species e.g. var. *israelensis* from the mud of mosquito pools. In Australia, a semi-selective medium has been used to isolate the insect pathogenic hyphomycete, *Metarhizium anisopliae* (Metschnikoff) Sorokin, from soil and termite mound material. Isolates vary enormously in colony morphology but this character rarely correlates with pathogenicity. Other more sensitive methods such as the analysis of nuclear DNA using polymerase chain reaction (PCR) technology is showing promise for identification of individual isolates (strains). A three tiered screening strategy which has been adopted to select the most promising isolates, firstly for control of sugarcane scarabs and more recently for termites, is described. Two isolates pathogenic for a wide range of sugarcane scarabs and another, more specific, isolate have been successfully field tested and are now being commercialized. For termites, one isolate effective against both of the main Australian pest genera has been selected and is now being field tested.

Introduction

The world's most successful microbial pesticides are based on the bacterium *Bacillus thuringiensis* (B.t.), with annual sales estimated to be over US$40M. What lessons can be learnt from this success? Firstly, success has been and continues to be, a slow process, with the first products on the market as long ago as 1935. Secondly, and central to this workshop, success has been based on the discovery of effective isolates, in particular, the discovery by Dulmage of the HD1 strain which is highly pathogenic for *Trichoplusia ni* (Hübner) (Lepidoptera: Noctuidae) (Dulmage, 1970). This transformed the product from a curiosity to a significant commercial product, and the HDI strain still forms the basis of products such as Dipel today. Subsequent searches in the habitat of the target pest revealed firstly B.t. var. *israelensis* Goldbert & Margarlit (Goldberg & Margarlit, 1977), then B.t. var. *tenebrionis* Krieg, Huger, Lagenbruch & Schnetter (Kreig *et al.*, 1983), now both successful commercial products, and very recently in New Zealand, isolates effective against the New Zealand grassgrub, *Costelytra zealandica* (White) (Coleoptera: Scarabaeidae) (Chilcott & Wigley, 1990). This search for new isolates with novel activities has become almost obsessive, with well over 25,000 isolates now in culture collections around the world. Finally, bioassay against the target insect is still the only way to determine the activity of these new isolates. I suggest that the task of developing an effective microbial pesticide for locusts and grasshoppers is going to be slow, and that a large number of isolates will have to be bioassayed before success is achieved.

In this short paper I will describe the work undertaken in my laboratory in Canberra to identify, and to characterize, isolates of the hyphomycete fungus *Metarhizium anisopliae* (Metschnikoff) Sorokin, for control of scarab pests of sugarcane (Milner, in press) and termites. In both cases it was necessary to find isolates which were highly pathogenic to the target under field conditions, effective against several related species of target pest, and had temperature profiles which matched the prevailing field conditions. Our approach has been firstly to assemble as large a library of isolates as possible, mostly from the target pest or its immediate environment, then to bioassay them against the pest using a three tiered strategy, and finally to compare the other relevant characteristics, such as temperature profiles, of a small number of effective isolates. It is rarely possible to evaluate more than about three (ideally just one) isolates in large-scale field trials.

Isolate acquisition

There are three main sources of isolates: culture collections such as the American Type Culture Collection or that of the International Mycological Institute (CABI); isolation from the environment of the target insect; and direct isolation from the target insect itself. If one is lucky enough to find a field epizootic and to isolate the fungus directly then this isolate(s) is likely, but not certain, to show a high degree of pathogenicity. For soil insects, this medium is the reservoir for all pathogens and not just *M. anisopliae*; thus it seems logical that effective isolates can be obtained in this manner. Effective isolates are rarely to be obtained from culture collections, in my experience.

We have found 'Veens Medium' (Milner & Lutton, 1976) to be extremely effective as a semi-selective isolation medium. It is able to detect levels of conidia down to 10^3/g soil and when compared with other selective media recovers a wider variety of isolates (A. Rath, pers. comm.). We generally isolate from a composite soil sample taken from 2–6 cm below the surface, the depth at which most conidia are found under natural conditions. A 1 g sample of soil is sonicated briefly in a 0.05% Tween 80 solution and 100 μl of the resulting suspension is spread over the surface of a Veens medium plate. The characteristic colonies of *M. anisopliae* start to sporulate after 2 or 3 weeks' incubation at 25°C. These can then be removed and subcultured into SDAYE for testing.

M. anisopliae is surprisingly easy to find in a wide range of habitats. Undisturbed pastures in wet climatic zones where Scarabaeidae are common certainly provide large numbers of isolates (Table 1). Under these conditions it is not unusual to find fields where the average density of conidia exceeds 10^6/g of soil. The fungus is much more scarce in frequently cultivated fields in relatively dry hot climates such as groundnut fields in Queensland and Myanmar. Under these conditions it is rare to find more than 2×10^3/g. Similarly in termite mounds the fungus is not uncommon but is always at a low density.

Table 1. Summary of the results of selective isolation of *Metarhizium anisopliae* from soil in natural habitats in Australia and Myanmar (Burma).

Area	Crop	No. sites	No. positive sites
Mackay, Qld	sugar	17	9
Bundaberg, Qld	sugar	11	8
Cairns, Qld	sugar	21	19
Yeppoon, Qld	pineapple	4	3
Busselton, WA	potatoes	11	10
Pemberton, WA	potatotes	20	9
Ebor, NSW	pasture	9	8
Kingaroy, Qld	peanuts	20	8
Myanmar	peanuts	21	10
Australia	termites	469	65

Isolate variability

The most obvious feature of *M. anisopliae* on isolation is the extreme diversity of colony types, viz. the colour of the conidia, the pattern of conidiation, the degree of sporulation, the colour and the texture of the aerial mycelium, the rate of growth, the level of pigmentation of the medium, and so on. It is possible to erect different morphological types and designate each isolate to a particular type. However, other characteristics (in particular pathogenicity) do not correlate with colony morphology and as the number of isolates to be so designated increases so does the difficulty of placing each isolate into a category.

Spore size also varies, but apart from the well-established (and extreme) difference between *M. anisopliae* var. *majus* (Johnston) Tulloch and *M. anisopliae* var. *anisopliae* Tulloch, this characteristic is not particularly useful. Isozymes have been extensively used to identify isolates and can be extremely useful in separating isolates which are otherwise very similar. However, this technique has two serious drawbacks. Firstly, the banding, especially for esterases which are the most useful marker enzymes, can be unstable with some bands absent for no apparent reason in some runs. Secondly, while differences are important and genuine, similarities are not. Thus, two distinct pathotypes can have identical isozyme patterns.

The most powerful and reliable way to characterize isolates is by means of DNA analysis using modern polymerase chain reaction (PCR) technology (see Clarkson, these proceedings). Recent unpublished work in my laboratory (F. Driver, J. Curran & R. Milner, unpublished data), has revealed significant sequence variation within *M. anisopliae*, and this has been used to develop a probe specific to some isolates of var. *anisopliae*. It is expected that, as our knowledge and understanding of the genome increases, we will be able to produce probes which have a greater degree of specificity.

Screening against scarabs

The first tier is a maximum challenge test which is extremely rapid and uses very few of the pest insects – an important factor because scarabs cannot be reared in the laboratory and are laborious to collect from the field. The larvae were rolled in pure dry conidia and incubated on moist tissue paper in individual chambers at 25°C for about 14 days. Under these extreme conditions 'good' isolates will kill 100% of the grubs and the majority of infected grubs will produce copious quantities of new conidia. Surprisingly, many isolates from the soil fail to kill under these conditions while some isolates obtained from the target pest do not kill more than 50% of the insects.

Isolates which were most effective in the Tier 1 test were then assessed using a quantitative bioassay. The larvae were dipped into suspensions of different concentrations of conidia and then incubated on moist tissue paper for 2 to 4 weeks at 25°C (Tier 2). Under these conditions the 'good' isolates had an LC_{50} (lethal concentration) below 10^5 conidia/ml.

Finally, a few really promising isolates were compared under simulated field conditions using soil treated with conidia or dosed with formulated fungus. The disease develops more slowly in soil and these tests usually continued for 7 weeks. The most promising isolates from this Tier 3 test were used for field trials.

In our work on sugarcane scarabs, this scheme was not applied rigorously because new isolates, often from field epizootics, became available during the testing and so were included in the then current Tier 3 tests without any prior testing. However a total of 115 isolate/target combinations were tested in Tier 1, 26 in Tier 2 and 40 in Tier 3 (Table 2). As a result two isolates with high pathogenicity for a wide range of sugarcane scarabs (FI147 and FI153) and one with a more restricted hose range (FI114) were selected for field trials. These isolates are now being commercialized under licence by Incitec Ltd.

Screening against termites

Termites are fragile insects, sensitive to handling and wetting. Thus, a dosing technique was devised to reduce these problems and to take advantage of the termites' natural grooming behaviour. For this method, a single worker termite is rolled in a dust of conidia of *M. anisopliae* and then placed in a 70 ml plastic container with 50 healthy workers. The treated carrier termite is groomed by the test termites and the mortality of this test group is determined after 4–10 days at about 27°C. By diluting the fungal conidia with talc this bioassay can be made quantitative. The dose is estimated from haemocytometer counts of conidia washed off the carrier termite.

In these termite assays, the Tier 1 testing consisted of both a high dose (1:10, conidia: talc) and a low dose (1:1000) together with controls. There are large numbers of termites available from the field consequently 150 workers (3 replicates of 50) could be tested per treatment. The most promising isolates progressed to a Tier 2 test which was a quantitative bioassay with 5 decimal doses. Finally, the best 10 isolates were tested against both soldiers and workers under more realistic conditions (25 g colonies in glass jars). In these Tier 3 tests, the termite colonies were dosed by adding 250 carrier termites treated with pure conidia, and the mortality was evaluated after 4 weeks at 26°C.

It was found that all isolates were at least moderately pathogenic and a large number of isolates were promising in Tier 1 tests (Table 3). In general the 'lower' termites, of the genus *Coptotermes*, were more susceptible than the 'higher' termites, *Nasutitermes*. Some 26 isolates were retested in Tier 2 bioassays and these also showed only small differences (Table 4). The final selection of 10 isolates for Tier 3 testing was somewhat arbitrary and the results varied depending on the particular colony of termites used for the testing. However, isolate FI610, derived originally from termite mound material, has generally performed well and has thus been chosen for the field trials which are currently in progress.

Table 2. Summary of Tier testing of isolates of *Metarhizium anisopliae* against seven species of cane grub (Coleoptera: Scarabaeidae).

	No. isolates tested			
Species	Tier 1	Tier 2	Tier 3	Best isolates
1 yr life cycle				
Lepidiota consobrina Girault	1	4	2	FI147;153
L. squamulata Waterhouse	10	0	0	
Antitrogus mussoni (Blackburn)	18	4	21	FI147;153
2 yr life cycle				
A. parvulus Britton	27	4	2	FI114;147
L. frenchi Blackburn	34	8	2	FI147;153
L. negatoria Blackburn	25	3	13	FI147
L. noxia Britton	0	3	0	FI147(?)

Table 3. Summary of results of Tier 1 testing of isolates of *Metarhizium anisopliae* against 3 species of pest termites.

Termite species	No. isolates	High dose mort. >80%	Low dose mort. >40%
Nasutitermes exitiosus (Hill)	93	33	16 (7)*
Coptotermes frenchi (Hill)	26	24	7 (7)
C. acinaciformis (Froggatt)	49	48	19 (19)
	24	16	0 (0)

*figures in brackets assessed after 4 days; others assessed after 8 days.

Table 4. Summary of results of Tier 2 testing of isolates of *Metarhizium anisopliae* against 2 species of pest termites.

Species tested	No. isolates	$LD_{50} \times 10^3$ spores/termite		
		1–15	<15–30	<30
Nasutitermes exitiosus (Hill)	26	11	9	6
Coptotermes acinaciformis (Froggatt)	26	26	0	0

Conclusions

The first priority in developing mycoinsecticides is to select an isolate which is highly pathogenic to the target pest or pests. In many situations, such as control of scarab larvae in Australian sugarcane fields, it is certainly desirable, and perhaps essential, that an isolate is found which controls a number of species from related genera. In order to find the best isolate, it is important that as wide a library of isolates as possible is tested and that this testing is by bioassay, ultimately under conditions as close as possible to those in the field. Isolates obtained directly from field epizootics on the target pest(s) have been found to be best, although isolates may vary in their pathogenicity even from the same epizootic.

The three tiered assay strategy has been found to be very useful in quickly assessing the efficacy of a large number of isolates. Three isolates (FI114, FI147 and FI153) with promise for control of sugarcane scarabs have been identified, and these are now being commercialized following successful field trials. Termites were found to be less variable than scarabs in their responses to various isolates. However, one isolate, FI610, which is highly pathogenic for both *Coptotermes* spp. and *Nasutitermes* sp., has been selected for detailed study and field trials. It has been found that DNA analysis using PCR technology is a valuable and sensitive technique for determining genetic differences between isolates. The isolates selected for field trials are all distinct and it is hoped to develop specific DNA probes for use in field trials.

References

Chilcott, C. & Wigley, P. (1990) Toxicity of *Bacillus thuringiensis* against grass grubs (Coleoptera: Scarabaeidae). *Proceedings of the Vth International Collo-*

quum on Invertebrate Pathology and Microbial Control, Adelaide, August 1990, 342.

Dulmage, H.T. (1970) Insecticidal activity of HD-1, a new isolate of *Bacillus thuringiensis* var. *alesti. Journal of Invertebrate Pathology* **15**, 232–239.

Goldberg, L. & Margarlit, J. (1977) A bacterial spore demonstrating rapid larvicidal activity against *Anopheles sergentii, Uranotaenia unguiculata, Culex univittatus, Aedes aegyptyi* and *Culex pipiens. Mosquito News* **37**, 355–358.

Kreig, A., Huger, A.M., Langenbruch, G.A. & Snetter, W. (1983) *Bacillius thuringiensis* var. *tenebrionis*: ein neuer, gegenuber Larven von Coleoptera wirksame Pathotyp. *Zeitschrift für Angewandte Entomologie* **96**, 505–508.

Milner, R.J. (in press) The selection of strains of *Metarhizium anisopliae* for control of Australian sugarcane white grubs. In: Jackson, T.J. & Glare, T.R. (eds), *The Use of Pathogens in Scarab Pest Management.* Intercept, London.

Milner, R.J. & Lutton, G.G. (1976) *Metarhizium anisopliae*: survival of conidia in soil. *Proceedings of the 1st International Colloquium on Invertebrate Pathology*, Kingston, Canada, 428–429.

Exploration for locust and grasshopper pathogens

C. Kooyman[1] & P. Shah[2]

[1]*Département de Formation en Protection des Végétaux, Niger:*
[2]*International Institute of Biological Control.*

Abstract
Current availability of pathogens from Orthoptera, particularly entomopathogenic fungi, and knowledge of their impact on field populations are very limited. The exploration methods for insect pathogens used in the IIBC/IITA/DFPV collaborative research programme for the biological control of locusts and grasshoppers are described. A combination of direct and indirect methods is used, including point surveys, site monitoring and networking. Yield is maximized in several ways, for example by stressing insects in cages at high densities, by exposing insects to infection from soil and by using selective media for isolation from soil. Monitoring of mortality factors over time will reveal the extent of pathogen impact on acridid populations.

Introduction

In the IIBC/IITA/DFPV collaborative research programme for the biological control of locusts and grasshoppers, the biological agents which are considered to have the greatest potential for development for control are entomopathogenic fungi in the genera *Metarhizium* and *Beauveria* (see Greathead; Prior; Lomer *et al.*, these proceedings). Much emphasis has been placed on the need to search for suitable genotypes in the environments where the target pest species occur, despite the apparent unsuitability of such hot and arid conditions for the existence of fungi. The reasons for this are two-fold.

Firstly, it is believed that isolates obtained from these environments will be better able to tolerate the harsh climatic conditions, especially high temperatures and high levels of damaging radiation, which occur in many of the areas where control must be carried out. Secondly, there are no clear guidelines at present on quarantine protocols for the movement of isolates of these fungi around the very wide geographical range over which desert locust (*Schistocerca gregaria* (Forskål)) control may be required, and it is therefore desirable to have isolates available from as wide a range of potential user countries as possible.

Although the climate in the more arid areas of Africa and Asia where grasshoppers and locusts are a problem is extremely dry for a large part of each year, favourable conditions for fungal growth do occur during the brief rainy season. These areas have been little explored for insect pathogens, and even short surveys may result in new discoveries. For example, during a six week study near Mourdiah, Mali, in 1990, a *Sorosporella* sp. (Deuteromycotina: Hyphomycetes) was found causing significant mortality in *Kraussaria angulifera* (Krauss). This fungus had not been recorded previously at this site despite several years' observations and may be a new species (P. Shah, unpublished data). Thus during a survey it is possible, and indeed likely, that new species will be discovered and it is also possible to study the impact of pathogens on populations.

Search range

The need for exploration is obvious if the first reason (above) is accepted because few isolates of entomopathogenic fungi which meet these requirements are available from existing collections. The isolates available from two major collections, the USDA Agricultural Research Service Collection of Entomopathogenic Fungi (ARSEF) and the International Mycological Institute (IMI) are listed in Table 1. The number of isolates of *Metarhizium* spp. and *Beauveria* spp. in these collections from the major outbreak areas of locusts and sahelian grasshoppers was extremely small when the project began, even if all hosts, including non-orthopterans, were included and the number of available isolates from orthopteran hosts world-wide was also very low. Although much of the sahelian zone is under-recorded in mycological collections, the same cannot be said of such habitats as rice fields where extensive collections have been made and grasshoppers are common. This suggests that infections by entomopathogenic deuteromycetes in orthopterans are either genuinely rare, or difficult to find.

The current surveys are attempting to concentrate on the areas where desert locusts are found during recession, despite the political difficulties involved in carrying out research in many of these areas: the Red Sea coast of Eritrea, Sind Province on the Pakistan–India border, the Tibesti

Table 1. Total numbers of isolates of *Metarhizium* and *Beauveria* spp. held in the collections of the United States Department of Agriculture and the International Mycological Institute (sources: Anon., 1988; Humber & Soper, 1986)

	Number of isolates held			
Species	All locations	Africa	Arabia	Pakistan/India
USDA (ARSEF)* **				
M. anisopliae var. *anisopliae* Tulloch	265	0	0	6*
Orthoptera	16	0	0	0
M. flavoviride W. Gams & J. Roszypal	45	0	0	0
Orthoptera	1	0	0	0
B. bassiana (Balsamo) Vuillemin	410	32**	0	0
Orthoptera	6	0	0	0
IMI* **				
M. anisopliae var. *anisopliae*	30	1****	0	1
Orthoptera	1	1****	0	0
M. flavoviride	0	0	0	0
Orthoptera	0	0	0	0
B. bassiana	14	0	0	0
Orthoptera	0	0	0	0

*From *Nilaparvata lugens* (Stål) (Homoptera: Delphacidae)
**From *Sitona discoideus* Gyllenhall (Coleoptera: Curculionidae)
***Only those isolates listed in Humber & Soper (1986) and Anon. (1988) are considered here: other isolates are held in Reserve (restricted access) at IMI including IMI 330189, collected by DFPV Niger in 1988 from *Ornithacris cavroisi* (Finot) (Orthoptera: Acrididae) and IMI 324673, collected by B. Nyambo in 1987 in Tanzania from *Zonocerus elegans* (Thunberg) (Orthoptera: Acrididae).
****From *Schistocerca gregaria* (Forskål) (Orthoptera: Acrididae), collected by F.L. Balfour-Browne in Ethiopia in 1959.

Mountains on the Libya–Chad border and the Tamesna region of the Ahaggar Mountains on the Niger–Algeria border have all been difficult or impossible to visit during recent years. The reasons for seeking pathogens in these areas have been discussed elsewhere (see Prior, these proceedings); it is hoped that genotypes of entomopathogenic fungi from these areas will combine virulence with the necessary ecological adaptations for survival.

Direct survey methods

Point surveys

This is the classical method of stopping at intervals along a road or a transect. Infected orthopterans are often slow and easy to catch. Those killed by fungus can occasionally be found attached to the tips of grass stems or branches: those infected by 'summit disease' (*Entomophaga grylli* (Fresenius) Batko) are commonly found in this position. Areas for survey are chosen on the grounds of previous rainfall and/or reports of high population densities. In this way, many sites can be visited increasing the chance of finding diseased insects. On the other hand, pathogen incidence is transient and there is a danger of not finding any infected cadavers.

Site monitoring

Regular sampling of chosen sites over a longer period allows a study of the development of pathogens and other natural enemies in a host population, thereby combining collection of pathogens with studies on their ecology and impact. The method is intensive and complementary to the extensive nature of point surveys: it can only be effective if prior knowledge of the site, gained by point surveys, indicates a high host population is likely.

Indirect survey methods

Networking

A network has been created within the sahelian countries and some other countries in West Africa. In each country, the national crop protection service has designated a co-ordinator from their staff, who organizes the search for pathogens by field staff and farmers (village brigades). He makes regular field trips and distributes information about collecting, preserving and sending specimens. In the beginning, there was a lack of interest in contributing to this network and this was addressed in 1991 by offering cash incentives. The co-ordinators are paid an allowance plus money to buy fuel for the field trips. People who find grasshoppers infected by a fungus are paid a reward of CFA FN 10,000 or equivalent in appropriate local currency.

Articles

A short article requesting people to send diseased grasshoppers has been sent to a number of journals with a distribution in the survey and network areas. So far, this has been published in SAS (Surveillance des Acridiens du Sahel) Bulletin of PRIFAS and by the newsletter Nouvelles de PRONAT, Dakar, Senegal. A reward is again offered to those people sending in specimens with suitable pathogens.

Maximizing the yield of pathogens

All of the methods outlined above have their shortcomings. Therefore, different methods are combined as far as possible. Obviously, the two indirect methods can be employed together with the direct ones. The extent to which one or the other of the direct methods is employed depends on local circumstances. For example, in known breeding grounds such as the Tokar Delta of Sudan where there is a high probability of finding breeding populations of desert locust, the emphasis would be on site monitoring. On the other hand, in West Africa where grasshopper populations must be examined over a very wide area, point surveys are necessary first, followed by site monitoring only when areas with a high potential for pathogen development are discovered.

Methods for improving pathogen yield include:

1. choosing sites with a history of high and/or diverse populations
2. concentrating on the more humid areas within these sites, and during the wetter parts of the year
3. capturing many grasshoppers at a site, keeping them in cages and checking for the development of symptoms of disease. By keeping densities and humidity artificially high in cages, stress will be increased and the development of incipient infections will occur more rapidly
4. baiting pathogens from the soil, using either well-proven susceptible insects such as greater wax moth larvae *Galleria mellonella* (Linnaeus) (Lepidoptera: Pyralidae) (Zimmermann, 1986) or local grasshoppers. The latter are more likely to yield pathogen genotypes with useful levels of virulence to orthopteran pests
5. direct isolation from soil, using one of the many selective agar media available (Veen & Ferron, 1966; Doberski & Tribe, 1980; Beilharz *et al.*, 1982; Chase *et al.*, 1986; Bååth, 1991; Sneh, 1991).

Conclusions

Very few methodical and extensive surveys for entomopathogenic fungi have been reported in the literature, and those isolates available in the world's collections have been obtained largely by chance. The majority of isolates have come from insects living in humid conditions, where fungal infections may often be common and the outgrowth of the sporulating mycelium on the exterior of the cadavers makes them obvious to collectors. By comparison, in dry environments no external growth occurs, and the fungal origin of infections is concealed unless the cadaver is examined internally. This lack of external symptoms may have led to an underestimation of the importance of fungal infections in dry environments. For example, two isolates of *M. flavoviride* W. Gams & I. Rozyspal held by IIBC are highly virulent to desert locusts and are under investigation in the current programme. Both were obtained from grasshoppers collected in the field (in Niger and Tanzania) where only internal growth and sporulation were observed. In the current survey programme the mortality due to these fungi in field populations in arid environments will be investigated and may be found to be higher than previously expected.

References

Anon. (1988) *Catalogue of the Culture Collection.* 9th edition. International Mycological Institute, Kew, UK.

Bååth E. (1991) Tolerance of copper by entomogenous fungi and the use of copper-amended media for isolation of entomogenous fungi from soil. *Mycological Research* **95**, 1140–1142.

Beilharz, V.C., Parbery, D.G. & Swart, H.J. (1982) Dodine: a selective agent for certain soil fungi. *Transactions of the British Mycological Society* **79**, 507–511.

Chase, A.R., Osborne, L.S. & Ferguson, V.M. (1986) Selective isolation of the entomopathogenic fungi *Beauveria bassiana* and *Metarhizium anisopliae* from an artificial potting medium. *Florida Entomologist* **69**, 285–292.

Doberski, J.W. & Tribe, H.T. (1980) Isolation of entomogenous fungi from elm bark with reference to ecology of *Beauveria bassiana* and *Metarhizium anisopliae. Transactions of the British Mycological Society* **74**, 95–100.

Humber, R.A. & Soper, R.S. (1986) *USDA-ARS Collection of Entomopathogenic Fungal Cultures: Catalogue of Strains.* USDA-ARS Plant Protection Research Unit, Boyce Thompson Institute, Ithaca, NY.

Sneh, B. (1991) Isolation of *Metarhizium anisopliae* from insects on an improved selective medium based on wheatgerm. *Journal of Invertebrate Pathology* **58**, 269–273.

Veen, K.H. & Ferron, P. (1966) A selective medium for the isolation of *Beauveria tenella* and *Metarrhizium anisopliae. Journal of Invertebrate Pathology* **8**, 268–269.

Zimmermann, G. (1986) The '*Galleria*' bait method for detection of entomopathogenic fungi in soil. *Journal of Applied Entomology* **102**, 213–215.

Panel discussion: precis

Following Dr Prior's talk, Dr Raina asked about the host range of pathogens in general compared with chemical pesticides. Dr Prior replied that there was no real comparison, as chemical pesticides are usually general poisons, whereas pathogens have an inherently much greater specificity.

Dr Milner asked Dr Charnley about the role of destruxins in host death. Dr Charnley replied that Lepidoptera muscle reacts by paralysis which can lead to death, but that this effect appears to be confined to Lepidoptera. In response to a question from Dr Goettel about synergism between insect growth regulators (IGRs) and pathogens, Dr Charnley replied that this was the subject of an ongoing research programme at Bath University, and commented that during moults the gut flora was not lost although the gut lining was replaced. Dr Charnley further commented that the activity of cuticle-degrading enzymes varied with temperature; thus any insect control systems which relied on these enzymes would be temperature-dependent in their effect. Concerning IGRs, Dr Matthews commented that the diflubenzurons were originally developed as fungicides. Was there any effect on fungal control agents? Dr Charnley replied that the second generation chitin synthesis inhibitors had very little effect on fungal spores.

Dr Lomer asked for clarification from Dr Streett of the doses of poxvirus used to kill *Oedaleus senegalensis* and he replied that 10^6 virus particles per insect caused 90% mortality, while 10^3 caused 30–50%, both in 10 days. The viruses were found in early season populations in most places searched. Infection rates varied from below 1% to 8%. Answering a question from Mr Mouhim, Dr Streett gave more details of the conditions under which the entomopox viruses were tested. Mainly US grasshopper species, not *Oedaleus senegalensis*, were used. Insects were treated in the third instar at 30°C. The virus survived for up to 8 h at 50°C.

Dr Prior called for comments on Mr Kooyman's efforts to set up a network of collaborators to look for grasshopper pathogens. Dr Castleton was very much in favour, and mentioned the SAS (Surveillance des Acridiens au Sahel) network established by PRIFAS. Network identity can be strengthened by tee-shirts, caps, etc. He also suggested the preparation of training materials to enable village brigades to be involved.

Dr Henry asked about the feasibility of infecting grasshoppers in locust breeding grounds during recessions, which could then act as reservoirs of infection. Mr Shah replied that no grasshopper or locust species were sufficiently dense in recession areas to support pathogens. Dr Milner commented that locust outbreak areas in Australia were as dry as Oman, but that rains were often dramatic and could lead to outbreaks of *Entomophaga grylli.* This implies that the spores must persist 5–7 years between rains in desert conditions. Although it is difficult to isolate spores from the soil, they must be present. Dr Goettel stressed the importance of variation in isolates, and that different isolates would be needed in different situations. He called for a free exchange of isolates between researchers. Dr Prior endorsed this, and noted the poor representation of African isolates in the world culture collections. Dr Matthews commented that most locust experts agreed that disease epidemics in swarming locusts were very rare, but that in some areas of grassland in Malawi, where small residual locust populations persist, epidemics of fungal diseases had been observed.

Section IV

Mass Production, Application and Formulation

Mass production, formulation and application of fungi as biocontrol agents

B.A. Auld

Agricultural Research & Veterinary Centre, NSW, Australia.

Abstract

Mass production, formulation and application methods are vital steps in downstream development of biopesticides but surprisingly little work has been done in these areas. While submerged culture fermentation is usually regarded as the most economical and convenient method for mass production of biopesticides by industry, it may not necessarily be so in developing countries. Various methods of liquid and solid state culture for fungi as biopesticides are described. Formulation of fungal spores or mycelium as dry powders for shelf life is well established. However the development of rehydrated propagules in liquid formulations for spraying is in the formative stages of research. The use of oils as spray supplements appears a promising means of overcoming dew or high humidity requirements for many fungi. Because of their small size fungal spores can usually be applied with conventional equipment and the range of application techniques is virtually unlimited.

Introduction

The greatest research effort in biocontrol of insects has been with viruses and bacteria although the entomopathogenic fungi are the largest group of insect pathogens. There appears to have been some reluctance to pursue fungi as biocontrol agents because of environmental limitations to their successful use (National Academy of Sciences, 1969). Such difficulties may be overcome with suitable formulations. The inability to produce many biocontrol fungi en masse has also hindered their development as biocontrol agents.

Fungi have been used in attempts to control weeds since the 1950s. Commercial mycoherbicides were produced in the USA in the early 1980s. Several candidate products are now at various stages of development.

Mass production

Submerged culture fermentation

In the developed world at least, industrial fermentation provides the simplest and most economical way to produce large numbers of fungal spores, as existing equipment can be used without modification. The commercial biocontrol agents for weed control, Collego® and Devine® are produced by this method (see Churchill, 1982; Stowell, 1991) as well as *Verticillium lecanii* (Zimmermann) Viégas (as blastospores) for control of aphids (Aphididae) (Mycotal®) and whitefly (Aleyrodidae) (Vertalec®) (Latge *et al.*, 1986) and some strains of *Beauveria bassiana* (Balsamo) Vuillemin for insect control (Thomas *et al.*, 1987).

Some fungi may sporulate even in liquid culture in flasks. Generally agitation is required to dissolve oxygen; the type of agitation may be important and the air/liquid ratio as well as the surface contact area may need to be high. Conical flasks of 50–2,000 ml may be used; the medium is sterilized with the flask, relying on a porous closure, such as cotton wool, to act as a depth filter. Flasks with side indentations to act as baffles will encourage greater turbulence and aeration. Reciprocating shakers are inferior to orbital shakers which can give high oxygen transfer rates. Reciprocating shakers tend to splash the closure, increasing the danger of contamination. Sophisticated shakers in which temperature and light are controlled may be necessary.

A pilot shaker represents the next stage up from shake flasks; it allows greater oxygen input and control as well as control of temperature, pH, agitation and foaming. Oxygen mass transfer is a major problem for aerobic processes as the solubility of oxygen in water is only about 6 ppm. Oxygen transfer can be increased by agitation which minimizes boundary layer resistance and maximizes the surface area for transfer, thus the speed and diameter of the impellor has a big influence on oxygen transfer. The diameter of the impellor should be about one-third the diameter of the reactor. Baffle plates assist turbulence, breaking up the liquid; they should be about one-tenth the diameter of the reactor. Standard industrial reactors are from 1,000 l to 800,000 l. Smaller pilot reactors cannot mimic exactly what larger reactors will do; for instance there is a marked increase in shear at impellor tips but longer mixing times as volume increases. The minimum size of pilot fermentors generally available is 1 l.

Fermentor (or Bioreactor) operation may be batch culture, semi-batch or continuous culture (e.g. see Trinci & Wiebe, 1990). Batch culture is the simplest procedure with less likelihood of contamination. The output of a product such as fungal spores generally follows a sigmoidal curve with lag, exponential, stationary, and perhaps decline, phases. The growth of product can be affected by substrate limitation and inhibition, product inhibition as well as temperature and pH. If growth is limited by the rate of solubility of an essential nutrient it will be linear; for filamentous organisms, growth in the exponential phase is reduced compared to unicellular organisms. For the latter the exponential growth phase can be described by:

$$\frac{dx}{dt} = \mu x$$

where μ is the specific growth rate (h^{-1})
x is the cell (biomass) concentration (g/l)
t is time
for filamentous organisms it is:

$$\frac{dx}{dt} = \mu x^{2/3}$$

as the cell growth is essentially in two dimensions.

Although maximum total number of product – say fungal spores – may be obtained in the stationary phase, spores harvested during the exponential phase may have a higher percentage viability. If this is the case, semi-batch (or fed batch) culture may be worthwhile.

Possibly one of the greatest problems encountered with fermentation will be contamination. Sterilization is a vital part of the process but the degree of sterility required is a function of the end use.

Media for growth of the biocontrol organism should be as simple as possible, utilizing a standard set of inorganic salts and sources of carbon and nitrogen. Production of spores in the fermentor may be enhanced by changes in media components or simply by diluting the medium (Auld *et al.*, 1988). Production may also be increased by beginning the fermentation process with a larger volume or concentration of starter culture than normal. (See Latge & Moletta (1988) for an extended treatment of the production of entomopathogenic fungi in submerged culture).

It may be necessary to screen isolates for spore productivity under fermentation conditions. The most virulent isolates may not be the most productive *in vitro*. Quantities of original single spore isolates should be stored for continued use in larger scale production because of possible loss of virulence through sub-culturing.

Recovery of spores from bioreactors may be a problem with filamentous fungi, requiring large centrifuges to spin off spores. Filtration methods often leave a large number of spores behind in the mycelial mass.

Following recovery of spores from a production process it is usually necessary to dry them for long term storage. It is not always possible to do this and retain viability of the organism. It is for this reason that the mycoherbicide Devine® is sold in liquid form like fresh milk. Drying should be done as quickly as possible under 'clean' conditions to prevent bacterial contamination. Spores may be washed during the collection process but this may reduce infectivity by removing enzymes in the matrix which surrounds many spores (McRae & Stevens, 1990). Inert materials such as kaolin, diatomaceous earth, or silica gel, may be suitable to hasten drying and to act as carriers. Contamination of the spore slurry during this stage may be a problem, so it is preferable to dry spores as quickly as possible.

Some fungi which do not sporulate in submerged culture may produce mycelium which can be dried (Pereira & Roberts, 1990) and applied as fragments or pellets in the field; among them is *Metarhizium anisopliae* (Metschnikoff) Sorokin produced by Bayer, Munich, Germany, as BIO 1020®. Such fungi may sporulate following dew (Roberts & Wraight, 1986; Rombach *et al.*, 1986; Roberts *et al.*, 1987). Walker & Connick (1983) describe the production of sodium alginate pellets of dried mycelium for a mycoherbicide.

Solid substrate fermentation

Solid substrate fermentation is widely used to produce fermented foods in Japan and elsewhere in eastern Asia. Media used contain some liquid; the 'solid' substrate itself may be relatively inert (e.g. paper, wood, vermiculite) allowing for use of defined nutrient levels. On the other hand, some nutritive solid substrates may be available locally at low costs (e.g. coffee pulp, sorghum, straw, groundnut shells). Particle size, moisture content and temperature may all need to be controlled for successful production. Equipment used may be bags, trays or rotating drums.

Industrial submerged culture fermentation production requires considerable capital investment. Production on solid media may be relatively costly in terms of labour and materials in the western industrial environment but not necessarily where labour is less costly and suitable raw material is freely available.

Beauveria bassiana has been produced on solid substrates such as heat sterilized grains in the USSR and the People's Republic of China. In the latter system 500 ml flasks of substrate are used to 'seed' 5 kg lots of steamed grain which is mixed with ten times the amount of wheat bran for fermentation in flat trays or in outdoor pits (Bartlett & Jaronski, 1988). The fungus is produced in liquid surface culture in large inflated plastic bags in Czechoslovakia (Kybal & Vilcek, 1976; Samsinakova *et al.*, 1981). Goettel (1984) has also described a technique for producing fungi using cellophane sheets on bran in autoclave bags. Abbott Laboratories in the USA have made commercial scale up tests for the fungus, using solid substrate to produce either a wettable powder or granular formulation (Bartlett & Jaronski, 1988). R.J. Milner (pers. comm. 1991) has developed a solid substrate fermentation system for *M. anisopliae* using rice, inoculating with conidia and harvesting conidia by a washing technique (Australian Patent PK3451/90).

Two phase systems

A two phase system has been used for *B. bassiana* and *M. anisopliae* production in the USSR, where mycelium produced in deep tank fermentation is allowed to sporulate in shallow open trays (Goral & Lappa, 1973; Roberts & Yendol, 1981). Walker & Riley (1982) described a similar preparation method for *Alternaria cassiae* Jurair & Khan for control of the weed *Cassia obtusifolia.* In Brazil *M. anisopliae* is produced on autoclaved rice or wheat bran in autoclavable plastic bags following inoculation with blastospores produced in liquid shake culture (Aquino *et al.*, 1975, 1977).

Bartlett & Jaronski (1988) highlight the problem of production volume. They cite typical application rates for *Beauveria* conidia per hectare as being about 1×10^{14} (however, Johnson *et al.* (these proceedings) suggest 1×10^{13} conidia/ha for *Beauveria* against grasshoppers); yields for *Beauveria* conidia obtainable from liquid surface culture are 1×10^{14} m^2, submerged liquid fermentation 3×10^{11}/l and 7×10^{12}/kg for solid substrate fermentation. Thus, if submerged liquid production were used a fermentation capacity of over 300 l would be required for each hectare treated. Apart from research on maximizing production per unit volume or area, improved formulation and application techniques may reduce the density of spores required in the field.

Formulation

Formulation has two main aims: to provide an economical and easily useable form of the active ingredient with long shelf life, and if possible to enhance the effectiveness of active ingredient. In many circumstances an aim will also be to minimize the quantity of water required. (Devisetty (1988) has recently reviewed formulations for *Bacillus thuringiensis* Berliner).

An active ingredient may be applied in the dry state as dust or granules or as a liquid or in the presence of liquid. This may be as a wettable powder, in oil, as aqueous concentrate, or emulsifiable concentrate. These concentrates are diluted by the addition of water. Other techniques such as microencapsulation will not be dealt with here, although they may have scope in the application of biocontrol agents.

Given that a biocontrol fungus can be produced en masse and dried, it can be applied as dry material or formulated as a wettable powder. In both cases clays such as kaolin, silica gel or diatomaceous earths can be used as fillers or carriers. Dusts are prepared so that particle sizes are between 3 and 50 μm in diameter; dusts are, however, vulnerable to wind. Granular formulations are less so, being mostly within the range of 0.3 to 1.0 mm diameter. Granules have been used for mycoherbicide applications by Walker & Connick (1983). Wettable powders may contain dispersing or suspending agents as well as inert fillers and wetting agents. Sodium alginate at 0.2–0.5% of final volume, for instance, will help keep some spore/clay powders in suspension. Wettable powders have been the most common form of microbial formulation (most *Bacillus thuringiensis* is sold in this form); they have advantages of each of storage and transport as well as minimal interaction between spores and other components. Moreover, given that most fungi used for plant and insect control require free water or very high humidity for infection, the provision of water at application is a logical tactic.

Spray supplements

The most important group of spray supplements are surface active agents (surfactants), which include wetting agents, emulsifiers and dispersing agents. They are characterized by having hydrophobic and hydrophilic moieties in their molecular structure. The hydrophobic moieties are generally lipophilic. The relative effect of these two parts of the molecule are described by its hydrophilic – lipophilic balance (HLB). Some examples of extreme HLB values are oleic acid (1) (lipophilic) and sodium lauryl sulphate (40) (hydrophilic). The following gives an indication of HLB values and their application: water in oil emulsifier (3–6), wetting agents (7–9), oil in water emulsifiers (8–18), detergent (13–15) (Becher, 1973). There are thousands of surface active agents produced by hundreds of manufacturers. The choice of surface active agents is apparently limitless but governed by appropriate HLB values.

In addition, sticking agents may be used to improve the adhesion of the spray. Materials used include oils, gelatine and gums. Humectants may also be used to decrease the rate of evaporation. Any solute in water will decrease its rate of evaporation, but propylene glycol and polyethylene glycol have been used specifically for this purpose. It should be noted that a supplement may act in more than one way, say as a humectant, as well as a dispersing agent.

Because many plant pathogenic fungi have a requirement for free water (or dew period) for infection, recent efforts by many mycoherbicide researchers have been directed towards overcoming this dew requirement via formulation; in particular, formulating fungal spores within the aqueous phase of an invert emulsion in oil (or oil mixtures) (Quimby *et al.*, 1989). Although the technique has been shown to overcome the need for dew in some fungi there are serious disadvantages with the method: the amount of oil required adds greatly to the cost of the product, non target contamination by oil, and the difficulty of application of the viscous material.

The lower limit for spore germination for Deuteromycetes infecting terrestrial insects is probably about 92% R.H. (Payne, 1988). The microenvironment of the surface of the insect may provide sufficiently favourable conditions in an otherwise unfavourable environment. The use of non-aqueous carriers such as oil based suspensions has been investigated by some workers (Agudelo & Falcon, 1983) and may show promise for low volume applications of *B. bassiana* (Prior *et al.*, 1988). Prior *et al.* cite work which demonstrated that *B. bassiana* does not actually require high humidity for infection but rather for the production/dispersal of conidia. Glare & Milner (in press) cite evidence for a similar situation with *M. anisopliae.*

The use of oils of vegetable origin at lower concentrations with appropriate emulsifying agents may be a profitable line of investigation. Various oils have been found to decrease inoculum thresholds for fungal infection (Rowell & Olien, 1957) and enhance mycoherbicide performance (Boyette *et al.*, 1991). The resulting mixture of oil, spores, inert carrier and water would be a suspension emulsion.

The use of microemulsions, which are thermodynamically stable transparent emulsions of very fine droplet size (< 0.1 μm), may also have a place in biocontrol formulations. Several surfactants are used to achieve low interfacial tensions. Some microemulsion formulations have already been shown to increase pesticide efficacy (Skelton *et al.*, 1988).

The sensitivity of spores to any ingredient will override other considerations and viability tests must be made continually as a formulation is developed. For instance, Soper & Ward (1981) report variation in the tolerance of *M. anisopliae* to various kaolins and Daoust *et al.* (1982) record the effect of a variety of formulations on the virulence of *M. anisopliae* against mosquito (Diptera: Culicidae) larvae.

Application

Because of their small size, fungal spores can usually be applied in suspension with conventional equipment. Matthews (1983, 1985) has discussed some particular problems and requirements for spray application in the tropics and developing regions. Obviously equipment will need to be free of residues of fungicides and any other harmful chemicals. Notwithstanding this there may be scope for the addition of low concentrations of conventional insecticides or herbicides to increase the efficacy of a fungus.

The range of techniques available for application therefore is as broad as those available for conventional pesticides and herbicides. These include high volume (about 1000 l/ha), medium (350 l/ha), low to very low volumes (3–150 l/ha), ultra low volumes (0.5–3 l/ha), controlled droplet application and electrostatic spraying. With medium and lower volumes, high powered fans are usually required; with ultra low volumes centrifugal energy may be employed. Symmons *et al.* (1989) describe a vehicular mounted spinning disc sprayer for ultra low volume applications of bendiocarb to desert locust (*Schistocerca gregaria* (Forskål)) nymphs.

Mycoinsecticides, unlike mycoherbicides, can be applied as baits. Bran baits have been a successful method for application of the protozoan *Nosema locustae* Canning for control of rangeland grasshopper (Miller, 1984). Novel methods for application of *B. bassiana* in China have been reported by Soper (1982). These included the use of mortar shells, firecrackers and landmines.

Conclusion

While there are aspects of both mass production and application of fungal pathogens for biocontrol which require a great deal of further work, it is evident that formulation is the area requiring greatest attention. The need for very high humidity or free water for many fungi to infect currently militates against their widespread use. However this requirement should be carefully checked experimentally; it does not appear necessary in *B. bassiana* and *M. anisopliae.* In any event, improved formulations might also mean that lower production per unit volume were required, and lower application concentrations could be used.

Acknowledgments

I wish to express my appreciation to IITA for the invitation to this workshop and to Dr R.J. Milner for his comments on the manuscript.

References

Agudelo, F. & Falcon, L.A. (1983) Mass production, infectivity, and field application studies with the entomogenous fungus *Paecilomyces farinosus. Journal of Invertebrate Pathology* **42**, 124–132.

Aquino, de L.M.N., Calvalcanti, V.A., Sena, R.C. & Queiroz, G.F. (1975) A new technique for the production of the fungus *Metarhizium anisopliae. Boletim Tecnico* CODECAP **4**, 1-31.

Aquino, de L.M.N., Vital, A.F., Calvalcanti, V.A. & Nascimento, M.G. (1977). Culture of *Metarhizium anisopliae* (Metchn) Sorokin in polypropylene bags. *Boletim Tecnico* CODECAP **5**, 7–11.

Auld, B.A., McRae, C.F. & Say, M.M. (1988) Potential for *Xanthium spinosum* control by *Colletotrichum orbiculare* as a mycoherbicide. In: Delfosse, E.S. (ed.) *Proceedings of the VII International Symposium on Biological Control of Weeds*, 6–11 March, Rome, Italy, pp. 435–443.

Bartlett, M.C. & Jaronski, S.T. (1988) Mass production of entomogenous fungi for biological control of insects. In: Burge, M.N. (ed.), *Fungi in Biological Control Systems*, Manchester University Press, Manchester, pp. 61–85.

Becher, P. (1973) The emulsifier. In: Van Valkenburg, W. (ed.), *Pesticide Formulations*, Marcel Dekker, New York, pp. 65–92.

Boyette, C.D., Quimby, P.C., Connick, W.J., Daigle, D.O. & Fulgham, F.E. (1991) Progress in the production, formulation and application of mycoherbicides, In: Te Beest, D.P. (ed.), *Microbial Control of Weeds*. Routledge, Chapman and Hall, New York, pp. 209–222.

Churchill, B.W. (1982) Mass production of microorganisms for biological control, In: Charudattan, R. & Walker, H.L. (eds), *Biological Control of Weeds with Plant Pathogens*. Wiley, New York, pp. 134–156.

Daoust, R.M., Ward, M.G. & Roberts, D.W. (1982) Effect of formulation on the virulence of *Metarhizium anisopliae* conidia against mosquito larvae. *Journal of Invertebrate Pathology* **40**, 228–236.

Devisetty, B.N. (1988) Microbial formulations – opportunities and challenges. *Pesticide Formulation and Application Systems* **8**, 46–64.

Glare, T.R. & Milner, R.J. (in press) Ecology of entomopathogenic fungi, In: Arora, D.K., Mukerji, K.G. and Agello, L. (eds) *Handbook of Applied Mycology* Vol II. Marcel Dekker, New York.

Goettel, M.S. (1984) A simple method for mass culturing entomopathogenic hyphomycete fungi. *Journal of Microbiological Methods* **3**, 15–20.

Goral, V.M. & Lappa, N.V. (1973) In-depth and surface culture of the green muscardine fungus. *Zashchita Rastyeni* **1**, 19.

Kybal, J. & Vilcek, V. (1976) A simple device for stationary cultivation of microorganisms. *Biotechnology and Bioengineering* **18**, 1713–1718.

Latge, J.-P. & Moletta, R. (1988) Biotechnology. In: Sampson, R.A., Evans, H.C. and Latge, J.-P. (eds). *Atlas of Entomopathogenic Fungi*. Springer-Verlag, Berlin, pp. 152–164.

Latge, J.-P., Hall, R.A., Cabrera Cabrera, R.I. & Kerwin, J.C. (1986) Liquid fermentation of entomogenous fungi, In: Sampson, T.A., Vlak, J.M. & Peters, D. (eds) *Fundamental and Applied Aspects of Invertebrate Pathology*. 4th International Colloquium of Invertebrate Pathology, Wageningen, pp. 603–606.

McRae, C.F. & Stevens, G.R. (1990) Role of conidial matrix of *Colletotrichum orbiculare* in pathogenesis of *Xanthium spinosum. Mycological Research* **94**, 890–896.

Matthews, G.A. (1983) Pesticide application technology. In: *Proceedings of the Seminar 16 Nov. 1982 Serdang, Malaysia.* MAPPS, Kuala Lumpur, pp. 163–170.

Matthews, G.A. (1985) Appropriate spraying technology for third world farmers. *World Crops* **37**, 84–85.

Miller, L.A. (1984) Recent developments in the use of insect pathogens for pest control. *Proceedings of the Fourth Australian Applied Entomological Research Conference*, Adelaide, pp. 394–404.

National Academy of Sciences (1969) *Insect Pest Management and Control. Vol. 3. Principals of Plant and Animal Pest Control.* Publication 1645, Washington, D.C.

Payne, C.C. (1988) Pathogens for the control of insects: where next? *Philosophical Transactions of the Royal Society of London* B **318**, 225–248.

Pereira, R.M. & Roberts, D.W. (1990) Dry mycelium preparations of entomopathogenic fungi *Metarhizium anisopliae* and *Beauveria bassiana*. *Journal of Invertebrate Pathology* **56**, 39–46.

Prior, C., Jollands, P. & Le Patourel, G. (1988) Infectivity of oil and water formulations of *Beauveria bassiana* (Deuteromycotina: Hyphomycetes) to the cocoa weevil pest *Pantorhytes plutus* (Coleoptera: Curculionidae). *Journal of Invertebrate Pathology* **52**, 66–72.

Quimby, P.C., Fulgham, F.E., Boyette, C.D. & Connick, W.J. (1989) An invert emulsion replaces dew in biocontrol of sicklepod – a preliminary study. *Pesticide Formulations and Application Systems* **8**, 264–270.

Roberts, D.W. & Wraight, S.P. (1986) Current status on the use of insect pathogens as biocontrol agents in agriculture: fungi. In: Sampson, T.A., Vlak, J.M. & Peters, D. (eds), *Fundamental and Applied Aspects of Invertebrate Pathology.* 4th International Colloquium of Invertebrate Pathology, Wageningen, pp. 510–513.

Roberts, D.W. & Yendol, W. (1981) Use of fungi for microbial control of insects. In: Burges, H.D. & Hussey, N.W. (eds), *Microbial Control of Insects and Mites.* Academic Press, New York, pp. 125–149.

Roberts, D.W., Dunn, H.M., Ramsay, G., Sweeney, A.W., Dunn, N.W., McCabe, B. & Soper, R.S. (1987) A procedure for preservation of the mosquito pathogen. *Culicinomyces clavisporus. Applied Microbiology and Biotechnology* **26**, 186–188.

Rombach, M.C., Aguda, R.M. & Roberts, D.W. (1986) Biological control of the brown planthopper, *Nilaparvata lugens* (Homoptera: Delphacidae) with dry mycelium applications of *Metarhizium anisopliae* (Deuteromycotina: Hyphomycetes). *Philippine Entomologist* **6**, 613–619.

Rowell, J.B. & Olien, C.R. (1957) Controlled inoculation of wheat seedlings with uredospores of *Puccinia graminis* var. *tritici*. *Phytopathology* **47**, 650–655.

Samsinakova, A., Kalalova, S., Vlcek, V. & Kybal, J. (1981) Mass production of *Beauveria bassiana* for regulation of *Leptinotarsa decemlineata* populations. *Journal of Invertebrate Pathology* **38**, 169–174.

Skelton, P.R., Munk, B.H. & Collins, H.M. (1988) Formulation of pesticide microemulsions. *Pesticide Formulation and Application Systems* **8**, 36–45.

Soper, R.S. (1982) Commercial mycoinsecticides. *Proceedings 3rd International Colloquium on Invertebrate Pathology*, 98–102.

Soper, R.S. & Ward, M.G. (1981) Production, formulation, and application of fungi for insect control. In: Papavizas, G.E. (ed.), *Biological Control in Crop Production.* Allanheld and Osmun, Totowa, pp. 161–180.

Stowell, L.J. (1991) Submerged fermentation of biological herbicides. In: Te Beest,

D.O. (ed.), *Microbial Control of Weeds.* Routledge, Chapman & Hall, New York, pp. 225–261.

Symmons, P.M., Boase, C.J., Clayton, J.S. & Gorta, M. (1989) Controlling desert locust nymphs with bendiocarb applied by a vehicle-mounted spinning disc sprayer. *Crop Protection* **8**, 324–331.

Thomas, K.C., Khachatourians, G.G. & Ingleden, W.M. (1987) Production and properties of *Beauveria bassiana* conidia cultivated in submerged culture. *Canadian Journal of Microbiology* **33**, 12–20.

Trinci, A.P.J. & Wiebe, M.G. (1990) Production of fungal biomass and fungal spores in continuous and fed-batch culture. *Aspects of Applied Biology* **24**, 255–261.

Walker, H.L. & Connick, W.J. (1983) Sodium alginate for production and formulation of mycoherbicides. *Weed Science* **31**, 333–338.

Walker, H.L. & Riley, J.A. (1982) Evaluation of *Alternaria cassiae* for the biocontrol of sicklepod (*Cassia obtusifolia*). *Weed Science* **30**, 651–654.

Mass production, formulation and field application of entomopathogenic fungi

M.S. Goettel[1] & D.W. Roberts[2]

[1]*Agriculture Canada Research Station, Lethbridge, Alberta:*
[2]*Insect Pathology Resource Centre, Boyce Thompson Institute, USA.*

Abstract
Successful use of entomopathogenic fungi as microbial control agents of insects will ultimately depend on the use of the right propagule, formulated in an optimum fashion and applied in the field at the right time. For this to be accomplished, detailed knowledge of the host-pathogen interactions and epizootiology is critical. Research and development must then concentrate on developing a method of mass production, formulation, and application, that retains the ability of the pathogen to kill its host. In this brief review, the presently available methods for mass production, formulation, and field application of entomopathogenic fungi are presented. Methods for mass production are *in vivo*, submerged culture, and surface culture. A major current limitation is the lack of readily available formulation technology. Consequently, formulation is frequently simple or nonexistent. Since fungal propagules are microscopic, most can be applied as conventional chemical insecticides; however, since we are dealing with a system involving two living organisms, application methods have to take into consideration the multitude of factors that may affect host-pathogen relationships.

Introduction

Successful development of a pathogen as a microbial insecticide depends on many factors. Not only must the pathogen be virulent against its intended host, but it must also be produced in large quantities, formulated in a way so as to optimize its storage, application, and virulence characteristics, and it must be applied in the field in an economical and efficacious way. For *Bacillus thuringiensis* Berliner, the attributes of the pathogen have made development relatively easy; fungi on the other hand, are proving more difficult.

Recent reviews on development of fungi for pest control include those of Hall & Papierok (1982), Lisansky & Hall (1982), Latge & Moletta (1988), McCoy *et al.* (1988) and McCoy (1990); reviews on mass production include Soper & Ward (1981) and Bartlett & Jaronski (1988); and reviews on formulation include Soper & Ward (1981), Sawicka & Couch (1983), Most & Quinlan (1986) and Baker & Henis (1990).

In the present paper, we review the production, formulation, and application of entomopathogenic fungi with particular emphasis on how these relate to grasshopper control.

Mass production

Although some potentially useful entomopathogenic fungi are difficult to mass produce, the great majority grow profusely on very simple, inexpensive media. There are several methods available for the mass production of entomopathogenic fungi; *in vivo*, surface, and submerged culture. The method used depends largely on the growth requirements of the fungus in question and the end product desired.

Production *in vivo*

Many obligate entomopathogenic fungi have complex nutritional requirements and are very difficult, if not impossible, to grow in artificial culture. Therefore, the only alternative is to propagate these fungi *in vivo* (Ignoffo & Hink, 1971). However, *in vivo* production is relatively expensive and it is doubtful this method could ever be used economically for mass production of a fungus for use as a microbial insecticide. It must not be disregarded altogether, as commercial production of several grasshopper microbial insecticides is based on the *in vivo* production of *Nosema locustae* Canning.

In vivo production could be used for dissemination of a fungus in a programme of classical or inoculative control; *in vivo* produced inoculum could be introduced into an area where it does not occur or to induce an epizootic at a time when it would not normally occur. For instance, there is still potential for classical biological control through introduction of fungal strains or species from other geographical areas.

Entomophaga grylli (Fresenius) Batko, a fungus responsible for numerous epizootics in grasshoppers worldwide (Skaife, 1925; Pickford & Riegert, 1964; Roffey, 1968; Milner, 1978; Erlandson *et al.*, 1988), is an example of a fungus which, although it can be grown *in vitro* as protoplasts (MacLeod *et al.*, 1980), produces infective stages only *in vivo.* Successful use of this fungus as a microbial insecticide would require mass production *in vivo.* However, there is still potential in using *E. grylli* for classical biological control; recent work by Carruthers *et al.* (1991) is aimed at exploiting in the USA a particularly virulent pathotype of *E. grylli* imported from Australia.

Submerged culture

Most technology for mass culture of fungi has been developed towards harvesting fungal metabolites using submerged liquid fermentation; however, few entomopathogenic fungi produce infectious propagules in submerged culture. Some exceptions are *Culicinomyces clavisporus* Couch, Romney & Rao (Roberts & Sweeney, 1982), and selected strains of *Aspergillus ochraceus* Wilhelm (Vezina *et al.*, 1965), *Beauveria bassiana* (Balsamo) Vuillemin (Thomas *et al.*, 1987; Rombach *et al.*, 1988; Hegedus *et al.*, 1990) and *Hirsutella thompsonii* Fisher (Van Winkelhoff & McCoy, 1984) which produce conidia in submerged culture; however, these conidia are usually less virulent and are shorter-lived than surface-produced ones (Roberts & Sweeney, 1982). Much more research is needed before this method can be adopted for mass production of conidia of many entomopathogenic fungi.

Most hyphomycetous fungi produce blastospores in submerged culture. Blastospores are short-lived and, consequently, have generally not been adopted for field application (Ferron, 1981; Roberts & Humber, 1981). An exception is *Verticillium lecanii* (Zimmermann) Viégas which has been used successfully as a dried blastospore preparation for control of greenhouse whiteflies and aphids (Lisansky & Hall, 1982). In this case, much of the mortality actually occurs from infection by conidia which develop after the formulation has been applied to the plant surface.

A recent breakthrough has been the development of a method for producing dry, viable mycelium which can be stored under refrigeration (McCabe & Soper, 1985; Andersch *et al.*, 1990). When introduced in the field, particles of dry mycelium rapidly produce infectious conidia following rehydration from dew, rain, or soil moisture. This method can be used with many species of fungi including *Metarhizium anisopliae* (Metschnikoff) Sorokin and *B. bassiana* (Pereira & Roberts, 1990) and has been successfully field tested (Rombach *et al.* 1986a, 1986b, 1988), and a commercial product, Bayer 1020, developed.

Submerged fermentation is most often used in a diphasic method of production; blastospores and mycelia are produced in submerged culture and then transferred to surface culture for production of conidia.

Surface culture

Many fungi grow profusely on damp solid media and produce conidia aerially. Surface culture on solid or semi-solid media is usually best suited for these fungi which include many species in the class Hyphomycetes. *M. anisopliae* is produced commercially in Brazil for control of the sugar spittle bug (*Mahanarva posticata* (Stål)). The fungus is grown on sterilized rice in autoclavable polyethylene bags for 15 to 20 days, dehydrated at 25°C and 35% RH for 72 h, and then milled to obtain a conidial powder (Aquino *et al.*, 1975, 1977; Mendonça, these proceedings). Surface culture methods were developed by Goettel (1984) to produce conidia of several Hyphomycetes, including *B. bassiana*, on bran and by Daoust & Roberts (1983) to produce conidia of *M. anisopliae* on rice.

Mass production of *B. bassiana* using surface culture has been in progress for many years in the USSR and the People's Republic of China. For example, 22 t of Boverin (*B. bassiana* plus inert ingredients) has been produced in a year from a pilot plant in the USSR (Ferron, 1981). In the People's Republic of China conidia are produced on wheat bran, rice powder, compost, or ground corn stalks in flat trays, glass crocks or shallow outdoor pits (Hussey & Tinsley, 1981).

A unique method of surface culture using liquid media has been developed for *B. bassiana* in Czechoslovakia (Kybal & Vlcek, 1976; Samsinakova *et al.*, 1981). Sporulation takes place on the liquid surface in large, inflated plastic tubes. The conidia are harvested by draining the liquid once conidiation is completed.

In the western world, there has been relatively little commercial interest in mass production of *B. bassiana* despite many research programmes involved in the development of this fungus as a microbial control agent. Abbott Laboratories was developing methods for commercial scale-up of *B. bassiana* in the USA, but this programme has recently been abandoned (S.T. Jaronski, pers. comm.).

A recent breakthrough has been the development of a solid culture process for *B. bassiana* by Mycotech Corporation, Butte, MT, (Bradley *et al.*, in press). The process uses a packed bed, solid culture system. A liquid phase is absorbed in a starch-based culture substrate. The gaseous phase remains in the interparticle spaces and the fungus growing on the substrate particles is aerated directly from the gas phase. Using this technique, Mycotech has produced *B. bassiana* at small pilot scale with yields of 10^{13} conidia with fermentor volumes of less than 1 l. Dry conidia powders contain up to 10^{11} spores/g. This process has also been used for production of *Paecilomyces farinosus, P. canadensis, Nomuraea rileyi* (Farlow) Samson, and *H. thompsonii* and could probably be used for production of most species of hyphomycetous entomopathogenic fungi.

Formulation

A major current limitation in the development of fungi for insect control is the lack of readily available formulation technology. Formulation is frequently simple or nonexistent. Yet, it is through formulation that improved shelf life, persistence, efficacy, and field targeting could be achieved. However, formulating entomopathogenic fungi is in its infancy and poses a very complex challenge. The little technology that does exist is usually proprietary information.

Formulations of fungi may incorporate additives such as wetters, stickers, humectants, UV protectants, and thixotropic agents. Types of formulation include dust, granular, wettable powder, liquid, and flowable formulations. The choice of formulation must ultimately be chosen on the basis of mode of infection, target host habitat, and application method.

B. bassiana has been successfully formulated for grasshopper control in wheat bran baits and oil. However, field results are inconsistent and further studies of formulation effects on host pathogen relationships are needed (see Johnson *et al.*, these proceedings).

Application

Since fungal propagules are microscopic, most can be applied as conventional chemical insecticides. It is somehow perceived that, if enough inoculum is applied, ultimately the hosts will succumb. However, this may be reason why we have not progressed sufficiently in successful field application of entomopathogenic fungi; too much emphasis has been placed on formulating products which can be applied using methodology developed for chemical insecticides and not enough attention has been placed on host-pathogen relationships. Since we are dealing with a system involving two living organisms (i.e. the host and its pathogen), application methods have to take into consideration the multitude of factors that may affect host-pathogen relationships, sunlight, temperature, humidity, host age, inoculum targeting, etc. The method of application is, of course, dependent on the type of formulation available. Since very few formulations are available, most preliminary field testing is done with an unformulated, or crudely formulated active ingredient. However, it is difficult to justify allocating many resources to formulation development unless the active ingredient has been shown to be effective in the field.

Field application must target the inoculum to the host. Since, for the most part, entomopathogenic fungi infect via the external cuticle, the propagule must come into contact with the insect cuticle. Consequently, even subtle differences in host behaviour may greatly affect the efficacy of an application method. For instance, two species of aphid, *Myzus persicae* (Sulzer) and *Aphis gossypii* Glover, are equally susceptible to *V. lecanii*; however, control of *A. gossypii* was markedly less than that of *M. persicae* when *V. lecanii* was applied according to the manufacturer's recommendations (Hall & Papierok, 1982). This effect was attributed to the higher mobility of *M. persicae* resulting in contact with the fungal spores. This lack of adequate control of *A. gossypii* was overcome by the application of the fungus using a low-volume electrostatic rotary atomizer which optimized deposition of spores on the aphids (Sopp *et al.*, 1989).

B. bassiana produced using Mycotech's surface culture method has been formulated as bran bait or oil formulation (Johnson *et al.*, these proceedings). Oil-formulated conidia can be dispersed in 30–300 μm droplet sizes using hand-held low-volume spinning disc sprayers. Microscopic observation confirmed even distribution of viable conidia in oil droplets. Application rate of 10^{13} spores/ha can be applied in a total volume of 3 l. Although grasshoppers succumb to both formulations in laboratory assays, field trials have given inconsistent results (Johnson *et al.*, these proceedings).

Conclusions

Successful use of entomopathogenic fungi will ultimately depend on the use of the right propagule, formulated in an optimum fashion, and applied in the field at the right time. For this to be accomplished, detailed knowledge of the host-pathogen interactions and epizootiology is critical. Research and development must then concentrate on developing a method of mass production, formulation, and application that retains the ability of the pathogen to kill its host.

References

Andersch, W., Hartwig, J., Reinecke, P. & Stenzel, K. (1990) Production of mycelial granules of the entomopathogenic fungus *Metarhizium anisopliae* for biological control of soil pests. *Proceedings of the 5th International Colloquium on Invertebrate Pathology and Microbial Control*, Adelaide 20–24 August 1990, 2–5.

Aquino, de M., Cavalcanti, V.A., Sena, R.C. & Queiroz, G.F. (1975) Nova técnologia de multiplicacao do fungo *Metarhizium anisopliae. Boletim Técnico CODE-CAP, Recife* **4**, 1.

Aquino, de M., Vital, A.E., Cavalcanti, V.A. & Nascimento, M.G. (1977) Cultura de *Metarhizium anisopliae* (Metsch.) Sorokin em sacos de polipropileno. *Boletim Tecnico Executivo do Defesa Fitossanitaria da Lavoura Canaviera de Pernambuco* **5**, 11.

Baker, C.A. & Henis, J.M.S. (1990) Commercial production and formulation of microbial biocontrol agents. In: Baker, R.R. (ed.), *New Directions in Biological Control: Alternatives for Suppressing Agricultural Pests and Diseases.* Alan R. Liss, New York, pp. 333–344.

Bartlett, M.C. & Jaronski, S.T. (1988) Mass production of entomogenous fungi for biological control of insects. In: Burge, M.N. (ed.), *Fungi in Biological Control Systems.* Manchester University Press, Manchester, pp. 61–85.

Bradley, C., Black, W., Kearns, R. & Woods, P. (in press). The role of production technology in mycoinsecticide development. *Mycological Society of America Symposium on Industrial Mycology,* Madison, WI, June 1990.

Carruthers, R.I., Humber, R.A. & Ramos, M.E. (1991) Development of *Entomophaga grylli* as a biological agent of grasshoppers. In: *Cooperative Grasshopper Integrated Pest Management Project 1990 Annual Report.* USDA, APHIS TPQ-Boise, Idaho, Boise, Idaho, pp. 220–231.

Daoust, R.A. & Roberts, D.W. (1983) Studies on the prolonged storage of *Metarhizium anisopliae* conidia: effect of temperature and relative humidity on conidial viability and virulence against mosquitoes. *Journal of Invertebrate Pathology* **41**, 143–150.

Erlandson, M.A., Johnson, D.L. & Olfert, O.O. (1988) *Entomophaga grylli* (Fresenius) infections in grasshopper (Orthoptera: Acrididae) populations in Saskatchewan and Alberta, 1985–1986. *Canadian Entomologist* **120**, 205–209.

Ferron, P. (1981) Pest control by the fungi *Beauveria* and *Metarhizium.* In: Burges, H.D. (ed.), *Microbial Control of Pests and Plant Diseases 1970–1980.* Academic Press, London, pp. 465–482.

Goettel, M.S. (1984) A simple method for mass culturing entomopathogenic Hyphomycete fungi. *Journal of Microbiological Methods* **3**, 15–20.

Hall, R.A. & Papierok, B. (1982) Fungi as biological control agents of arthropods of agricultural and medical importance. *Parasitology* **84**, 205–240.

Hegedus, D.D., Bidochka, M.J. & Khachatourians, G.G. (1990) *Beauveria bassiana* submerged conidia production in a defined medium containing chitin, two hexosamines or glucose. *Applied Microbiology and Biotechnology* **33**, 641–647.

Hussey, N.W. & Tinsley, T.W. (1981) Impressions of insect pathology in the People's Republic of China. In: Burges, H.D. (ed.), *Microbial Control of Pests and Plant Diseases 1970–1980.* Academic Press, London, pp. 785–795.

Ignoffo, C.M. & Hink, W.F. (1971) Propagation of arthropod pathogens in living systems. In: Burges, H.D. & Hussey, N.W. (eds), *Microbial Control of Insects and Mites.* Academic Press, New York, pp. 541–580.

Kybal, J. & Vlcek, V. (1976) A simple device for stationary cultivation of microorganisms. *Biotechnology and Bioengineering* **18**, 1713–1718.

Latge, J.-P. & Moletta, R. (1988) Biotechnology. In: Samson, R.A., Evans, H.C. & Latge, J.-P. (eds), *Atlas of Entomopathogenic Fungi.* Springer-Verlag, Berlin, pp. 152–164.

Lisansky, S.G. & Hall, R.A. (1982) Fungal control of insects. In: Smith, J.E., Berry, P.R. & Kristonson, B. (eds), *The Filamentous Fungi,* Edward Arnold, London, pp. 127–345.

McCabe, D. & Soper, R.S. (1985) Preparation of an entomopathogenic fungal insect control agent. United States Patent 4, 530, 834.

McCoy, C.W. (1990) Entomogenous fungi as microbial pesticides. In: Baker, R.R. (ed.), *New Directions in Biological Control: Alternatives for Suppressing Agricultural Pests and Diseases.* Alan R. Liss, Inc., New York, pp. 139–159.

McCoy, C.W., Samson, R.A. & Boucias, D.G. (1988) Entomogenous fungi. In: Ignoffo, C.M. & Bushan Mandava, N. (eds), *CRC Handbook of Natural Pesticides: Vol. V, Microbial Insecticides: Part A, Entomogenous Protozoa and Fungi.* CRC press, Boca Raton, pp. 151–236.

MacLeod, D.M., Tyrrell, D. & Welton, M.A. (1980) Isolation and growth of the grasshopper pathogen, *Entomophthora grylli. Journal of Invertebrate Pathology,* **36**, 85–89.

Milner, R.J. (1978) On the occurrence of *Entomophthora grylli*, a fungal pathogen of grasshoppers in Australia. *Journal of the Australian Entomological Society* **17**, 293–296.

Most, B.H. & Quinlan, R.J. (1986) Formulation of biological pesticides. In: Samson, R.A., Vlak, J.M. & Peters, D. (eds), *Fundamental and Applied Aspects of Invertebrate Pathology.* Foundation of the 4th International Colloquim of Invertebrate Pathology, Wageningen, pp. 624–627.

Pereira, R.M. & Roberts, D.W. (1990) Dry mycelium preparations of entomopathogenic fungi, *Metarhizium anisopliae* and *Beauveria bassiana. Journal of Invertebrate Pathology* **56**, 39–46.

Pickford, R. & Riegert, P.W. (1964) The fungous disease caused by *Entomophthora grylli* Fres., and its effects on grasshopper populations in Saskatchewan in 1963. *Canadian Entomologist* **96**, 1158–1166.

Roberts, D.W. & Humber, R.A. (1981) Entomogenous fungi. In: Cole, G.T. & Kendrick, B. (eds), *Biology of Conidial Fungi.* Vol. 2. Academic Press, Inc., New York, pp. 201–236.

Roberts, D.W. & Sweeney, A.W. (1982) Production of Fungi Imperfecti with vector control potential. In: *Invertebrate Pathology and Microbial Control. Proceedings 3rd International Colloquium on Invertebrate Pathology,* University of Sussex, 6–10 September 1982, pp. 409–413.

Roffey, J. (1968) The occurrence of the fungus *Entomophthora grylli* Fres. on locusts and grasshoppers in Thailand. *Journal of Invertebrate Pathology* **11**, 237.

Rombach, M.C., Aguda, R.M. & Roberts, D.W. (1986a) Biological control of the brown planthopper, *Nilaparvata lugens* (Homoptera Delphacidae) with dry mycelium applications of *Metarhizium anisopliae* (Deuteromycotina: Hyphomycetes). *Philippine Entomologist* **6**, 613–619.

Rombach, M.C., Aguda, R.M., Shepard, B.M. & Roberts, D.W. (1986b) Infection of rice brown planthopper, *Nilaparvata lugens* (Homoptera: Delphacidae), by field application of entomopathogenic hyphomycetes (Deuteromycotina). *Environmental Entomology* **15**, 1070–1073.

Rombach, M.C., Aguda, R.M. & Roberts, D.W. (1988) Production of *Beauveria bassiana* (Deuteromycotina: Hyphomycetes) in different liquid media and subsequent conidiation of dry mycelium. *Entomophaga* **33**, 315–324.

Samsinakova, A., Kalalova, S., Vlcek, V. & Kybal, J. (1981) Mass production of *Beauveria bassiana* for regulation of *Leptinotarsa decemlineata* populations. *Journal of Invertebrate Pathology* **38**, 169–174.

Sawicka, E.M. & Couch, T.L. (1983) Formulations of entomopathogens. In: Kaneko, T.M. & Akesson, N.B. (eds), *Pesticide Formulations and Application Systems: Third Symposium, ASTM STP 828.* American Society Testing and Materials, Philadelphia, pp. 5–11.

Skaife, S.H. (1925) The locust fungus *Empusa grylli* and its effect on its host. *South African Journal of Science,* **22**, 298–308.

Soper, R.S. & Ward, M.G. (1981) Production, formulation and application of fungi for insect control. In: Papavizas, G.C. (ed.), *Biological Control in Crop Protection,* Allanheld & Osmun, Totowa, pp. 161–180.

Sopp, P.I., Gillespie, A.T. & Palmer, A. (1989) Application of *Verticillium lecanii* for the control of *Aphis gossypii* by a low-volume electrostatic rotary atomiser and a high-volume hydraulic sprayer. *Entomophaga* **34**, 417–428.

Thomas, K.C., Khachatourians, G.G. & Ingledew, W.M. (1987) Production and properties of *Beauveria bassiana* conidia cultivated in submerged culture. *Canadian Journal of Microbiology* **33**, 12–20.

Van Winkelhoff, A.J. & McCoy, C.W. (1984) Conidiation of *Hirsutella thompsonii* var. *synnematosa* in submerged culture. *Journal of Invertebrate Pathology* **43**, 59.

Vezina, C., Singh, K. & Seghal, S.N. (1965) Sporulation of filamentous fungi in submerged culture. *Mycologia* **57**, 722.

Mass production, application and formulation of *Metarhizium anisopliae* for control of sugarcane froghopper, *Mahanarva posticata*, in Brazil

A.F. Mendonça

Alagoas State Federal University, Brazil.

Abstract

The fungus *Metarhizium anisopliae* (Metschnikoff) Sorokin is used for the control of sugarcane froghopper, *Mahanarva posticata* (Stål) (Homoptera; Cercopidae), on a large scale in Brazil. The present article discusses the background to early work on the fungus, current mass production, substrates and techniques, quality control, formulation, and application.

Introduction

Epizootics of the fungus *Metarhizium anisopliae* (Metschnikoff) Sorokin on the sugarcane froghopper, *Mahanarva posticata* (Stål) (Homoptera: Cercopidae) were first reported in the region of Campos, Rio de Janeiro, in 1964 by Guagliumi (1973).

In the 1960s, with the spread of *M. posticata*, the Commission for the Control of the Cane froghopper in the states of Alagoas and Pernambuco (CCCEAP) was set up to deal with this pest, principally using insecticides. In 1969, during a search for biological control agents, a natural epizootic of *Metarhizium anisopliae* in the root froghopper, *Mahanarva fimbriolata* (Stål) was observed by the author and E.J. Marques. With the collaboration of Maria de Lourdes Aquino of the Agronomical Research Institute (IPA), the first isolation, laboratory culture and experimental applications were carried out.

In 1970, mass production and large-scale application were begun in Alagoas and Pernambuco. Several other Brazilian research organizations became involved in research on the utilization of *Metarhizium anisopliae* including IAA-PLANALSUCAR and EMBRAPA/CENARGEM.

Mass production – substrates

Liquid media

The use of liquid media for mass production of entomopathogenic fungi is still at an experimental stage. A medium based on molasses, soya flour and mineral salts gave low spore yields (Alves, 1983). Cruz *et al.* (1983) demonstrated satisfactory sporulation in media containing bean broth. In Cuba, 10^{11} spores/l of *Beauveria bassiana* (Balsamo) Vuillemin have been produced in floating cultivation on a medium containing the following ingredients;

Molasses	20–50 g/l
Ammonium phosphate	3 g/l
Copper sulphate ($7H_2O$)	0.5 g/l

Solid media

Rice has been the most commonly used substrate for the mass production of *M. anisopliae* and *B. bassiana* in Brazil. Yields of fungus vary from 10 to 14% of the substrate weight, depending on the quality of the rice. Corn (raw and triturated), potato, beans, sorghums and soya were also tested; all gave lower yields than rice.

Mass production techniques

Various mass production methods have been investigated in Brazil; in this paper, we will only consider those methods currently in use, or likely to be used in the future.

Production in wide-mouthed glass bottles

This method has been widely used in the north-east of Brazil since 1969 for the mass production of *M. anisopliae*, and, on a smaller scale, *B. bassiana.* Currently, this method is not so widely used due to the high cost and difficulty of replacing the bottles.

The following stages are followed:

1. isolation, purification and characterization of the fungus to be produced
2. preparation of the fungus strain inoculum
3. preparation of the inoculum suspensions in 800 ml Roux flasks
4. preparation of the rice medium
5. inoculation of the 500 ml flasks for mass production
6. germination and growth
7. sifting and storage of spores.

This method usually gives a final yield of 10% conidia, but it can be as high as 16%. Contamination does not normally exceed 5% of the bottles. The residual rice is not used again in the laboratory; it is often used in the field in granulated form as an additional source of inoculum (Marques *et al.*, 1981; Mendonca & Rocha, 1987).

Production in plastic bags

This method, using polypropylene plastic bags, is currently the most widely used means of producing *M. anisopliae.* It is also used for the production of *B. bassiana*; in both cases, rice is used as the substrate.

Stages 1 to 4 are identical to those mentioned above:

5. preparation and inoculation of plastic bags
6. germination and growth
7. storage of the bags with fungus.

This method yields 10% of fungus, up to 10^{10} spores/g (Aquino *et al.*, 1977; Mendonca & Rocha, 1987).

With the intention of reducing costs, Biotech (Controle Biologico Ltda) in the state of Alagoas, introduced some innovations in the plastic bag technique, as follows:

1. use of pre-soaked rice instead of dry rice. Yield is increased by enlarging the rice grains and thus increasing their surface area, resulting in economies of up to 50% in the amount of rice used
2. reduction in the size of bags from 40 × 25 × 0.1 cm to 35 × 22 × 0.1 cm with an economy of 20%
3. use of 300 or 400 g of rice per bag instead of 200 g, providing a gain of 50% in the number of bags used.

With these changes, and using the isolate PL 43 of *M. anisopliae*, an average yield of at least 10^{10} spores/g of rice is obtained.

Production in trays (Biomax method)

Developed by the Labormax Produtos Quimicos Ind. e Com. Ltda., in São Paulo, this method is no longer used due to the serious problem of contamination. In Cuba, a similar system is used for the production of *B. bassiana* on barley substrate.

Stages 1 to 4 are the same as those mentioned above (Alves, 1983).

5. preparation and inoculation of the trays
6. germination
7. sifting in vibratory sieve
8. quality control and formulation.

This system shows an average yield of around 8.5%.

Quality control

The mass production of a pathogen requires rigorous quality control. The following factors need to be taken into account when selecting a strain for production; pathogenicity (LD_{50}), conidia production, ultra-violet resistance, conidia viability, etc.

During production, the following quality control tests are carried out at IAA-PLANALSUCAR.

Conidial concentration

Weigh 0.1 or 1 g of the end product; prepare an aqueous suspension containing a dispersant. The number of conidia/ml is determined using a Neubauer chamber. The number of conidia/ml times the volume of dilution will give the number of conidia/g.

Conidial viability

PDA petri dishes plus antibiotic are prepared, conidial suspension is added and the plates incubated for 18–20 hours. 500 spores are checked in two dishes. This test is carried out 0, 30, 45, 60, 75 and 90 days after the fungus is produced. The result is given as a germination percentage.

Purity

Ten microlitres of conidial suspension at a known dilution (500 to 1,000 conidia/10 ml is pipetted on to five dishes of PDA with antibiotic and five without. After four to five days incubation at 27 to 28°C, the colonies of *M. anisopliae* are counted as well as those of contaminating bacteria. The result is given as a percentage of purity.

Virulence (relative dose response)

The LT_{50} of the test strain and the standard is determined by bioassay in the test insect. The relative response (RDR) is determined as follows:

$$RDR = \frac{LT_{50} \text{ of standard}}{LT_{50} \text{ of test fungus.}}$$

Formulation and application

The application of *M. anisopliae* for the control of *Mahanarva posticata* froghopper has generally been carried out using an aqueous suspension obtained by washing the rice and fungus with water. The application rate is 200 g of conidia/ha, corresponding to approximately 10^{12} conidia/ha.

Around 1975, a product called Metaquino was developed in the state of Pernambuco, in which the rice and conidia were ground to a powder. This product was suspended in water at the time of application (Aquino *et al.*, 1975).

Biotech recommends an application rate of 10^{13} conidia/ha. This corresponds to the average production from 10 plastic bags, and this higher dose gives better control in a shorter time (Mendonca & Rocha, 1988).

The volume of suspension applied/ha varies according to the application equipment used:

Ground application	
— back-pack sprayer	400 l/ha
— animal-drawn sprayer	200 l/ha
— motorized sprayer	50 l/ha
Aerial application	20 l/ha

During periods of high fungus production, the residual rice following conidial separation is commonly used as an additional source of inoculum, applied by plane.

The production programme installed in the north-east of Brazil has produced over 50 t of *Metarhizium anisopliae* since 1977. More than 600,000 ha of sugarcane has been treated with this material, making this the biggest microbial control project in the world using *M. anisopliae.*

References

Alves, S.B. (1983) Producao de fungos entomopatogenicos. In: Alves, S.B. (ed.), *Controle Microbiano de Insectos* Manole Ltd., São Paulo, Cap. III - 17, pp. 311–323.

Aquino, M.L.N., Cavalcanti, V.A.L.B., Sena, R.C. & Queiros, G.F. (1975) Nova technologia de multiplicacao do fungo *Metarhizium anisopliae. Boletim Technico CODECAP, Recife* **no. 4**, 29 pp.

Aquino, M.L.N., Vital, A.F. & Cavalcanti, V.L.B. (1977) Cultura de *Metarhizium anisopliae* (Metsch.) Sorokin em sacos de polipropileno. *Boletim Técnico CODECAP, Recife,* **no. 5**, 11 pp.

Cruz, B.P.B., Abreu, O.C., Oliveira, D.A. & Chiba, S. (1983) Crescimento de *Metarhizium anisopliae* (Metsch.) Sorok. em meios de cultura naturais, liquidos. *Biologico (São Paulo)* **49**, 111–116.

Guagluimi, P. (1973) *Pragas da Cana d-Acucar: Nordeste do Brasil.* Rio de Janeiro, IAA. (Colecão canavieira, 10).

Marques, E.J., Vilas Boas, A.M. & Pereira, C.E.F. (1981) Orientacoes technicas para a producao do fungo entomogeno *Metarhizium anisopliae* (Metschn.) em laboratorios setoriais. *Boletim Tecnico PLANALSUCAR,* Piracicaba **3**, 5–23.

Mendonça, A.F. & Rocha, I.C.B. (1987) Laboratorio de producao de fungo *Metarhizium anisopliae* – Usina Vassoura, Sergipe. *BIOTECH – Maceio,* pp. 22. (Projeto Tecnico).

Mendonça, A.F. & Rocha, I.C.B. (1988) Inovaciones technológicas en la produción de fungo *Metarhizium anisopliae* utilizando bolsas plasticas. *Jornada Internacional de Lucha Biologica en el Cultivo de la Cana de Azucar,* 2, La Habana, Cuba, 23–24 Nov. 1988, pp. 1 (Abstract only).

The principles of ultra-low volume spraying in relation to the application of microbial insecticides for locust control

G.A. Matthews

International Pesticide Application Research Centre, Imperial College of Science, Technology and Medicine, UK.

Abstract

Droplet size needs to be optimized at 70–100 μm VMD to drift spray locusts using aerial or ground equipment to apply ultra-low volumes (1 l/ha). The concentration of conidia is determined by the dose per insect and number of droplets expected to be deposited on the locusts. Rotary atomizers are appropriate to achieve the narrow droplet spectrum required.

Introduction

Aerial and ground ultra-low volume spraying began with research on application technology for locust control, and especially with the concept of vegetation baiting using a persistent insecticide, notably dieldrin (Courshee, 1959). Using an exhaust gas nozzle to provide a plume of oil-based spray which is deposited over a swath downwind, it was estimated that as a fifth instar hopper could eat approximately 10 cm^2 foliage per day, so a lethal dose of insecticide would be accumulated if there were an insecticide deposit of 4 $\mu g/cm^2$.

Successive track spacings of 200 m have been recommended with the exhaust nozzle drift spraying technique, with droplets having a volume median diameter of the order of 100 μm. The actual distribution of droplets downwind depends on their size and movement relative to the air turbulence, but the aim is to have droplets falling at an angle of 5–7° to the horizontal so that a high proportion of the insecticide is deposited on vertical surfaces, such as the clumps of grass on which the locusts are feeding, rather than wasting chemical on the exposed soil surface. A peak deposit occurs at a particular distance downwind from a single swath, but with a persistent stomach poison accumulated by the locust hopper, the variability in deposit is relatively unimportant. However, if a contact insecticide is applied the track spacing needs to be adjusted to provide overlapping swaths that overall produce a more uniform deposit.

Johnstone (1991) has developed a computer model to predict the dose received by settled locusts, for example, it predicts that a 100 m track spacing is justified for a spray emitted at 15 l/min flow rate containing droplets with a volume median diameter of 120 μm or less released at a height of 10 m in a wind speed not exceeding 2 m/s.

This paper discusses the relevance of the earlier studies on ultra-low volume spraying to the requirements for efficient transfer of a fungal pathogen to settled locusts.

Droplet size

Theoretical studies on the impaction of droplets on flying locusts suggested that the optimum droplet size was 50 μm (Townsend, 1948), and other studies have confirmed the importance of aerosol droplets (< 50 μm) for direct collection on insects. However, the smallest droplets are more prone to dispersal in air currents and can be lifted away from vegetation under hot convective conditions. It was for this reason that the drift spraying technique compromised on a volume median diameter of about 100 μm droplets. This avoided excessively large droplets which wasted chemical and yet had a large number of droplets below 100 μm, filtered out by the vegetation and insects provided the sprays were applied early in the day, preferably under adiabatic or inversion conditions.

Recent studies of deposits on grasshoppers have confirmed that better control was obtained with droplets with a vmd of 76 μm rather than 44 μm. (Symmons *et al.*, 1991).

Formulation

When small droplets are used, rates of evaporation can be high as both the convective and radiation heat transfer coefficients are inversely proportional to droplet size (Courshee, 1959). In consequence, relatively involatile oil-based formulations are preferred, although in agricultural work, water-based formulations have been used successfully if an involatile component is used to restrict the effect of evaporation on droplet size to prevent their shrinking too small.

Spray volume

This is determined on the basis of droplet size (d) and the number of droplets (n) required per unit area. Thus when spraying a flat surface the number of litres per hectare (Q):

$$Q = \frac{n\pi}{60} \div \frac{(100)^3}{(d)}$$

For example if you require 19 droplets of 100 μm per cm^2 you need to apply one litre per hectare. The number of droplets needed is affected by the amount of the insecticide that can be carried in individual droplets, and, taking into consideration that the carrier liquid needs to be relatively involatile, adhere to the insect surface on impaction, and spread and transfer the toxicant.

Spray concentration

With particulate suspensions it is necessary to have the appropriate concentration of particles in each droplet. Several studies have considered this in relation to the application of baculoviruses; thus, against *Panolis flammea* (Denis & Schiffermüller) (Lepidoptera: Noctuidae) Entwistle (1986) required a delivery of 10–20 polyhedral inclusion bodies (PIB) per droplet with $1.1–2.2 \times 10^{10}$ droplets per hectare. They obtained the best results with the lowest number of PIBs per droplet, but more droplets per unit area (Entwistle *et al.*, 1990).

If a practical optimum droplet size of 70–100 μm is selected, each droplet will have a volume of 180–524 picolitres. Thus if 1,000–40,000 conidia per insect are required to cause mortality of *Schistocerca gregaria* (Forskål), the concentration in the spray can be varied in relation to the number of droplets that might be expected to deposit on the locusts. Assuming 20 droplets of 500 picolitres impact, i.e. 10,000 picolitres, 20,000 conidia would need to be suspended in this volume of oil, i.e. 2×10^{12} conidia per litre. The chances of more droplets impacting directly on locusts will increase if the volume is increased, and the concentration of spores kept to a minimum. However the cost of the carrier oil and the logistics of maintaining a high work rate over the extensive areas with locusts, necessitate that the volume per hectare is between 0.5 and 2.0 l/ha and preferably about 1 l/ha.

Conclusion

Regardless of whether the application technique involves aerial, vehicle-mounted or hand-held equipment, locust control with liquid formulations is normally carried out at ultra-low volume application rates. Rotary atomizers are most commonly used for this purpose, and in order to be most effective it is important to optimize the rotational speed and physical characteristics and flow rate of the formulation, to achieve a narrow droplet spectrum of an appropriate size.

References

Courshee, R.J. (1959) Drift for vegetation baiting. *Bulletin of Entomological Research* **50**, 355–370.

Entwistle, P.F. (1986) Spray droplet deposition patterns and loading of spray droplets with NPV inclusion bodies in the control of *Panolis flammea* in pine forests. *Proceedings of the IVth International Colloquium of Invertebrate Pathology*, Veldhoven, The Netherlands, 613–615.

Entwistle, P.F., Evans, H.F., Cory, J.S. & Doyle, C. (1990) Questions on the aerial application of microbial pesticides to forests. *Proceedings of the Vth International Colloquium on Invertebrate Pathology and Microbial Control*, Adelaide, Australia, 159–163.

Johnstone, D.R. (1991) Variations in insecticide dose received by settled locusts – a computer model for ultra-low volume spraying. *Crop Protection*, **10**, 183–194.

Symmons, P.M., Dobson, H.M. & Sissoko, M. (1991) Pesticide droplet size and efficacy: a series of trials on grasshoppers. *Crop Protection* **10**, 136–144.

Townsend, A.A. (1948) Theoretical effects of drop size on the collection of spray by flying insects. In: Kennedy, J.S., Ainsworth, M. & Toms, B.A. *Laboratory Studies on the Spraying of Locusts at Rest and in Flight. Anti-Locust Bulletin* **2**, 62–64.

Controlled droplet application of mycopesticides to locusts

R.P. Bateman

International Institute of Biological Control.

Abstract

Oil-based ULV formulations containing conidia of *Metarhizium flavoviride* have been prepared which are compatible with equipment for controlled droplet application and are toxic to *Schistocerca gregaria*. The numerical aspects of mycoinsecticide sprays are discussed and compared with the activity of chemical pesticides.

Introduction

Application of entomopathogenic fungus spores has in the past usually involved hydraulic spraying techniques. These have the advantages of versatility and familiarity, and aqueous media have often been selected in the belief that a humid environment is required for the survival and germination of fungi. Prior *et al.* (1988) demonstrated that *Beauveria* conidiospore suspensions applied to *Pantorhytes plutus* (Oberthür) (Coleoptera: Curculionidae) had lower LD_{50} values when formulated in oil than when they were water-based. The IIBC group in the Locust & Grasshopper Biological Control Programme (LGBCP) has subsequently established that locusts can become infected by topical oil-based applications even under dry conditions. However horizontal transmission is believed to be unlikely without a humid environment, therefore good spray coverage of each insect is necessary. Maximization of coverage at low volume application rates of spray mixture essentially requires the production of large numbers of small droplets – however not so small that they do not deposit on their target (Matthews, these proceedings). This paper gives an outline of the approach taken to formulation and application in our research, and describes some initial findings.

Formulation

It is relatively straightforward to prepare oil-based ultra-low volume (ULV) formulations containing suspensions of conidia in the deuteromycete genera *Beauveria* and *Metarhizium*. Their lipophilic cuticles enable conidia to suspend easily after vigorous agitation of suitable carrier oils poured over the sporulating culture. Oils are preferred in ULV formulations since evaporation of the carrier liquid must be minimized when using small droplets, especially under dry conditions. Oils also readily stick and spread on insect exocuticles, and may assist in transport of conidia to the more susceptible intersegmental membranes and subsequent hyphal penetration (Prior *et al.*, 1988).

Wrigley (1973) gives a useful review of the properties required of mineral oils for ULV formulation. Special emphasis has been placed on substances (usually vegetable oils) that are readily available in tropical countries, and early work in this project involved their screening for toxicity to conidia. Vegetable oils have a high viscosity which must be adjusted by mixing with light paraffins so that satisfactory flow characteristics are obtained for existing equipment. The restrictor-airbleed combination for the Micron 'Micro Ulva' has been used in these tests; it should be relatively easy to 'scale up' for larger equipment used in acridid control.

Bioassays using drops placed under the posterior lip of locust pronota have been used for initial screening. Volumes of 2 μl are satisfactory, although this can be reduced to 500 nl with some increase in experimental variability. Even the latter is still several orders of magnitude larger than the volume of typical insecticide spray droplets. Preliminary bioassays have indicated that the *Metarhizium flavoviride* W. Gams & J. Rozsypal strain IMI 330189 has an LD_{50} of approximately 2×10^4 spores/adult *Schistocerca gregaria* (Forskål) after 5 days, and 10^3 spores after 8 days. At approximately 18 pg per spore, this **tentative** five day mortality appears to compare well with most other insecticides used against locusts (Table 1).

Using the LD_{50} measurements given above, a formulation containing 10^9 spores/ml would have a theoretical 5 day toxicity coefficient of 24 million*, compared with 5.5–10.9 million for dieldrin at field rates (MacCuaig & Watts, 1963). Toxicity coefficients based on LD_{50} data may

*Estimated number of insects which could be killed by uniformly dosing 1 l of spray formulation (half number of LD_{50}s/l).

Table 1. Contact toxicity of insecticides to adult locusts (mostly *S. gregaria*: from MacCuaig, 1983).

Insecticide	Type	LD_{50} µg/g	LD_{99} µg/g	Rate (if not LD_{99})	Time for action (>90% mortality)
Bendiocarb	ca	1.0– 2.1	1.4– 3.8		22 h
Carbaryl	ca	25–>100	69–>100		8–18 h
Chlorpyrifos	op	3.0– 3.2	6.2	5µg/g	3 d (100%)
Deltamethrin	py	0.5	13.2		5 d
DDVP	op	1.7– 8.7	6.3–27		<1 d
Diazinon	op	3.4– 6.5	7.9–17.8		3½ d
Dieldrin	oc	3.7– 6.9	8.6–25		7–21 d
Fenitrothion	op	3.7– 8.4	9.1–35		1–6 d
γ-HCH	oc	5.5–14.5	13–30		5–10 d
Metarhizium flavoviride IMI 330189	**fp**	**≈0.2**	**≈1.1**	**LD_{95}**	**<6 d**
Lambdacyhalothrin	py	0.4– 0.6	0.8– 1.9	LD_{95}	<24 h*
Malathion	op	25–38	73–110		3–9 d
Propoxpur	ca	1.0– 2.6	4– 8		5 h

Key: ca – carbamate; fp – fungal pathogen; oc – organochlorine; op – organophosphate; py – pyrethroid;
* – data for lambdacyhalothrin using *Locusta migratoria migratorioides* (Reiche & Fairmaire) which is often slightly more susceptible to insecticides than *S. gregaria* (from Alcantra Santos, 1987).

be misleading however, since the slope of the dose response curve for fungus pathogens is often much shallower than for that of chemical pesticides. The data in Table 1 show 2–3 times differences between LD_{50} and LD_{99} for chemical insecticides. In the test described above the difference was six-fold, however Lai *et al.* (1982) measured 12–62 times differences with various fungus strains active against termites, and Prior *et al.* (1988) calculated LD_{95} values that were 3–4 orders of magnitude higher than the LD_{50}s.

Controlled droplet application (CDA)

Atomizers that can produce monodisperse (uniformly sized) sprays include rotating discs, cups and cages. The centrifugal force acting on a liquid fed to the centre of the rotor causes relatively uniform disintegration at the periphery under suitable operating conditions. When spinning discs are used for applying insecticides, the usual form of atomization is via the formation and break-up of ligaments. One way of defining CDA is that a high proportion (80% or more) of the spray liquid volume should be atomized within limits of a required size band (illustrated in Fig. 1). 50–100 μm (65–254 pl) is considered a range appropriate for ULV insecticide spraying, and represents an eight-fold dose variation between the limits.

Frequently the number distribution of sprays produced by ligament disintegration has been shown to be bimodal – this is confirmed by studies using high speed photography, where the ligaments break up into principal and 'satellite' droplets. Droplet size may be adjusted most readily by changing the disc speed; the nature of the formulation itself and the flow rate of liquid has a smaller effect, however large variations in droplet size take place under conditions where transitions may occur between single droplet and ligament formation.

The 'Malvern' laser particle size analyser has been used to check that the atomization of formulations is suitable for ULV application (i.e. essentially similar to the atomization of existing ULV formulation with commonly used equipment). Fig. 1 shows the distribution of spray droplets produced with a spore formulation atomized by a spinning disc sprayer of the type used in early field trials. The average droplet volume (ADV)* is nearly 90 pl, but the distribution is bimodal with two approximately equal modes by droplet *number*; these represent volumes of approximately 10

*The volume in pl represented by the volume average diameter (VAD) or $D_{(3,0)}$. It is an estimate of the:

$$\frac{\text{Total volume of spray}}{\text{Total number of droplets}} \text{ of the sample measured.}$$

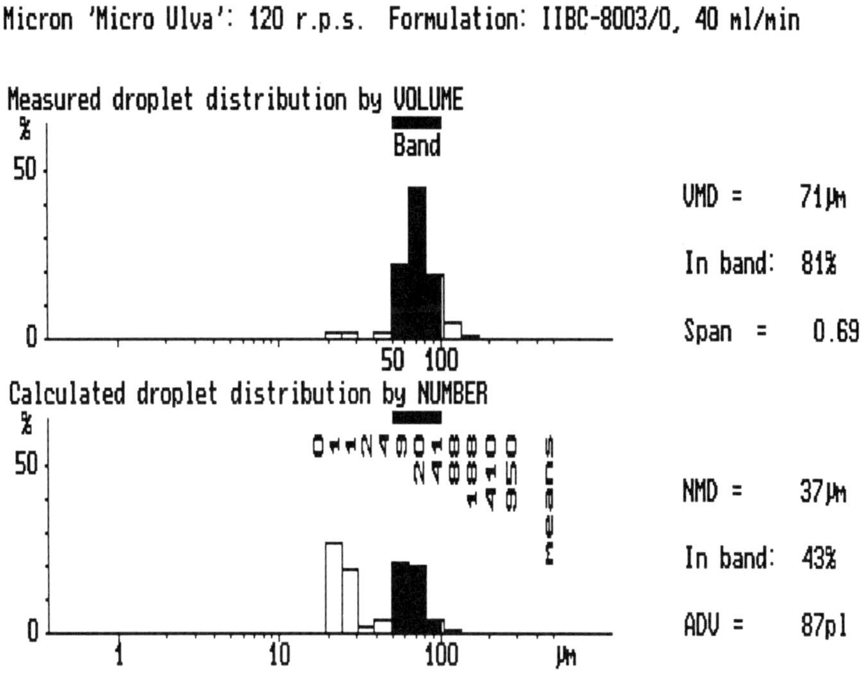

Figure 1. An example of droplet size measurement with a Malvern 2,600 particle size analyser. 'Means' indicate predicted average number of spores/droplet in each size class, for a formulation containing 10^8 spores/ml.

and 200 pl respectively. The computer programme used to illustrate these measurements also displays the theoretical number of suspended particles in each size class (in this case representing spores at a relatively low concentration for ULV spraying). It has of course been assumed that spore numbers are proportional to the volume of each droplet; this may not be the case, and is the subject of current research.

It is the larger droplets however that constitute by far the greatest *volume* of biopesticide in a spray, and droplets in this mode are also more likely to impact on stationary acridids, vegetation, and artificial targets used in field trials. At ≈ 200 pl (70+ µm diam) such droplets should typically contain approximately 200 spores at 10^9 spores/ml. Thus, 105 droplets of 200 pl on each insect might be expected to achieve a 50% mortality in 5 days with a formulation containing 10^9 spores/ml; to achieve the same result in 8 days would require only about 6 droplets.

There has been evidence that contact insecticides applied as small (≈ 20 µm) droplets are intrinsically more insecticidal for a given dose than larger ones (e.g. Himel, 1969), however MacCuaig (1962) found no significant differences in organochlorine insecticide toxicity to adult locusts with droplets ranging from 68–250 μm. Much depends on the precise nature of the acridid target: Symmons *et al.* (1991) achieved better control of grasshoppers in the field with bendiocarb sprays of volume median diameter (VMD) ≈ 76 μm, than with a VMD of ≈ 44 μm. This is clearly a complex subject, and constitutes another line of research for the LGBCP, both in the field and using an experimental track sprayer in the laboratory.

Acknowledgements

This work has been carried out under a collaborative programme between IIBC, IITA-BCP and DFPV on the biological control of locusts and grasshoppers, which was funded by the Canadian International Development Agency (CIDA), the Directorate General for Development Cooperation of the Netherlands (DGIS), the Overseas Development Administration of the UK (ODA), and the United States Agency for International Development (USAID). The author would also like to thank Ms M.J. Carey for the bioassay data and Drs G.A. Matthews and C. Prior for help in preparing this paper.

References

Alcantara Santos, L.M.K. (1987) *Studies on the Toxicity of Three Insecticides to the Migratory Locust,* Locusta migratoria migratoriodes (*R & F*). MSc thesis, University of London.

Himel, C.M. (1969) The optimum size for insecticide spray droplets. *Journal of Economic Entomology* **62**, 919–925.

Lai, P.Y., Tamashiro, M. & Fujii, J.K. (1982) Pathogenicity of six strains of entomogenous fungi to *Coptotermes formosanus. Journal of Invertebrate Pathology* **39**, 1–5.

MacCuaig, R.D. (1962) The toxicity of some insecticidal sprays to adult locusts. *Bulletin of Entomological Research* **53**, 597–608.

MacCuaig, R.D. (1983) *FAO Insecticide Index.* (2nd edition). Food and Agriculture Organization of the United Nations, Rome.

MacCuaig, R.D. & Watts, W.S. (1963) Laboratory studies to determine the effectiveness of DDVP sprays for the control of locusts. *Journal of Economic Entomology* **56**, 850–859.

Prior, C., Jollands, P. & le Patourel, G. (1988) Infectivity of oil and water formulations of *Beauveria bassiana* (Deuteromycotina: Hyphomycetes) to the cocoa weevil pest *Pantorhytes plutus* (Coleoptera: Curculionidae). *Journal of Invertebrate Pathology* **52**, 66–72.

Symmons, P.M., Dobson, H.M. & Sissoko, M. (1991) Pesticide droplet size and efficacy: a series of trials on grasshoppers. *Crop Protection* **10**, 136–144.

Wrigley, G. (1973) Mineral oils as carriers for ultra-low-volume (ULV) spraying. *Pest Abstracts and News Summaries* **19**, 54–61.

Development of a novel field bioassay technique for assessing mycoinsecticide ULV formulations

R.P. Bateman[1], I. Godonou[2], D. Kpindu[2], C.J. Lomer[1] & A. Paraïso[2]

[1]*International Institute of Biological Control.* [2]*IITA Biological Control Programme.*

Abstract

An experimental design is presented which allows close simulation of field conditions while retaining a degree of control more typical of laboratory situations. Oil-based ULV sprays containing conidia of *Metarhizium flavoviride* W. Gams & J. Rozsypal have readily killed locusts at humidities lower than previously considered necessary for infection by fungus pathogens.

Introduction

Different application strategies are likely to be required for the various locust and grasshopper biological control problems, but most techniques involve ULV spraying with rotary atomizers (Bateman, these proceedings). Small-scale grasshopper control may be carried out using hand-held spinning disc sprayers such as the Micron Micro-Ulva or the Berthoud C8. Larger-scale treatments for application to several hectares may be carried out with the Micron X15, a stacked array of 88 mm spinning discs mounted on a vehicle, and ultimately, aerial application using rotary cage atomizers could be envisaged for treatment of areas of greater than 10 ha.

The number of larger droplets impacting directly on insects in the field typically spans orders of magnitude, but is lower than numbers that can easily be achieved in the laboratory. This has been revealed in pilot studies using a fluorescent tracer dye (Staniland, 1959) mixed with a pyrethoid, then counting droplets on the cuticle of dead insects recovered after spraying. It is possible that an important mode of entry for conventional insecticides might be via the smaller droplets or secondary pick-up from vegetation. The work of Symmons *et al.* (1991) suggests, however, that hand-held spinning disc sprayers should be adjusted to produce medium-sized rather than small droplets to achieve optimal performance.

Before carrying out full scale field trials, a step by step approach has been taken to the development of spray application, as recommended by Matthews (1983). This paper describes a novel technique which has been developed to spray acridid targets under controlled conditions, with droplet numbers commensurate with those encountered following normal field applications.

Materials and methods

Figure 1 is a diagram of treatment arenas used in these tests. An area larger than 50 × 50 m was mown and sixteen 3 × 3 m sampling zones were cleared of all vegetation, in four lines situated at 5, 10, 20, and 30 m downwind of a marked spray path. Four sets of samples were taken during each test, consisting of columns of sampling zones positioned parallel to the

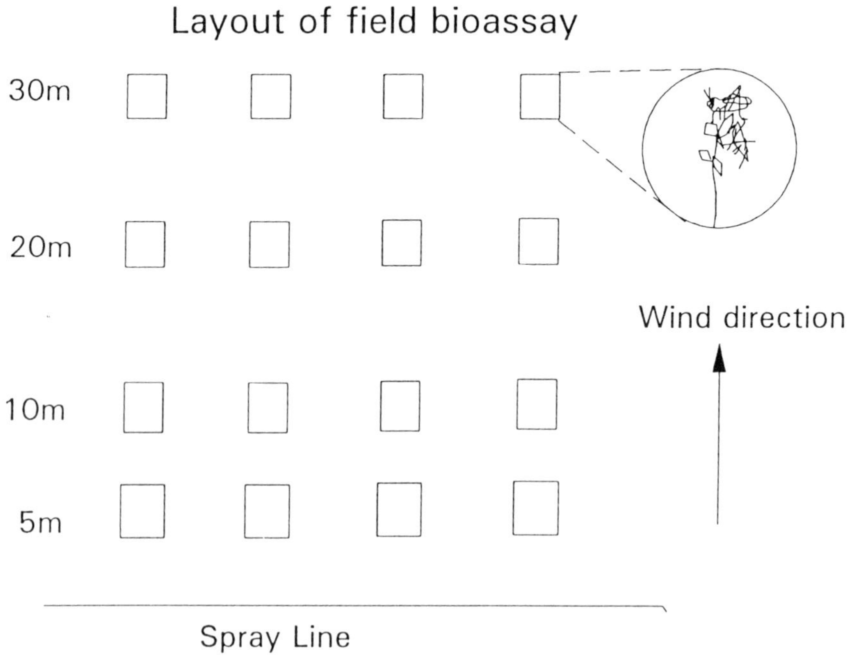

Figure 1. Layout of arena trial.

prevailing wind. Vegetation was placed in the centre of each arena to attract the locusts; in the test illustrated cassava leaves sprayed with sugar solution were used. 20 newly fledged *Schistocerca gregaria* (Forskål) adults were released onto the plants, and more than half of these could usually be recaptured immediately after spraying; locusts are usually highly active, but can be restrained using paper clips to hold their wings together. A sampling post was also sited in each arena, and droplet deposits were assessed using oil-sensitive cards pinned to it.

This design was developed after analysis of swath pattern data (Figs 2 and 3) which has also proved useful for determining practical swath widths with different application techniques. The method was first developed by Picken (in Heinrichs *et al.*, 1981) and has been modified by Bateman (1989) with faster ways of assessing and analysing droplet data. There is an initial peak in deposit, the position of which is dependent on droplet size, emission height, wind-speed, air turbulence and formulation characteristics (Johnstone, 1991). After this there is a progressive diminution of droplet numbers deposited per unit area, with increasing distance downwind of a spray line.

The spray formulations consisted of spores of *Metarhizium flavoviride*

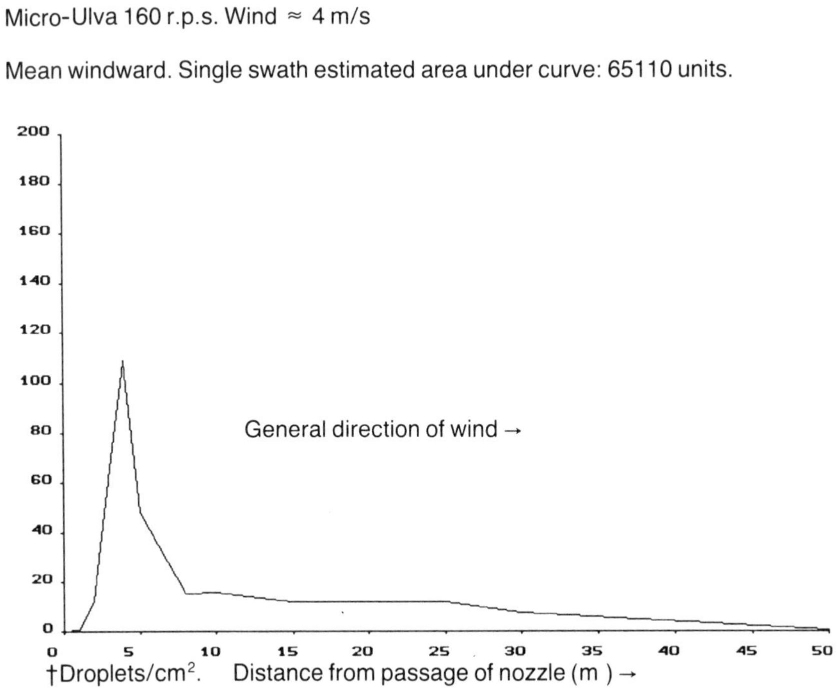

Figure 2. Droplet deposits down-wind: single swath.

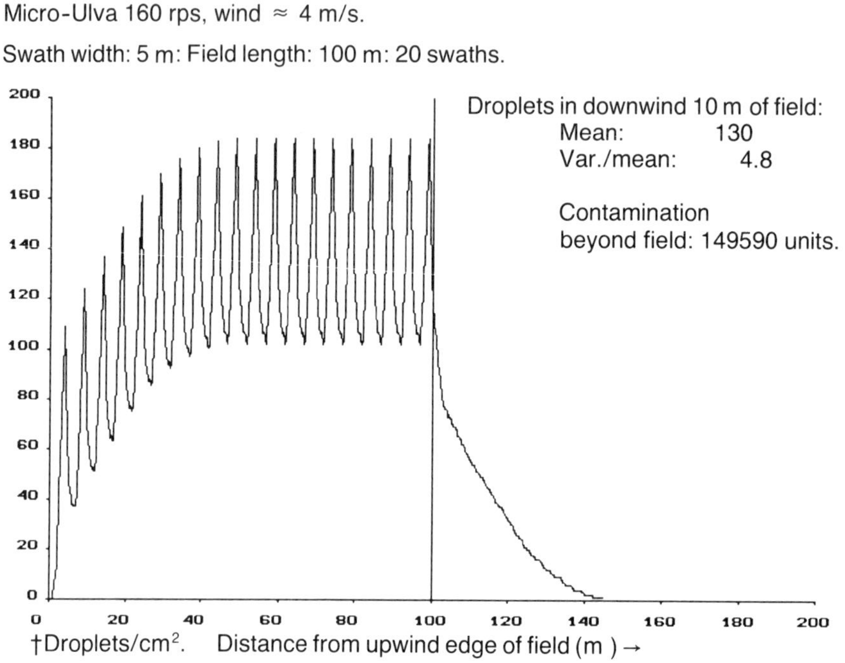

Figure 3. Incremental droplet deposition: computer simulation, from data in Fig. 2.

W. Gams & J. Rozsypal strain IMI 330189, grown on Molisch's agar and suspended in a mixture of raw groundnut oil and kerosene. Spore concentration was determined with a Neubauer haemocytometer; it was often necessary to increase spore concentration by allowing the suspension to stand and pouring off excess oil. Before spraying the spore formulation, a similar oil-based mixture containing Saturn Yellow fluorescent tracer was applied to the arena, with locusts placed along one column only (i.e. 4 sampling zones, at each distance from the spray line).

After spraying, the locusts were returned to a different rearing room from the original cultures for evaluation, since mortality can be very high with cages left in the field (J. Langewald, pers. comm.). Dead insects were placed in boxes containing moistened paper and were checked for signs of fungus sporulation.

Results

The results of two tests that were successfully carried out in Cotonou are summarized in Table 1; two others were less conclusive, in the one because

Table 1. Results of two arena tests carried out on 7/2/91 and 4/3/91 with *Schistocerca gregaria* at IITA, Cotonou.

				Formulation				Sampling position					
Test	Temp (°C)	RH (%)	Wind m/s	Spores /ml	Rates of emission[1]	% germination after spraying	Results	5m	10m	20m	30m	Control	
A	31	73	2–4	5.9×10^8	2.5 ml/m	62%	**10 days:**						
							% mortality	44	48	29	32	12	
							% sporulation	28	15	10	0	0	
							18 days:						
							% mortality	81	85	52	44	29	
							% sporulation	56	22	26	7	3	
							Mean numbers of droplets counted on:						
							Oil sensitive cards	161	101	44	32		
							($numbers/cm^2$) s.e.	45	12	7	4		
							insects sprayed in control (total counts):						
							head	7	7	4	1		
							thorax	26	25	18	7		
							abdomen	15	15	6	2		
							wings	44	37	33	8		
							legs, antennae	21	25	17	5		
B	32	80	4–5	1.5×10^9	2.3 ml/m	85%	**10 days:**						l.s.d.
							% mortality	87**	59	58	24	29	33
							% sporulation	48***	22*	20*	7	0	17
							18 days:						
							% mortality	95***	83**	73*	48	36	27
							% sporulation	55**	42**	29	28	3	27

1: total estimated volume (ml) emitted per 1 m of spray path.
Asterisks indicate significant differences between sampling positions and controls (*: $P < 0.05$; **: $P < 0.01$; ***: $P < 0.001$).

of premature spore germination in the formulation, and in the other due to excessive parasitism of locust stocks with *Malamoeba.* A consistent pattern of mortality, decreasing in the order of 5, 10, 20 and 30 m downwind is usually observed. Detailed results of one of these tests are given in Fig. 4, which shows the total mean mortality at the four downwind sampling positions over a three week period after spraying. Figure 5 shows the proportion of insects for which infection was confirmed by fungus sporulation.

Discussion

The experimental layout is designed to provide a variety of mean droplet numbers at sampling stations, from which it should be possible to correlate mortality with numbers of droplet impactions. The distances from the spray line have no particular significance in themselves, apart from providing an ordinal ranking of probability of spray deposit levels. The droplet coverage on locusts can be evaluated with ultra-violet lamps.

Winds in Cotonou are relatively consistent in speed and direction and therefore it is easy to lay out tests ahead of spraying. It may be less easy to carry out similar experiments elsewhere since such consistency is exceptional away from coastal regions. Unreliable winds are a common problem

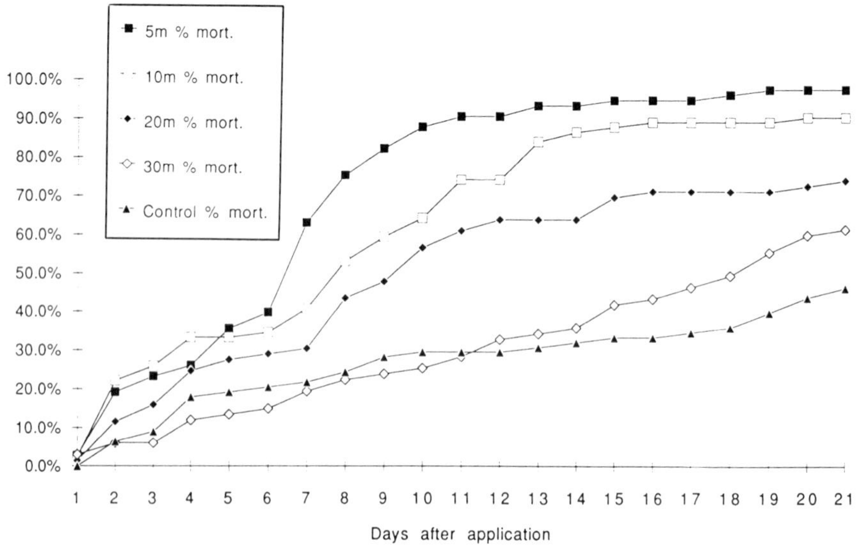

Figure 4. Results of second arena test on *Schistocerca gregaria* : *Metarhizium flavoviride* spores (@ 10^9 spores/ml).

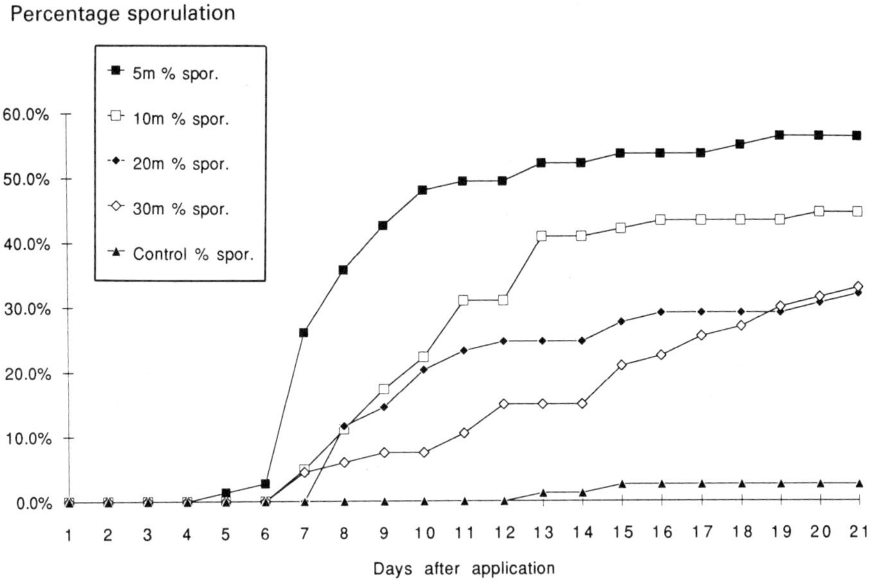

Figure 5. Same experiment as Figure 4: percentage of insects with positive identification of sporulation.

during tests and spray operations that rely on wind drift; this problem has been inadequately addressed to date by research and extension personnel.

Acknowledgements

This work has been carried out under a collaborative programme between IIBC, IITA-BCP and DFPV on the biological control of locusts and grasshoppers, which was funded by: the Canadian International Development Agency (CIDA), the Directorate General for Development Cooperation of the Netherlands (DGIS), the Overseas Development Administration of the UK (ODA), and the United States Agency for International Development (USAID). The authors would also like to thank all their colleagues in the UK and Benin who helped carry out the research, and to Drs G.A. Matthews and C. Prior, for help in preparing this paper.

References

Bateman, R.P. (1989) *Controlled Droplet Application of Particulate Suspensions of a Carbamate Insecticide.* PhD Thesis, University of London.

Heinrichs, E.A., Chelliah, S., Valencia, S.L., Arceo, M.B., Fabellar, L.T., Aquino, G.B. & Pickin, S.R. (1981) *Manual for Testing Insecticides on Rice.* IRRI Publications, Los Baños, Philippines.

Johnstone, D.R. (1991) Variations in insecticide dose received by settled locusts: a computer model for ultra-low-volume spraying. *Crop Protection* **10**, 183–194.

Matthews, G.A. (1983) Evaluation of novel pesticide application techniques. *EPPO Bulletin* **13**, 525–529.

Staniland, L.N. (1959) Fluorescent tracer techniques for the study of spray and dust deposits. *Journal of Agricultural Engineering Research* **4**, 42–81.

Symmons, P.M., Dobson, H.M. & Sissoko, M. (1991) Pesticide droplet size and efficacy: a series of trials on grasshoppers. *Crop Protection* **10**, 136–144.

Equipment

'Micro-Ulva' and 'X15' atomizers obtainable from:
Micron Sprayers Ltd.,
Three Mills,
Bromyard,
Herefordshire,
HR7 4HU, UK.

Berthoud 'C8' obtainable from Technoma S.A.
54, Rue Marcel Paul,
B.P. 195 F 51206,
Epernay, FRANCE.

Panel discussion: precis

Replying to a question by Mr Abdalla, Captain Kitenda said that fenitrothion was the pesticide used which gave an unusually delayed effect against immature adult desert locusts during operations in 1988 in Sudan. Dr Auld commented on the cost of biological agents in Australia.

Dr Prior asked how bacterial contamination is avoided in the Chinese method for mass production of *Beauveria* in trenches and if the method had been attempted with *Metarhizium.* Dr Roberts stated that the *Beauveria* isolate used is aggressive and rapidly colonizes substrate material, thus circumventing the need for anti-bacterial compounds. The method has been repeated in the USA but not with *Metarhizium.*

Dr Cardwell wondered what area of rangeland had been treated in the USA with *Nosema locustae* and whether it was persistent. Dr Evans said that 1.2 million hectares have been treated with the bait formulation, and persistence varied from none to confirmed reports of seven years. Some ranchers were adding carbaryl to extend residual activity.

Dr Zelazny asked whether fungal spores are inactivated at high temperatures of around 35 to 45°C and if human allergies were a problem during the production and application of fungal spores. Dr Goettel responded by saying that although conidia are unlikely to be killed, germination and infection could be inhibited. Production, formulation and application technologies should be developed which minimize the possible risks of human allergies.

Section V

Biology, Ecology, Field Experimentation and Environmental Impact

Introduction: biology, ecology, field experimentation and environmental impact

D.L. Johnson

Agriculture Canada Research Station, Lethbridge, Alberta.

Abstract
Investigations into the effects of biological agents on target organisms under field conditions, and also their impact on the environment, can only be carried out effectively if due attention is paid to precise experimental design and methodology. Many biological agents are slower-acting and have less obvious effects than chemical pesticides and particular attention must be paid to sampling procedures if their full impact is to be measured. Plot sizes will vary according to target mobility, the variable under investigation and the time scale of the experiment, but due attention must always be paid to established principles of statistical design. Methods which could play a greater role in analysis of experimental and observational data are discussed and particular attention is given to analysis of covariance and to competing risk theory. Principles and techniques discussed in the paper are illustrated by reference to two field investigations on the use of pathogens for locust and grasshopper control: a field trial on the use of *Nosema locustae* Canning for control of Canadian grasshoppers and a laboratory trial on the interaction of two *Nosema* spp. infecting the migratory locust, *Locusta migratoria migratorioides* Reiche & Fairmaire.

Introduction

Although the topic of this technical session may at first seem quite wide-ranging, the organizers have selected four areas which are indeed closely linked. Field experimentation is the required proving ground of any of the results of our laboratory experiments or computer models concerned with the biological agents that have been discussed during this workshop.

Potential biological control agents must pass repeated and carefully designed testing before researchers proceed to development of the agent for applied use, and during this period numerous questions arise, while some of the earlier questions are answered. One of the crucial questions waiting for any new agent of insect control that reaches the field testing stage is whether any adverse environmental impact is likely, and ultimately this question also must be examined in the field. Thus, biology and ecology are the matrix within which effectiveness and non-target safety must eventually be studied, and the search for improved efficacy and safety are linked by a mutual reliance on precise experimental design and methodology.

Part I: design

After reviewing the published literature on the agents that could provide successful biological control of grasshoppers and locusts (examples include *Entomophaga grylli* (Fresenius) Batko, *Beauveria bassiana* (Balsamo) Vuillemin, other fungi, *Nosema locustae* Canning, *Farinocystis* sp., parasitic Diptera and mites), it is clear that although field experiments must be designed to suit the special attributes of each agent and its relationship to the host target, some common attributes of field experimentation are required for valid hypothesis testing and decision making. The impact of biological control is often not as clear as in the case of field experimentation with chemical insecticides, nor are biological control studies limited to measurement of mortality alone. Therefore, there exists in this area of research an even greater need for correct experimental design and for useful application of powerful new methods of analysis. Before reviewing past results in the panel discussion, or attempting to standardize our research protocols, it is worth our time to review proven practices and new developments, and consider applications. Speakers have been asked to draw on their own experience, so I will use some examples with which I am familiar.

The basic steps in field experimentation are design, execution, analysis and interpretation. Each of the attributes of the overall design is based on or composed of considerations regarding the questions and measurements of interest (Table 1). Our field results from planned experiments in biological control of grasshoppers should be weighed in the context of these attributes.

When testing biological control agents, for example fungal spores applied as a microbial insecticide against grasshoppers, ecological attributes of both the target and the pathogen must be considered in the context of the particular hypotheses to be examined. The particular attributes of

Table 1. Fundamental considerations in field experimentation.

Hypotheses
— Include both research hypotheses and those required for statistical tests
— Determine the measured variables and suggest design attributes

Experimental design
— Demands for repeatability
— Restrictions on randomization
— Choice of variables to be controlled and monitored
— Method of measurement and sampling

Concomitant and nuisance variables

Experimental and sampling error

Analyses and tests
— Interpretation, may lead to revision of hypotheses; new subsets take precedence
— Lead to redesign and implementation of subsequent experiments
— Communication of results

acceptable field trials depend on the questions being asked. For example, it is quite valid to conduct a microbial treatment in cages of 1 m^2 when the questions of interest concern interaction of synergistic agents with the spores over a short period, or when precise measurements of reproduction or feeding are to be made, or when only small amounts of inoculum are available for a first outdoor test of pathogenicity (for example, cage trials – Johnson *et al.*, 1988). It is, however, also valid to conduct treatments with an agent in larger plots, each 10 to 20 ha, for timing trials that presume limited movement of the target insect over less than one season (e.g., Johnson, 1989c), and even larger plots are required in cases in which problems with movement are anticipated (e.g., the fifteen 200 ha plots used in Mali in 1989 by Van der Paauw *et al.*, 1990). Very large plots, such as in the treatment of plots of thousands of hectares per plot by Henry & Onsager (1982) are required to ask other, equally valid but different questions. There is no single plot size, application method, or even sampling method that is always right (or always wrong) for a particular biocontrol agent or target pest species, but there are of course standards of design that are universal requirements, such as the employment of replication, randomization, adequate sample sizes, and well-tested assay methods. Even enormous plot size does not guarantee a useful test if the need for replication and randomization are ignored.

Sometimes field experiments must appear to break the rules in order to test them. For example, it has been generally accepted that the microsporidan *Nosema locustae* should be targeted at the peak modal density of the third instar. A recent field test in Alberta of this hypothesis dispelled this notion, and will serve here to illustrate some of the basic principles involved in field experimentation involving biological control of grasshoppers.

An experimental example: the effects of timing and frequency of application of *Nosema locustae* on the infection rate and activity of grasshoppers

Introduction

The ability of *Nosema locustae* to debilitate grasshoppers and locusts by attacking the fat body and other internal organs has suggested that, although it is slow-acting, this entomopathogen may have application as an environmentally safe, long-term management tool for grasshopper control (Henry, 1971, 1972).

Although the detrimental effects of *N. locustae* on grasshopper growth and survival can be demonstrated easily in laboratory experiments, the results of field experiments designed to measure its effectiveness vary widely. Field results have varied from no discernable impact up to 60–70% mortality with infection of 95–100% of the surviving grasshoppers (although the experiment in which this best result was observed (Ewen & Mukerji, 1980) was unreplicated, having only one plot of each treatment, and assessment of the change in population density was not based on actual counts of grasshopper density). More typical results fall between these two extremes, attaining 30–50% grasshopper mortality caused by *N. locustae*, and infection of 20–50% of the survivors. In atypical situations, such as application against roadside grasshopper populations, only about 10% are infected (Johnson & Henry, 1987).

Because the primary goal of both experimental and practical field application of *N. locustae* has been to reduce the number of grasshoppers in the treated area, the more susceptible third and fourth nymphal instars are targeted (Henry *et al.*, 1973; Henry & Onsager, 1982). Late-season application is considered inadequate, or at best inferior to earlier application, because the larger and more robust adults are less likely to succumb to the disease. Application too late in the season is a common explanation given for poor field results. However, the nonlethal symptoms of infection include significant suppression of feeding (Johnson & Pavlikova, 1986) and of reproduction. It is also reasonable to assume that higher rates of infection of the adults would increase the rate of transmission of the pathogen to the next generation. In the interest of maximizing the percentage of the grasshopper population successfully infected, the effects of the timing and frequency of *N. locustae* application were examined without the constraint of following the methods aimed at attaining maximum grasshopper mortality. Because of the controversy surrounding demonstrations of efficacy, the comparisons were made as part of a rigorous field experiment.

Methods

The *N. locustae* bait spores used in this experiment were produced and formulated on wheat bran as described by Johnson (1989a). The spore concentration of the formulated bait was 1.3×10^9 spores/kg bait (wet weight).

Four blocks of native and improved grass pasture near Taber, Alberta, Canada, were each divided into four 16 ha plots. Each plot measured 200 × 800 m. This was considered to be a minimum size for a 9 week trial. A complete set of the following four treatments was randomly assigned to the plots in each block: early-season bait application (June, when younger instars 2–4 predominate), late-season application (July, when a majority of grasshoppers are in the adult stage), double application (both early and late application to the same plot), and no bait application (control). The treated plots received wheat bran bait containing 3.3×10^9 spores/ha at each application in 2.5 kg of wheat bran bait/ha.

Measured variables were: the infection rate, defined as the percentage of grasshoppers collected during the experiment that were found to contain *N. locustae* spores; and the grasshopper population density, estimated by making counts of grasshoppers observed in 320 permanent quadrats and by collection of grasshoppers with sweepnets. The two methods were employed because under typical field conditions the first provides an unbiased estimate of population density of active and lethargic insects alike, while the latter method depends on grasshopper condition and activity (Johnson *et al.*, 1986).

The $\log_e$-transformed count data and the number of sweeps per 100 grasshoppers were analysed separately for each post-treatment sampling date, using analysis of covariance. Since the quadrat positions did not change during the experiment, the pre-treatment observation (week 0) was the concomitant variable. Treatment effects were tested with experimental error (block by treatment interaction), experimental error was tested with subplot error, and subplot error was tested with sampling error among quadrats. Orthogonal contrasts were used to compare the following treatment combinations: early vs late treatment, single vs. double treatment, and treated vs. untreated.

Results and discussion

Grasshopper population mean density in the plots at the time of treatment ranged from 5.0 to 7.5/0.25 m^2. Table 2 indicates how the early and late treatments differed in age structure. The results were surprising: although

Table 2. Grasshopper species and age structure at the time of application of *N. locustae* bait in the timing experiment. (The total number collected and the percentage of each species is shown.)

Species	% Adult and species sample size			
	Early application[a]		Late application[b]	
Melanoplus infantilis Scudder	1.1	2584	83.1	2468
Camnula pellucida (Scudder)	6.6	1341	97.0	1914
Melanoplus sanguinipes (Fabricius)	3.5	935	69.5	902
Melanoplus packardii Scudder	3.2	155	92.2	192
Ageneotettix deorum (Scudder)	0.0	107	89.3	177
Spharagemon campestris (McNeill)	0.0	85	58.3	175
Trachyrhachys kiowa (Thomas)	0.0	80	49.0	98
Rare species (combined)	1.0	102	47.3	188
All species	2.9	5389	83.6	6114

[a] 25 June 1986.
[b] 16 July 1986.

the mortality rates did not differ, the later application, when older grasshoppers predominated, resulted in significantly higher infections.

Although the infection rate that resulted from the early application of *N. locustae* bait was initially higher than that caused by the late application, the late application of spores infected more individuals by the end of the experiment ($\chi^2 = 7.97$, $P < 0.01$). The effect occurred consistently: later treatment resulted in a higher rate of infection at all four block locations (Table 3). The degree of infection also differed between the early and the late treatments. The early season infections were not more advanced or dense.

On no date did early application result in a greater or lesser decline in grasshoppers than resulted from later application (up to 8 weeks, $P < 0.2$). At 4 weeks, the overall adjusted mortality (Abbott, 1925) in the treated plots was 39% or 8%, 44-, 35- and 14% in blocks 1–4, respectively. This is typical of the range of response to *Nosema* treatment. We can conclude that timing is not as critical a factor as was believed, relative to other variables affecting virulence and efficacy.

The number of sweeps required to collect a fixed number of grasshoppers increased significantly in the plots treated with *N. locustae.* The estimates of the reduction in density from the quadrat samples were less than the estimates based on sweepnet samples. The greater sweeping effort required in the plots treated with *N. locustae* reflects symptoms of the disease which are expressed as reduction in activity or a change in position of the grasshoppers. This second result indicates the importance of careful selection of sampling methods.

Table 3. Repeatability of the greater infection rate resulting from late treatment. The values are percentages of grasshoppers infected 9 weeks after the early and 6 weeks after the late bait application (n = 240 grasshoppers assayed per block) (Johnson, 1989a).

Timing	Block 1	Block 2	Block 3	Block 4
Untreated	6.7	8.3	3.3	5.0
Early	16.7	33.3	23.3	18.3
Late	46.7	35.0	30.0	26.7
Early & Late	36.7	43.3	41.7	33.3

Part II: results and analysis

Before we look at the results of more field trials, it is helpful to list and review some accepted and new methods that are useful in interpretation. Data that require such interpretation include:

Measured variables

- Population dynamics of target
- Survival and activity of agent
- Direct and indirect effects
- Primary and secondary impact

Impact

- Primary
  - infection
  - predation
  - parasitism
- Secondary
  - crop protection
  - synergism with other agents
  - target reproduction
  - short- vs. long-term impact

Some useful methods for tests on trials of entomopathogens and the applications of results of these trials include the following:

- Analysis of covariance
- Probits, logits, logistic regression
- Discrete multivariate analysis counts

- Simulation and other non-statistical modelling
- Competing risks theory
- Spatial and geographic analysis
- Expert systems

This list is a mix of often overlooked standard methods, and some new methods that would benefit field tests of microbial pesticides. The application of analysis of covariance in field experimentation on biological control of locusts and grasshoppers is an obvious but neglected tool that has been mentioned in the preceding example. If the sampling sites (quadrats, for example) are uniquely identified from start to finish in assessments of impacts of a treatment on grasshopper population density, the pre-treatment density can be profitably used as a covariate. 'Profitably' means that a sufficient portion of the variability is accounted for by the initial densities to make up for the loss of the one degree of freedom required for inclusion of the pre-treatment density in the model. The user may also be alerted to different degrees of effect under conditions of high and low grasshopper density, because analysis of covariance adjusts the result on the scale of the initial number. Adjustment of the post-treatment counts by the pre-treatment densities is often necessary, but is less preferred because no variation (SS) is accounted for in this way.

Probit-type models can be of use in cases in which we find a dose-mortality relationship (LD), or in which estimation of the rate of accumulation of mortality is important (LT), although these methods are more generally applicable to carefully controlled laboratory trials. Discrete multivariate methods (Bishop *et al.*, 1980) are of value, because our data often consist of counts for which we wish to compare and assess interactions, to which this method of analysis is well-suited. Computer simulation, usually based on difference equations and numerical integration, is a powerful method of formalizing our conception of the system and determining how the system might behave.

A less well-known method that is useful in this particular area of research is the application of competing risks theory. This is a body of statistical theory which seems to have been overlooked by entomologists but which may have important applications in insect experimentation and population modelling. The theory is not new, but has been used mainly by demographers and medical statisticians concerned with analysis of data involving death due to one of several possible causes. Competing risks theory deals with situations in which there is interest in the failure (or exit) times of individuals, where the subjects are susceptible to two or more causes of failure, and where the failure occurs over time. Questions for which competing risks theory is designed to provide solutions include:

1. inference on the effects of treatments or other covariables on specific types of failure

2. inference on the ways in which the failure types are related under specific conditions
3. estimation of failure rates for some causes if some or all other causes were eliminated.

You will recognize the last point as a variation of a question sometimes asked during the interpretation of the often murky results of biological control field experiments: 'considering the circumstances, do we have something here or don't we?'.

Competing risks theory is useful in analysing the results of biological control trials because the models used in analysis of this type of experiment, where the impact on the insects may take more time than mortality caused by insecticide, are based on stage-frequency data. The models or concepts are built around the idea that upon entering a growth stage, insects spend a certain amount of time in a stage and then exit from it either by dying or maturing to the next growth stage. The theory allows assessment of the simultaneous action of the agent on mortality and on developmental success and rate. Explanation of the models involved and several formulations of the theory with application to insect experimentation are given by Schaalje *et al.* (1989).

An interesting example of application of the value of competing risks theory occurred in an experiment designed to determine and compare the effects of *Nosema locustae* and *Nosema cuneatum* Henry on development and mortality of African migratory locusts *Locusta migratoria migratorioides* Reiche & Fairmaire (G.B. Schaalje, D.L. Johnson & H.R. van der Vaart, unpublished data).

Information was desired not only on the rates of successful maturation as a function of inoculation rate, but also on the distributions of the maturation times.

Third instar locusts (N=720) were inoculated *per os* with spores of either *N. locustae* or *N. cuneatum* at one of the following rates: check (0 spores), 1×10^2, 1×10^3, 1×10^4, 1×10^5, or 1×10^6 per disk. After a 24 hour feeding period, the treated hoppers were transferred to individual 500 ml plastic cages for observation until reaching adulthood. Initial weight, sex (roughly equal numbers were used) and condition were recorded. They were fed daily, and dates of moulting, date of death, final weight, and level of infection were recorded.

The observed locust maturation time did not increase with increasing dosage of *N. locustae*, even though percentage mortality did increase with increased dosage. One might erroneously conclude that *N. locustae* did not affect development, but competing risks analysis and proportional hazards analysis indicated that this seemingly obvious conclusion would be incorrect. The 'force of maturation function' indicated that maturation decreased significantly as dosage increased, but that the effect had been obscured by mortality. *N. cuneatum* appeared to have only a slight impact on maturation, but the estimated hazard functions clearly showed that maturation is severely affected by high doses of *N. cuneatum*. I will not spend more time on this particular method of analysis here, but it shows that one can be misled by looking for only the 'obvious' effects when two competing results, such as maturation and death, are measured in the same experiment.

Field experimentation on the biological control of grasshoppers may benefit from spatial and geographic analysis. New technology in this area has allowed the assessment of the role of large-scale geographic factors in determining changes in grasshopper distribution and abundance (Johnson, 1989b). The same technology allows the user to determine and map the environmental conditions that may allow a biological control agent to operate effectively, or to at least determine the regions that allow survival of a pest. An example of the latter use is the CLIMEX system developed by CSIRO Division of Entomology, Australia. Other modern geographic information systems are in use for forecasting grasshopper abundance, in Alberta since 1987, and also recently in Montana (Kemp *et al.*, 1989), and Saskatchewan, and by FAO and other agencies interested in forecasting African grasshopper and locust appearance (Cherlet, 1990). Adaptation of the software and database to include natural enemies is likely to be completed within the next few years. An example of a geographic-scale application would be to monitor the occurrence of entomopathogens over a large area, for example *Entomophaga grylli* in the Canadian Prairies (Erlandson *et al.*, 1988).

Part III: environmental impact

There have been several detailed reviews of the impact of possible microbial control agents of grasshoppers. Burges (1981) summarized the ways in which microbial pesticides may present a hazard to health, infection of non-targets including people, effects of toxins on human health, allergic reaction, carcinogenesis, and mutagenic effects. Other possible hazards include ecological impact resulting from removal of pests with complex ecological relationships, and the impact on non-target arthropods. The former is a rare but interesting possibility, but the latter is a more likely hazard, especially when applying microbial pesticides with a wide range of hosts, e.g. *Beauveria bassiana*. However, it has been noted (Prior, 1990) that even these non-specific fungi are limited by environmental restrictions and probably do not present insurmountable problems. The host range, specificity, and registration status of fungi that could affect nontarget invertebrates are reviewed in detail by Goettel *et al.* (1990).

References

Abbott, W.S. (1925) A method of computing the effectiveness of an insecticide. *Journal of Economic Entomology* **18**, 265–267.

Bishop, Y.M.M., Fienberg, S.E. & Holland, P.W. (1980) *Discrete Multivariate Analysis: Theory and Practice.* The MIT Press, Cambridge, Mass.

Burges, H.D. (1981) Safety, safety testing and quality control of microbial pesticides. In: Burges, H.D. (ed.), *Microbial Control of Pests and Plant Diseases, 1970–1980*, Academic Press, London, pp. 737–767.

Cherlet, M. (1990) Remote sensing in locust control. In: *Proceedings of a Symposium on Practical Applications of Agrometeorology in Plant Protection.* Firenze, Italy, Dec. 4–6, 1990.

Erlandson, M.A., Johnson, D.L. & Olfert, O.O. (1988) *Entomophaga grylli* infections in grasshopper (Orthoptera: Acrididae) populations in Saskatchewan and Alberta, 1985–1986. *Canadian Entomologist* **120**, 205–209.

Ewen, A.B. & Mukerji, M.K. (1980) Evaluation of *Nosema locustae* (Microsporida) as a control agent of grasshopper populations in Saskatchewan. *Journal of Invertebrate Pathology* **35**, 295–303.

Goettel, M.S., Poprawski, T.J., Vandenberg, J.D., Li, Z. & Roberts, D.W. (1990) Safety to nontarget invertebrates of fungal biocontrol agents. In: Laird, M., Lacey, L.A. & Davidson, E.W. (eds) *Safety of Microbial Insecticides.* CRC Press, Boca Raton, pp. 209–231.

Henry, J.E. (1971) Experimental application of *Nosema locustae* for control of grasshoppers. *Journal of Invertebrate Pathology* **18**, 389–394.

Henry, J.E. (1972) Epizootiology of infection by *Nosema locustae* Canning (Microsporida: Nosematidae) in grasshoppers. *Acrida* **1**, 111–120.

Henry, J.E. & Onsager, J.A. (1982) Large-scale test of control of grasshoppers on rangeland with *Nosema locustae. Journal of Economic Entomology* **75**, 31–35.

Henry, J.E., Tiahrt, K. & Oma, E.A. (1973) Importance of timing, spore concentrations, and levels of spore carrier in applications of *Nosema locustae* (Microsporida: Nosematidae) for control of grasshoppers. *Journal of Invertebrate Pathology* **21**, 263–272.

Johnson, D.L. (1989a) The effects of timing and frequency of application of *Nosema locustae* (Microspora: Microsporida) on the infection rate and activity of grasshoppers (Orthoptera: Acrididae). *Journal of Invertebrate Pathology* **54**, 353–362.

Johnson, D.L. (1989b) Spatial analysis of the relationship of grasshopper outbreaks to soil classification. In: *Estimation and Analysis of Insect Populations. Lecture Notes in Statistics*, 55, 347–359. Springer-Verlag, New York.

Johnson, D.L. (1989c) Spatial autocorrelation, spatial modelling, and improvements in grasshopper survey methodology. *Canadian Entomologist* **121**, 579–588.

Johnson, D.L. & Henry, J.E. (1987) Low rates of insecticides and *Nosema locustae* (Microsporidia: Nosematidae) on baits applied to roadsides for grasshopper (Orthoptera: Acrididae) control. *Journal of Economic Entomology* **80**, 685–689.

Johnson, D.L. & Pavlikova, E. (1986) Reduction of consumption by grasshoppers (Orthoptera: Acrididae) infected with *Nosema locustae* Canning (Microsporidia: Nosematidae). *Journal of Invertebrate Pathology* **48**, 232–238.

Johnson, D.L., Hill, B.D., Hinks, C.F. & Schaalje, G.B. (1986) Aerial application of the pyrethroid deltamethrin for grasshopper (Orthoptera: Acrididae) control. *Journal of Economic Entomology* **79**, 181–188.

Johnson, D.L., Huang, H.C. & Harper, A.M. (1988) Mortality of grasshoppers (Orthoptera: Acrididae) inoculated with a Canadian isolate of the fungus *Verticillium lecanii. Journal of Invertebrate Pathology* **52**, 335–342.

Kemp, W.P., Kalaris, T.M. & Quimby, W.F. (1989) Rangeland grasshopper (Orthoptera: Acrididae) spatial variability: macroscale population assessment. *Journal of Economic Entomology* **82**, 1270–1276.

Prior, C. (1990) The biological basis for regulating the release of micro-organisms, with particular reference to the use of fungi for pest control. *Aspects of Applied Biology* **24**, 231–238.

Schaalje, G.B., Stinner, R.L. & Johnson, D.L. (1989) Modelling insect populations affected by pesticides with application to pesticide efficacy trials. *Ecological Modelling* **47**, 233–263.

Van der Paauw, H., Johnson, D.L. & Maiga, B. (1990) Nosema locustae *against African Grasshoppers.* USAID, Washington.

The *Beauveria–Melolontha* project: experiences with regard to locust and grasshopper control

S. Keller

Federal Research Station for Agronomy, Zürich.

Abstract

A project on the use of the fungus *Beauveria brongniartii* (Saccardo) Petch to control the soil inhabiting larvae of *Melolontha melolontha* Linnaeus, which has been running in Switzerland for nearly 20 years, is summarized. Parallels to the possible use of fungi for the control of locusts and grasshoppers are pointed out and discussed. Emphasis was put on strain selection, mass production, formulation, application and monitoring the trials.

Introduction

In the early 1970s a project was started at the Federal Research Station for Agronomy at Zürich to control *Melolontha melolontha* Linnaeus (Coleoptera: Scarabaeidae) with the fungus *Beauveria brongniartii* (Saccardo) Petch (Deuteromycetes: Moniliales). This pathogen was chosen mainly for the following reasons:

1. it is considered as one of the most important antagonists (Keller, 1986)
2. it proved to be the most promising candidate of all tested pathogens (Hurpin & Robert, 1972)
3. it is easy to produce
4. it is a specific pathogen of *Melolontha* spp. (Baltensweiler & Cerutti, 1986).

Biology and ecology of the host

In the research area *M. melolontha* develops in three years. The larvae live in the soil and feed on roots of nearly all cultivated plants including trees. The adults swarm mainly in May and concentrate at the borders of forests. After a feeding/egg maturation period of about 7–10 days the females fly back to the breeding sites (mainly meadows and orchards), burrow into the soil and deposit egg batches. A female may produce up to three egg batches. Development of the individuals is regionally synchronized so that swarming of adults takes place every three years.

Periodic fluctuations characterize the population dynamics. In the past, population outbreaks occurred every 9–15 generations (27–45 years) and lasted 4–5 generations. The length of the periods of low density was more flexible and lasted 4–10 generations (Keller, 1986). There are three theories to explain this fluctuation:

1. climatic conditions (Richter, 1966)
2. availability of food for the larvae (Schütte, 1976)
3. diseases (Keller, 1986).

About 40 micro-organisms and nematodes are reported to be associated with *Melolontha* spp. About 10 can be considered as primary pathogens. Some are very rare (e.g. viruses), others occur regionally (e.g. *Rickettsiella melolonthae* Krieg); fungi and protozoans seem to occur throughout the distribution area.

The use of the fungus *Beauveria brongniartii* to control *M. melolontha* in Switzerland

Strain selection and quality control

Nearly 300 strains of fungi attacking *M. melolontha* have been isolated from larvae, pupae and adults, originating from different geographic regions of Switzerland. They show a wide variation in growth patterns as well as in virulence. Also the susceptibility of larvae from different regions varies widely.

Strains used for blastospore production and aerial application were selected by virulence tests on larvae and adults. Those used for conidia/mycelium production and soil treatment were selected by virulence tests on larvae only. In all cases, re-isolates from infected hosts were used for the field trials to prevent an eventual decrease of virulence by too long cultivation on artificial media.

The use of blastospores

Blastospores were used for helicopter application to treat the swarming adults. In this method the egg depositing females are used to carry the disease into the breeding sites. Precise timing of spray application is necessary since feeding/egg maturation and incubation period last about the same length of time. Furthermore, the blastospores used in these treatments cannot be stored for more than 4 weeks. Consequently the time between the end of production procedure and application should be kept as short as possible, which may cause problems.

For the field trials we selected two to five strains pathogenic for both adults and larvae. The strains were first multiplied separately but later mixed for the final production steps which took place in a 5,500 l fermenter (Keller *et al.*, 1989). The final broth contained about 2×10^9 spores/ml.

The suspension was applied at a concentration of 4×10^8 to 2×10^9 spores/ml. Skimmed milk was added as a sticker and UV-protectant. The spray flights took place in the late afternoon and evenings to reduce inactivation by sunlight. The dosage amounted to $2\text{–}4 \times 10^{14}$ spores/ha.

The use of conidia/mycelium

The fungus was cultivated on barley kernels in autoclavable polyamide bags (Aregger, in press). After a growth time of about 4 weeks at 18–23°C the kernels were dried and cooled. At that time the fungus had completely colonized the kernels and started to produce conidia. At 2°C the material can be stored for about a year. The strain and the mode of storage strongly influence the length of storage (Aregger, in press).

The kernels colonized with *B. brongniartii* were applied with a drill machine which allowed their deposition at a soil depth of about 3–5 cm, i.e. in the habitat of the white grubs. In the soil under normal conditions the fungus grows on the kernels and produces conidia. The fungal masses on the kernels remain clearly visible for 2–5 months depending on the season. In the first two field trials under practical conditions 90–120 kg kernels/ha were applied.

Monitoring the trials

Blastospore trials

The following parameters were checked:

1. viability (germination rate) of the blastospores by samples taken immediately before spraying

2. the effect of spraying on the adults by samples taken before and after the treatments
3. the reproduction rate (ratio of the density of the larvae after the treatment to the density of the adults before the treatment)
4. the feeding damage of the adults in the generations before and after the treatment
5. population dynamics was monitored by soil samples taken each year. Samples of larvae were taken to determine the infection rate. Both samplings were started usually two years before the treatment. The efficacy is expressed as change of the population density after the treatment in comparison to the situation before.

Conidia/mycelium trials

Population density was monitored by soil samples, the first one taken before the treatment, the second one about 2–5 months after the treatment and the following ones in intervals of a year. The efficacy is expressed as above (5).

Results

The results were published in detail (Keller *et al.*, 1986, 1989; Keller, 1989, 1991). They can be summarized as follows.

Blastospore trials

Treatment of the adults resulted in mean infection rates between 63 and 96% and in a reduction of reproduction rate from 5.1 to 2.15 second instar larvae/adult in the trials of 1988. At all sampling sites the fungus established in the *M. melolontha* populations during the generation after the treatment. The disease developed epizootically in the second generation after the treatment but only at densities greater than 20 larvae/m^2. At 11 treated sites we followed the development of the populations for at least two generations. At four sites the efficacy was good (more than 80% density reduction), at three other sites it was sufficient (50–80% reduction). No effect was observed at three sites. This failure is attributed to the low population density.

In this method the fungus acts slowly and probably depends on the population density. It is therefore unsuitable for achieving rapid, overall control; it seems rather to be a method for long-term regulation of the populations, as is demonstrated by the trial carried out in 1976 (Fig. 1).

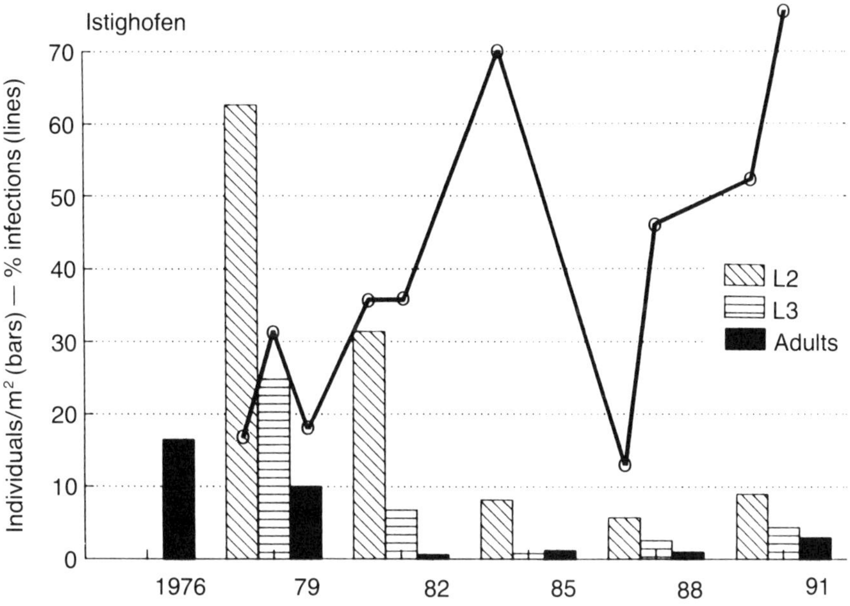

Figure 1. Development of the population density (individuals/m²) and of the percentage of individuals succumbed to *B. brongniartii* (% infection) following the treatment of the swarming adults with blastospores in 1976. The 3 connected columns represent a generation. Infection rates are given only in years marked with a circle.

Conidia/mycelium trials

Five months after the treatment, the treated and the untreated populations did not differ remarkably in their densities but in their infection rates. The fungus needed one more year to distinctly reduce the densities (Fig. 2). The efficacy amounted to 84% in an orchard and 98% in a meadow. Control of the pest insect in the orchard was sufficient, better than with chemicals, and clearly visible by the health of the trees.

Comparisons and connections with locust and grasshopper control

Biology and ecology of the pest insects

M. melolontha spends most of its life in the soil whereas locusts and grasshoppers only have their eggs there. Both have periodic population outbreaks during which *M. melolontha* increases densities and enlarges the

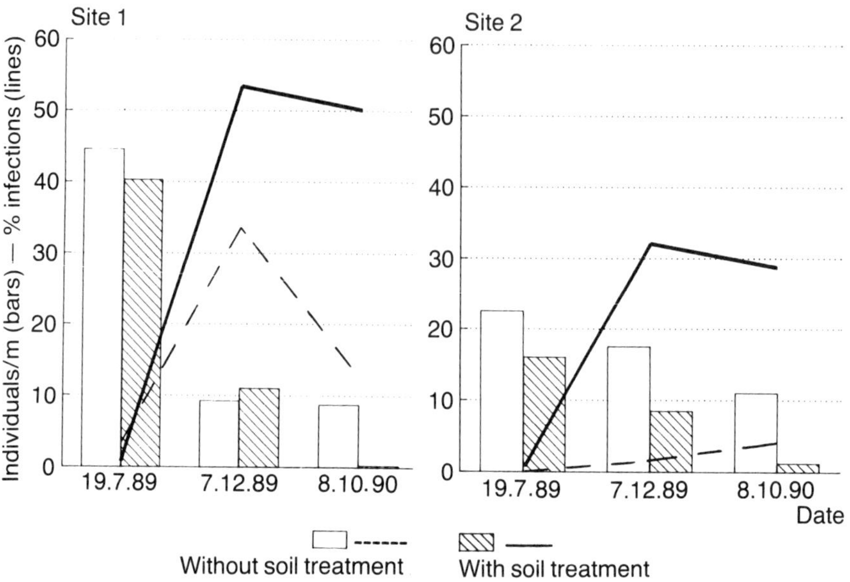

Figure 2. Development of the population densities and of the infection rates at two sites following a soil treatment carried out on 13.6.1989. Site 1: natural meadow, adults treated with blastospores by helicopter in May 1988; site 2: apple orchard with usual chemical treatment of the white grubs.

breeding areas, whereas locusts migrate. The collapse of *M. melolontha* populations is often initiated by diseases.

M. melolontha keeps its breeding sites and feeding places for generations and even over several cycles. This site-fidelity makes it easy to survey the populations and to plan eventual control measures well in advance.

Considerations on the use of fungi

B. brongniartii was selected as the control agent mainly for the following reasons, it occurs naturally and often causes epizootics, in laboratory and field trials it proved to be more virulent than other pathogens, it can be produced in large quantities on solid or inexpensive liquid media, and it is host specific.

The submersed production requires expensive equipment and experienced staff. *B. brongniartii* produces blastospores which cannot be stored for a longer period without special formulation. Other fungi (e.g. *B. bassiana* (Balsamo) Vuillemin) produce blastospores and/or conidia in liquid media. The type of the resulting spores may be influenced by the fermentation procedure. A new fermentation technique makes it possible to produce mycelial globules, which can be dried and stored. After rehydration the mycelium produces conidia (Andersch *et al.*, 1990).

A surface production of *Beauveria* spp. and *Metarhizium anisopliae* (Metschikoff) Sorokin can be done with less expensive equipment and less experienced staff. But it requires more time, staff and space. Such a product, however, can be stored under cool and dry conditions for many months.

The strains to be used must be carefully selected. Fungal strains vary considerably in respect of pathogenicity, virulence, production patterns and other characteristics. The target insects as well may vary in their susceptibility, depending not only on age and instar, but also on population density and geographic origin. It is, therefore, important to search for the best host-pathogen combination. The fungal strains must be stored or maintained in a manner to preclude loss or reduction of virulence.

Since locusts and grasshoppers live on the soil surface and are distributed over a vast area, only an aerial treatment makes sense. Many questions remain, for example, dosage, type of fungal material, formulation (sticker, UV-protectant, hygroscopic additives, oils, baits, combinations of different pathogens), application time in respect of both climatic conditions and stage of development (individual, population), area to be treated, self-propagation, distribution of the fungus, etc.

The aims of the treatments are to define:

1. killing the animals
2. protection of crops
3. prevention of forming swarms
4. limitation (regulation) of the population growth.

The field application must be adjusted to these aims and be monitored in a way which allows conclusions about success or failure, and about why and how to improve the method.

When setting up a schedule we must be aware that many time consuming attempts have to be made and many methods and approaches have to be tested to draw final conclusions on the feasibility of the use of fungi to control locusts and/or grasshoppers.

References

Andersch, W., Hartwig, J., Reinecke, P. & Stenzel, K. (1990) Production of mycelial granules of the entomopathogenic fungus *Metarhizium anisopliae* for biological control of soil pests. *Proceedings of the Vth International Colloquium on Invertebrate Pathological & Microbiological Control*, Adelaide, 2–5.

Aregger, E. (in press) Culture and storage of *Beauveria brongniartii. Journal of Invertebrate Pathology.*

Baltensweiler, W. & Cerutti, F. (1986) Bericht über die Nebenwirkungen einer Bekämpfung des Maikäfers (*Melolontha melolontha* L.) mit dem Pilz *Beauveria brongniartii* (Sacc.) Petch auf die Arthropodenfauna des Waldrandes. *Mitteilungen der Schweizerischen Entomologischen Gesellschaft* **59**, 267–274.

Hurpin, B. & Robert, P.H. (1972) Comparison of the activity of certain pathogens of the cockchafer *Melolontha melolontha* in plots of natural meadowland. *Journal of Invertebrate Pathology* **19**, 291–298.

Keller, S. (1986) Biologie/Populationsdynamik. In: *Neuere Erkenntnisse über den Maikäfer.* Beiheft zu den Mitteilungen Thurgauische Naturforschende Gesellschaft, Frauenfeld, pp. 12–40.

Keller, S. (1989) The use of blastospores of *Beauveria brongniartii* to control *Melolontha melolontha* in Switzerland. Pp. 91–97 in *Proceedings of an International Conference. Biopesticides, Theory and Practice.* Ceske Budejovice, CSFR.

Keller, S. (1991) Pilzkrankheiten bei Schädlingen und ihre praktische Bedeutung. *Landwirtschaft Schweiz* **4**, 219–230.

Keller, S., Keller, E. & Auden, J.A.L. (1986) Ein Grossversuch zur Bekämpfung des Maikäfers (*Melolontha melolontha* L.) mit dem Pilz *Beauveria brongniartii* (Sacc.) Petch. *Mitteilungen der Schweizerischen Entomologischen Gesellschaft* **59**, 47–56.

Keller, S., Keller, E., Schweizer, C., Auden, J.A.L. & Smith, A. (1989) Two large field trials to control the cockchafer *Melolontha melolontha* L. with the fungus *Beauveria brongniartii* (Sacc.) Petch. In N.R. McFarlane (ed.) *Progress and prospects in insect control.* (BCPC Monograph No. 43) pp. 183–190.

Richter, G. (1966). Prognose zum Massenwechsel des Maikäfers. *Archiv für Phytopathologie und Pflanzenschutz* **2**, 195–216.

Schütte, F. (1976) Begründung von Untersuchungen zur Populationsdynamik der Maikäfer (*Melolontha melolontha* L. und *M. hippocastani*: F). *Zeischrift für Pflanzenkrankheiten und Pflanzenschutz* **83**, 146–158.

Biological control of grasshoppers in the Cape Verde Islands

M.L. Lobo Lima[1], J.M. Brito[1] & J.E. Henry[2]

[1] *National Institute for Agricultural Research, Cape Verde:* [2] *Montana State University.*

Abstract

Beauveria bassiana (Balsamo) Vuillemin was tested against *Oedaleus senegalensis* (Krauss) and *Diabolocatantops axillaris* (Thunberg) in Cape Verde. Formulations in mineral oil and oil-water emulsions were applied in the field to 1 ha plots and also to the vegetation in cage trials before grasshoppers were introduced. *Nosema locustae* Canning and *B. bassiana* were also tested as baits. *B. bassiana* caused a statistically significant mortality when sprayed directly on to the insects in the field but application to vegetation in cages was less effective. Infection occurred in the *N. locustae* trials but was insufficient for control. Studies with the entomopox viruses of *Oedaleus* and *Melanoplus* and a survey of pathogens in Cape Verde grasshoppers are reported.

Introduction

During the past ten years, the National Institute for Agricultural Research (INIA) in Cape Verde has been investigating integrated control of major crop pests. This research into biological control methods has concentrated on the use of predators and parasites of insect pests of irrigated crops. Research into biological control of grasshoppers began in 1989 when INIA in collaboration with Montana State University (USA) and with financial support from USAID, initiated research on grasshopper pathogens. The entomopathogens *Beauveria bassiana* (Balsamo) Vuillemin, *Nosema locustae* Canning and the entomopoxviruses OPV (*Oedaleus* entomopox-virus) and MPV (*Melanoplus* entomopoxvirus) have been tested against

Oedaleus senegalensis (Krauss), *Diabolocatantops axillaris* (Thunberg) and other species. Also, surveys are being conducted for endemic pathogens in the native grasshopper fauna of Cape Verde.

Current research situation and prospects

Beauveria bassiana

The strain of *Beauveria bassiana* used against *Oedaleus senegalensis* in trials in Cape Verde on the island of Santiago, was provided by Mycotech Corporation (Butte, Montana, USA), which has developed production techniques for this entomopathogenic fungus and which participated in conduct of the trials. The spores of *B. bassiana* were formulated to produce a dry powder containing 4×10^{10} spores/g. Two field trials were conducted involving both general field applications and field cages and which were supervised by INIA research scientist, F. Delgado.

Field dosage evaluation

Dosages of 5×10^{12} and 2×10^{13} conidia/ha were applied by spraying 5 l/ha of an oil suspension using Micro-Ulva sprayers. For each dosage, three plots of 1 ha, distributed in three blocks, were treated. The same number of plots was used for controls. The evaluation of results was by assessing variation in population density measured with rings (Johnson *et al.*, these proceedings), and by the percentage mortality of grasshoppers collected 24 and 72 hours after treatment and held in the laboratory to observe the development of infection.

The infectivity of this *B. bassiana* strain to *O. senegalensis* was clearly demonstrated. For grasshoppers collected 24 hours after treatment, significant mortality was noted compared with the control, with infection of 30% for the highest dosage (Fig. 1). Mortality in grasshoppers collected 72 hours after was not significant (Fig. 2) although, for the higher dosage, mortality was higher than the control in all plots treated.

Estimation of the population density of *O. senegalensis* based on counts of grasshoppers in rings showed a very large variation, and accordingly, it was not possible to demonstrate significant differences between treatments and controls (Fig. 3). However, in two of the plots treated with the higher dosage, a very high reduction in the population was noted.

Formulation trials in cages

In this trial three formulations were evaluated at dosages of 5×10^{12} and 2×10^{13} conidia/ha. The formulations were as follows:

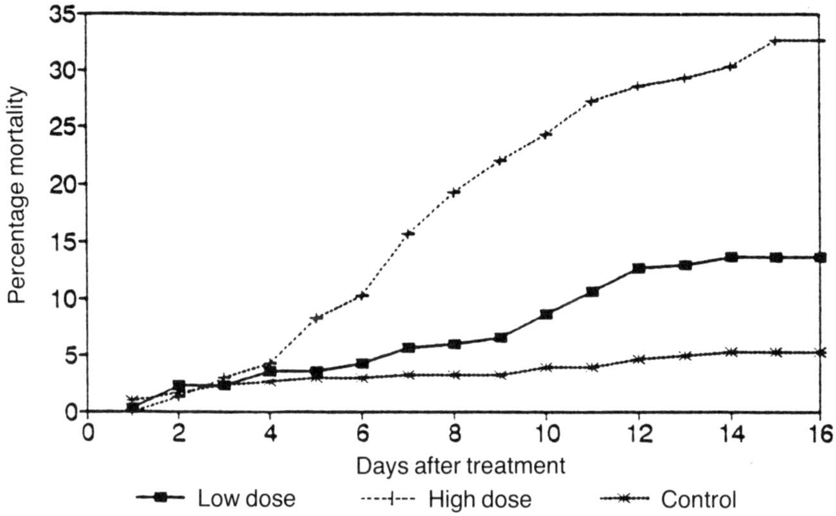

Figure 1. Mortality of grasshoppers collected from the field 24h after treatment with *Beauveria bassiana* and held in the laboratory.

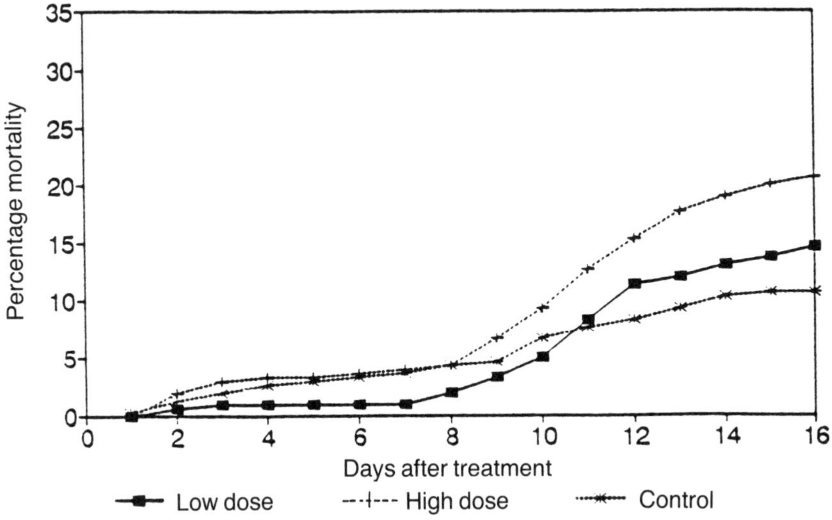

Figure 2. Mortality of grasshoppers collected from the field 72h after treatment with *Beauveria bassiana* and held in the laboratory.

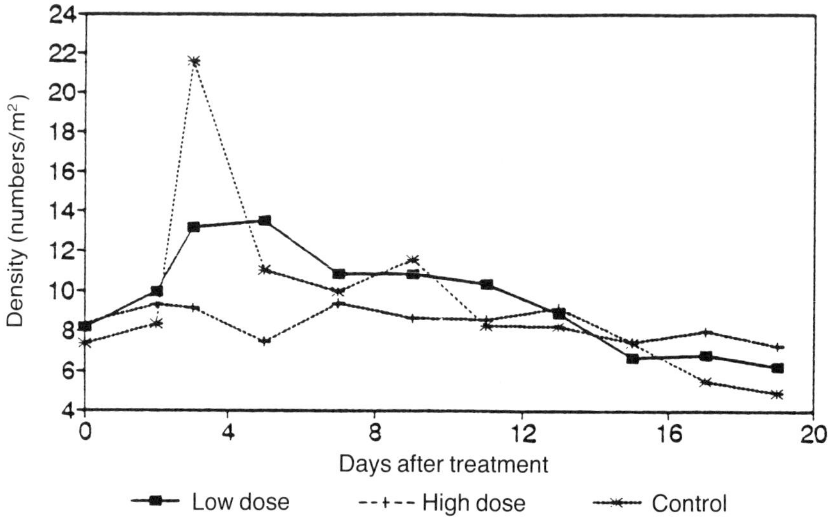

Figure 3. Population density of grasshoppers in plots treated with *Beauveria bassiana*.

1. suspension of conidia in oil
2. suspension of conidia in oil mixed with water (10:1)
3. conidia in a bran bait.

The suspensions were applied using Micro-Ulva sprayers. For the 5×10^{12} dose, 5 l/ha of liquid were applied and 10 l/ha for the 2×10^{13} dose. The bait was applied at 0.1 g and 1 g per cage. Fifty grasshoppers were introduced into each cage after treatment of the plots. Infection of the grasshoppers was by both contact and consumption of vegetation and bait. Grasshoppers were counted on each of 20 days after treatment in each cage. Dead grasshoppers were removed and placed in incubation chambers for diagnosis of the infection.

The results were based on the average number of live grasshoppers for each formulation and each dosage. There were no significant differences between treatments with conidia in oil suspension and control. However, the percentages of grasshoppers still alive at 12 and 20 days after treatment with *B. bassiana* as bait were 12 and 5%, respectively, compared to 50% still alive in control groups (Fig. 4). It was not possible to assess results for the oil and water formulation, because several cages were destroyed by animals. Both bait treatments caused significantly greater mortality than that which occurred in the control cages.

The results of these field cage trials indicated that formulation was an important factor in the use of *B. bassiana* as a bio-insecticide. The application of spores in the oil suspension to vegetation was not effective in Cape

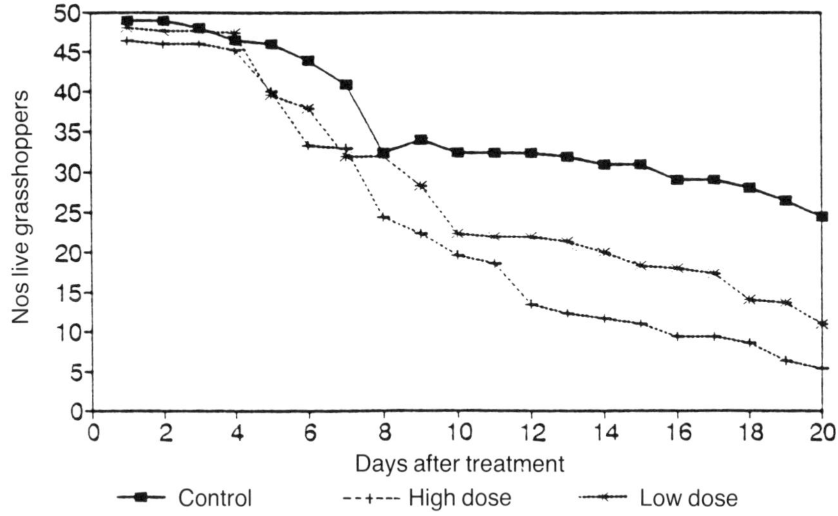

Figure 4. Results of the application of *Beauveria bassiana* as a bait.

Verde, contrary to the results obtained in Montana (Delgado *et al.*, 1990). The type of vegetation, climatic conditions and the species of grasshoppers may all be factors contributing to this difference. Based on these results further research should address the following:

1. formulation and application protocols
2. mode of infection
3. specificity of *B. bassiana* to certain species of grasshopper.

Nosema locustae

The spores of *N. locustae* used in the trials carried out in Cape Verde were produced by Evans-Biocontrol in the USA. After bioassay in the laboratory in Cape Verde to demonstrate viability of the spores, trials were set up in the field on Santiago island in September 1989, involving two doses of *N. locustae*: 2.5×10^9 spores/ha and 5×10^9 spores/ha. For the lower dose, six plots of 500 ha each were established in areas infested by grasshoppers, three treated and three controls. The dose of 5×10^9 spores/ha was applied to two plots, one of 200 ha and another of 100 ha with appropriate controls. Spores of *N. locustae* were applied in a bran-bait formulation with aerial application equipment provided by GTZ. In 1989, the assessment of results was based on evaluation of population density, using the ring method (0.1 m^2) and disease prevalence. The assessment of population density was begun two to three days before application and continued for 41 days. Disease prevalence was based on percentage of grasshoppers infected in collections of 100–150 grasshoppers each week near the centre of each plot. These samples also were used to determine the species composition of the grasshopper populations, the age structure of the grasshoppers and infection by other micro-organisms. Only *O. senegalensis* and *D. axillaris*, which were the most common grasshoppers, were examined for *N. locustae* and other micro-organisms. The observations were continued during the rainy season in 1990 (August–November).

Results and conclusions

The evaluation of population composition and density did not show any significant differences between treatments and controls. However, analysis of data on population composition and density of *O. senegalensis* showed a significant difference ($P < 0.05$) on the 27th day in 1989. Also, in the 100 ha plot in the north of the island that was treated with 5×10^9 spores/ha we noted a distinct reduction in population in the treated plot compared with the control. However, the difference was not significant.

Since *O. senegalensis* was the predominant species in plots treated with 2.5×10^9 spores/ha, representing about 90% of all grasshoppers, observations in 1989 for prevalence of *N. locustae* were restricted to this species. Approximately 10,000 grasshoppers were examined. The first cases of infection by *N. locustae* were noted 27 days after treatment. As indicated in Fig. 5, the maximum prevalence of infection was about 18%. Infections were not observed in grasshoppers from control plots which demonstrates that infections resulted from treatments.

For the plots treated at 5×10^9 spores/ha, observations were made on *O. senegalensis*, and *D. axillaris*. The level of infection in *O. senegalensis* by *N. locustae* was, on average, over 28% (Fig. 6). Infections were not observed in *D. axillaris*.

Observations were made one year after treatment (1990), both in plots treated with 2.5×10^9 spores/ha and in control plots, both of which showed general decrease in grasshopper population density from the previous year. There were no significant differences between treated and untreated plots.

The level of infection of *N. locustae* one year after treatment was lower than that in 1989 when the trial was begun.

The results obtained show that the dosages of 2.5×10^9 and 5×10^9 spores/ha of *N. locustae* did not significantly reduce population density of *O. senegalensis*. One of the reasons for this may be the very rapid development of *O. senegalensis* compared with the time necessary for *N. locustae* to reach a level sufficient to kill the insect. These results have however confirmed, that *O. senegalensis* is sensitive to *N. locustae*, as previously

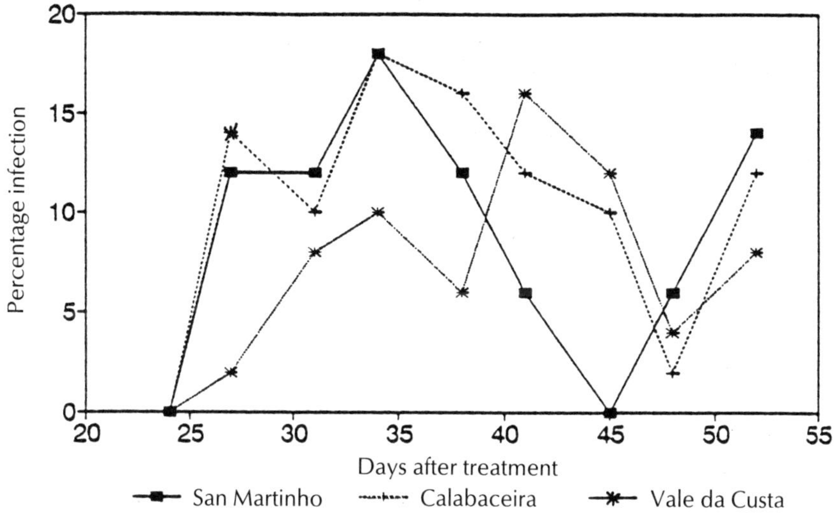

Figure 5. Infection levels of *Nosema locustae* in *Oedaleus senegalensis* (dose 2.5 × 10^9 spores/ha)

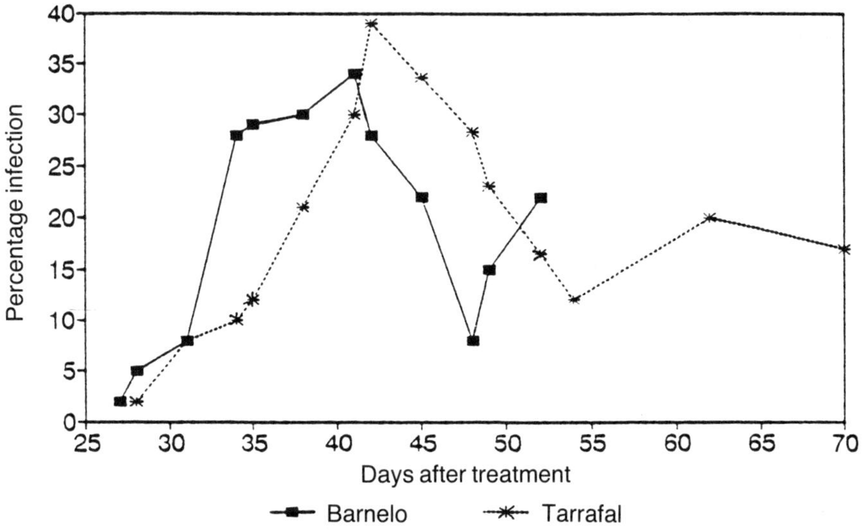

Figure 6. Infection levels of *Nosema locustae* in *Oedaleus senegalensis* (dose 5 × 10^9 spores/ha)

described by Henry *et al.* (1985a). The absence of infection in *D. axillaris*, which is also sensitive according to Henry (1991) and Henry *et al.* (1985a), was probably due to the unacceptability of the baits to this species.

In conclusion, large scale applications of *N. locustae* resulted in infections in *O. senegalensis* which possibly reduced densities, but the reductions are not sufficient for control of *O. senegalensis* in Cape Verde.

Viruses: evaluation of infection of *O. senegalensis* and *D. axillaris* with entomopoxviruses

Towards the end of 1990 two shipments containing cadavers of grasshoppers infected with OPV or MPV viruses were received from Montana State University (USA).

In the laboratory, extractions of these micro-organisms from the cadavers provided inoculum for bioassays in Cape Verdian grasshoppers and for mass production of these viruses to produce inoculum for subsequent field and laboratory tests.

Bioassays

Third instar nymphs were separated, placed individually in small glass tubes and starved for 24 hours. The inoculum in an aqueous suspension was placed on 7 mm discs of maize (or bean) leaves, using a 10 ml syringe. When the drops were dry, the leaf discs were fed to the grasshoppers. Only those grasshoppers which completely consumed the leaf disc were used in bioassays.

The following dosages were used in the bioassays: 10^6, 10^5, and 10^4 spores/insect (three replicates). After inoculation, the grasshoppers were placed in tubes in groups of five nymphs. The dead grasshoppers were removed daily from the tubes, titrated and homogenized in 5 ml of distilled water and the homogenate examined under the microscope for virus inclusions.

After 21 days, the remaining live grasshoppers were sacrificed and each was examined as above. The prevalence of infection noted at 10^6 varied between 16% and 35%, which established that *O. senegalensis* is susceptible to OPV infections. However, the high level of mortality provoked by other factors considerably reduced the number of grasshoppers at the beginning of the experiment, in treatments as well as in controls. Accordingly, another trial in the laboratory using other methodology is needed to obtain more conclusive results.

An identical study was tried with MPV against *D. axillaris*. However, the fact that infections were not evident, suggested the MPV does not infect this species.

In addition to the bioassays, grasshoppers were inoculated in order to mass produce these viruses. These inoculations resulted in production of a considerable quantity of OPV in *O. senegalensis.* However, again no infections occurred among the *D. axillaris* inoculated with MPV.

Isolation and evaluation of endemic organisms in grasshoppers in Cape Verde

A considerable number of grasshoppers (over 7,000 specimens) were collected on the islands of Santiago, Maio, Boavista and Santo Antao for disease diagnosis. Infection was observed in *O. senegalensis, D. axillaris* and other species by eugregarines (Protozoa) as previously observed by Henry *et al.* (1985b). These organisms exert little influence on grasshopper mortality. Some grasshoppers, especially *O. senegalensis* and *D. axillaris,* were parasitized by the protozoan *Malamoeba locustae* (King & Taylor). This protozoan causes debilitative effects that reduce the reproductive capacity of grasshoppers. A small number of *O. senegalensis* collected from different locations were infected with various fungi, which in one case was tentatively determined as *Metarhizium anisopliae* (Metschnikoff) Sorokin. Also, a fungus has been isolated from *D. axillaris* from Santo Antao island which is being studied for species determination. A microsporidian has been isolated from *Pyrgomorpha cognata* Krauss from Santo Antao and Santiago islands which is possibly an undescribed species. Also, endemic infections by an entomopoxvirus, which probably is the same as OPV that is being tested, has been observed in *O. senegalensis* from Santiago island. In addition, infections by the bacterium *Bacillus* (probably *B. cereus* Frankland & Frankland) have been diagnosed in grasshoppers from Santiago island.

References

Delgado, F., Bradley, C. & Henry, J. (1990) *Beauveria bassiana* grasshopper bioinsecticide field trial. Cape Verde. Special report included in final project report submitted to US-AID.

Henry, J.E. (1991) Results of field trials with *Nosema locustae* against grasshoppers in Cape Verde. Special report included in final project report submitted to US-AID.

Henry, J.E., Fowler, J.L., Wilson, M.C. & Onsager, J.A. (1985a) Infection of West African grasshoppers with *Nosema locustae* Canning (Protozoa: Microsporida: Nosematidae). *Tropical Pest Management* **31**, 144–147.

Henry, J.E., Wilson, M.C., Oma, E.A. & Fowler, J.L. (1985b) Pathogenic microorganisms isolated from West African grasshoppers (Orthoptera: Acrididae). *Tropical Pest Management* **31**, 192–195.

Field trials with the entomopathogenic fungus *Beauveria bassiana* against grasshoppers in Mali, West Africa, July, 1990

D.L. Johnson[1], M.S. Goettel[1], C. Bradley[2], H. van der Paauw[3] & B. Maiga[4]

[1]Agriculture Canada Research Station, Lethbridge, Alberta: [2]Mycotech Corporation: [3]Ciba-Geigy AG: [4]Service Nationale de la Protection des Végétaux Ministère de l'Agriculture, Mali.

Abstract

Spores were applied to open field sites and field cages near Mourdiah, Mali. Hand-held spinning disk nozzles (Micro-Ulva) were used to spray spores in dormant oil. For the field trials, grasshoppers were sprayed in replicated plots in 5 randomized complete blocks. Fifteen plots of 0.5 ha each were established, sampled for grasshopper age and density, and treated with spores and oil, oil alone or no treatment. Excellent spore viability (averaging 88%), grasshopper densities of 30 or more immatures per m^2, and optimum application conditions favoured a useful test. Grasshoppers were successfully infected in the field plots, although post treatment hatching and rainfall tended to obscure detection of infection and impact on population density.

Incubation of dead hoppers at high humidity confirmed the presence of *B. bassiana* in insects dying 4–14 days after treatment. Two weeks after field treatment, total mortality in cages of grasshoppers from plots sprayed was 72%. Hoppers collected from control plots had a total mortality of 22% when held in cages over the same period.

Cage trials included sprayed and unsprayed hoppers, collected and treated at the site, that were monitored in 60 field cages and assayed for infection. The results of these cage trials indicated that, over the 19 days following treatment application, mortality of grasshoppers sprayed with spores was approximately double the natural mortality experienced by control groups. Spores sprayed directly onto vegetation before grasshoppers were added to the cages did not result in significant mortality on most sampling dates. Direct contact spray treatment, resulted in significant mortality in samples of grasshoppers caged after spraying. However, no direct reduction in population was noted in this trial.

Introduction and background

Locusts and grasshoppers have caused considerable losses to African crops in both modern and traditional agricultural systems. Existing control strategies rely on chemical insecticides to prevent damage to vegetation (Table 1), and these methods, though often effective, are not always appropriate. Effective alternatives that offer improved safety could have rapid and favourable environmental and economic impact.

The use of pathogens may offer an environmentally sound method for the management of grasshoppers and locusts. Hyphomycete fungi are the most promising candidates (Prior & Greathead, 1989) because in addition to causing mortal diseases in many insects, they are usually cheap to produce and are available from commercial sources in quantities large enough for experimental purposes, and they are generally not pathogenic to non-target organisms (Goettel *et al.*, 1990). They can penetrate directly through the cuticle and do not necessarily need to be ingested in order to initiate disease. Recent research at Lethbridge and Butte indicates that grasshoppers are highly susceptible to some isolates of the fungus *Beauveria bassiana* (Balsamo) Vuillemin.

There are several records of *B. bassiana* infecting Orthoptera (MacLeod, 1954; Humber & Soper, 1986; Li, 1987; Moore & Erlandson, 1988). Some recent experimental studies have also demonstrated its pathogenicity to grasshoppers under laboratory conditions (Marcandier & Khachatourians, 1987; Moore & Erlandson, 1988). Other recent research has shown that grasshoppers are highly susceptible to a strain of *B. bassiana* isolated from a dead grasshopper in Montana (Johnson *et al.*, 1988). Grasshoppers that were fed wheat leaves treated with spores died within 10 days. In subsequent laboratory dose-mortality tests, spores of *B. bassiana* sprayed in water or applied on lettuce disks were found to infect and kill grasshoppers of other species and ages at economically reasonable levels of application. Experiments in which third-instar grasshoppers were

Table 1. Amounts and value of insecticide used for control of grasshoppers and locusts in Mali, 1986. (Rachadi (1986) cited by Kawasaki (1990)).

Product	Value (1,000 FFr)	Quantity
Diazinon 960	4,130	56,400 l
Fenitrothion ULV 500	11,379	199,625 l
Fenitrothion ULV 960/1000	2,637	35,400 l
γ-HCH 25 (BHC)	5,140	514 t
Malathion ULV 960	367	10,000 l

fed lettuce disks treated with droplets of spores indicated mortality of over 60% at one million spores per hopper. Reasonable field application rates (such as in the Mali field trial described below) would result in an average of over 1,000 times this quantity of spores per m^2. Economic analysis by Mycotech has indicated that, if successful, an application rate of 10^{13} conidia per ha can be competitive in price with chemicals currently used for grasshopper control.

The development of methods for the mass production of this strain by Mycotech Corporation has allowed preliminary field trials to be conducted against grasshoppers in Alberta, Montana, and Saskatchewan (Bradley, M.A. Erlandson, Goettel & Johnson, unpublished data). These applications included treatment of caged grass and crop, and also treatment of whole fields, using bran bait and spray formulations.

Objectives of Mali trials

Development of *B. bassiana* as a microbial insecticide effective for grasshopper control in Africa is a complex undertaking that will require an extended development and testing programme. The 1990 trials in Africa were a first step in this development programme and had several objectives:

1. to evaluate formulation and application methods under African conditions in field and cage trials
2. to test effectiveness against mixed species population of African grasshoppers
3. to gain experience in use of hand-held ULV sprayers for the purpose of fungal spore application.

Materials and methods

Conidia production and formulation

The *B. bassiana* isolate used in this study was originally obtained from a migratory grasshopper (*Melanoplus sanguinipes* (Fabricius)) collected near Three Forks, MT, USA, and is being developed by Mycotech Corporation, Butte, MT, for control of grasshoppers. Conidia were produced according to solid culture technology developed by Mycotech Corporation (Bradley *et al.*, in press; Goettel & Roberts, these proceedings). Conidia yields and concentrations were consistent, ranging from 1 to 3 $\times$ 10^{13} conidia per kg of dry substrate, and producing conidia powders ranging from 2 to 7 $\times$ 10^{10} conidia per g. Final blended conidia powders contained 4 $\times$ 10^{10} viable conidia per g. The conidia were transported to Africa as dry powder in screw cap plastic bottles. The powder was held in refrigeration in Bamako and Mourdiah, Mali, but was otherwise held at ambient temperatures when taken to the field.

Conidia powders were formulated in oil on site immediately prior to field application. The oil (Sunspray, Sun Refining and Marketing Co., Philadelphia) is an inert paraffinic type and is registered with the EPA as an insecticide carrier. The oil formulation had been previously tested as a concentrate diluted in water, but to achieve ultra-low volume (ULV) application, it was necessary to use a suspension of undiluted oil and conidia. Greater infectivity of oil over water formulations was previously demonstrated by Prior *et al.*, 1988. The conidia were suspended in the oil at a rate of 100 g/1(w/v).

Conidia viability

Both the dry conidia powder and the formulated oil suspensions were assayed before and after application. To determine viability of the raw spore product, conidia powder was suspended and diluted in sterile water. Oil formulated conidia were diluted in oil. Aliquots of 0.1 ml containing approximately 1×10^4 conidia were spread onto the surface of Sabouraud's dextrose agar supplemented with 2% yeast extract, streptomycin (50 μl/ml) and penicillin (25 I.U./ml) in a 10 cm petri dish with a sterile glass rod and incubated at room temperature. After 7–10 h, the numbers of germinated and non-germinated spores were counted using a compound microscope. Conidia in oil were first stained by placing a drop of lacto-fuchsin (Carmichael, 1955) onto the surface of the agar and covering with a glass cover slip.

Ultra-low volume spray application tests

Preliminary application tests were conducted in Lethbridge to evaluate ULV application of the oil formulation. Micro-ulva sprayers manufactured by Micron Sprayers Ltd, Bromyard, England, were provided by Ciba Geigy AG, Basel. These sprayers are hand-held, and use a battery-powered spinning disc fed by gravity, from a 500 or 1,000 ml reservoir. Flow rate is determined by the orifice size of the nozzle that feeds the disc. Droplet size is determined by disc rotation speed, controlled by the number of batteries and by the viscosity of the formulation. Using the largest available nozzle size and a mid-range of 7,000 rpm (red nozzle, 4 batteries), the flow rates of oil containing various concentrations of conidia powder were determined. Droplet size and conidia dispersion were determined using oil sensitive spray cards and microscopic examination of droplets on glass slides. The cards and slides were treated by walking a 2 m swath in still air, using 70 g/l conidia suspension.

Mali field trial

Site description and experimental design

The field trial site was approximately 5 km from the village of Mourdiah, about 250 km north of Bamako. The terrain was flat and vegetation consisted of areas of trees and scrub intermixed with open areas. Open areas were a mix of grass cover and sandy areas without vegetation.

The trial was replicated in 5 complete blocks. Each block contained three 0.5 ha plots. The blocks occupied open areas, with the exception of the first block which was a mixture of trees with interspersed grass and open, sandy areas. Plots measured 70 m × 70 m and were laid out on compass bearings using a measuring wheel. The plots were separated from each other by a minimum barrier strip of 30 m. In each block, one plot was an untreated control, one plot was sprayed with formulation oil only, and the third plot received a spray application of spores in oil.

Field application

Application volume was 1.5 l/0.5 ha plot, giving an application rate of 1.2×10^{13} conidia/ha. Application rates were verified by collecting the formulated oil from the sprayer and counting spore density by using a haemocytometer. Oil only control plots were treated at the same spray volume. All plots were sprayed using Micro-ulva sprayers, with 4 batteries, with 1-3 sprayers in use simultaneously. Swath width was approximately 5 m. Wind speed was measured at the time of application, and plots were sprayed only if wind speed was less than about 2 m/s. All plots were sprayed in the evening between 17.00 and 19.00 h, with the exception of plot 3B which was sprayed beginning at 10.00 h. Control and test plots were sprayed on successive evenings on 14–17 July. Because of rainfall after treatment application (30 mm and 6 mm received on 14 and 16 July, respectively), plots were resprayed on 21 and 22 July. (In the results, these are referred to as the first and second spray applications.) An additional 38 mm of rain was recorded 23 July. Air temperatures during the trial ranged between 23 and 33°C.

Grasshopper population monitoring and mortality assessment

Grasshopper population species composition was determined from sweepnet samples taken prior to spraying. Grasshopper densities were determined using sample rings of 0.1 m^2 each, with 25 rings arranged diagonally across each plot. Population estimates were recorded by approaching and counting grasshoppers in each of the 25 rings, and an additional confirmative measure was made by counting the number observed in 25 visual m^2 quadrats. Sample rings were counted prior to spraying and at three-day intervals after spraying. Because of problems with passing livestock herds, it was not possible to keep track of the identity and position of individual ring counts. The pre-treatment means for each of the 15 plots were calculated, and this value was subtracted from each individual post-treatment observation to adjust the data to absolute changes from the original mean population density for the respective plots. The result was a set of DELTAs, where

for date i, block j, plot k, ring l, the deviation is
$$\text{DELTA(ijkl)} = \text{COUNT(ijkl)} - \text{COUNT(0jk.)},$$

that is, the lth count minus the initial kth plot mean. COUNT is the mean number of grasshoppers counted per 0.25 m^2 ring, and DELTA is the mean deviation from the pre-treatment ring count mean (date 0). A positive DELTA indicates a population increase; a negative DELTA indicates a decline relative to the initial grasshopper density. The DELTAs were subjected to analysis of variance, with F-tests against appropriate experimental error and sampling error mean squares.

Plots were searched for samples of dead grasshoppers beginning three days after application. *B. bassiana* infection was confirmed by incubating cadavers collected from the plots in petri dishes with moist cotton and observing for conidiation of the fungus. In addition, grasshopper samples were collected from test and control plots 0-3 days after spraying (using sweepnets) and held for daily observation in screened cages.

Vegetation and soil samples were collected from the site before treatment, and screened for *B. bassiana,* using a selective growth medium (Dodine Oatmeal Agar) (Beilharz *et al.*, 1982)

Cage trials

Montana

A preliminary cage trial was conducted by Mycotech Corporation near Three Forks, Montana, in late June, 1990. The objectives were to test the undiluted conidia preparations under field conditions and to test conidia preparations and formulation oil to be used in Mali trials.

Two application rates and two methods were tested. Application rates were equivalent to 1×10^{13} and 2×10^{13} conidia in 3 ha, applied to plots of 20 m^2 each. To assess direct contact, plots containing grasshoppers were sprayed. Grasshoppers were removed from these plots and placed in cages on unsprayed vegetation. Secondary contact was tested by placing unsprayed grasshoppers in cages on previously sprayed vegetation. There were replicate cages for each conidia application rate and application method.

Cages were observed daily by Mycotech personnel for seven days. At seven days after application the remaining living grasshoppers were removed to laboratory containment for continued observation and confirmation of *B. bassiana* infection.

Mali

Cage trials were conducted to evaluate direct contact versus contact with sprayed vegetation. The conidial suspension was made to be approximately equivalent to suspensions used in field trials. The suspension contained 2.3×10^9 conidia/ml, determined by microscopic count. Grasshoppers were field-collected and were of mixed species composition and age. Cages covered 1.0 m^2 of ground surface and were 0.5 m high. They were constructed at the site from cloth netting over wooden frames. The netting could be opened at the top for introducing grasshoppers and for purposes of observation. Stakes and a soil berm around the bases held the cages in place and prevented grasshoppers from escaping under the netting.

The cage trials each included 4 treatments and two controls as shown below:

1. Cage 1 Control – no spray
2. Cage 2 Control – grasshoppers sprayed with oil only
3. Cage 3 Grasshoppers sprayed, vegetation unsprayed
4. Cage 4 Grasshoppers sprayed, vegetation sprayed
5. Cage 5 Grasshoppers unsprayed, vegetation sprayed
6. Cage 6 Grasshoppers unsprayed, vegetation sprayed, 4x dose.

Each set of six cages was replicated 5 times, resulting in a total of 30 cages. Each cage held 25 grasshoppers. For contact spray, treatment 3, grasshoppers were released on a large rectangular sheet of plastic and sprayed in one pass with a Micro-ulva sprayer. Grasshoppers were recaptured and placed in cages on unsprayed vegetation.

For the 'vegetation spray' treatment, one pass with the Micro-ulva sprayer was made over the wooden frames of the cages before the netting was put in place. Unsprayed grasshoppers were then placed in the cages on the sprayed vegetation. Treatment 4 consisted of sprayed grasshoppers confined with sprayed vegetation. In treatment 6, a four-fold higher dose was sprayed on vegetation, by two passes over the cages, using a double concentration of conidia suspension containing 4.9×10^9 conidia per ml.

The cage trial was set up and sprayed on 18 July between 18.00 and 19.30 h. High wind with light rain (16.5 mm) occurred at about midnight. Cages withstood the wind but in the morning were found to contain water. The experiment was continued as planned, but to confirm the results the entire cage trial was repeated with a new set of hoppers and treatments on 19 July (referred to in the results as Trial 2).

Results

Conidia viability and application rates

Conidia in powder were determined to be 90% viable at packaging in Butte, Montana. Viability of oil formulated conidia in Mali at time of field application ranged from 85 to 95% with a weighted average of 88%. There was no apparent effect on viability of conidia held in oil during the spraying operation (approximately 1–2 h).

Flow rates decreased with increasing spore concentration (Table 2). At 170 g/l significant plugging of the valve occurred. Consequently, the concentration adopted for field trials was 100 g/l requiring application of 3 l/ha to obtain an application rate of 10^{13} viable spores per ha. At this concentration, most droplets varied from 30 to 300 microns diameter, and conidia were dispersed in droplets with little evidence of clumping.

Examination of spore droplets on microscope slides placed in the sprayer swath indicated a typical density of 20–40 spores per oil droplet.

Mali field trials

At the time of application of the spores in oil, the dominant grasshopper species in the site east of Mourdiah were *Kraussella amabile* (Krauss), *Cataloipus cymbiferus* (Krauss) and *Hieroglyphus daganensis* (Krauss), more than 95% as first to third instars. Less common species, also primarily represented by first to third instars, included *Acorypha glaucopsis* (Walker), *Acrida bicolor* (Thunberg), *Kraussaria angulifera* (Krauss), *Oedaleus senegalensis* (Krauss), *Diabolocatantops axillaris* (Thunberg), and *Zacompsa festa* (Karsch).

Population density just prior to treatment application was 4.2 immature grasshoppers/0.25 m^2 (17 July, n = 150). Although some post-treatment hatching obscured detection of levels of infection, and ants were seen to remove dead and dying hoppers, some dead hoppers that produced *Beauveria bassiana* hyphae were found at the site. High variation, eclosion,

Table 2. Flow rates of conidia oil suspensions in Micro-ulva sprayers.

Conidial Powder in Oil (g/l)	Flow Rate (ml/min)
0 (oil only)	33
33	32
67	24
170	intermittent (plugging)

and only moderate impact of the treatment resulted in no significant discernable decline in abundance following spray application. Three days after the second application the increase in mean grasshopper density (DELTA) was higher in the untreated plots than in the plots sprayed with either spores (lowest increase) or oil only (Table 3, Tukey's HSD, $P < 0.05$), indicating a somewhat greater population increase in the untreated plots. Only Block 5 had lower DELTA in the control plot. After this date even this limited impact in the field plots was not evident. The effects of spraying oil only vs. spraying spores in oil did not differ significantly ($P > 0.05$). Evidence of recent eclosion and large numbers of newly-hatched hoppers (mostly *C. cymbiferus*, *H. daganensis*, and *K. angulifera*) were observed within days after both the first and second spray dates. After this first post-treatment sampling date, the differences among treatments were not significant.

Field-collected hoppers from *B. bassiana*-treated plots held in cages confirmed infection by *B. bassiana.* Incubation of dead hoppers at high humidity resulted in fungal growth and sporulation in cadavers dying between 4 and 14 days after treatment. Two weeks after field treatment,

Table 3. Mean grasshopper count in each plot 3 days after the second application. COUNT is the mean number of grasshoppers counted per 0.25 m^2 ring. DELTA is the mean deviation from the ring count mean at the beginning of the experiment. A positive DELTA indicates a population increase.

			COUNT		DELTA	
Block	Treatment	n	Mean	S.D.	Mean	S.D.
1	untreated	25	9.84	3.44	5.08	3.44
1	oil only	25	7.16	3.21	−0.72	3.21
1	spore spray	25	8.20	3.55	4.40	3.55
2	untreated	25	6.20	3.52	3.00	3.52
2	oil only	25	11.12	4.24	5.56	4.24
2	spore spray	25	7.40	3.45	1.64	3.45
3	untreated	25	12.96	5.57	8.12	5.57
3	oil only	25	13.84	6.55	6.20	6.55
3	spore spray	25	11.00	3.54	3.88	3.54
4	untreated	25	11.32	5.71	1.36	5.71
4	oil only	25	4.72	4.37	0.84	4.37
4	spore spray	25	11.24	3.97	0.84	3.97
5	untreated	25	9.32	3.48	7.12	3.48
5	oil only	25	9.92	4.07	6.40	4.07
5	spore spray	25	10.08	3.96	7.28	3.96

total grasshopper mortality in all treated blocks was 72%. Hoppers collected from control plots had a total mortality of 22% when held in cages over the same period.

Vegetation and soil samples were collected from the site before treatment, and screened for *Beauveria* spp., using selective growth media. Colonies subsequently examined turned out to be other taxa. No native *Beauveria* spp. were found at the site.

Cage trials

Montana

All treatments in the trials conducted in Montana by Mycotech Corporation showed significant infection and 80 to 100% mortality in 7 to 14 days. Infection occurred equally from both direct contact spray and contact with sprayed vegetation. The Mycotech trial confirmed the compatibility of the conidia preparation with the oil formulation to be used in Africa.

Mali

Sprayed grasshoppers confined in the cages suffered significantly higher mortality than the control groups (Table 4). The average percentage of the grasshoppers that remained over 19 days following treatment application is plotted in Figs 1 and 2 (Trials 1 and 2). Even though the rains may have interfered with Trial 1, the impact of the direct spraying of spores is evident in both trials. In both trials, spores sprayed onto hoppers provided significant mortality ($P < 0.05$) one week after application.

The pattern, but not the statistical significance, persisted in the later dates.

Discussion

The conidia powder was stable and did not lose viability over the course of the experiments; although there were no extended periods of extreme (greater than 35°C) temperatures during transport and storage, this indicates that the spores are not highly sensitive to environmental conditions while kept in dry form. Formulation in oil did not adversely affect viability. The oil provides a stable, liquid formulation in which conidia do not germinate. The hydrophobic conidia were also found to disperse well in the oil, assisting in evenness of application.

The oil provided a means of easy application via hand-held sprayers. Based on discussions with Ciba Geigy and plant protection staff in Mali

Table 4. Analysis of variance and comparison of mean percentages of hoppers remaining alive in the treatment cages. The F-tests indicate overall block and treatment differences (tested against experimental error, block*treatment interaction). Means with the same letter, within a particular trial and date, are not significantly different (Tukey's HSD, $P > 0.05$).

TRIAL = 1 DAYS = 7 (Block $P = 0.028$, Treatment $P = 0.002$)

Test	Treatment	n	% alive	S.D.
a	check	5	73.6	21.47
ab	oil on hoppers	5	58.0	12.33
b	spores on hoppers	5	36.8	21.61
ab	spores on veg 1x	1	60.0	—
ab	spores on veg 4x	5	48.0	15.23
b	spores on hop & veg	5	31.2	11.10

TRIAL = 1 DAYS = 9 (Block $P = 0.060$, Treatment $P = 0.009$)

Test	Treatment	n	% alive	S.D.
ab	check	5	41.6	2.19
a	oil on hoppers	5	56.4	13.45
ab	spores on hoppers	5	32.8	20.67
ab	spores on veg 1x	1	52.0	—
ab	spores on veg 4x	5	29.6	16.64
b	spores on hop & veg	5	24.0	8.00

TRIAL = 2 DAYS = 7 (Block $P = 0.249$, Treatment $P = 0.062$)

Test	Treatment	n	% alive	S.D.
a	check	5	68.8	20.86
ab	oil on hoppers	5	58.4	21.84
b	spores on hoppers	5	22.4	11.17
ab	spores on veg 1x	5	41.6	22.38
ab	spores on veg 4x	5	39.2	27.77
ab	spores on hop & veg	5	45.6	31.57

TRIAL = 2 DAYS = 9 (Block $P = 0.331$, Treatment $P = 0.002$)

Test	Treatment	n	% alive	S.D.
a	check	5	56.8	18.42
ab	oil on hoppers	5	45.6	8.76
c	spores on hoppers	5	15.2	9.12
abc	spores on veg 1x	5	30.4	13.15
bc	spores on veg 4x	5	25.6	15.13
abc	spores on hop & veg	5	38.4	17.80

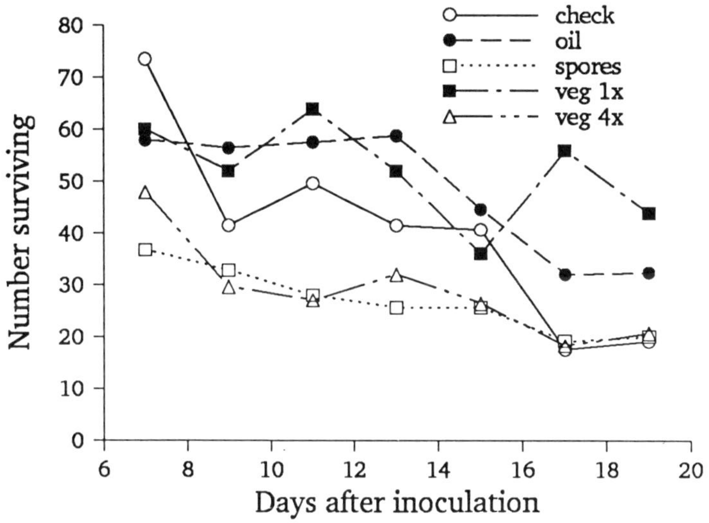

Figure 1. The average percentage of the grasshoppers that remained over 19 days following treatment application, Trial 1.

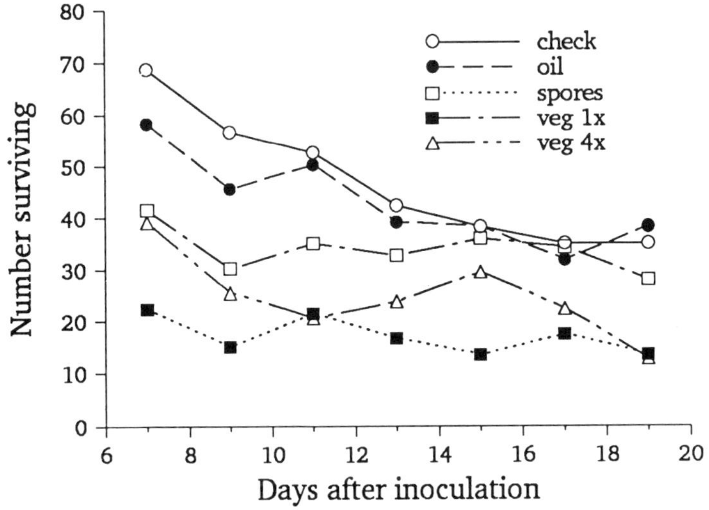

Figure 2. The average percentage of the grasshoppers that remained over 19 days following treatment application, Trial 2.

and Cape Verde, it was determined that ULV spinning disc sprayers would be the best application method for these initial trials. This type of sprayer is in widespread use in Africa, and they are also a model for ULV aerial application. The oil formulation was easily applied using this technology, although some difficulties were encountered due to variable winds and ground convection currents that occasionally hampered uniform application.

Pilot production data were evaluated by Mycotech Corporation in an economic model. The expected costs of solid culture technology production of spores to treat 1 million h at an application rate of 1×10^{13} conidia per ha are such that *B. bassiana* conidia could be profitably marketed. For example, the cost of 1×10^{13} conidia would be approximately US$5.00/ha, competitive with the midrange price of chemicals now used for grasshopper control.

Although no discernable decline in abundance of hoppers following field-spray application could be detected, indications were that infections were established and that there were greater population increases in the untreated plots. Post-treatment hatching, aggravated by movement of livestock herds through the experimental fields, obscured detection of any differences in population density between treatment and control plots beyond the initial sampling dates. On the other hand, 72% of the hoppers collected from treated plots 0–3 days after treatment died within 2 weeks of the treatment date, with confirmed *B. bassiana* occurring between 4 and 14 days. Although this may be an indication of actual mortality in the field, it must be taken into consideration that caged hoppers may be stressed and were possibly more susceptible to infection. In any case, these results demonstrate that the hoppers were at least exposed to the inoculum in sufficient quantity for infection to occur.

Results of cage trials confirmed that grasshoppers sprayed directly were susceptible to infection by the fungus. The results from the sprayed vegetation and vegetation plus hoppers are not as clear, but the direct spray treatment was significantly superior in most cases.

Results of subsequent trials in Cape Verde using the same conidia and oil preparations as in Mali (Delgado *et al.*, 1991) indicate that formulation attributes are very important. The Mali trials used only the oil formulations in field and the corresponding cage trials, whereas separate Cape Verde cage trials also included a wheat bran bait formulation. Sweep net samples from field plots taken 24 h after spraying showed a significant infection rate. In their trials, wheat bran bait in cage trials also showed significant mortality with greater than 90% kill in 14 days. However, field plot sweep net samples taken 72 h after spraying and cage trials of sprayed vegetation showed no significant mortality. The Cape Verde results agreed with our suggestion that grasshoppers did not become infected from contact with sprayed vegetation, but did become infected when contacted directly by spray and through consumption of spores on wheat bran bait. Preliminary cage trials in Montana showed that contact with sprayed vegetation was effective. A possible explanation for this discrepancy is that conidia may be less viable on vegetation surfaces in Africa than in Montana, for environmental reasons, such as intensity of sunlight. Another explanation is that grasshoppers may have avoided sprayed vegetation. This hypothesis is supported by preliminary laboratory bioassays in Lethbridge: 30% of *Melanoplus sanguinipes* starved for 24 h and presented with a lettuce disk treated with 5 µl of a conidia suspension in oil did not consume the lettuce whereas 100% accepted unsprayed control leaves (Bradley, Goettel & Johnson, unpublished data).

At this time, there is no explanation for the ineffectiveness of sprayed vegetation. Laboratory and environmental chamber studies will be necessary to determine differences between conditions in Montana and Africa. If further laboratory studies are pursued, they will be aimed at determining mode of pathogenesis and virulence as affected by formulation, inoculum targeting, host species and fungal strain.

Acknowledgements

The authors acknowledge the co-operation of Walter Knausenberger, US Agency for International Development; C. Omar Daffe and Sekou Coulibaly, SNPV; and Pauline Wood, Mycotech Corporation. They are also grateful for assistance from Houcine Hadj, Dahmaine, Eric Marinot and Olivier Berthelier, Ciba-Geigy; Souliman Coulibali, Boye Diallo and Amadou Toure, SNPV; and Craig Andrews, Grant Duke, Robyn Russell and Barb Nemeth, Agriculture Canada.

References

Beilhaz, V.C., Parbery, D.G. & Swart, H.J. (1982) Dodine: a selective agent for certain soil fungi. *Transactions of the British Mycological Society* **79**, 507–511.

Bradley, C., Black, W., Kearns, R. & Woods, P. (in press) The role of production technology in mycoinsecticide development. In: *Mycological Society of America Symposium on Industrial Mycology.* Madison, WI. June 1990.

Carmichael, J.W. (1955) Lacto-fuchsin: a new medium for mounting fungi. *Mycologia* **47**, 611.

Delgado, F., Bradley, C. & Henry, J. (1991) Beauveria bassiana *Grasshopper Bioinsecticide Field Trial, Cape Verde, August, 1990.* Report to USAID.

Goettel, M.S., Poprawski, T.J., Vandenberg, J.D., Li, Z & Roberts, D.W. (1990) Safety to nontarget invertebrates of fungal biocontrol agents. In: Laird, M., Lacey, L.A. & Davidson, E.W. (eds), *Safety of Microbial Insecticides.* Boca Raton, CRC PRESS, pp. 209–231.

Humber, R.A. & Soper, R.S. (1986) USDA-ARS collection of entomopathogenic fungal cultures. Catalog of strains. USDA. Agricultural Research Service, Ithaca, NY, 56 pp.

Johnson, D.L., Pavlik, E. & Bradley, C. (1988) Activity of *Beauveria bassiana* sprayed onto wheat against grasshoppers. Expert Committee on Pesticide Use in Agriculture, Pesticide Research Report, Ottawa, p. 140.

Kawasaki, S. (1990) Country report: locust control in West Africa. *Japan Pesticide Information* **56**, 15–16.

Li, Z. (1987) A list of the insect hosts of *Beauveria bassiana. In* First National Symposium on Entomogenous Fungi, Gongzhuling, Jilin, People's Republic of China.

MacLeod, D.M. (1954) Investigations on the genera *Beauveria* Vuill. and *Tritirachium* Limber. *Canadian Journal of Botany* **32**, 818–890.

Marcandier, S. & Khachatourians, G.G. (1987) Susceptibility of the migratory grasshopper, *Melanoplus sanguinipes* to *Beauveria bassiana*: influence of relative humidity. *Canadian Entomologist* **119**, 901–907.

Moore, K.C. & Erlandson, M.A. (1988) Isolation of *Aspergillus parasiticus* Speare and *Beauveria bassiana* (Bals.) Vuillemin from melanopline grasshoppers (Orthoptera: Acrididae) and demonstration of their pathogenicity in *Melanoplus sanguinipes* (Fabricius). *Canadian Entomologist* **120**, 989–991.

Prior, C. & Greathead, D.J. (1989) Biological control of locusts: the potential for the exploitation of pathogens. *FAO Plant Protection Bulletin* **37**, 37–48.

Prior, C., Jollands, P. & le Patourel, G. (1988) Infectivity of oil and water formulations of *Beauveria bassiana* (Deutermycotina: Hyphomycetes) to cocoa weevil pest *Pantorhytes plutus* (Coleoptera: Curculionidae). *Journal of Invertebrate Pathology* **52**, 66–71.

Field cage trials on the effects of enriched neem oil, insect growth regulators and the pathogens *Beauveria bassiana* and *Nosema locustae* on desert locusts in the Republic of Niger

O.M. Nasseh, T. Freres, J. Wilps, E. Kirkilionis & S. Krall

Deutsche Gesellschaft für Technische Zusammenarbeit GmbH.

Abstract

Field trials in large cages of 2 m^2 base area were carried out in the Tamesna area, northern Niger, in 1990–91, to test various spray and bait treatments against *Schistocerca gregaria* (Forskål). The insect growth regulator teflubenzuron was compared with a standard dieldrin treatment by direct application to *S. gregaria* adults and nymphs and *Anacridium wernerellum* (Karny) adults and also by application to the main food plant, *Schouwia thebaica* (Cruciferae) bushes. Pure and enriched neem oil sprays were tested for insecticidal and anti-feeding properties. Oil formulations of commercial preparations of *Beauveria bassiana* (Balsamo) Vuillemin were applied by spraying and *B. bassiana* and *Nosema locustae* Canning were also tested as baits with wheat bran. Teflubenzuron caused less adult mortality than dieldrin but completely prevented development of third and fourth instar nymphs. Neem oil caused no mortality by topical application but showed strong anti-feeding effects: however, severe burning of *S. thebaica* foliage by neem oil was also observed. None of the treatments involving spraying with *B. bassiana* or baiting with *B. bassiana* or *N. locustae* caused any mortality.

Introduction

Prior to the 1980s, organochlorines and other persistent pesticides were used extensively for locust control. Environmental and ecological problems were not seriously discussed until 1985 when swarms of *Schistocerca gregaria* (Forskål) reappeared in Africa and the Near East. Analysis of this recent outbreak showed that climatically favourable conditions in conjunction with neglect of the warning services and the inaccessibility of some areas due to armed conflict had all contributed to the sudden increase. The countries affected were largely unprepared and poorly equipped to cope with the plague (Krall & Nasseh, 1991).

Since the use of pesticides is rigorously controlled in most temperate countries, but less so in many tropical ones, GTZ initiated a project to investigate and develop more acceptable alternative methods of controlling locusts and grasshoppers. In parallel with this, GTZ requested that trials should be initiated on the side effects of the new products on the environment and on non-target organisms. The first environmental study was performed in Cape Verde in 1989 and the second, on locusts, in Niger in September–October 1990 (Peveling & Weyrich, 1991 and these proceedings).

Field cage trials on alternative methods of locust control were carried out in Niger (Tamesna area) October 1990–January 1991 (Freres & Nasseh, 1991). Their purpose was to investigate the efficacy of the insect growth regulator teflubenzuron, neem oil and pathogens against desert locust.

Neem, *Azadirachta indica*, has been found to be a promising source of natural pesticides. Extracts possess distinct insecticidal and antifeedant effects against several species of insects including locusts (Wilps *et al.*; Langewald & Schmutterer, these proceedings). Since neem trees grow in Niger, it was decided to investigate the influence of enriched neem oil on adults of *S. gregaria*. The reasons for using neem are to minimize the contamination of the environment, to encourage the use of locally available plant material, to identify sources of botanical insecticides for commercial use and to replace or supplement existing synthetic insecticides against pests.

As early as the 1950s, *Beauveria bassiana* (Balsamo) Vuillemin has been field-tested on a small scale against a wide range of insects, and since the early 1970s it has been mass-produced in USSR and eastern Europe, mainly for control of Colorado potato beetle (*Leptinotarsa decemlineata* (Say) (Coleoptera: Chrysomelidae). The fungal biomass is usually ground and made into dusts or granules and in recent years separators have been used to collect pure conidia from dried cultures. Such products contain up to 1×10^{11} conidia/g and have usually been applied in water suspensions at high volumes. However, the possibility also exists for formulation into oil emulsion preparations for spraying at low or ultra-low volumes (Bateman; Bateman *et al.*; Johnston *et al.*; Matthews; Prior *et al.*; all these proceedings). The purpose of the oil would be to act as a 'carrier', ensuring sufficient spray volume to cover the target area adequately and to reduce evaporation of the droplets, which usually have a diameter of 70–90 μm. It has also been claimed that oils may reduce the rate of inactivation of the fungus.

Nosema locustae Canning, a microsporidian, has been developed as an insecticidal bait and tested extensively against grasshopper populations in the northern part of USA and also in Cape Verde. It is pathogenic to a wide range of acridids and infection has been shown to reduce feeding (Johnson & Pavlikova, 1986).

Methods

Site details

The trial area, at In-Sinkat, was 300 km north-west of Agadez and 40 km south of the GTZ base in Tamesna, northern Niger. This area is well-known as a recession area for *S. gregaria* during the dry season. The area is classified as between Sahelian and Saharan savanna with rainfall of 50–100 mm per annum (Freres & Nasseh, 1991). Vegetation occurs in discrete 'islands', surrounded by large tracts of sand. These islands provide shade, food, oviposition sites, protection from birds and also cover from extremes of temperature. The vegetation includes *Acacia* spp. (Leguminosae), *Panicum turgidum* (Gramineae), *Aerva javanica* (Amaranthaceae), *Tribulus* spp. (Zygophyllaceae) and *Citrullus colocynthis* (Cucurbitaceae). However, the dominant vegetation is the bush *Schouwia thebaica* (Cruciferae) which reaches a height of 1.5–2.5 m. A few of these vegetation islands harbour desert locusts during the recession time.

Adult *S. gregaria* collected from the field were counted, checked for abnormalities and kept under observation for one week. The population of *S. gregaria* in the collecting area was fairly stable (800–1000/ha). None were parasitized. The only other locust species seen in the trial plots was *Anacridium wernerellum* (Karny) which was much less numerous than *S. gregaria.*

Construction of cages

Experiments were carried out in 2 × 2 × 2 m cages with removeable sides. All the sides and the top were covered with removeable wire mesh (8 meshes/cm^2) which was fixed to the cross members. The cages were designed to avoid crowding, assist in counting and allow easy access (Nasseh & Freres, 1991). The lower 30 cm of the cage was made out of sheet metal and was sunk into the sand to a depth of 20 cm. In each cage there were two thinned *Schouwia thebaica* plants of uniform growth. The trials were replicated four times, using 30 adult desert locusts.* Assessments were made at daily intervals during the cooler morning time.

*No statistical analysis of the results was presented (eds).

Treatments

Insect growth regulators

Teflubenzuron ULV formulation was used at a rate equivalent to 50 g a.i/ha, a dose derived from previous trials in 1989 in Sudan where a dose of 25–50 g a.i./ha, was indicated. Where treatments were applied to the insects, the pesticide was applied outside the cages and the insects were transferred into the cages 30 min later. Where treatments were applied to the plants the insects were placed in the cages 30 min after spraying. Dieldrin ULV at 20 g a.i./ha was used as a standard insecticide and an untreated control was also included.

Enriched neem oil

This was obtained from Prof. H. Schmutterer, Justus-Liebig Universität Giessen, Germany. It was coded AZT-VR-K and originated from Togo and Tanzania. Pure neem oil from Niger was also tested. In the first trial, adult locusts were sprayed with enriched neem oil AZT-VR-K, enriched neem oil from Benin and pure neem oil from Niger at a rate equivalent to 10 1/ha. Thirty locusts were used in each treatment and the treatments were replicated four times.

In two other unreplicated trials on antifeeding effects, adult locusts were added to cages in which, in one trial, one *S. thebaica* plant had been sprayed with enriched neem oil at a rate equivalent to 10 1/ha 30 l min previously but the other had not, and in the other trial only one, sprayed plant was present. Assessments in all trials were made daily.

Pathogens

The *Beauveria bassiana* product (1×10^{13} conidia/kg) was obtained from Mycotech Inc. Butte, Montana, USA, (by courtesy of Dr C. Bradley) and was applied at two rates of 320 g and 960 g/ha in 3 litres mineral oil. *Nosema locustae* Canning (2.5×10^{9} spores on 1 kg of wheat bran/ha) was obtained from Durango Inc., Bayfield, Colorado, USA, and was compared with *B. bassiana* in a feeding trial where the latter was also applied on bran at rates for both pathogens equivalent to 320 and 960 g/ha. In these bait trials the locusts were starved for 24 or 48 h before treatment to enhance feeding. All these dosages refer to products, applied as received from the producers except the rate of 960 g/ha.

Application techology

A solar operated Micro-Ulva (Micron Sprayers Ltd., UK) was used for application in the early morning. Droplet distribution was assessed using oil sensitive paper.

Results

Insect growth regulators

Analysis of oil sensitive papers showed that the droplet deposition density was 20 ± 12 droplets/cm^2. The mortality caused by the treatments to *Schistocerca gregaria* (adults and third and fourth instars) and *Anacridium wernerellum* (adults) are shown in Tables 1–3.

The best control was obtained with dieldrin. Teflubenzuron gave better results when applied to the vegetation than to the insects.

The results obtained by applications of teflubenzuron to third and fourth instars of solitarious *S. gregaria* and by treatment of their food plant (*Schouwia thebaica*) are shown in Table 2.

Table 2 shows the number of surviving, dead and deformed (abnormal wings and tarsae) and the number of so called mini adults (inhibition of normal adult development) resulting from application of teflubenzuron at 50 g a.i./ha.

Mean body weight of male larvae treated with teflubenzuron was approximately half that of untreated larvae. None of the deformed larvae developed normally and none were able to complete development. Thus teflubenzuron appeared more effective in controlling the larval stage of desert locust than the adults under these conditions.

Table 1. Effect of teflubenzuron and dieldrin on adult *Schistocerca gregaria*.

Product	Application rate	No. of *S. gregaria* at application	No. of *S. gregaria* after 17 days
Teflubenzuron (topical)	50 g a.i/ha	120	78
Teflubenzuron (vegetation)	50 g a.i/ha	120	38
Dieldrin	20 g a.i/ha	120	19
Control		120	119

Table 2. Effect of teflubenzuron on third and fourth larval stages of *Schistocerca gregaria*.

Product	Application rate	Initial no. insects	No. alive after 12 days	No. of 3rd/4th larval stages after 12 days		
				No. dead	No. deformed	No. mini
Teflubenzuron (topical)	50 g a.i/ha	120	30	77	13	0
Teflubenzuron (vegetation)	50 g a.i/ha	120	11	84	21	15
Control		118	118	2	0	0

Table 3. Effects of teflubenzuron on adults of *Anacridium wernerellum*.

Product	Application rate	Initial no. of insects	No. of insects after 17 days
Teflubenzuron (topical)	50 g a.i/ha	51	21
Teflubenzuron (vegetation)	50 g a.i/ha	51	10
Control		51	50

The data in Table 3 suggest that the intake of teflubenzuron from treated *Schouwia thebaica* plants was more effective against the adults of *A. wernerellum*, than topical application. Treatment of the vegetation reduced the population from 51 to 10.

Enriched neem oil

The results shown in Table 4 demonstrate that there was no effect of pure and enriched neem oil on adults of *Schistocerca gregaria* up six weeks after treatment.

In the unreplicated anti-feeding trial, the locusts consumed 100% of the leaves of the *Schouwia thebaica* in the untreated control but on the

Table 4. Effect of neem oil on adult *Schistocerca gregaria.*

Product	Application rate	No. of *S. gregaria* after treatment	No. of *S. gregaria* after 6 weeks
Neem oil Giessen*	10 l/ha	120	116
Neem oil Benin*	10 l/ha	120	117
Neem oil Niger	10 l/ha	120	117
Control		120	118

*enriched neem oil

plants sprayed with neem oil at 10 1/ha there was no feeding until day 11, by which time 100 out of the 120 adults had starved to death. After four weeks there was severe phytotoxic burning of the leaves of *S. thebaica* treated with enriched neem at 10 1/ha.

Pathogens

The results for all treatments with *B. bassiana* and *N. locustae* are given in Tables 5–7. Analysis of oil sensitive paper distributed during the application of *B. bassiana* showed an average droplet coverage of 20 $\pm$12 droplets/cm^2.

Table 5 presents the results of direct spraying of the desert locust adults. Only the combination of *B. bassiana* and neem oil had any effect within six weeks and this was only slight.

Table 6 indicates that all the adult locusts which fed on *Schouwia thebaica* treated with 3 1 mineral oil/ha or on the non-treated controls survived, but the *B. bassiana* treatments also had very little effect up to six weeks after treatment.

In other experiments also, the application of *B. bassiana* in either neem or mineral oil at a rate of 320 g in 3 1/ha had no effect on adult *Schistocerca gregaria* up to six weeks after treatment when it was sprayed directly on *Schouwia thebaica* bushes.

Adult desert locusts were fed on wheat bran mixed with *B. bassiana* or *Nosema locustae.* The results are presented in Table 7 and indicate that neither treatment caused any mortality within the six week period of recording.

Table 5. Effect of *Beauveria bassiana* on *Schistocerca gregaria* adults.

Product	Application rate	No. of *S. gregaria* at application	No. of *S. gregaria* after 6 weeks
B. bassiana + mineral oil	320 g in 3 l/ha	120	117
B. bassiana + mineral oil	960 g in 3 l/ha	120	114
B. bassiana + Neem oil	320 g in 3 l/ha	120	98
Mineral oil	3 l/ha	120	119
Control		120	119

Table 6. Effect of *Beauveria bassiana* on adults of *Schistocerca gregaria* after feeding on treated plants.

Product	Application rate	No. of *S. gregaria* after application	No. of *S. gregaria* after 6 weeks
B. bassiana + mineral oil	320 g in 3 l/ha	120	115
B. bassiana + mineral oil	960 g in 3 l/ha	120	111
Mineral oil	3 l/ha	120	120
Control		120	120

Conclusions

The results of the teflubenzuron experiments demonstrated a significant effect on development and mortality became obvious on treated plants. A similar trend was observed in the mortality of sprayed *A. wernerellum.* However, mortality was higher in the dieldrin treatments. Treatment of larval stages of desert locusts with teflubenzuron in the field has promise. Larvae of *A. wernerellum* were not included in the experiments but further tests will be carried out.

Enriched neem oil caused no mortality but was effective as an anti-feedant. Neem is known to alter locust behaviour in several ways (Wilps *et al.*, these proceedings). For 10 days after treatment, no adult locusts fed on

Table 7. Effect of *Beauveria bassiana* and *Nosema locustae* on adults of *Schistocerca gregaria* after being fed with treated wheat bran (results of 2 experiments.

Product	Application rate	Starvation period (h)	No. of *S. gregaria* at treatment	No. of *S. gregaria* after 6 weeks
B. bassiana + wheat bran	320 g in 2 kg/ha	–	120	118
B. bassiana + wheat bran	960 g in 3 kg/ha	–	120	116
Control			120	120
(*B. bassiana* treatment)				
N. locustae + wheat bran	2 kg/ha	24	120	120
N. locustae + wheat bran	2 kg/ha	48	120	119
Control (*N. locustae* treatment)	2 kg/ha		120	118

neem-treated plants and the majority died in this period, although the survivors did begin to feed on the eleventh day. Neem oil therefore shows some promise as a treatment within programmes for the integrated management of desert locusts and could help to reduce dependency on chemical pesticides. It can also be produced locally in sahelian countries, which would help to reduce control costs. Other vegetable oils such as cottonseed have also been used with encouraging results as repellants against *Myzus persicae* (Sulzer) and *Brevicoryne brassicae* (Linnaeus) (Homoptera: Aphididae), *Spodoptera exigua* (Hübner) (Lepidoptera: Noctuidae) and also thrips pests (Butler & Henneberry, 1990). However, the severe phytotoxic effects of enriched neem on *Schouwia* indicate a need for further investigations on the feasibility of using neem in this way.

Six weeks after application of treatments to caged locusts in the field, nearly all locusts survived in the controls. Survival was not significantly less in all *B. bassiana* treatments, either applied in mineral oil to the plants or to the insects, nor was any effect demonstrated when locusts were fed wheat bran treated with *B. bassiana* or *N. locustae.*

The results show that *N. locustae* and *B. bassiana* were not effective biological control agents against *Schistocerca gregaria* under the conditions of these trials. The question of whether or not these two pathogens could contribute to reducing the larval population densities of desert locusts could not be answered because larvae were not included in the experiments but tests will be continued with larvae. The viability of the *B. bassiana* conidia was not checked.

References

Butler, G.D. & Henneberry, T.J. (1990) Cottonseed oil and safer insecticidal soap; effects on cotton and vegetable pests and phytotoxicity. *Southwestern Entomologist* **15**, 257–264.

Freres, T. & Nasseh, O.M. (1991) Versuchs zur Bekämpfung der Wüstenheuschrecke, *Schistocerca gregaira* Forskål in der Republik Niger. Report submitted to GTZ, 22 pp.

Johnson. D.L. & Pavlikova, E. (1986) Reduction of consumption by grasshoppers (Orthoptera: Acrididae) infected with *Nosema locustae* Canning (Microsporida: Nosematidae). *Journal of Invertebrate Pathology* **48**, 232–238.

Krall, S. & Nasseh, O.M. (1990) Erforschung biologisch-integrieter Methoden zur Bekämpfung schädlicher Heuschrecken – ein Projekt der GTZ. *Plant Protection Information Tropics/Subtropics* **8**, 215–223.

Nasseh, O.M. & Freres, T. (1991) Käfigfreilandversuche zur Bekämpfung der Larvenstadien und Adulten Tiere von *Schistocerca gregaria* Forskål mit biologischen und chemischen Präparaten in der Republik Niger. Report submitted to GTZ, 33 pp.

Peveling, R. & Weyrich, J. (1990) Non-target Wirkungen von Heuschreckenbekämpfungsmitteln in Niger. Report submitted to GTZ, 24 pp.

Effects of neem oil, *Beauveria bassiana* and dieldrin on non-target tenebrionid beetles in the desert zone of the Republic of Niger

R. Peveling & J. Weyrich

Universität des Saarlandes.

Abstract

Field trials on the impact of locust control agents on non-target arthropods were carried out in Tamesna, southern Sahara, Republic of Niger, in September/October 1990. The study was conducted within the framework of the GTZ-Project 'Integrated Biological Control of Grasshoppers and Locusts'. The effects of neem oil (0.1% and 0.2% azadirachtin), *Beauveria bassiana* (Balsamo) Vuillemin and dieldrin on the tenebrionid beetle *Pimelia angulata tschadensis* Koch were studied in standardized *in situ* cage trials. Additionally, neem oil and *B. bassiana* were tested in small scale field trials in typical *Schistocerca gregaria* (Forskål) (Orthoptera: Acrididae) habitats (*Schouwia thebaica* vegetation islands). Dieldrin and neem (0.1%) caused high mortalities in the cage trials. Neem (0.2%) induced an increase, dieldrin a decrease in activity of the beetles. Neither in the cage trials nor within additional laboratory tests could *B. bassiana* infections be observed in *P. angulata tschadensis.* Only topically inoculated *Trachyderma hispida* (Forskål) (Tenebrionidae) were infected. The field applications did not appear to cause any side-effects on the tenebrionid fauna, i.e., neither alteration of activity pattern nor lethal effects. The final results of these investigations (effects on other non-target arthropods) will be presented in subsequent publications. As key components of arid ecosystems Tenebrionidae could be useful indicator organisms to study ecotoxicological risks of insecticides prior to large scale field applications.

Introduction

For decades locust control has relied almost exclusively on the application of chemical insecticides. However the increasing knowledge about their potential hazardous side-effects (related to their non-specificity and persistence) has recently promoted the search for environmentally sound alternatives and adoption of the conceptual approach of integrated pest control, which incorporates biological and biotechnological methods, has received increasing attention from experts.

The application of alternative locust control agents can by no means be considered *a priori* to be environmentally sound. As with chemical pesticides, they must undergo a careful and thorough evaluation of potential side effects prior to large scale field application.

This ecotoxicological risk assessment involves both laboratory and field trials, the former to work out principal physico-chemical and toxicological (or pathogenic) properties of the respective control agent, the latter being indispensable to study its field behaviour, and thus preferably carried out at an early stage of risk assessment programmes.

Because most alternative insecticides are not selective, adverse effects on non-target organisms are to be expected. The assessment of the impact on non-target organisms is one of the prime objectives of ecotoxicology. An in-depth risk assessment can only be achieved if non-target-specific ecological processes are understood. This is a formidable task in tropical and subtropical ecosystems, where many species have not yet been taxonomically described. For ecological monitoring of (large scale) conventional applications, when a prompt assessment is required, it is common practice to confine ecotoxicological studies to higher taxonomic categories (mostly order or family). This simplification ignores the fact that there are significant differences in ecology, behaviour and susceptibility to pesticides even between closely related taxa. As a result, severe effects at lower taxonomic levels might be camouflaged. The search for sensitive *species* as indicators of undesirable side-effects (e.g. incorrect applications) in further routine field applications of the same insecticide in the same area should therefore receive more attention Grant, 1989; Everts, 1990.

In the first phase of environmental impact studies, investigations should focus on identifying non-target species either directly 'ecologically linked' to the target (competitors and natural enemies such as parasites or predators) or occupying key positions within the respective ecosystem (e.g. pollinators, reducers). However, it has to be emphasized that the importance of certain species may be underestimated or overlooked simply because the structure of the ecosystem, the underlying ecological processes and inter-specific relations are not sufficiently understood. Once identified, key species could undergo further standard laboratory testing (toxicity tests) in order to predict ecotoxicological risks of the application of a variety of agents in the same area. These indication methods should not be understood as substitutes for synecological approaches and will have to be worked out together with appropriate field scale assessments during field operations.

In the southern Saharan recession areas of the desert locust (*Schistocerca gregaria* (Forskål)), tenebrionid beetles are characteristic elements of the ground dwelling coenosis. Isolated plant and animal communities, low species density and diversity, and simple food webs are specific attributes of these ecosystems. Due to their high abundance and their omnivorous trophic function Tenebrionidae dominate the flow of organic matter. Moreover, they are direct food competitors of desert locusts and, as Popov (1980) demonstrated for the Senegalese grasshopper (*Oedaleus sengalensis* (Krauss)), potential predators of locust eggs due to their partly hypogaeic way of life. Therefore, in the first phase of the study, tenebrionids were chosen for studying non-target effects of alternative acridicides. The following agents were tested:

1. two formulations of neem oil (seed extract of *Azadirachta indica*)
2. *Beauveria bassiana* (Balsamo) Vuillemin, an entomopathogenic fungus
3. dieldrin as a reference.

The potential of neem oil for the control of *S. gregaria* has so far been tested only in the laboratory. Schmutterer & Freres (1990) demonstrated its larvicidal effects. Furthermore, laboratory reared gregarious hoppers developed the typical anatomical and ethological characteristics of solitary locusts. *B. bassiana* was field tested against *Nomadacris septemfasciata* (Serville) as early as the 1930s in South Africa (Schaefer, 1936). Prior & Greathead (1989) recommended additional investigations of the potential of *B. bassiana* and other entomopathogens as alternative acridicides. Dieldrin used to be the most commonly applied insecticide during locust control operations. The environmental hazards of its use are still controversial (Müller, 1988; Everts, 1990) despite an almost universal ban on its use. Further field investigations of its ecotoxicological effects should therefore be carried out.

Study sites

The studies were conducted in the Iguidi region about 15 km south-west of the CINA (Centre National de Lutte Antiacridienne) station 'In-Abangharhit' (south-east Tamesna, 18°03'N/6°02'E). The landscape can be described as more or less flat gravel and sand deserts, which are quite regularly separated by lines of dunes up to 20 m high. The vegetation consists of low-growing herbs, which are distributed in isolated patches between the dunes. Vegetation cover is dense along the dunes where patches of *Schouwia thebaica* (= *purpurea*)* (Cruciferae) up to 70 cm high

*Taxonomy in dispute (eds).

(cover ≈ 80% can often be found; smaller, less dense patches are found between the dunes. *S. thebaica* is dominant and constitutes the major food of *Schistocerca gregaria* in this area. Hemming & Symmons (1969) studied the germination and growth of this annual cruciferous plant. Other species such as *Fagonia* sp. and *Tribulus ochroleucus* (Zygophyllacease), *Citrullus colocynthis* (Cucurbitaceae), *Aerva javanica* (Amaranthaceae), *Pergularia tomentosa* (Asclepiadaceae) and *Aristida* sp. (Gramineae) are loosely scattered within the *Schouwia* stands. Similarly, the macrofauna is characterized by a small number of species, most of them birds such as *Hirundo obsoleta buchanani* (pale crag martin), *Cursoprius cursor* (cream-coloured courser) and *Corvus ruficollis* (brown-necked raven) or reptiles such as *Acanthodactylus boscianus.*

As an adaptation to the dry and hot conditions, most arthropod species are active during the night or at dusk. Tenebrionid beetles make up the largest part of the zoomass. *Blaps bifurcata mirei* Gredelli, *Prionotheca coronata coronata* (Olivier) and *Pimelia subquadrata chudeaui* Koch occur frequently, but are less abundant than *Pimelia angulata tschadensis* Koch and *Trachyderma hispida* (Forskål). As with *S. gregaria,* they feed mainly on *Schouwia thebaica.*

The cage trials were conducted in a plains area of about 5 ha mainly covered with *S. thebaica.* For the field applications three dense *S. thebaica* fields of about 500 to 1500 m^2 were selected on the lee side of sand dunes. For logistical reasons, the trial sites were chosen near each other.

Materials and methods

Spraying operation

In the cage trials the oral and residual effects of the following agents were tested:

1. neem oil (0.075% ≈ 0.1% AZA (azadiractin) (Inst. f. Phytopathologie, Giessen/FRG))
2. neem oil (0.22% ≈ 0.2% AZA (IITA, Benin))
3. *Beauveria bassiana* (oil-formulated suspension (Mycotech, USA))
4. dieldrin (Shell-Agro).

Neem oil (0.1%) and *B. bassiana* were applied in the field trials. Spraying was conducted between 06.00 and 10.00 h (windspeed < 2 m/sec, temperature ≈ 25°C) with a Micro-Ulva-spinning disc sprayer (dieldrin: ULV, other agents LV application) (see Table 1).

Table 1. Application parameters.

Formulation	a.i.	Dosage rate	Flow rate	Nozzle	NB
Neem oil	0.1 % (AZA)	10.0 l/ha	60 ml/min	red	4
Neem oil	0.2 % (AZA)	10.0 l/ha	34 ml/min	red	4
B. bassiana	4 * 10^9 sp/ml	1 * 10^{13} sp/ha	61 ml/min (*)	red (*)	5
Dieldrin	18 %	0.4 l/ha	22 ml/min	yellow	4

NB = number of batteries/sprayer; sp = spores; (*) = a constant flow of the suspension could only be achieved when widening the nozzle diameter and shaking the sprayer continuously during application; AZA = azadiractin.

Cage trials

In the *Schouwia thebaica* field 20 suitable 2 m quadrats with at least 15% vegetation cover were selected (minimum buffer zone between the plots = 15 m). After treatment (four replicates per insecticide, randomized cage order) the cages (steel frame, galvanized iron netting, 2 × 2 × 2 m size; cage design see Krall & Nasseh, 1990) were dug into the ground 20–30 cm deep. All arthropods in the cages were removed. Subsequently, each cage was stocked with 30 *P. angulata tschadensis.* Over a period of 16 days the following parameters were recorded:

1. mortality (M) (twice daily at 07.00 and 18.00 h.)
2. relative activity (RA) (i.e. percentage of beetles captured in one pitfall trap per cage; the traps were covered with a lid during the day and opened for one hour starting at 18.30 h).

At the end of the trial all remaining beetles were collected to assess potential losses by cannibalism or escape.

The calculations of mortality and activity correspond to the sum (S) of dead (D) or alive (A) test beetles collected until the end of the trial. The cumulative mortality on day *i* is calculated as:

$$Mi\,(\%) = \frac{Di}{S} \times 100$$

(Di = number of dead animals collected up to day i).

The effects of the agents were calculated according to Schneider-Orelli (Krall & Nasseh, 1990). The relative activity on day *i* is calculated as:

$$\mathrm{RA}i\,(\%) = \frac{\mathrm{G}i}{\mathrm{S} - \mathrm{D}i} \times 100$$

($\mathrm{G}i$ = number of animals collected on day i).

Prior to statistical treatment all data were arc-sine transformed. In particular the following statistical calculations were performed:

1. mortality at the end of the trial (day 16): single classification ANOVA and Newman-Keuls-multiple comparison among means
2. RA of all days: cross correlation; days 3–15: Friedman-ANOVA and Wilcoxon-Wilcox-multiple comparison among means.

Small-scale field trials

In each *Schouwia thebaica* field 4 permanent 1 m^2 plots were randomly established to survey potential mortalities of non-target organisms. To study effects on the activity abundance AA (= 'Aktivitätsdichte' *sensu* Heydemann (1953), 'availability' *sensu* Southwood (1978)) of ground-dwelling arthropods, four pitfall traps were placed in each test plot (conservation fluid: 5% formol) for a period of 15 days (3 days pre- and 11 days post-spray interval).

Mortality (M) was recorded daily between 07.30 and 08.30 h, 17.30 and 18.30 h in the permanent plots, and pitfall traps were emptied daily between 17.30 and 18.30 h.

At present only effects on the abundant tenebrionid species, *Pimelia angulata tschadensis*, *P. subquadrata chudeaui*, *Trachyderma hispida*, *Blaps bifurcata mirei*, and *Prionotheca coronata coronata*, can be given.

All data were transformed as : $A_T = 10 \times (\ln \mathrm{AA} + 1)$ [A_T = AA transformed]. The mean catches of days 2 and 1 (pre-spray) were compared to the catches of days 2–4, 6–7 and 9–11 (post-spray) (Kruskal-Wallis). The effect of the agents is calculated as

$$\mathrm{E}\,(\%) = \left[\frac{D_T}{D_C} - 1\right] * 100$$

D_T = mean difference between pre- and post-spray catches in the treated plot

D_C = mean difference between pre- and post-spray catches in the control plot

For the calculation of standard error see Everts *et al.* (1985).

Additional trials

To study the contact effects of *B. bassiana* on several tenebrionid beetles field tests and bioassays were conducted:

1. LV-application in an arena: 1 ml spore suspension/m^2 (as specified in Table 1) applied with a Micro-Ulva
2. topical application in the laboratory: approximately 1 μl suspension applied dorsally between thorax and abdomen by micro caps.

The test animals were analysed by the BBA Darmstadt–Germany for infection by *B. bassiana.*

Results

Cage trials

91.3% of the original stock of *P. angulata tschadensis* were recollected. The 8.7% beetles undetected must be attributed to cannibalism. One out of four replications in the control group was proved significantly to be an outlier (Outlier text of Dixon as described by Snedecor & Cochran (1980)) and was treated as missing (statistical analysis for unbalanced design).

All test agents had an adverse effect (Table 2 and Figs 1 & 2), but only dieldrin ($P < 0.001$) and neem 0.1% ($P < 0.05$ caused significantly increased mortalities. Surprisingly, neem 0.1% finally caused higher mortalities than neem 0.2%, which is probably due to the different additives used in both formulations. No infection could be detected in the *B. bassiana*-treated beetles.

The activity of the beetles is cyclical (Fig. 3). Data from days 1 and 2 are slightly biased due to a prolonged sampling period (day 1: 90 min; day 2: 110 min). The periodicity of the data, although biologically important, is irrelevant for assessing the effects of the agents. This becomes evident when comparing the pattern of the activity of cage-tested tenbrionids in all replications (Table 3) and that of field-tested tenebrionids in all plots, respectively (see small-scale field trials, below). Differences in the effects of the agents are indicated by level of activity (Table 4) as compared to that of the control. Neem-treated beetles exhibit insecticide-caused hyperactivity whereas the dieldrin- and *B. bassiana*-treated groups exhibit hypoactivity.

Table 2. Mean mortality at the end of the trial.

Agent	Control	Neem (0.1%)	Neem (0.2%)	Dieldrin	*B. bassiana*
Mortality	14%	56%	48%	78%	37%
Corrected effect	–	49%	40%	74%	27%

Control ≠ dieldrin & neem (0.1%) ($P < 0.05$; ANOVA & Newman-Keuls multiple comparison among means); other differences not significant.

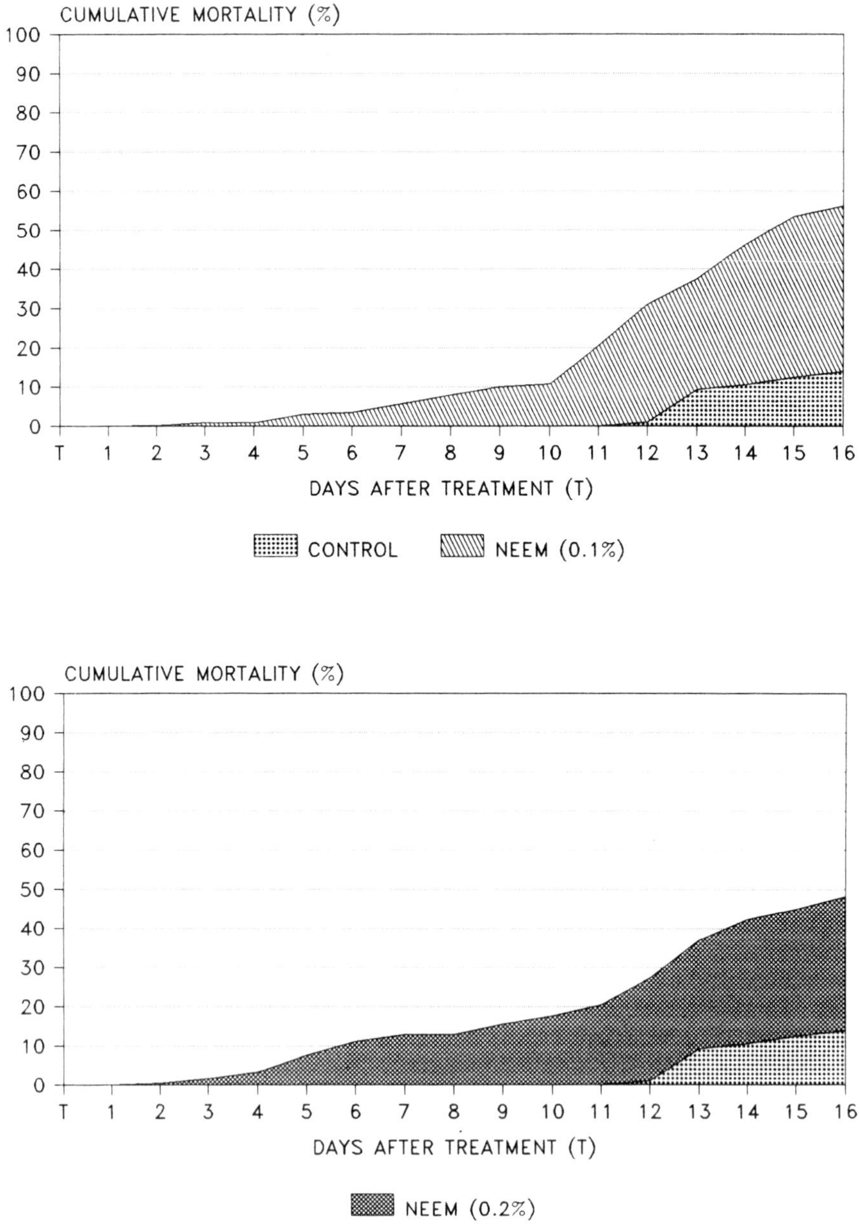

Figure 1. Cumulative mortality (M) of *Pimelia angulata tschadensis*; neem (0.1%) and neem (0.2%).

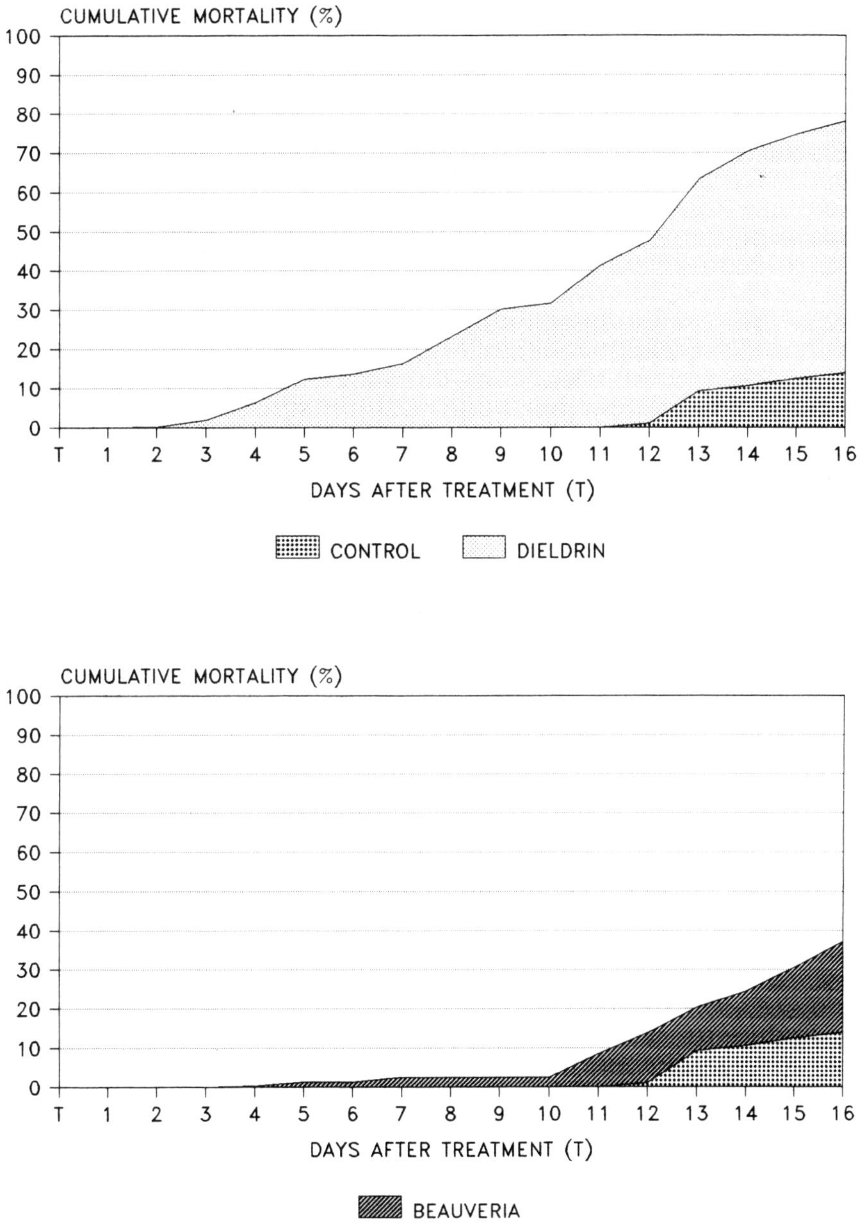

Figure 2. Cumulative mortality (M) of *Pimelia angulata tschadensis*; dieldrin and *Beauveria bassiana*.

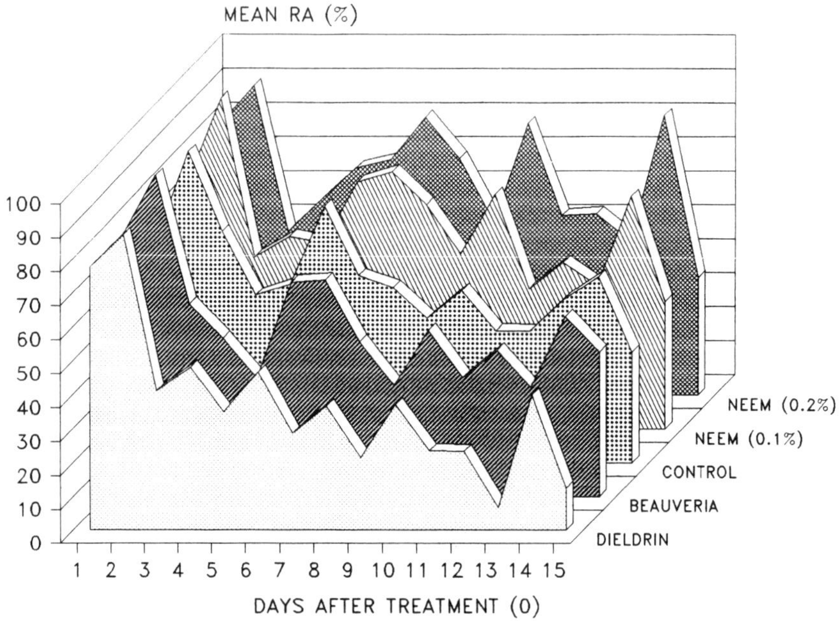

Figure 3. Mean relative activity (RA) of *Pimelia angulata tschadensis.*

Table 3. Correlation matrix (Pearson's r) of the mean relative activity (RA) (all days).

	Control	Neem (0.1%)	Neem (0.2%)	Dieldrin	*B. bassiana*
Control	1.00				
Neem (0.1%)	0.82***	1.00			
Neem (0.2%)	0.67**	0.95***	1.00		
Dieldrin	0.84***	0.82***	0.74**	1.00	
B. bassiana	0.87***	0.86***	0.75**	0.89***	1.00

Correlation coefficient significant at: ** $P < 0.01$; *** $P < 0.001$.

Small-scale field trials

The field trials did not indicate any adverse effects of neem oil (0.1%) and *Beauveria bassiana* on tenebrionid beetles. No dead animals, neither tenebrionids nor other arthropods, could be found on the permanent plots.

There was no difference in the activity of tenebrionid beetles (species group listed in small-scale field trials, above) between pre- and postspray periods (Table 5). As with the RA of the beetles in the cage trials, the

Table 4. Mean relative activity (RA) of *P. angulata t. schadensis* on days 3–15 (retransformed data).

Agent	Control	Neem (0.1%)	Neem (0.2%)	Dieldrin	*B. bassiana*
Activity	51%	56%	60%	32%	46%

Control ≠ Neem (0.1%), Neem (0.2%) & *Beauveria* ≠ Dieldrin; Neem (0.2%) ≠ *Beauveria* ($P < 0.05$; Friedman-ANOVA & Wilcoxon-Wilcox multiple comparison among means with days 3–15 as replicates); other differences not significant.

Table 5. Effect of the agents on the activity abundance (AA) in the field trials.

Agent	P	A(1)	E	SE	A(2)	E	SE	A(3)	E	SE
Control	62	49			41			38		
Neem (0.1%)	40	58	18.7	9.3	33	6.8	7.8	30	5.5	3.7
Beauveria	44	42	5.4	3.5	34	4.7	5.4	28	−0.6	3.2

Mean AA (number tenebrionids/trap) on days −2 & −1 (P), 2 to 4 (A(1)), 6 to 8 (A(2)) and 9 to 11 (A(3)); all differences not significant. (Kruskal-Wallis-ANOVA); E = effect, SE = standard error.

activity of the tenebrionids in the field tests is phased sequentially (Fig. 4; maximum on days -3, 1, 5, 8/9). This phenomenon can be shown clearly by a correlation matrix. A period of 5 days between the peaks is evident (Fig. 5 & Table 6).

The synchronous pattern of activity of the beetles is evident not only *within* the cage or the field trials, but also *between* these as illustrated in Fig. 6 and Table 7 (simultaneous testing period). Only during days 11–13 are the curves not synchronous (probably due to increased silting of the pitfall traps in the *Schouwia thebaica* fields).

The activity abundance of the tenebrionids in the control area (field tests) is higher on most days than in the treated plots (Table 8, Fig. 4).

Biotests

Both in the laboratory (constant 35°C test temperature) and in *in situ* topical application tests, *Pimelia angulata tschadensis* showed no *B. bassiana* infection (analysis by BBA, Darmstadt). Only in *Trachyderma hispida* could sporulation be detected (the beetles had died 4 to 8 days after treatment without showing any specific symptoms; also, under

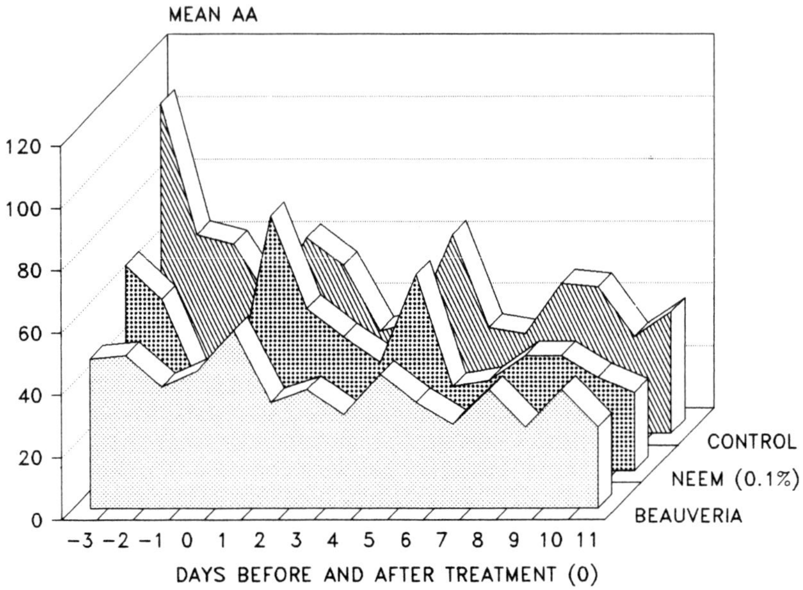

Figure 4. Mean activity abundance (AA) of tenebrionids (number of beetles/trap).

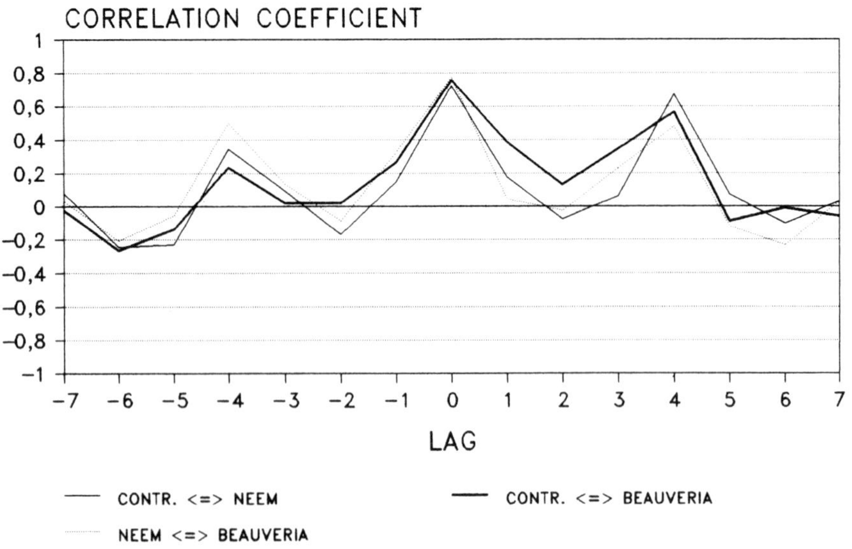

Figure 5. Correlation of the AA of tenebrionids in treated and untreated plots (LAG = 0, 1, 2, ..., 7 means, that the AA in plot *a* on day *x* is correlated with the AA in plot *b* on day $x + 0, 1, 2, \ldots, 7$; for negative LAGs the same applies: $x - 0, 1, 2, \ldots, 7$); correlation coefficient > 0.6 or < −0.6 are significant at $P < 0.05$.

Table 6. Correlation matrix (Pearson's r) of activity abundance (AA) (all days).

	Control	Neem (0.1%)	*Beauveria*
Control	1.00		
Neem (0.1%)	0.73**	1.00	
Beauveria	0.76**	0.77***	1.00

Correlation coefficient significant at: ** $P < 0.01$; *** $P < 0.001$.

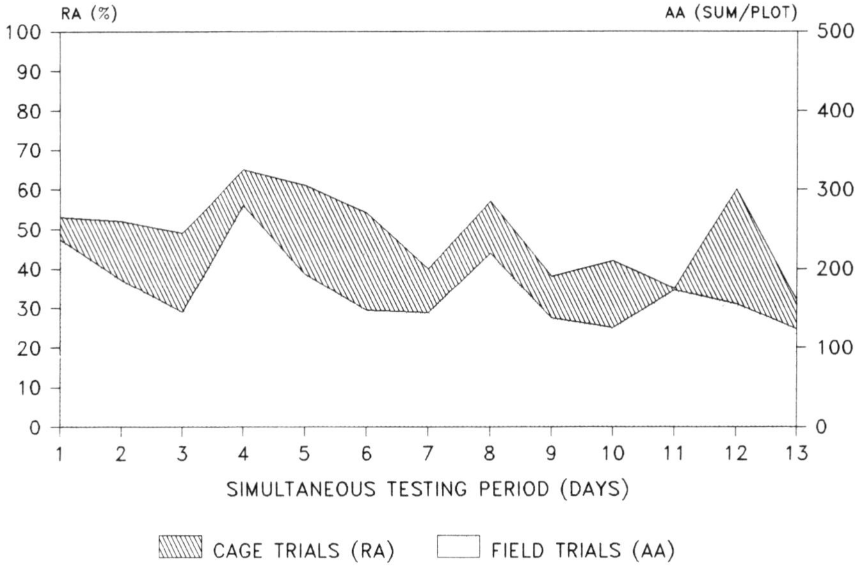

Figure 6. Mean AA in the field trials (total catch/day & plot) and mean RA in the cage trials (all replicated and treatments pooled) on simultaneous days.

Table 7. Matrix (Pearson's r) between relative activity (RA) (cage trials) and activity abundance (AA) (field trials) on simultaneous days.

AA RA	Control	Neem (0.1%)	Neem (0.2%)	Dieldrin	*Beauveria*
Control	0.77**	0.52	0.38	0.63*	0.67*
Neem (0.1%)	0.86***	0.58*	0.34	0.46	0.75**
Beauveria	0.79**	0.35	0.15	0.53	0.54

Correlation coefficient significant at: * $P < 0.05$; ** $P < 0.01$; *** $P < 0.001$.

Table 8. Mean activity abundance (AA) of tenebrionid beetles (retransformed data).

Trial plot	Control	Neem (0.1%)	*B. bassiana*
AA	47%	39%	37%

Control ≠ Neem (0.1%) & *B. bassiana* ($P < 0.05$; Friedman-ANOVA & Wilcoxon & Wilcox multiple comparison among means, days 1–15 as replications); other differences not significant.

increased post-treatment humidity conditions the fungus did not break out within an 8-week observation period; only when beetles were kept in wet chambers did mycelia and spores develop).

It is remarkable that the oil-formulated spore suspension remained virulent for more than 10 days even under extremely arid conditions.

Discussion

The assessment of the impact of alternative locust control agents on non-target fauna requires a sound knowledge of the structural and functional components of the native ecosystem. Investigations of deleterious effects on parasitoids or predators of the target and on ecological key-species should be part of the risk assessment studies. With regard to the control of *Schistocerca gregaria* tenebrionid beetles can be defined as characteristic elements of the epigeal arthropod fauna of Saharan *S. gregaria* recession areas. It is not yet clear whether they are regulators of the density of desert locusts. However, they are both competitors for food and potential egg predators (Popov, 1980). Moreover, they represent a high percentage of the native zoomass. Their population reduction or, at worst, their extinction would probably cause severe disruptions of the mass and energy balances.

The cage trials indicated the ecologically hazardous potential of dieldrin. None of the other agents tested had comparable effects on *P. angulata tschadensis.* The significant effects of neem oil (0.1%) in the cage trials could not be verified in field tests. However, as with the cage trials, the activity level in the neem applied field test plot increased directly after treatment (see Table 5). This hyperactivity might indicate a repellent effect of neem (H. Schmutterer, pers. comm.). Over the whole observation period, the activity abundance in the control plot was higher than in the treated plots. This might be attributed to the different size of the *Schouwia thebaica* fields (control-plot ≈ 1500 m^2, neem-plot ≈ 1000 m^2 & *B.*

bassiana-plot ≈ 500 m^2), the larger ones having a higher carrying capacity. *Beauveria bassiana* did not have any effect on the tenebrionids. Even topical applications led only to infection of *T. hispida.* Tests on desert locusts which were carried out at the same time (Nasseh & Freres, 1991) gave just as little evidence of *B. bassiana* virulence. The low virulence may have been caused by the arid and hot conditions, by specific non-susceptibility, or by both factors together. The *B. bassiana* formulation tested does not seem to be fully developed. In addition, because of flocculation the suspension is not suitable for ULV applications. Periodic fluctuations of the activity are superimposed on potential treatment effects. Because of the periodicity (5-day intervals) and the consistent curve pattern of activity of the cage- and the field-tested beetles, these must be explained by external influences (for example, wind or humidity) and not by population dynamic factors in a narrow sense such as birth or death rates, gains from immigration, and losses from emigration. Insecticide-induced effects, even if statistically proved, should be interpreted with careful evaluation of ecosystem-specific characteristics. Consequently, a proper risk assessment can only be achieved if basic ecological research is included.

In recent ecotoxicological studies, due to a low susceptibility, Tenebrionidae did not appear to be good indicators of early effects of pesticide impacts (Müller, 1988; Van der Valk, 1990). Nevertheless, we believe that because of their high abundance and important ecological function in arid ecosystems as well as their potential for predating *Schistocerca gregaria,* the tenebrionids *Pimelia angulata tschadensis* and, to a lesser extent, *Trachyderma hispida* are appropriate test animals in early step laboratory investigations to assess the ecotoxicological risk of a wide range of chemicals in sahelian ecosystems.

Acknowledgements

We are grateful to Mrs F. Casci (Ministry of Agriculture, Fisheries and Food, London), Mrs B. Fliedner (Institut für Biogeographie, Univ. Saarbrücken, FRG) and Dr P. Matteson (Dept. of Entomology, Iowa State University) for reviewing the text.

References

Everts, J.W. (1990) Methods for monitoring the impact of chemical control of locust and grasshoppers in Africa. *Proceedings of the Workshop on Health and Environmental Impacts of Alternative Control Agents for Desert Locust control, 14–17 January 1990, Oslo, 45–54.*

Everts, J.W., Kortenhoff, B.A., Hoogland, H., Vlug, H.J., Jocqué R. & Koeman, J.H. (1985) Effects on nontarget terrestrial arthropods of synthetic pyrethroids used for the control of tsetse fly (*Glossina* spp.) in settlement areas of the southern Ivory Coast, Africa. *Archives of Environmental Contamination and Toxicology* **14**, 641–650.

Grant, I.F. (1989) Monitoring insecticide side-effects in large-scale treatment programmes: tsetse spraying in Africa. In: Jepson, P.C. (ed.), *Pesticides and Non-target Invertebrates.* Intercept, Wimborne, Dorset, 43–69.

Hemming, C.F. & Symmons, P.M. (1969) The germination and growth of *Schouwia purpurea* (Forsk.) Schweinf. and its role as a habitat of the desert locust. *Anti-Locust Bulletin* **46**, 38 pp.

Heydemann, B. (1953) Agrarökologische Problematik (dargetan an Untersuchungen über die Tierwelt der Bodenoberfläche der Kulturfelder). Dissertation, Kiel.

Krall, S. & Nasseh O. (1990) *Versuchsplan für die Feldversuche in Niger.* GTZ, Eschborn.

Müller, P. (1988) Ökotoxikologische Wirkungen von chlorierten Kohlenwasserstoffen, Phosphorsäureestern, Carbamaten und Pyrethroiden im nordöstlichen Sudan. Unpublished report to the GTZ.

Nasseh, O. M. & Freres, T. (1991) Käfigfreilandversuche zur Bekämpfung der Larvenstadien und adulten Tiere von *Schistocerca gregaria* Forskal mit biologischen und chemischen Präparaten in der Republik Niger. Unpublished report to the GTZ.

Popov, G.B. (1980) *Studies on Oviposition, Egg Development and Mortality in Oedaleus senegalensis (Krauss), (Orthoptera, Acridoidea) in the Sahel.* Centre for Overseas Pest Research, London.

Prior, C. & Greathead, D.J. (1989) Biological control of locusts: the potential for the exploitation of pathogens. *FAO Plant Protection Bulletin* **37**, 37–48.

Schaefer, E.E. (1936) The white fungus disease (*Beauveria bassiana*) among the red locusts in South Africa, and some observations on the grey fungus disease (*Empusa grylli*). *Science Bulletin, Department of Agriculture and Forestry Union of South Africa* **47**, 167–177.

Schmutterer, H. & Freres T. (1990) Beeinflussung der Metamorphose, Färbung und Verhalten der Wüstenhauschrecke *Schistocerca gregaria* (Forsk.) und der Afrikanischen Wanderheuschrecke *Locusta migratoria migratorioides* (R. & F.) durch Niemsamenöl. *Zeitschrift für Pflanzenkrankheiten und Pflanzenschutz* **97**, 431–438.

Snedecor, G.W. & Cochran, W.G. (1980) *Statistical Methods.* 7th edition. Iowa State University Press, Iowa, USA.

Southwood, T.R.E. (1978) *Ecological Methods.* Methuen & Co Ltd, London.

Van der Valk, H.C.H.G. (1990) Beneficial arthropods. In: Everts, J.W. (ed.) *Environmental Effects of Chemical Locust and Grasshopper Control* FAO, Rome.

The effect of various neem products on the survival and flight activity of adult *Schistocerca gregaria*

H. Wilps[1], O. Nasseh[2] & S. Krall[2]

[1]Forstzoologisches Institut, Universität Freiburg; [2]GTZ-Projekt Biologisch Integrierte Heuschreckenbekämpfung, Eschborn.

Abstract

Schistocerca gregaria (Forskål) adults were collected in the Tamesna desert (Republic of Niger) and treated topically with various neem product formulations. Depending on the application method, untreated controls and locusts sprayed with palm oil did not show any mortality, but the treatment with neem oil usually decreased the flight performance by up to 70%. Recovery from this reduction could not be observed in flight experiments repeated at day 6 after application.

Injection of synthetic adipokinetic hormone did not raise the blood lipid concentration of neem-treated *S. gregaria* nearly as much as it did in untreated controls. Therefore, it can be inferred that compounds from neem seed kernels inhibit the lipid mobilizing system of *S. gregaria.* Consequently, the locusts treated with neem products have insufficient reserves to fly long distances.

Introduction

Energy metabolism of the locust is regulated by hormones stored in the corpora cardiaca (cc). The adipokinetic hormones (AKH) synthesized and released by the cc increase the concentration of energy-rich metabolites (lipids) in the haemolymph to provide flight muscle with energy required for long-distance flights. Release of the hormones is initiated at the onset of flight activity and the lipids originating from the fat body are completely oxidized by the flight muscle cells (Beenakkers *et al.*, 1984).

In various insect species neem products, as well as injected azadirachtin, interfered with the hormonal regulation of flight metabolism and reproduction (Schulz, 1985a, 1985b; Rembold *et al.*, 1986, 1988,

1989; Dorn *et al.*, 1988; Subrahmanyam *et al.*, 1989), and led to reduced or completely inhibited flight ability and fertility (Steffens & Schmutterer, 1982; Wilps, 1989; Schmutterer, 1990).

Most of the investigations on the effect of neem products as well as the mode of action of azadirachtin have been done under laboratory conditions. Additionally, there is no information on the effect of neem products on the adults of *Schistocerca gregaria* (Forskål).

In our experiments, adult *S. gregaria* collected and kept in field cages were used in tests carried out at In-Abangharit (Tamesna desert, Republic of Niger). The studies aimed to elucidate the fitness reduction of *S. gregaria* following the application of various neem products by different methods. The mortality rate and flight performance were chosen as the measured variables.

Materials and methods

The locusts were collected in Arabigou (Tamesna desert, Niger), an area of about 3.5 km^2 covered with *Schouwia thebaica* (= *purpurea*)* (Cruciferae), located 100 km to the north-west of In-Abangharit. The locusts were caught between October and November 1990 and reared in cages (2 x 2 x 2 m) set up in a field, also covered with *S. thebaica*, located near the base of In-Abangharit. When the locusts were caught, most of them were immature and showed an intermediate phase status. After three weeks, however, most had changed to the gregarious phase and also were fully developed. In the experiments only adult males were used.

Application on resting locusts (ground treatment)

Neem and palm oil were applied at a rate of 1 ml/m^2 (10 l/ha) by using an ultra-low volume (ULV) hand sprayer. To prevent *S. gregaria* from flying away they were exposed to cold (20 min at 6°C) before experimentation, and subsequently transferred into an area of 16 m^2 bordered with a plastic fence 1.5 m high.

Application during flight activity (flight treatment)

The locusts were fixed on a flight mill immediately before treatment with a dosage of 1 ml/m^2. The volume applied was calculated from the flow rate of the sprayer, the spraying time, and the ground area which was covered

*Taxonomy in dispute (eds).

by the spraying cloud. After application, flight activity continued for at least 3 min, at an average speed of 7.7 ± 0.4 km/h.

Measurement of flight activity

Six locusts were attached to a flight mill and, utilizing the fact that insects without ground contact show permanent flight activity, the number of revolutions was counted by a mechanical counter to obtain an average for all six. All experiments were carried out at temperatures between 28°C and 32°C. Flight was measured for periods of 30 or 60 min.

Concentration of lipids in the haemolymph

The change in haemolymph lipid concentration in treated and untreated locusts was measured following flight activity and injection of adipokinetic hormones. Haemolymph samples were obtained by pricking the membrane between hindleg and thorax. The hormone was injected in 10 µl distilled water through the intersegmental cuticle between thorax and abdomen. Haemolymph lipid concentration was measured spectrophotometrically using the method described by Zöllner & Kirsch (1962).

Substances tested and controls

1. Neem oil enriched with methanolic extracts of pressed neem seed kernels to a final concentration of 0.075% azadirachtin (prepared at the University Giessen = Neem Giessen)
2. Neem oil enriched with an azadirachtin content of 0.25% (prepared at IITA, Benin = Neem Benin)
3. Pure neem oil pressed from neem seeds (origin: Republic of Niger)
4. Pure palm oil as control (origin: Republic of Nigeria)
5. Adipokinetic hormone (synthetic *Schistocerca* adipokinetic hormone I, Peninsula Laboratories, Belmont, USA).

The neem products used were a gift from Prof. Schmutterer, University of Giessen, FRG, Dipl.-Biol. J. Langewald, IITA, Cotonou, Benin, and Dipl.-Biol. H. Ostermann, Protection des Végétaux, Niamey, Republic of Niger.

Statistical analysis

After confirming that the data were normally distributed, statistical significance was tested by Student's t-test. If not mentioned otherwise, significance was calculated on a 95% level ($P \leq 0.05$).

Results and discussion

Mortality rate and flight activity of *S. gregaria* treated during the resting phase

In initial ground application trials neither the treated population nor the untreated control showed a significant increase in mortality rate during the observation period of 15 days. Nevertheless, two days after application the flight performance of these locusts was tested. The flight distance was measured every five minutes to control the uniform course of the flight activity (Fig. 1).

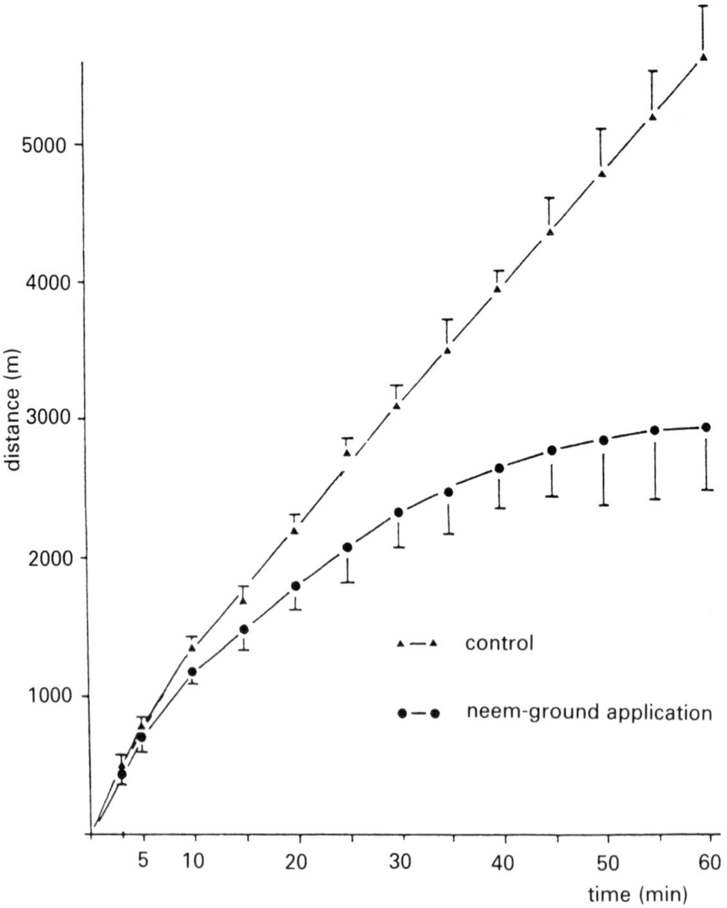

Figure 1. Flight performance of treated and untreated *S. gregaria* (distance in m/h). The data are the mean ± SD of 3 replicates with 6 locusts for each experiment.

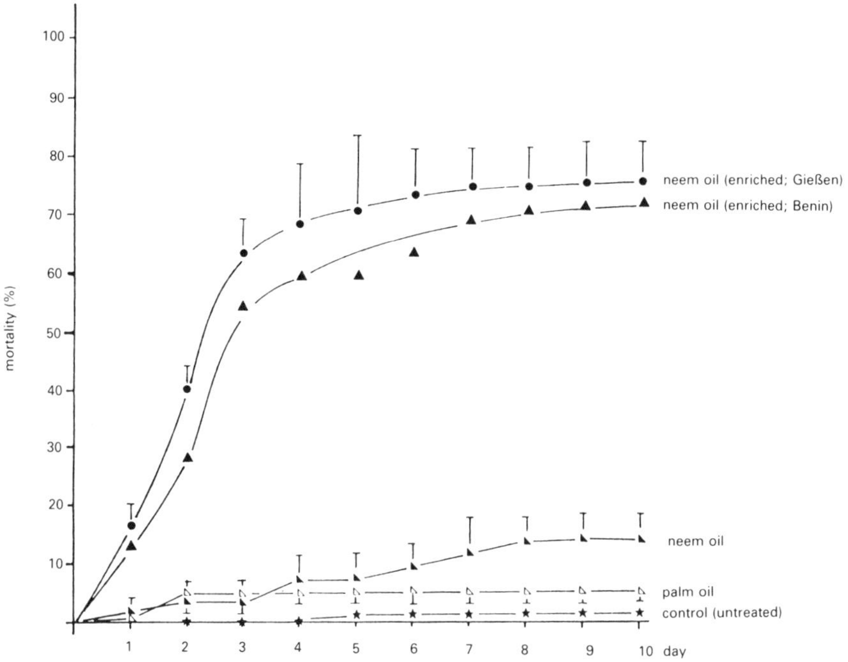

Figure 2. Mortality rate of *S. gregaria* treated during flight activity. The curves demonstrate the increase in mortality expressed as % of the initial population size. The data are the mean ± SD of 4 to 5 replicates for each experiment, except the application of neem Benin (unreplicated).

Although enriched neem oil applied during a resting phase did not affect the life span of *S. gregaria*, it reduced the flight performance by more than 50%. With respect to locust control these results are interesting because they demonstrate that neem oil can influence the migration behaviour of *S. gregaria*. If it is possible to treat locusts in the desert, far from agriculture, reduction of flight activity might be a useful effect because treated locusts may be more susceptible to predators.

This reduction is not sufficient to combat locusts that have reached cultivated areas. In this case, an increase in the mortality rate of the treated locusts is necessary. Therefore neem products were also tested against flying locusts. This technique was attempted for the following two reasons:

1. to produce an effect on *S. gregaria* neem oil has to pass the cuticle but the most sensitive parts of the insect body (such as intersegmental membranes or wing joints) are covered by the wings during resting periods
2. the dispersal of a substance in an insect body is correlated with the metabolic rate. According to the findings of Weis-Fogh (1952), the

metabolic rate of *S. gregaria* increases during flight activity by a factor of about 50 and the effect of neem might therefore be enhanced during flight.

The effect of various neem products and palm oil applied during flight activity on the mortality rate of *S. gregaria* is presented in Fig. 2.

Neem Giessen and neem Benin increased the mortality rate to up to 70% of the initial population within 3 to 4 days and even pure neem oil caused a slightly increased mortality rate. This was in contrast to the natural mortality of the untreated and palm oil controls which remained below 10%. The comparable results of neem Benin and neem Giessen were surprising because these products differ in azadirachtin content by a factor of nearly 3. This may be of importance when developing new neem products since azadirachtin is said to be the most effective neem compound, but also the most difficult component to extract.

The flight performance of neem Benin- and neem Giessen-treated locusts did not differ significantly in the various measurements. Therefore only the flight performance of neem Giessen-treated *S. gregaria* is presented in Fig. 3.

After treatment with neem oil, the flight performance of *S. gregaria* decreased by more than 60% (Fig. 3). The fact that the flight performance improved slightly at day six after spraying does not point to a recovery of the insects but was caused by the fact that by this time only the less contaminated locusts survived (mortality rate more than 70%).

The flight periods were measured for only 30 min, because about 60% of the treated *S. gregaria* did not sustain a continuous flight activity longer than 30 min; 30–40% of the insects had already stopped flying after 10 to 20 min and furthermore, nearly 30% of the locusts treated with enriched neem oil were completely incapable of any flight activity.

The flight performance of *S. gregaria* sprayed with pure neem oil was only slightly affected (data not shown).

Migrating locusts utilize lipids stored in the fat body as fuel for long distance flights. The onset of flight activity is registered by the brain and leads to the secretion of AKH, which are synthesized and stored in the corpora cardiaca. The hormones are released into the haemolymph and transported to the fat body. In this organ the hormones initiate the activation of the lipid mobilizing system. Lipids in the form of fatty acids are secreted into the haemolymph and transported to the flight muscle, where a complete oxidation to water and carbon dioxide yields energy. Therefore the haemolymph lipid profile depends on the physiological state of the insect, and furthermore can be influenced by the injection of synthetic AKH. Thus changes in blood lipid concentration in treated and untreated locusts may be mediated by flight activity or hormone injection and allow conclusions about the mode of action of neem products and the physical capacity of treated and untreated locusts to be drawn. The differences in

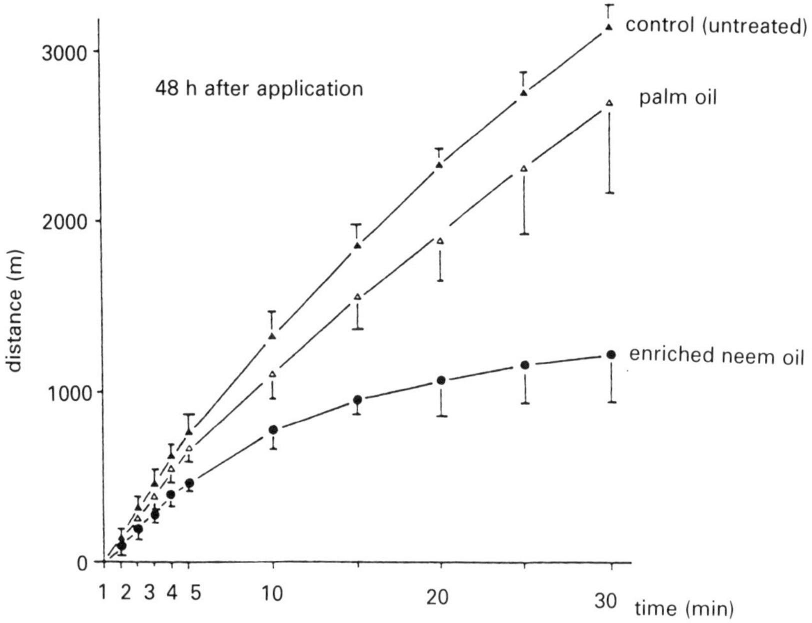

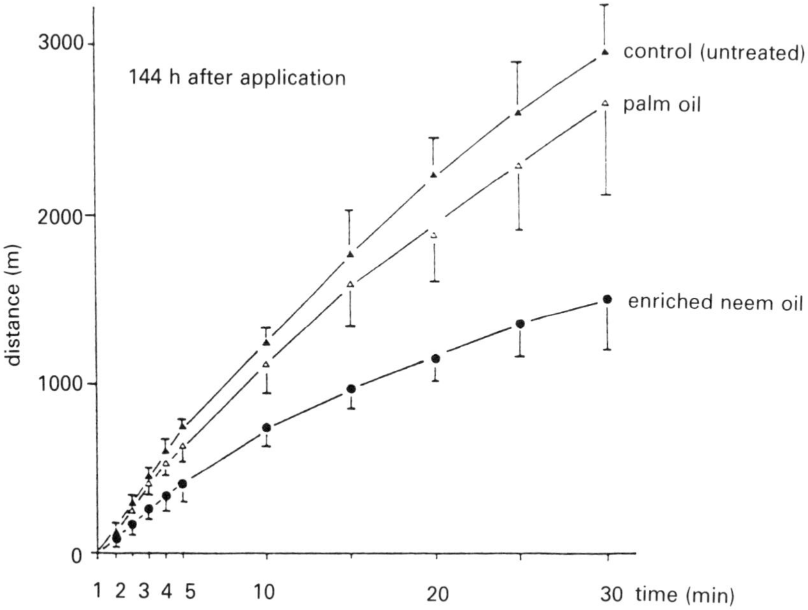

Figure 3. Flight performance of *S. gregaria* 48 h and 144 h after flight treatment. The curves present the flight performance given in m/30 min for *S. gregaria* untreated and treated with enriched neem oil (0.075% azadirachtin) or palm oil. The data are the mean ± SD of 3 to 4 replicates with 6 locusts each.

blood lipid concentration before and after flight or AKH injection of control and neem treated locusts are shown in Fig. 4.

In untreated locusts, flight activity decreased the blood lipid level, whereas the injection of AKH increased the lipid content. The lower lipid concentration resulting from flight activity indicated that the lipids released by the fat body were oxidized immediately to provide the energy needed for this physical activity. The increase in lipids after AKH injection demonstrated the hormone induced activation of the lipid mobilizing system, and the fact that these lipids were not oxidized because the animals were not allowed to fly. In ground-treated locusts comparable observations were made, but the lipid content after flight as well as AKH injection was reduced, indicating that the energy mobilizing system was affected by the neem products. In flight-treated *S. gregaria* a complete disruption of the energy providing system can be observed. Neither the flight activity nor the

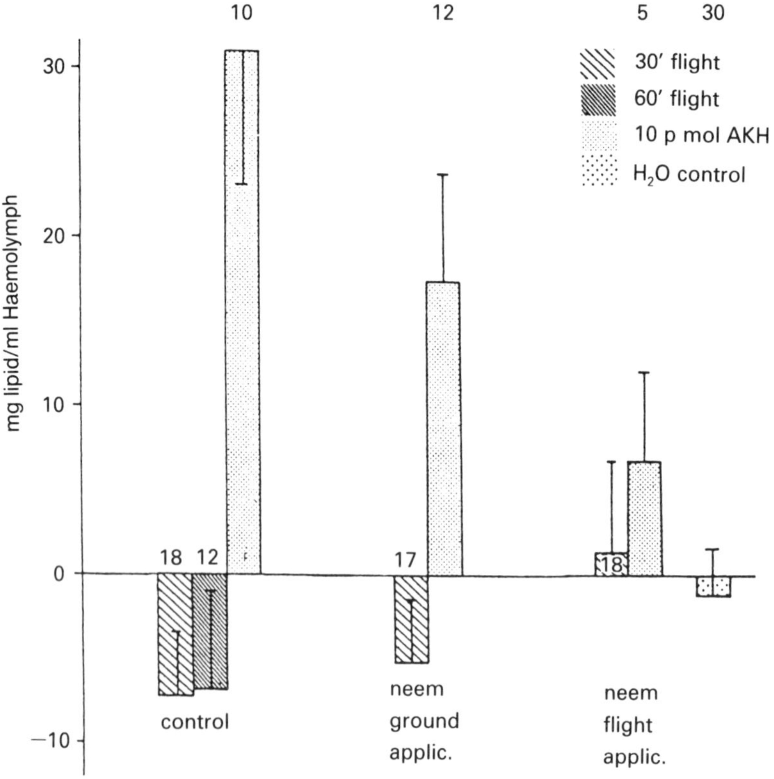

Figure 4. The columns represent the difference in blood lipid concentration before and after flight activity and AKH injection, respectively and were expressed in mg lipid/ml haemolymph. The data are the average ± SD of 5 to 30 estimates for each column, indicated by the number above each column.

AKH injection led to a large change in blood lipid concentration. Therefore one may assume that these locusts were completely unable to provide their flight muscles with the energy necessary for long distance flights.

Conclusions

Ground treatment with enriched neem oil did not affect the mortality rate of *S. gregaria* but decreased the flight performance, and influenced the lipid mobilizing system. The same products applied during flight increased the mortality rate up to 70% and led to a complete inability to sustain flight activity, also induced a disruption of the energy mobilizing system. Flight treatment promises a successful strategy for the use of neem products against *S. gregaria*, but further investigations are necessary. The goals of these investigatons must be oriented toward:

1. varying the formulation to obtain higher concentrations of the effective compounds in neem (to reduce the application volume and to test the feasibility of a ground application)
2. further dose-response experiments involving various application methods in order to minimize the dosage needed
3. a better understanding of the mode of action of the neem products. This must include the identification of the most effective compound in the seed kernel extracts.

Acknowledgements

The authors wish to thank their counterparts on the station, particularly Mr Ali Ayouba, for their technical help.

We also sincerely thank Prof. Dr H. Schmutterer, Dipl.-Biol. J. Langewald and Dipl.-Biol. H. Ostermann for generous samples of neem oil. Last but not lease, financial support of our studies and logistic assistance during field work in the Republic of Niger by the Deutsche Gesellschaft für Technische Zusammenarbeit (GTZ) and the support of J. Haag (Protection des Végétaux, in Niamey) as well as productive collaboration with Dr E. Kirkilionis and Dipl.-Agr. T. Freres, are acknowledged gratefully.

References

Beenakkers, A.M.T., Van der Horst, D.J., & Van Marrewijk, W.I.A. (1984) Insect flight muscle metabolism. *Insect Biochemistry* **14**, 243–260.

Dorn, A., Rademacher, J.M. & Sehn, E. (1988) Effects of azadirachtin on reproductive organs and fertility in the large milk weed bug, *Oncopeltus fasciatus.* In: Schmutterer, H. & Ascher, K.R.S. (eds), *Natural Pesticides from the Neem Tree and other Tropical Plants.* GTZ, Eschborn, pp. 273–288.

Rembold, H., Foster, H., Czoppelt, C.H., Rao, P.J. & Sieber, K.-P. (1966) The azadirachtins, a group of insect growth regulators from the neem tree. In: Schmutterer, H. & Ascher, K.R.S. (eds), *Natural Pesticides from the Neem Tree and other Tropical Plants.* GTZ, Eschborn, pp. 153–161.

Rembold, H., Uhl, M. & Müller, T. (1988) Effect of azadirachtin A on hormone titers during the gonadotrophic cycle of *Locusta migratoria.* In: Schmutterer, H. & Ascher, K.R.S. (eds), *Natural Pesticides from the Neem Tree and other Tropical Plants.* GTZ, Eschborn, pp. 289–298.

Rembold, H., Subrahmanyam, B. & Müller, T. (1989) Corpus cardiacum-a target for azadirachtin. *Experientia* **45**, 361–363.

Schmutterer, H. (1990) Properties and potential of natural pesticides from the neem tree, *Azadirachta indica. Annual Review of Entomology* **35**, 271–297.

Schulz, W.-D. (1985a) Histologische Untersuchungen zur Wirkung von Extrakten aus Samen des Neem-Baumes *Azadirachta indica* auf weibliche Imagines von *Epilachna varivestis* (Coleoptera, Coccinellidae). I. Schädigungen von Ovarentwicklung und Oogenese. *Zoologische Jahrbücher Anatomie und Ontogenie der Tiere* **113**, 193–214.

Schulz, W.-D. (1985b) Histologische Untersuchungen zur Wirkung von Extrakten aus Samen des Neem-Baumes *Azadirachta indica* auf weibliche Imagines von *Epilachna varivestis* (Coleoptera, Coccinellidae). II. Schädigungen von neuroendokrinem System und Corpora allata. *Zoologische Jahrbücher Anatomie und Ontogenie der Tiere* **113**, 267–287.

Steffens, R.J. & Schmutterer, H. (1982) The effect of a crude methanolic neem (*Azadirachta indica*) seed kernel extract on metamorphosis and quality of adults of the Mediterranean fruit fly, *Ceratitis capitata* Wied. (Diptera, Tephritidae). *Zeitschrift für Angewandte Entomologie* **94**, 98–103.

Subrahmanyam, B., Müller, T. & Rembold, H. (1989) Inhibition of turnover of neurosecretion by azadirachtin in *Locusta migratoria. Journal of Insect Physiology* **35**, 493–500.

Weis-Fogh, T. (1952) Fat combustion and metabolic rate of flying locusts (*Schistocerca gregaria* Forskål). *Philosophical Transactions of the Royal Society of London B Biological Science* **237**, 1–36.

Wilps, H. (1989) The influence of neem seed kernel extracts (NSKE) of the neem tree *Azadirachta indica* on flight activity, food ingestion, reproduction rate and metabolism in the Diptera *Phormia terraenovae* (Diptera, Muscidae). *Zoologische Jahrbücher Allgemeine Zoologie und Physiologie der Tiere* **93**, 271–282.

Zöllner, N. & Kirsch, K. (1962) Über die quantitative Bestimmung von Lipoiden (Mikromethode) mittels der vielen natürlichen Lipoiden (allen bekannten Plasmalipoiden) gemeinsamen Sulfophospho-vanillin Reaktion. *Zeitschrift für die Gesamte Experimentelle Medizin* **135**, 545–561.

A review of field studies of the environmental impacts of locust/grasshopper control programmes in Africa

P.C. Matteson

Department of Entomology, Iowa State University.

Abstract

The desert environment may be adversely affected by the application of chemical pesticides for desert locust control and microbial pesticides must also be monitored for environmental side effects. Locusts concentrate to feed and reproduce in areas of vegetation which are also richest in non-target species. The microecology of these habitats is very important in determining the effects of pesticides, as is the application method used. The effects on pollinators have caused particular concern and methods have been evolved to study impact on honey bees. Effects on other non-target organisms are best studied by time series analysis, since the large areas and long time scales required for conventional analysis are not usually practical. The results of some preliminary studies on non-target effects of locust control indicate significant effects on terrestrial arthropods, aquatic organisms and birds. More work is needed on methodology and on criteria for judging the acceptability of pesticide side-effects.

Introduction

The plague of desert locust (*Schistocerca gregaria* (Forskål)) that afflicted Africa and the Middle East from 1986–9, coupled with a simultaneous grasshopper outbreak in the West African Sahel, triggered a massive emergency response from the international community. The problem was countered with the same method employed during the last major plague, 25 years previously: insecticide application to acridid swarms and their feeding and breeding sites. Extensive land areas were treated. Nearly 14 million ha in Africa were sprayed for locusts, and insecticides were applied to additional millions of hectares in the Sahel for grasshopper control (Everts, 1990b; OTA, 1990).

Also, as in the past, little or no environmental monitoring was done in connection with the acridid control campaign. Insufficient data were available to estimate the campaign's impact on non-target species, or for informed decision making on controversial questions such as the relative environmental costs of dieldrin and less persistent chemicals that were proposed as substitutes (Van der Valk, 1988). The assumption that pesticide applications in the desert cause scant or no environmental damage is being questioned. USAID's Programmatic Environmental Assessment of the locust/grasshopper control programme in Africa and the Middle East (TAMS/CICP, 1989) underlined the importance of avoiding treatment of fragile habitats, of developing alternative control methods to replace the current unilateral dependence on synthetic insecticides, and of making environmental monitoring a central element of acridid control activities.

USAID and other agricultural development organizations are acting on those recommendations. Since insecticides are the main locust/grasshopper control method available for Africa in the near future and will probably remain part of integrated control programmes, field researchers have begun to investigate insecticide impact on non-target species. Experimental findings will help to develop safe and selective application guidelines as well as environmental monitoring methods.

Microbial insecticides must undergo scrutiny just as synthetic and botanical ones do. They may harm non-target species which are rare or which are pollinators, scavengers, important food sources for insectivores, or predators and parasitoids of insect pests (Laird *et al.*, 1990). Much of the following applies to entomopathogens, should field tests be required.

Characteristics of locust/grasshopper control campaigns that affect pesticide hazard to non-target species

Certain characteristics of locust/grasshopper control campaigns and the arid environments in which they operate affect the hazard to non-target species. Most of these characteristics increase hazards (de Visscher *et al.*, 1988; Everts, 1990a).

Seasonality

Locusts and grasshoppers are attracted to moist, green habitats to eat and reproduce. In the desert this means oases, wadis with permanent vegetation, or restricted areas where rainfall has produced temporary plant cover and the desert is in bloom for a brief period. These habitats are rich in species taking advantage of favourable conditions for their annual period of activity and reproduction, not only acridids, but other vertebrate and invertebrate herbivores and their predators, as well as human nomads with their livestock. Thus, locust/grasshopper insecticide applications are made when and where they can do the most damage to non-target species.

On the other hand, the extreme seasonal conditions in desert environments, particularly the irregularity of rainfall, have caused native flora and fauna to develop defences against a temporarily unsuitable environment. For example, many organisms are dormant during dry periods, with development and activity triggered by rainfall; however, in some species (including some of the major natural enemies of acridids) only a portion of the population is reactivated at any one time, with delays between emergences lasting months or years (Greathead, 1963). Such adaptations could protect part of non-target arthropod populations from exposure to a small number of insecticide applications (Grant, 1989), and it is important to consider the biologies of non-target organisms when interpreting risk.

Isolation of sensitive habitats

Many rich habitats, particularly oases, permanent springs and temporary pools, are isolated. Ephemeral and non-mobile animal populations are vulnerable to local extinction with poor prospects for recolonization.

Enhanced degradation of insecticides

High UV light intensity and high temperatures promote insecticide degradation, as does increased microbial activity during rainy periods (Grant, 1989). Thus the residual effect of insecticides applied in locust/grasshopper habitats may be much shorter-lived than in temperate zones.

Large scale insecticide application

Treatments generally cover large areas, up to 10 km^2 for locusts and 100+ km^2 for grasshoppers (Everts, 1990b). This slows or even prevents the recovery of non-target species through recolonization. However, prospects for population recovery in savannas are probably relatively good, since even a large treated parcel is surrounded by similar untreated grassland.

Application methods

Equipment used for large scale operations, especially fixed-wing aircraft, decreases the precision of applications and increases environmental risks. Water holes, water sources for treated cropland and other small or dispersed non-target habitats are frequently contaminated.

Insecticide dosages

The insecticide dosages used for locust control are generally higher than dosages applied in other crop protection campaigns. In practice, overdoses are common and can cause dramatic ecological damage.

Repetition of treatments

Repeated insecticide applications multiply the hazard to non-target species and may seriously delay the recovery of populations. A series of applications in a single location is frequently made to control grasshoppers, and sometimes for locust control.

Ecological importance of locusts and grasshoppers

Many vertebrate and invertebrate species use acridids as a food source. This increases the risk of secondary poisoning of insectivores and of sudden significant food deprivation for some non-target species after an insecticide application.

Field research methods for determining insecticide impact on non-target species

Pesticide hazard to a non-target species is evaluated by combining data on pesticide toxicity and exposure, and then interpreting the risk in the light of life history, application patterns, habitat and other factors that will determine the severity of effects and the ability of the population to recover. The epidemiology of entomopathogens may play a significant role where microbial pesticides are concerned. Predatory and parasitic arthropods can disseminate pathogens within host populations, sometimes with a serious negative effect on the beneficials (Vinson, 1990). It is not possible to estimate risk accurately without a field experiment to reflect genuine exposure (Grant, 1988, 1989; Jepson, 1988; Brown, 1989). Preliminary toxicity trials in the laboratory are useful for identifying susceptible non-target groups that should be the focus of field trials.

Honey-bees

Honey-bee (*Apis mellifera* Linnaeus) poisoning by insecticides has become the number one problem for bee-keepers on a worldwide scale (Atkins, 1975; Johansen, 1977), and honey-bees are customarily included in studies of pesticide impact on non-target species. Oomen (1986) and Felton *et al.* (1986) have proposed a sequential evaluation scheme that would start with laboratory screening, continue with cage trials and end with field studies.

Insecticide impact on honey-bees is measured in the field by observing exposed colonies for several days before and after the insecticide application. Queen and brood condition, the number of dead bees and foraging flights at colony entrances, and foraging activity on a treated crop can all be monitored (Gary, 1967; Gary & Mussen, 1984; Gary & Lorenzen, 1989). In addition, caged bees can be exposed to pesticide applications to determine direct effects. Dead bees may be analysed for insecticide residues to confirm cause of death. Experienced local beekeepers who inspect bee colonies before and after the insecticide application can evaluate the probable long-term impact of the insecticide as well as the resulting economic losses.

Other non-target species

Field experiments usually involve periodic sampling to compare changes in target and non-target species numbers or impact (percentage parasitism, predation) between treated and untreated areas before and after pesticide application. Ideally, an experiment would investigate the entire recovery phase of non-target species populations over the total area affected. Since the area affected is normally much larger than the largest possible experimental plots and recovery may require several years, limited experimental budgets and other constraints rarely permit studies of such extent. The failure to distinguish between the experimental and biological dimensions is one of the major flaws in the design and interpretation of pesticide side-effects studies (Jepson, 1989; Everts, 1990a).

Because of the potential for dispersal and redistribution of non-target species between plots, small-plot experiments are generally suitable only for short-term monitoring studies. Season-long investigations may require very large plots (many square kilometers) to be realistic, especially for birds and flying insects. Replication raises the likelihood of observing significant treatment effects, and means that the experimental results can be considered applicable to other similar habitats, not only to the specific plots used (Hurlbert, 1984). However, where large plot sizes are required it can be difficult or impossible to replicate (Sotherton *et al.*, 1988). In that case, a time series analysis is preferred. In order to obtain statistically analysable results, a period of pretreatment monitoring of all plots is required, as well as post-treatment monitoring (Stewart-Oaten *et al.*, 1986; FAO, 1989).

Birds, mammals, fish and aquatic and terrestrial invertebrates are the non-target groups most frequently observed to determine pesticide side-effects. Terrestrial arthropods, particularly pollinators and beneficial species associated with insect pests, would be the focus of studies on the non-target effects of microbial insecticides (EPA, 1989). Previous work has shown that entomopathogens can harm beneficial insects through direct infection and/or through a reduction in the availability or quality of their food sources. Parasitic Hymenoptera appear to be particularly vulnerable. While entomopathogens are known to reduce prey available to predators, they are decidedly less hazardous to predators than are synthetic broad-spectrum insecticides (Vinson, 1990).

Most arthropod experiments have involved extensive collecting using general sampling methods, and have analysed findings only at order or family level. Yet genus and species level information is usually necessary for a meaningful study. Species within a taxon that have particular ecological and/or economic significance may react much differently to a pesticide application than does the taxon as a whole (Sotherton *et al.*, 1988; Van der Valk, 1990).

To confirm the causal relationship between a pesticide application and an observed effect, at least two of the following observations should be made (FAO, 1989):

- Coincidence of treatment and effect
- Dose-response relationship
- Observed recovery from effect
- Additional information from residue or cholinesterase measurement
- Observations of effects in individual organisms.

Work to date and future directions

Reports have been published recently on initial experiments to determine the ecological impacts of locust/grasshopper insecticides in Africa (Ottesen, 1987; Ottesen & Sømme, 1987; Dynamac, 1988a, 1988b; Müller, 1988, 1990; Pinto *et al.*, 1988; Ottesen *et al.*, 1989; Everts, 1990b). Due to lack of time, resources and/or skilled personnel, few of the experiments followed the ideal experimental guidelines described above. Results are thus of limited applicability, but a general picture of the impact of some commonly used locust/grasshopper insecticides is emerging (Everts, 1990b). Terrestrial arthropods and aquatic animals (particularly crustaceans) are significantly affected, and severe effects on birds have been observed in some cases. Not nearly enough is yet known to designate 'indicator species' that can simplify the monitoring of pesticide impact (Everts, 1983), or to design practical environmental monitoring methods for insecticide application teams.

Consistent with their recent emphasis on integrated pest management and sustainable agriculture, international development organizations are continuing to increase their attention to the ecological effects of pesticides. Further work is needed to improve experimental methodology for studies of insecticide effect on non-target arthropods. Possibilities of supplementing field trials with laboratory or semi-laboratory approaches should be investigated. Statistical methods need to be improved for analysing time series data and indirect phenomena such as insecticide-induced pest resurgence, and for detecting small changes in non-target arthropod populations that exhibit wide natural fluctuations in population density. Appropriate time scales for observations must be determined and applied. There also remain considerable problems with interpreting field studies and establishing indicators of environmental quality (Sotherton *et al.*, 1988). This is especially true for Africa, where the taxonomic status and ecology of so many arthropod species are unknown.

Finally, there is the question of criteria for judging the acceptability of pesticide side-effects. What limits should be set on honey-bee mortality and reduction of populations of threatened or endangered species? Are perturbations in beneficial insect populations acceptable if detectable for only one season? Two seasons? These and similar questions merit careful investigation. Policymakers depend on scientists for defining key issues for proposing research and for advice on adequate environmental protection standards.

References

Atkins, E.L. (1975) Injury to honey bees by poisoning. In: *The Hive and the Honey Bee.* Dadant & Sons, Hamilton, Illinois, USA, pp. 663–696.

Brown, R.A. (1989) Pesticides and non-target terrestrial invertebrates: an industrial approach. In: Jepson, P.C. (ed.), *Pesticides and Non-target Invertebrates.* Intercept Ltd., Wimborne, Dorset, England, pp. 19–42.

de Visscher, M.N., Duranton, J.F., Launois, M. & Garcia, G. (1988) *Effets Directs et Indirects, Immediats et Differés de la Lutte Antiacridienne sur l'Environnement, Démarches Préliminaires.* CIRAD/PRIFAS, Montpellier, France.

Dynamac (1988a) *Results of the Mali Pesticide Testing Trials against the Senegalese Grasshopper. Final Technical Report.* Dynamac Corporation, Rockville, Maryland, USA.

Dynamac (1988b) *Results of the Locust Pesticide Testing Trials in Sudan. Technical Report.* Dynamac Corporation, Rockville, Maryland.

EPA (1989) *Subdivision M of the Pesticide Testing Guidelines: Microbial and

Biochemical Pest Control Agents. Part A, Microbial Pest Control Agents. PB89-211676. US Environmental Protection Agency, Washington, DC.

Everts, J.W. (1983) Animal indicators for side-effects of chemical vector control. *Environmental Monitoring and Assessment* **3**, 229–326.

Everts, J.W. (1990a) Methods for monitoring the impact of chemical control of locust and grasshoppers in Africa. *Proceedings of the Workshop on Health and Environmental Impact of Alternative Control Agents for Desert Locust Control,* Oslo, Norway, January 14–17, 1990, 45–54. (Development and Environment No. 5, NORAGRIC Occasional papers series C.)

Everts, J.W. (ed.) (1990b) Environmental effects of chemical locust and grasshopper control. A pilot study. *ECLO/SEN/003/NET Project Report.* FAO, Rome.

FAO (1989) *Report of the Working Group on Environmental Side-effects of Desert Locust Control, 14–16 February 1989.* FAO, Rome.

Felton, J.C., Oomen, P.A. & Stevenson, J.H. (1986) Toxicity and hazard of pesticides to honeybees: harmonization of test methods. *Bee World* **67**, 114–124.

Gary, N.E. (1967) A method for evaluating honey bee flight activity at the hive entrance. *Journal of Economic Entomology* **60**, 102–105.

Gary, N.E. & Lorenzen, K. (1989) Effect of methamidophos on honey bees (Hymenoptera: Apidae) during alfalfa pollination. *Journal of Economic Entomology* **82**, 1067–1072.

Gary, N.E. & Mussen, E.C. (1984) Impact of Mediterranean fruit fly malathion bait spray on honey bees. *Environmental Entomology* **13**, 711–717.

Grant, I.F. (1988) Environmental concerns and locust control. In: Steedman, A. (ed.), *The Locust Handbook.* ODNRI, London, pp. 155–159.

Grant, I.F. (1989) Environmental effects of desert locust control. *FAO Plant Protection Bulletin* **37**, 27–35.

Greathead, D.J. (1963) A review of the insect enemies of Acridoidea (Orthoptera). *Transactions of the Royal Entomological Society of London* **114**, 437–517.

Hurlbert, S.H. (1984) Pseudoreplication and the design of ecological field experiments. *Ecological Monographs* **54**, 187–211.

Jepson, P.C. (1988) Ecological characteristics and the susceptibility of non-target invertebrates to long-term pesticide side-effects. *In*: Greaves, B.D., Smith, B.D. & Greig-Smith, P.W. (eds), *Field Methods for the Study of the Environmental Effects of Pesticides.* British Crop Protection Council Monograph 40, Thornton Heath, England, pp. 191–200.

Jepson, P.C. (1989) The temporal and spatial dynamics of pesticide side-effects on non-target invertebrates. *In: Pesticides and Non-Target Invertebrates.* Jepson, P.C. (ed.) Intercept Ltd., Wimborne, Dorset, England, pp. 95–128.

Johansen, C.A. (1977) Pesticides and pollinators. *Annual Review of Entomology* **22**, 177–192.

Laird, M., Lacey, L.A. & Davidson, E.W. (eds) (1990) *Safety of Microbial Insecticides.* CRC Press, Boca Raton, Florida, USA.

Müller, P. (1988) *Ökotoxicologische Wirkungen von chlorierten Kohlwasserstoffen, Phosphorsäureestern, Carbamaten und Pyrethroiden im nordöstlichen Sudan.* Institut für Biogeographie der Universität des Saarlandes, Saarbrücken, Germany.

Müller, P. (1990) Target- und Nontarget-Wirkungen von *Nosema locustae* auf den Kapverden. Deutsche Gesellschaft für Technische Zusammenarbeit, Eschborn, Germany.

Oomen, P.A. (1986) A sequential scheme for evaluating the hazard of pesticides to bees, *Apis mellifera. Mededelingen van de Faculteit Landbowwetenschappen Rijksunversitat Gent* **51**, 1205–1213.

OTA (1990) *A Plague of Locusts.* US Congress Office of Technology Assessment, Special Report, OTA-F-450. US Government Printing Office, Washington, DC.

Ottesen, P. (1987) *The Mortality of* Oedaleus senegalensis *(Orthoptera) and other Invertebrates in Mali Using Reduced Dosages of Fenitrothion.* Department of Zoology, University of Oslo, Norway.

Ottesen, P. & Sømme, L. (1987) *Environmental Effects of Insecticides against Grasshoppers and Locusts.* Report to Royal Norwegian Ministry of Development Cooperation. University of Oslo, Norway.

Ottesen, P., Fossland, S. Johannessen, B. & Simonsen, J.H. (1989) *Reduced Rates of Fenitrothion: the Effect on* Oedaleus senegalensis *(Orthoptera) and Non-Target Arthropods in Mali, West Africa.* Report to the Royal Norweigian Ministry of Development Cooperation, Oslo.

Pinto, L.J., Mann, J.B. & Bottrell, D.G. (1988) *Analysis of Aerial Application of Fenitrothion ULV for Locust Control in Sudan. Environmental Assessment. Sudan Multi-donor Locust/Grasshopper Control Program.* Consortium for International Crop Protection, College Park, Maryland, USA.

Sotherton, N.W., Jepson, P.C. & Pullen, A.J. (1988) Criteria for the design, execution and analysis of terrestial non-target invertebrate field tests. In: Greaves, M.P., Smith, B.D. & Greig-Smith, P.W. (eds) *Field Methods for the Study of Environmental Effects of Pesticides.* British Crop Protection Council Monograph 40, Thornton Heath, England., pp. 183–190.

Stewart-Oaten, A., Murdoch, W.W. & Parker, K.R. (1986) Environmental impact assessment: 'pseudoreplication' in time? *Ecology* **67**, 929–940.

TAMS/CICP (1989) *Locust and Grasshopper Control in Africa and the Middle East. A Programmatic Environmental Assessment.* TAMS Consultants, Inc., Washington, DC. & Consortium for International Crop Protection, College Park, Maryland, USA.

Van der Valk, H.C.H.G. (1988) *Environmental Impact of Dieldrin Applications in Locust Control; a Hazard Assessment. Working Paper,* FAO/ECLO meeting 21 Oct 1988. FAO, Rome.

Van der Valk, H.C.H.G. (1990) Beneficial arthropods. In: *Environmental Effects of Chemical Locust and Grasshopper Control. A Pilot Study.* ECLO/SEN/003/NET Project Report. FAO, Rome, pp. 171–224.

Vinson, S.B. (1990) Potential impact of microbial insecticides on beneficial arthropods in the terrestrial environment. In: Laird, M., Lacey, L.A. & Davidson, E.W. (eds), *Safety of Microbial Insecticides.* CRC Press, Boca Raton, Florida, USA, pp. 43–64.

Environmental impact and safety of fungal biocontrol agents

M.S. Goettel & D.L. Johnson

Agriculture Canada Research Station, Lethbridge, Alberta.

Abstract

Compared with chemical insecticides, fungal microbial control agents offer, among other advantages, a method of insect pest control that has a very narrow host range, can usually be integrated with other biocontrol agents, may provide prolonged control by establishment in the host population, and is also biodegradable. A brief review of the potential environmental impact and safety of candidate fungal control agents is presented. There are indications that these organisms pose only a minimal risk to humans, domestic animals and wildlife. The wide host ranges of some species have caused concern regarding safety to non-target invertebrates. Results of a laboratory study on the safety of a grasshopper isolate of *Beauveria bassiana* Balsamo (Vuillemin) to alfalfa leafcutter bees are reported. No significant increase in bee mortality resulted from treatment of alfalfa with *B. bassiana* conidia. However, the limitations in our knowledge of fungal epizootiology make it impossible to extrapolate from such data to the field situation. Continuous monitoring during field use after preliminary laboratory and field safety testing is recommended to ensure safety to non-target invertebrates.

Introduction

Compared with chemical insecticides, fungal microbial control agents offer, among other advantages, a method of insect pest control that has a very narrow host range, can usually be integrated with other biocontrol agents, may provide prolonged control by establishment in the host population, and is also biodegradable. The best documented cases of detrimental environmental impact of fungal biocontrol agents are indirect effects on the predators and parasitoids of the target pest through host depletion (Goettel *et al.*, 1990). In certain instances, fungi may also adversely affect certain non-target invertebrates directly including predators and parasitoids (Goettel *et al.*, 1990; Vinson, 1990). In general, it is not possible to reduce a pest population without also affecting another component of the ecosystem. For instance, by depleting or even reducing a host population, it is inevitable that the host's predators and parasites will be adversely affected. In such situations, it is imperative that an integrated pest management programme be put into effect that would integrate fungal control with other available control methods.

Safety

A review of present knowledge of potential fungal control agents indicates that these organisms pose only a minimal risk to humans (Siegel & Shadduck, 1990), domestic animals and wildlife (Saik *et al.*, 1990), and non-target invertebrates (Goettel *et al.*, 1990). Nevertheless, the general consensus is that since fungi may pose inherent risks they should be regulated. Most guidelines for registration of entomopathogenic fungi require laboratory testing for infectivity to non-target organisms including mammals (Hall *et al.*, 1982; Aizawa, 1990; Betz *et al.*, 1990; Kandybin & Smirnov, 1990; Quinlan, 1990).

The potential hazards from fungal microbial control agents to higher animals including man, centre on direct exposure to high levels of inoculum. These hazards include toxicity, allergenicity, and infection, and are generally associated with improper handling and application of the product. As pointed out by Prior (1990), these do not generally pose new problems since the same types of hazards are present and dealt with in the use of chemical pesticides.

Host range and specificity

The most likely environmental risk of fungal microbial agents is that non-target invertebrates may be infected and killed. A 'safe' microbial insecticide is essentially one with a restricted host range under the conditions of use. Some fungal species are highly specific and pose a minimal threat to non-target invertebrates. For instance, *Entomophaga grylli* (Fresenius) Batko is restricted to Orthoptera even to the point of species specificity of pathotypes (MacLeod, 1963). Some other entomopathogenic fungi have very wide host ranges. For instance, *Beauveria bassiana* Balsamo (Vuillemin) has been recorded as infecting over 700 species of arthropods (Li, 1987).

However, laboratory studies have shown that different isolates of the same species with a wide host range are generally most virulent to the host from which they were first isolated (Goettel *et al.*, 1990). Prior (1990) points out that there are some exceptions; certain strains possess high pathogenicity to previously unencountered hosts.

Fungi with wide host ranges are frequently more specific under field conditions, especially during epizootics (Goettel *et al.*, 1990). There are several reports of fungi attacking only one host even though closely related species are present. Such resistance is thought to occur as a result of the complex biotic and abiotic interactions which occur in the field. Furthermore, some insects can be infected readily in the laboratory by fungi not known to attack them naturally.

Host specificity needs much further investigation, both from the point of view of the range of arthropods infected, and from that of the biotic and abiotic factors or interactions responsible for its restriction or extension. In view of the complexities of the field situation, great caution should be exercised when attempting to extrapolate laboratory results.

Safety testing

Even though the value of laboratory results on non-target susceptibility to fungal agents is dubious as far as establishing safety in the field is concerned, most requirements for registration and even limited field experimentation require laboratory safety testing to non-target invertebrates. Such requirements usually include the honey-bee (*Apis mellifera* Linnaeus) as a test organism, but laboratory testing of entomopathogenic fungi against social insects such as the honey-bee poses unique problems. For instance, Vandenberg (1990) demonstrated that a strain of *B. bassiana* caused mycosis among honey-bees treated with very high doses of conidia, although the result was obscured by the fact that mortality was not significantly different from the control. If a pollinator species must be included in safety testing, more suitable candidates should be used. The sustained viability of caged leafcutter bees would make these bees better candidates for pollinator safety testing requirements because caged honey-bees do not survive well.

Safety of *B. bassiana* to the alfalfa leafcutter bee

The alfalfa leafcutter bee, *Megachile rotundata* (Fabricius), is used extensively in North America for pollination of seed alfalfa (*Medicago sativa*). Although no records of *B. bassiana* infecting leafcutter bees in nature have been reported (Goettel *et al.*, 1990), recently Goerzen *et al.* (1990) demonstrated that prepupae were susceptible to the fungus. Caution is therefore warranted if applications include direct exposure of bee colonies or foragers.

We tested the effects to adult leafcutter bees of *B. bassiana* applied directly onto alfalfa. The *B. bassiana* isolate used is being developed by Mycotech Corporation, Butte, MT, for control of grasshoppers (Johnson *et al.*, these proceedings). The fungus was supplied as a dry conidial preparation containing starch. Conidial viability was determined to be 60%. Three 2 l pots of flowering alfalfa cv. Beaver, were placed in each of 10 cages, 1.32 m^2. The plants in five cages were sprayed with a conidial suspension in water at a rate of 1×10^9 viable conidia per cage. This is equivalent to 1×10^{13} conidia/ha, the target application rate for grasshopper control. Uniformity of spray application was verified through the use of water sensitive paper. Twenty-five male and 15 female leafcutter bees were added to each cage 12 h after the alfalfa had been sprayed. Equivalent numbers were added to five paired cages containing unsprayed alfalfa. Mortality of the bees was monitored daily for 14 days. Samples of dead bees were surface-sterilized with 40% ethanol and held in a chamber at 100% RH and room temperature to encourage fungus growth on the cadavers. At the termination of the experiment, a census was made of a number of bees remaining in each cage, and the initial cage counts were adjusted to account for a few bees that escaped.

After 14 days, there was no female mortality and male mortality averaged 9% in the treated cages. There were no significant differences in mortality between treatment and control bees; however, all surface-sterilized cadavers from treated cages produced *B. bassiana* hyphae and conidia within three days, indicating that the bees were infected with the fungus.

Conclusions

With few exceptions, fungi are generally safe and do not pose any serious threat to higher animals. The wide host ranges of some species have caused some concern regarding safety to non-target invertebrates, and this has hindered their field testing. Current recommendations for registration include laboratory infection tests on selected non-target invertebrates including bees. However, the limitations in our knowledge of fungal specificity and how it relates to epizootiology make it impossible to extrapolate such data to the field situation. Based on present knowledge of fungal epizootiology, a better approach for ensuring long-term safety to invertebrates would be continuous monitoring during and after field application following preliminary laboratory and field safety testing. It is imperative that excessive safety and registration requirements do not hinder the development of fungal insecticides, which will be generally much safer than the chemicals used at present.

References

Aizawa, K. (1990) Registration requirements and safety considerations for microbial pest control agents in Japan. In: Laird, M., Laccy, L.A., & Davidson, E.W. (eds), *Safety of Microbial Insecticides.* CRC Press, Boca Raton, pp. 31–39.

Betz, F.S., Forsyth, S.F. & Stewart, W.E. (1990) Registration requirements and safety considerations for microbial pest control agents in North America. In: Laird, M., Lacey, L.A. & Davidson, E.W. (eds), *Safety of Microbial Insecticides.* CRC Press, Boca Raton, pp. 3–10.

Goerzen, D.W., Erlandson, M.A. & Moore, K.C. (1990) Effect of two insect viruses and two entomopathogenic fungi on larval and pupal development in the alfalfa leafcutting bee, *Megachile rotundata* (Fab.) (Hymenoptera: Megachilidae). *Canadian Entomolgist* **122**, 1039–1040.

Goettel, M.S., Poprawski, T.J., Vandenberg, J.D., Li, Z. & Roberts, D.W. (1990) Safety to nontarget invertebrates of fungal biocontrol agents. In: Laird, M., Lacey L.A. & Davidson, E.W. (eds), *Safety of Microbial Insecticides.* CRC Press, Boca Raton, pp. 209–231.

Hall, R.A., Zimmermann, G. & Vey, A. (1982) Guidelines for the registration of entomogenous fungi as insecticides. *Entomophage* **27**, 121–127.

Kandybin, N.V. & Smirnov, O.V. (1990) Registration requirements and safety considerations for microbial pest control agents in the USSR and adjacent eastern European countries. In: Laird, M., Lacey, L.A. & Davidson, E.W. (eds), *Safety of Microbial Insecticides.* CRC Press, Boca Raton, pp. 19–30.

Li, Z. (1987) A list of the insect hosts of *Beauveria bassiana.* In: *First National Symposium on Entomogenous Fungi,* Gongzhuling, Jilin, People's Republic of China.

MacLeod, D.M. (1963) Entomophthorales infections. In: Steinhaus, E.A. (ed), *Insect Pathology: an Advanced Treatise.* Academic Press, New York, pp. 189–231.

Prior, C. (1990) The biological basis for regulating the release of micro-organisms, with particular reference to the use of fungi for pest control. *Aspects of Applied Biology* **24**, 231–238.

Quinlan, R.J. (1990) Registration requirements and safety considerations for microbial pest control agents in the European Economic Community. In: Laird, M., Lacey, L.A. & Davidson, E.W. (eds), *Safety of Microbial Insecticides.* CRC Press, Boca Raton, pp. 11–18.

Saik, J.E., Lacey, L.A. & Lacey, C.M. (1990) Safety of microbial insecticides to vertebrates – domestic animals and wildlife. In: Laird, M., Lacey, L.A. & Davidson, E.W. (eds), *Safety of Microbial Insecticides.* CRC Press, Boca Raton, pp. 115–132.

Siegel, J.P. & Shadduck, J.A. (1990) Safety of microbial insecticides to vertebrates – humans. In: Laird, M., Lacey, L.A. & Davidson, E.W. (eds), *Safety of Microbial Insecticides.* CRC Press, Boca Raton, pp. 101–113.

Vandenberg, J.D. (1990) Safety of four entomopathogens for caged adult honey bees: (Hymenoptera: Apidae). *Journal of Economic Entomology* **83**, 756–759.

Vinson, S.B. (1990) Potential impact of microbial insecticides on beneficial arthropods in the terrestrial environment. In: Laird, M., Lacey, L.A. & Davidson, E.W. (eds), *Safety of Microbial Insecticides.* CRC Press, Boca Raton, pp. 43–64.

Panel discussion: precis

Dr Bateman opened the discussion by asking whether replications can be achieved repeating the same experiment in sequence. Dr Johnson replied that this could be done but that the problems lie in designing replication in time and in its analysis. Asked about statistical treatment, Dr Johnson recommended using time in the model, for example using pre-treatment counts and time as co-variates or analysing weekly time-points separately.

Dr Prior wanted to know what sort of co-variate should be used. Dr Johnson suggested the pre-treatment population density. Each co-variate only loses one degree of freedom, and age and body weight can also be used as co-variates and tested in the model.

Dr Oomen asked how we should approach the problem of testing a slow acting agent such as a fungus. Migration in and out of the plots occurs during the incubation period; how big should the plots be and can we decrease the number of replicates as we increase the plot size? Dr Johnson suggested the marking and recapture of insects to allow following the insects and said that a good understanding of the ecology of each grasshopper species is essential. Migration can be treated as a variable, always remembering that treatment may affect migration. It is essential to concentrate on the individual insects and always maintain a rigorous approach.

Dr Matteson suggested time series analysis as a substitute for replication. To do this a long period of sampling before and after treatment is required. Dr Johnson agreed that replication in time can be a valuable approach, however the method is still controversial and should not be a substitute for replication in space in our experiments. Besides the statistical problems there are also logical problems in treating time as a variable.

Dr Cardwell indicated that it was necessary to know the time x treatment interaction and that sequential analysis would not give this interaction. Dr Johnson agreed that this may be better modelled by other means since times are not randomized.

Dr Mouhim asked about the population level of grasshoppers in trials in Mali with *Beauveria bassiana* and was told that the density varied between blocks but was about 15–22 individuals/m^2, but certainly not low.

Dr Magor asked whether migration could be ascertained from GIS data and Dr Johnson said that he was trying to build this element into the model and is sure that it can be done.

Dr Auld asked Dr Keller what the concentration of skimmed milk used in his formulation was. The reply was 1%. Dr Milner asked what the spore application rate was for *Beauveria* using cereal bait at a dose of 200 kg/ha. The spore production was not known, but the dose applied was 100 kg/ha which will be reduced to 30–50 kg/ha. The spore production from each infected larva was approximately 10^9 per larva.

Dr Bateman asked Dr Lobo Lima what sort of oil had been used in Cape Verde and how it was mixed with water. Dr Lobo Lima and Dr Henry said that it was a vegetable oil produced by Mycotech (Mycotech Corporation, Butte, MT) where the emulsion was produced by shaking oil and water together, and some problems with separation were experienced.

Dr Lomer wanted to verify the plot size used and was informed that it was 0.5 ha.

Dr Prior first expressed his gratitude to Dr Nasseh for presenting the rather disappointing results for *B. bassiana* and wanted to know why it hadn't worked. Was it perhaps the temperature? Dr Nasseh indicated that they had experienced a range of temperatures from 12°C to 42°C in the desert with a humidity between 15% away from the plant and 35% next to the plant. He thought that the combination of temperature and humidity might be a factor. Dr Prior then asked if the viability of the formulation had been checked prior to usage and both Dr Nasseh and Dr Wilps indicated that it had not.

Dr Oomen asked Dr Matteson how she could judge whether possible effects found in field trials were acceptable or not. Dr Matteson's reply was that these factors were almost always political. As an example, supposing you found 50% of an important parasitoid killed by a pesticide, the problem in interpreting the effect could be, will this level of mortality cause pest resurgence or affect the crop? What losses are people willing to tolerate in exchange for the benefits of using pesticides? None of these decisions are simple.

Dr Knausenberger asked Dr Matteson whether most of the recent work had been done in recession breeding sites. Are there possibilities for several teams in different areas to support work already being done? How relevant is the work done so far for ecotoxicological studies of remote sites which are poorly known but which may be important breeding sites? Dr Matteson replied that until now the assumption made has been that we are only treating the desert so why worry? The excellent work done by PRIFAS has shown conclusively that locusts need green plants to eat and humidity in order to breed – so they need the oases and wadis and other temporary green areas. Other invertebrates and vertebrates, including birds and other predators, also come to these places, as do nomads with their herds. Insecticide applications are inevitably made at a time and place where their impact is maximized. In an environment where there are irregular rainfall and harsh conditions the native species have developed strategies against harsh conditions. In the diapause staggered batches of eggs can mature months or even years apart. It is essential to understand the biology of species in order to assess the impact of potential solutions. With large application sites and the use of aeroplanes to apply treatments, the potential for contaminating water holes or the very sensitive environment of the desert is enormous. We must also remember that the locust is important in the diet of many local animals.

Dr Bateman asked whether safety tests for mycoinsecticides should be done on a species to species basis, to which Dr Goettel replied that he thought testing should be examined case by case. The scientist should provide necessary data on strain formulation and the authorities should decide on the basis of these data. For example, conidia do not reproduce in rabbit brain – but might they not do so if in an oil based formulation? The ramifications are endless. Safety regulators themselves have to be careful, since a poor decision could influence their jobs, but one of the problems in this area is that they don't know much about pathogens.

Dr Bateman also wished to know Dr Goettel's own opinion as to how regulation should be done and he replied that in his view low risk pathogenic species can be identified in the laboratory and then closely monitored under controlled conditions over a long period in the field. If there is an indication of an effect on mammals or humans then further tests will obviously be required, but it is difficult to justify the safety testing of each strain on mammals simply because each one has a slightly different specificity from an insect species.

Dr Evans then asked whether Dr Goettel was referring to Canadian, EPA or international regulations. Dr Goettel maintained that there is turmoil in regulation everywhere. For example, in certain states in the USA there are rules about testing from EPA, APHIS and the state to fulfill. Dr Evans felt that things were not quite so gloomy and that there are indications that officials of the EPA and USDA in the USA are trying to improve testing on a species to species basis, partly in order to save money, for example, *Bacillus thuringiensis* species, the first codling moth virus from California, or the granulosis virus, are test cases in this area. Dr Goettel mentioned that the EPA has just recently insisted on the re-registration of every *B. thuringiensis* strain. Despite the fact that they have all been in use for years, they all have to be tested again using 'good laboratory practice'.

Dr Goettel asked why neem oil had been chosen to mix with the spores, and Dr Nasseh replied that as mixing *Beauveria bassiana* with mineral oil had produced no conclusive results, they tried neem oil and obtained a slight mortality.

Dr Goettel was then asked, when using commercialized spore formulations, how often one should return to the original strain in order not to lose any virulence? He replied that it depends on the fungus – some lose their virulence after two cultures and others reproduce a sub-culture for years without losing virulence. It is important to deposit useful isolates in a recognised culture collection in liquid nitrogen so that the strain is available for years to come. It may be important to consider the substrate as an important factor in affecting the virulence of a strain.

Dr Lomer took this opportunity to point out that all the field experiments which had negative results using *Beauveria bassiana* had used the Mycotech formulation which had been specifically selected for productivity and not for virulence. Dr Nasseh agreed that this was the case, but Dr Goettel pointed out that results in the laboratory had been satisfactory and perhaps the answer lay instead in further work on the host range. The session chairman, Dr Johnson, pointed out that isolates can vary in their sensitivity to ultra-violet light and this might be one of the reasons why the fungus killed in the laboratory but not in the field. Dr Nasseh added that those desert locusts in humid conditions were affected by the fungus.

Mr Fousséni added a human dimension to the discussion, saying that farmers have been battling with the locust problem for centuries and have been using insecticides for 50 years. When did the panel think that the farmer might be able to use this ecologically sound product? The chairman passed the question to Dr Goettel who felt that because the technology is so new and innovative, it is difficult to give a precise idea – it could be very soon or many years. There are so many hypotheses still to test, results must be consistent and this is not the case at the moment where products work in the laboratory but not in the field. More work is needed on UV protectants. If a heavy concentration of fungal spores is applied in the field it might affect insect parasites, parasitoids and predators which all fluctuate with the pest. Natural epizootics of microbial pathogens occur very rarely and do not occur without the right environmental conditions. If we want to take a short cut to induce an epizootic artificially we have to do more than provide sufficient infective inoculum to start the epizootic. There is a big difference between microbial control and control by parasitoids

In reply to Mr Fousséni's original question Dr Prior stated that experiments on biological control of locusts have gone from unproven theory to proven kill within the short time of 18 months and that this can be consolidated within the next 18 months. He was of the opinion that the technology should be available after a further five years and that he would be surprised if it weren't possible within that time, so maybe in seven years from now the product would be available to the farmer.

Dr Johnson referred back to Dr Goettel's comments saying that in his opinion there was more to an epizootic than the lack of spores in the right conditions since it hasn't yet proved possible to trigger an epizootic as such. Dr Goettel responded that the interaction between the environment, the biology of the insect and the inoculum was still insufficiently understood. Dr Johnson maintained that what was needed was a host for the spore population since it seemed clear that the missing element was not a release of spore mass. Dr Goettel suggested that what was being done was the use of a microbial pathogen as an insectide to induce massive mortality and that we have to iron out the problems between the laboratory and the field first. Dr Johnson felt that maybe we were trying to measure something precisely without actually knowing what that something is.

Dr Gutierrez intervened at this point to ask whether it was not probable that environmental factors affect pathogens on the plants and plant pathologists have modelled these interactions, so it might be worth surveying what has already been done. Did Dr Goettel know of any specific examples of the effect of pathogens on population dynamics of species? Usually insects, host plant and parasitoids were present at the same time, but here they were not. Dr Goettel quoted *E. grylli* as a complex example where attempts are being made to model the epizootic. Dr Gutierrez wanted to know whether it is possible to model the effects using rainfall patterns to obtain the mortality without knowing the dynamics. Would a lot of inoculum be needed? Dr Goettel wondered whether conidia need humidity and if a rapid epizootic could be induced using a specific amount of conidia, for example as in aphids.

Section VI

Closing Session

Discussion: precis

Dr Knausenberger commented that the objectives of the meeting, i.e. to discuss achievements and future objectives, have been reached, with a concrete development in the form of international links between locust and grasshopper groups and he hoped that these links will grow stronger, as there is much expertise in North America and Europe to be tapped. There should be more work on fully involving African experts and including their initiatives and interests in research. It is important to involve Africans in field trials this season as GTZ and other groups, including the IITA/IIBC/DFPV axis, are already doing. There are many people in research systems all over the Sahel who are close to the problem and the country representatives should inform their people that there is a new tool on the horizon and a specific agent to be tried out this season. It is important that they identify the colleagues who can be of most help. In talking with Mme Ba-Diallo he had already got a list of two to three people per country who should be involved as entomologists or pathologists. The key is involvement. There is a long horizon for improvement. At the moment *Metarhizium* seems to be the most promising, but other solutions will come. The potential for *Beauveria* is high and we are working on a strain enhancement in Canada and the USA. Who knows what the entomopox virus research in Cape Verde will produce? We have achieved and surpassed the purpose of the workshop and he saw this programme as a viable and continuing area of activity and this is the message he would take back to USAID. The tensions during the workshop were helpful as there was no ill-will, rather a creative tension which is helpful in debates and insights from different approaches, which is good. He hoped that everyone feels the same – it may be discouraging for those who are involved in this kind of activity for the first time. The motivation for the workshop to arrive at an alternative to chemical pesticides is definitely going in the right direction, it may take us ten years but there may also be middle ways – the home cottage industry for example, as with producing neem, maybe local production of *Beauveria* and *Metarhizium* with bran using appropriate technology to involve the creativity of the individual. We should maintain this decentralized activity, spread knowledge and wealth and put it in the hands of the people who can then find their own solution to the problem.

Dr Henry presented some ideas on training. In order to help the evaluation of microbial pathogens of grasshoppers and other insects, a course in insect pathology is proposed which would concentrate on grasshoppers and locusts and would be a three month intensive course.

It could either be held at Montana State University or in collaboration with IIBC/IITA in Benin. The obvious advantage to holding the course in Benin is that it would be less expensive, while Montana has a well established grasshopper laboratory with a staff of 11 scientists, five of whom are grasshopper pathologists. There is also extensive literature available.

Candidates should be of university level with a BSc or equivalent and the course would be taught in French and English for African and Asian participants.

Syllabus:

1. microscopy including electron microscopy
2. histology
3. abiotic diseases
4. biotic diseases
   — bacteria
   — fungi
   — viruses
   — protozoa
5. disease epizootiology
   — natural
   — applied
6. bioassay protocol
   — laboratory
   — field – plot design
7. reporting results.

If there is enough interest a formal programme will be developed and the necessary funds sought.

Dr Smit asked whether Dr Henry thought that people educated in the techniques for experiments and trials would be able to do the experiments themselves. What about the great need for equipment? Dr Henry agreed that there was a real problem regarding equipment in many locations, but that for isolating and characterizing most microbial pathogens all that was needed was a good compound microscope. His intention was not to make instant experts, but to inform and communicate. Dr Smit stated that in the experience of DFPV in training field and laboratory technicians with a medium level of education, it is necessary to train them well, even though they are not graduates, as they are the backbone of much authoritative work in the difficult discipline of crop protection. Dr Henry agreed that technicians are important but suggested that this was not an appropriate level for Montana State University and that it might be better handled at local level. He also maintained that another benefit to training at a higher level was that the trainees can then train or help to train technicians themselves.

Dr Lomer wanted to put on record that insect pathology is not difficult and that any entomologist at the end of two months of microscope training should know enough pathology to do field experiments.

Dr Bani wanted the meeting to think very carefully about the African context, given that most African countries are poor and it is important that the training be given to those who will benefit most and can then pass on that benefit. For example, at the end of secondary level schooling in the Congo a student knows nothing about microscopes, fungi or viruses and would not be able to cope with training at the level described by Dr Henry, which would then not have the desired impact. It is better to train someone who has the right background and who can then explain and pass on his training to others.

Mr Maiga agreed with Dr Bani and Dr Henry, saying that the problem in Africa was that there are many entomologists but no phytopathologists or entomopathologists and that Africans have been saying this for a long time. We are looking for some ideas to help our people. Another delegate said that the training service of the plant protection services was the only way to perpetuate the work on biological control.

Mr Wodageneh said that all training is important and that it should be given priority. One of the most important aspects is the proper selection of candidates for training – and this must be done by consultation with officials at national level and by interviews with potential candidates. In this way officials value the training and we get the proper candidates. By building up this trust with officials we have a high success rate in retaining trainees in the jobs for which they were trained – 80% are still in place after 6–7 years. The level of education must be carefully screened – many people of a relatively low level of education make excellent field workers and technicians given the proper training, but there must also be appropriate training available to those with a higher level of education. We need to train more assistants than leaders. With some knowledge of entomology and pathology and an elementary knowledge of how to use a microscope the students can, with a little training use their sound basis to get a programme started.

Dr Herren agreed that it is essential to train at both technical and academic levels and said that in his view extension and research go hand in hand. He said that we need help from the national representatives because this is a new area for Africa and all levels of training are needed. We must start with academic training so that these people, once trained, can go home and teach or do research in their own right.

Dr Smit reiterated that DFPV train technicians for nine Sahelian countries and they have sent questionnaires out to these countries to try to assess the training needs. They find that they are getting fewer and fewer candidates for training and need to know why this is. By July they will hopefully have analysed the questionnaires. He emphasized that training technicians is important since you soon get enough high level people – but of course, both are important.

Mr Gallédou said that little had been heard about biological control by insect predators of grasshoppers. These are important, and there are interesting studies of egg pod parasites, for example. Might there also be other possibilities for biological control of other pests such as the mealybug of date palm? He mentioned that he was pleased to have come to the workshop and was delighted with what he had heard, as he regards the use of chemical insecticides as an attack on traditional lifestyles. Biological control of locusts could improve the farmer's lot and it would be a good thing to associate the farmer with such control measures. On the whole it was a better outlook for the environment.

Mr Hammond said that when trying to build a biological control capacity in Africa, we must be careful to use an integrated pest control approach. The technicians should only have a short training since they are not the people who will make research decisions. Technicians have other functions, are not specialized and often may not even be available to do the work they have been trained for. There should be an emphasis on training people with a basic university education to do a specific job. They should be able to handle biological control including parasites and microbial pathogens. Not all the available money for training should be spent on training technicians.

Dr Lomer affirmed that support was needed from the top to advance this type of research.

Dr Mushi remarked that plant protection experts were in short supply, and there are no experts in biological control. His experience suggests that short courses can be useful for technicians. To make a breakthrough in this field we need people who can influence the policy makers. Co-operation between the USA, Europe and Africans can convince donors. At this stage he requested that funds be made available to implement training recommendations. The first priority is high level manpower development and the second is the training of technicians for once they are trained they can, in turn, train local staff.

An American delegate said that we must work with the existing institutions at both levels. Advanced methodology in insect pathology can be given to Africans – as an example to strengthen the existing ICIPE programme through collaboration.

Mr Saizonou recommended training specialists in biological control and ecology along with technicians who will be in contact with the farmers. He recommended a programme which would include both extension and research aspects.

Dr Nkouka supported Dr Herren and Mr Wodageneh, saying that an army cannot function with only soldiers or only generals. There are important human resources in Africa involved in the national programmes and they should be clearly identified. There are many people working in national programmes who are not in the right places. Everyone wants to go on a course and when they return, many want to do everything except that which they learnt on the course. It is essential that the managers of national programmes go and look at their people and give their opinions of what is needed. It is often the case that the people who go to scientific conferences are not scientists but administrators who cannot properly benefit by the experience. Africa does not start from zero in this matter for there are many laboratories at national institutes of agronomy and in universities. We must look at the human resources – some university lecturers may know about microbiology. We are not about to remake the world but must reinforce what already exists. If it is necessary then we can send people abroad, but it does not matter where the basic techniques are acquired as long as they are learned and used. The research and techniques should be placed in their work situation and therefore in Africa. We must check what is already available.

Dr Lomer agreed that it was essential to identify available resources and this was supported by Dr Knausenberger who suggested an inventory of manpower such as DFPV already does for the Sahel. He went on to say that he looked to all the participants from UNDP, FAO, and IITA, for advice in this area. The exchanges had been very valuable in discussing the kind of training needed and the kind of people to train and he suggested setting up a committee to assess the training question. He noted the efforts in this area of PRIFAS, IITA, and DFPV, and the strong presence of the GTZ programme in Africa. There are many experts in biological control using pathogens and there is a network already involved in training – Dr Smit, Mr Wodageneh and others, who should meet and come up with a strategy.

Dr Herren recommended that Dr Nkouka be involved since FAO sponsor IITA's training UNDP/FAO programme. The consensus was that Drs Smit, Nkouka, Lomer and Wodageneh should meet within the next few days to devise a strategy with which to tackle the extensive research, technical and academic training needed, taking into account what is already available.

Dr Lomer thanked the interpreters Claire Lord, Oscar Hounvou, and Carol Moudachirou, the administrative staff, especially Jacob Quaye, Samson Nyampong, and Leo Sossou, and the drivers, for their help in running the workshop.

Dr Roberts concluded the meeting by thanking Dr Lomer and his wife for their part in organizing the workshop, despite their having been in Benin for only three months.

Acronyms and abbreviations

a.i.	active ingredient
ADV	average droplet volume
AGRHYMET	Agronomie Hydrologie Météorologie (CILSS)
AKH	adipokinetic hormones
ALRC	Anti-Locust Research Centre
APHIS	Animal and Plant Health Inspection Service (USDA)
ARSEF	Agricultural Research Service Collection of Entomopathogenic Fungi (USDA)
BBA	Biologische Bundesanstalt für Land- und Forstwirtschaft
BCP	Biological Control Programme (IITA)
CABI	CAB International
cc	corpora cardiaca
CDA	controlled doplet application
CEC	Commission of European Communities
CG	Management Committee (DFPV)
CHEF	contour-clamped homogeneous electric field
CIDA	Canadian International Development Agency
CILBA	Complexe International de Lutte Biologique Agropolis
CILSS	Comité Inter-Etats pour la Lutte contre la Sécheresse dans le Sahel
CINA	Centre National de Lutte Antiacridienne
CIRAD	Centre de Coopération Internationale en Recherche Agronomique pour le Développement
CNLA	Centre National de Lutte Anti-acridienne (Morocco)

CNRS	Centre National de la Recherche Scientifique (Montpellier)
COPR	Centre for Overseas Pest Research (UK)
CSIRO	Commonwealth Scientific and Industrial Research Organization (Australia)
CSP	Scientific and Pedagogical Committee (DFPV)
DFPV	Département pour la Formation en Protection des Végétaux
DGIS	Netherlands Directorate General for International Cooperation
DLCOEA	Desert Locust Control Organization for Eastern Africa
DPP	Directorate for Plant Protection (Senegal)
DTX	destruxins
EC	emulsifiable concentrate
EDTA	ethylenediaminetetra-acetic acid
ENSAM	Ecole Nationale Supérieure d'Agronomie de Montpellier
EPA	Environmental Protection Agency
FAO	Food and Agriculture Organization (United Nations)
GERDAT	Département de Gestion, Recherche, Documentation et Appui Technique
GHIPM	Grasshopper Integrated Pest Management
GTZ	Gesellschaft für Technische Zusammenarbeit (Germany)
HAN	heavy aromatic naphtha
I.U.	international unit
IAPSC	Inter-African Phytosanitary Council (OAU)
ICIPE	International Centre of Insect Physiology and Ecology (Kenya)
ICTZ	Inter-Tropical Convergence Zone
IGR	Insect Growth Regulator
IIBC	International Institute of Biological Control
IITA	International Institute of Tropical Agriculture
IMI	International Mycological Institute
INIA	National Institute for Agricultural Research (Cape Verde)
INRA	Institut National de la Recherche Agronomique
INSAH	Sahelian Institute (Bamako)
IPARC	International Pesticide Application Research Centre (Imperial College of Science, Technology and Medicine, London)
IPDR	Institute for Practical Rural Development (Niger)
IRLCOCSA	International Red Locust Control Organization for Central and Southern Africa

LD	lethal dose
LGBCP	Locust and Grasshopper Biological Control Programme
MPV	*Melanolpus* entomopoxvirus
NDVI	Normalized Difference Vegetation Index
NPV	nuclear polyhedrosis virus
NRI	Natural Resources Institute (ODA)
OAU	Organization for African Unity
OCLALAV	Office Centrale pour la Lutte Anti-acridienne et Anti-avaire
ODA	Overseas Development Administration (UK)
OPV	*Oedaleus* entomopoxvirus
ORSTOM	Office de la Recherche Scientifique et Technique Outre-Mer
OTA	Office of Technology Assessment (US Congress)
PAGE	polyacrimide gel electrophoresis
PCR	polymerase chain reaction
PFGE	pulsed field gel electrophoresis
PIB	polyhedral inclusion body
PPS	Plant Protection Service (Mali)
PRIFAS	Acridologie Opérationnelle - Ecoforce Internationale Programme de Recherche Interdisciplinaire Français sur les Acridiens du Sahel
PVP	polyvinyl pyrolidine
RAPD	randomly amplified polymorphic DNA
RESADOC	Sahelian Documentation Network (INSAH)
RFLP	restriction fragment length polymorphism
SAS	Surveillance des Acridiens du Sahel
SDAYE	Sabouraud's dextrose agar with yeast extract
SDS	sodium dodecyl sulphate
SNPV	Service Nationale de la Protection des Végétaux
SPC	Surveillance des Pathogènes des Criquets (DFPV)
TDRI	Tropical Development Research Centre
TRAIS	Tropical Agriculture Information Service (NRI)
TSPV	Training Course for Crop Protection Technicians (DFPV)
ULV	ultra-low volume
UNDP	United Nations Development Programme
USAID	United States Agency for International Development
USDA	United States Department of Agriculture
UV	ultra-violet
VAD	volume average diameter
VMD	volume mean diameter

Addresses of delegates

Mr A. Ali Abdalla
c/o Dr W.G. Mohamed
Head of Locust and Grasshopper
Control Unit
Plant Protection Department
PO Box 8192 Elamarat
Knartoum
Sudan
Tlx: 240565 GTZ

Mr L. de Abreu
Crop Protection Service
c/o USDA-APHIS
Guinea-Bissau

Dr J.B. Ackonor
Entomology Division
Cocoa Research Institute
Private Mail Bag
Kotoka International Airport
Accra
Ghana

Dr N. Aho
Directeur Général Adjoint
Centre Béninois de Recherche
Scientifique et Technique
BP 03-1665
Cotonou
Bénin
Tel: (229) 32 21 63

Ms G.O. Akpokodje
Department of Agricultural Biology
University of Ibadan
Oyo State
Nigeria

Dr B.A. Auld
Agriculture Research and Veterinary
Centre
Forest Road
Orange 2800
New South Wales
Australia
Fax: (61) 63 636799
Tel: (61) 63 636700

Dr D. Ba-Diallo
CILSS-INSAH-UCTR/PV
BP 1530
Bamako
Mali
Fax: (227) 73 33 37
Tel: (227) 73 21 81
Tlx: 55 45 DFPVNI

Dr J.W. Bahana
International Red Locust Control
Organisation for Central and Southern
Africa
PO Box 240252
Ndola

Zambia
Tel: (260) 2 614584/5; 615684
Tlx: ZA 30072

Dr G. Bani
Direction Générale de la Recherche Scientifique
BP 2499 Brazzaville
Congo

Prof. S. El Bashir
ICIPE
PO Box 30772
Nairobi
Kenya
Fax: (254) 2 80 33 60
Tel: (254) 2 80 25 01/3/9
Tlx: 22053/25066

Dr R.P. Bateman
International Institute of Biological Control
Silwood Park
Buckhurst Road
Ascot
Berks SL5 7TA
UK
Fax: (44) 344 872901
Tel: (44) 344 87299
Tlx: 93121022555

Mr E. Baumann
Ciba-Geigy
Agriculture Division
AG 714
CH-4002 Basel
Switzerland
Tel: (41) 61 697 71 60
Fax: (41) 61 697 39 70
Tlx: 926 355 CG CH

Mr M. Baumgart
Projet Neem GTZ
Institut für Phytophathologie und angewandte Zoologie
Universität Giessen
Ludwigstrasse 23
6300 Giessen
Germany
Tel: (49) 641 74596
Fax: (49) 641 74596

Mr J. Brito
CX Postal 128
Praia
Cabo Verde Islands
Fax: c/o (238) 612020
Tel: (238) 61570

Dr K. Cardwell
International Institute of Tropical Agriculture
Oyo Road
PMB 5320 Ibadan
Nigeria
Fax: (234) 611896/(229) 301466
Tlx: 31417

Dr C.W. Castleton
Area Director
USDA-APHIS
L'Ambassade des Etats Unis
BP 1712 Abidjan
Côte d'Ivoire 01
Fax: (225) 22 32 59
Tel: (225) 21 09 79
Tlx: 23660 AMEMBCI

Dr A.K. Charnley
School of Biological Sciences
University of Bath
Claverton Down
Bath
Avon BA2 7AY
UK
Fax: (44) 225 826779
Tel: (44) 225 826826
Tlx: 449097

Dr J. Clarkson
School of Biological Sciences
University of Bath
Claverton Down
Bath
Avon BA2 7AY
UK
Fax: (44) 225 826779
Tel: (44) 225 826826
Tlx: 449097

Mr A. Coffi
Chef, Division Protection des Végétaux
BP 648
Cotonou
Bénin

Dr G.L. Cunningham
USDA APHIS-PPQ
Grasshopper IPM Project
3380 Americana Terrace
Boise
Idaho 8370
USA
Fax: 208 384 3920
Tel: 208 334 9644

Prof. V. Delucchi
ETH
Institut für Pflanzenwissenschaften
Bereich Phytomedizin
Clausiusstrasse 21
8092 Zurich
Switzerland
Fax: (41) 262 2546
Tel: (41) 256 22 11/256 39 30

Dr J.S. Evans
1034 Spring Drive
Boulder
Colorado 80303
USA
Fax: (1) 303 673 0133
Tel: (1) 403 499 1413
Tlx: 023 40 18928

Mr A. Fousséni
Direction du Service de la Protection des Végétaux
BP 1263
Cacavali, Lomé
Togo

Dr. H. Franzen
ATSAF
German Council for Tropical and Subtropical Agricultural Research
Hans Böckler Strasse 5
D-5300 Bonn 3
Germany
Fax: (49) 228 4001 311

Dr K.S. Fischer
DDG Research
International Institute of Tropical Agriculture
Oyo Road
PMB 5320 Ibadan
Nigeria
Fax: (234) 611896/ (229) 301466
Tlx: 31417

Mr le Gall
ORSTOM
Brazzaville
Congo

Mr T. Galledou
Bureau OASIS/DA
BP 180 Nouakchott
Mauritania
Tel: 54769
Tlx: 5867 MTN

Mr S. Ganbobo
Directeur de la Protection des Végétaux
Minstere de l'Agriculture
BP 323
Niamey
Niger

Dr L. van der Geest
Department of Pure & Applied Biology
University of Amsterdam
Kruislaan 302
1098 SM Amsterdam
Netherlands
Fax: (31) 205 257754
Tel: (31) 205 257740
Tlx: 16460

Mr S. Glodjinon
Ciba-Geigy Services S.A.
BP 8123
Cotonou
Bénin

Dr M. Goettel
Agriculture Canada
Lethbridge Research Station
P.O. Box 3000 Main
Lethbridge
Alberta T1J 4B1
Canada
Fax: (1) 403 382 3156
Tel: (1) 403 327 4561

Dr D.J. Greathead
International Institute of Biological Control
Silwood Park
Buckhurst Road

Ascot
Berks SL5 7TA
UK
Fax: (44) 344 872901
Tel: (44) 344 872999
Tlx: 93121022555

Dr D. Greenland
CAB International
Wallingford
Oxon OX10 8DE
UK
Fax: (44) 491 33508
Tel: (44) 491 32111
Tlx: 847964

Prof. A.P. Gutierrez
Division of Biological Control
University of California, Berkeley
1050 San Pablo Avenue
Albany CA 94706
USA
Fax: (1) 415 642 08 75
Tel: (1) 415 642 71 91
Tlx: 910 366 7114

Mr J. Gwinner
GTZ/MGBPP
PO Box 49
Muzuzu
Malawi
Fax: 332 396
Tlx: 0222

Dr W.N.O. Hammond
West and Central Africa Regional Coordinator
IITA Biological Control Programme
Biological Control Centre for Africa
BP 08 0932
Bénin
Fax: (229) 301466
Tel: (229) 301994/360188
Tlx: 5329 Itaben

Ms K. Hell
Service Protection des Végétaux
DAGRI BP 58
Porto Novo
Bénin
Tel: (229) 21 32 90/93

Dr J.E. Henry
Montana State University
USDA Rangeland
Bozeman, MT 59717
USA
Fax: (1) 406 9946462

Dr H.R. Herren
Programme Director
IITA Biological Control Programme
Biological Control Centre for Africa
BP 08-0932 Cotonou
Bénin
Fax: (229) 301466
Tel: (229) 301994/360188
Tlx: 5329 Itaben

Son Excellence M.P. Houtoundji
Ministre de l'Education
BP 348 Cotonou
Bénin
Tel: (229) 31 06 81/19 91/16 93

Dr D.L. Johnson
Agriculture Canada
Lethbridge Research Station
P.O. Box 3000 Main
Lethbridge
Alberta T1J 4B1
Canada
Fax: 403 382 3156
Tel: 403 327 4561

Dr K. Jones
ODA Natural Resources Institute
Central Avenue
Chatham Maritime
Chatham
Kent ME4 4TB
UK
Fax: (44) 634 880066/77
Tlx: 263907/8

Dr S. Keller
Federal Research Station for Agronomy
Postfach 8046
Zürich
Switzerland
Fax: (41) 3777 201
Tel: (41) 3777 111

Captain R.A. Kitenda
Director for Operations
DLCO-EA
PO Box 30023
Nairobi
Kenya
Fax: (254) 2 50 51 37
Tel: (254) 505517

Dr W. Knausenberger
US Agency for International Development
Africa Bureau AFR/TR/ANR
Washington, DC 20523–1515
USA
Fax: (1) 703 235 3805
Tel: (1) 703 235 3826

Mr A. Kogo-Salaou
GTZ Service d'Administration des Projets
BP 10814
Niamey
Niger
Fax: (227) 73 26 29
Tel: (227) 72 25 51
Tlx: 5410 GTZ Ni

Mr S. Koné
Sockim / Ciba-Geiby
Division Agriculture
BP Abidjan
Côte d'Ivoire 01
Fax: (225) 35 08 00
Tel: (225) 35 56 25
Tlx: 43215

Ir C. Kooyman
DFPV
BP 12625
Niamey
Niger
Fax: (227) 73 22 37
Tel: (227) 73 21 81
Tlx: 5545 DFPVNI

Mr S. Krall
Plant Protection & International Agricultural Research
GTZ, Dag-Hammarskjöld-Weg 1–2
BP 5180
D-6236 Eschborn 1
Germany
Fax: (49) 6196 797150- 791115
Tlx: 4075010

Mr. J. Langewald
IITA Biological Control Programme
Biological Control Centre for Africa
BP 08 0932
Cotonou
Bénin
Fax: (229) 30 14 66
Tel: (229) 30 19 94/30 14 66
Tlx: 5329 Itaben

Dr M.H. Launois-Luong
CIRAD-PRIFAS
BP 5035
Avenue du Val de Montferrand
34032 Montpellier Cedex 1
France
Fax: (33) 67 41 09 58
Tel: (33) 67 61 58 00
Tlx: 480762F

Mr C. Lawani
Chef Service Protection des Végétaux
DAGRI B.P. 58
Porto Novo
Bénin

Dr M.L. Lobo Lima
President of INIA
CX Postal 128
Praia
Cape Verde Islands
Tel: (238) 61570
Fax: c/o (238) 612020

Dr C.J. Lomer
IIBC/IITA-BCP Locust Project
IITA Biological Control Programme
Biological Control Centre for Africa
BP 08 0932 Cotonou
Bénin
Fax: (229) 301466
Tel: (229) 301994/360188
Tlx: 5329 Itaben

Mr W. Luhanga
Lunyangwa Research Station
PO Box 59
Muzuzu
Malawi
Fax: 332396
Tlx: 0222

Dr J.I. Magor
Natural Resources Institute
Central Avenue
Chatham Maritime
Chatham
Kent ME4 4TB
UK
Fax: (44) 634 880066/77
Tlx: 263907/8 LDNG mark
attn Magor at NRI
Tel: 0634 883270

Mr B. Maiga
Service de la Protection des Végétaux
BP 1560
Bamako
Mali

Dr P. Matteson
Department of Entomology
Iowa State University
Ames
Iowa 50011–3140
USA
Fax: (515) 294 8027
Tel: (515) 294 4916

Dr G.A. Matthews
Director, IPARC
Imperial College of Science, Medicine & Technology
Silwood Park
Buckhurst Road
Ascot
Berkshire SL5 7TA
UK
Fax: (44) 344 294450/294339
Tel: (44) 344 23911
Tlx: 929484

Mr A.L. Mbiele
Secrétaire Scientifique
Conseil Phytosanitaire Interafricain
OUA
BP 4170 Nlongkak
Yaoundé
Cameroun
Tel: (237) 22 25 28
Tlx: 8460

Mr A. Meier
Ciba-Geigy
Agriculture Division
CH-4002 Basle
Switzerland
Tel: (41) 61 697 71 60
Fax: (41) 61 697 39 70
Tlx: 926 355 CG CH

Dr A. Mendonça
UFAL Campus Rio Largo
Caixa Postal 672
57001 Maceio, Al
Brazil
Fax: (55) 82 221 7876
Tlx: (55) 82 157 XPMCB BR

Dr R. Milner
CSIRO
Division of Entomology
PO Box 1700
Canberra ACT 2601
Australia
Fax: (61) 6 246 4000
Tel: (61) 6 246 4911
Tlx: AA 62309

Dr D. Moore
International Institute of Biological Control
Silwood Park
Buckhurst Road
Ascot
Berks SL5 7TA
UK
Fax: (44) 344 872901
Tel: (44) 344 872999
Tlx: 93121022555

Mr A. Mouhim
Centre National de la Lutte Anti-Acridienne
BP 125 Inezgane
Morocco
Fax: (212) 83 05 70
Tel: (212) 83 12 21/83 16 76
Tlx: 81741

Mr A. Mushi
Assistant Commissioner
Plant Protection Services
Ministry of Agriculture & Livestock Development

PO Box 9071
Dar es Salaam
Fax: (255) 51 38 428

Dr O.M. Nasseh
Plant Protection & International
Agricultural Research
GTZ, Dag-Hammarskjöld-Weg 1–2
BP 5180
D-6236 Eschborn 1
Germany
Fax: (49) 6196 797150/791115
Tel: (49) 6196 790
Tlx: 4075010

Mr A.B. Ndiaye
OCLALAV
BP 1066
Dakar
Sénégal
Fax: (221) 32 04 87
Tel: (221) 32 34 79/32 80
Tlx: 61 238 OLA

Dr P. Neuenschwander
IITA Biological Control Programme
Biological Control Centre for Africa
BP 08-0932 Cotonou
Bénin
Fax: (229) 301466
Tel: (229) 301994/360188
Tlx: 5329 Itaben

Mr A. Niassy
Chef du Laboratoire d'Entomologie
Direction de la Protection des
Végétaux
BP 20054 Thiaroye
Dakar
Sénégal
Fax: (221) 34 42 90
Tel: (221) 34 42 94

Dr N. Nkouka
OUA/ISTRC
Conseil Phytosanitaire Interafricain
BP 4170 Nlongkak
Yaoundé
Cameroun
Tel: (237) 20 25 28
Tlx: 8460 KN

Dr P.A. Oomen
Plant Protection Service
PO Box 9102
6700 HC Wageningen
Netherlands
Fax: (31) 8370 21701
Tlx: 45163 PD NL

Dr A. Paraïso
Locust Project
IITA Biological Control Programme
Biological Control Centre for Africa
BP 08-0932 Cotonou
Bénin
Fax: (229) 301466
Tel: (229) 301994/360188
Tlx: 5329 Itaben

His Excellency W.M. Pridun
Ambassador of Austria
Embassy of Austria
Olosa Street
Victoria Island
Lagos
Nigeria
Tlx: 21463 OENIGNG

Dr W.J. Primeau
Anglophone Africa Branch
CIDA
Promenade du Portage
Hull
Quebec
Canada K1A 0G4
Fax: (1) 403 819 953 6379
Tel: (1) 403 819 997 0984
Tlx: 053 4140

Dr C. Prior
International Institute of Biological
Control
Silwood Park
Buckhurst Road
Ascot
Berks SL5 7TA
UK
Fax: (44) 344 872901
Tel: (44) 344 872999
Tlx: 93121022555

Dr S.K. Raina
ICIPE

PO Box 30772
Nairobi
Kenya
Fax: (254) 2 80 33 60
Tel: (254) 2 80 25 01/3/9
Tlx: 22053/25066

Dr D. Roberts
Insect Pathology Resource Center
Boyce Thompson Institute for Plant Research
Cornell University
Tower Road
Ithaca
New York 14853–1801
USA
Fax: (1) 607 254 1242
Tel: (1) 607 254 1352

Mr S. Saizonou
Service Protection des Végétaux
DAGRI BP 58
Porto Novo
Bénin

Mr S. Sanyang
Department of Agricultural Services
Yundum Agricultural Station
Ministry of Agriculture
The Gambia
Tel: 82758/95420/95377

Mr E. Sayoum
International Institute of Biological Control
Silwood Park
Buckhurst Road
Ascot
Berks SL5 7TA
UK
Fax: (44) 344 872901
Tel: (44) 344 872999
Tlx: 93121022555

Dr F. Schulleri
BP 1073
Porto Novo
Bénin

Mr P. Shah
International Institute of Biological Control
Silwood Park
Buckhurst Road
Ascot
Berks SL5 7TA
UK
Fax: (44) 344 872901
Tel: (44) 344 872999
Tlx: 93121022555

Mr R. da Silva
PNUD
Cotonou
Bénin
Tel: (229) 32 30 45/46/79

Ir J.J. Smit
DFPV
BP 12625
Niamey
Niger
Fax: (227) 73 22 37
Tel: (227) 73 21 81
Tlx: 55 45 DFPVNI

Mr G. Stachel
Ministry of Foreign Affairs
Austrian Development Copperation
Ballhausplatz 3
A-1014 Vienna
Austria
Fax: (43) 222 5354530
Tel: (43) 222 9370295

Dr W.M. Steele
International Institute of Biological Control
Silwood Park
Buckhurst Road
Ascot
Berks SL5 7TA
UK
Fax: (44) 344 872901
Tel: (44) 344 872999
Tlx: 93121022555

Dr D. Streett
USDA/ARS
Montana State University
Rangeland Insect Laboratory
Bozeman MT 59717
USA
Fax: (1) 406 9946462

Dr L. White
Africa International Service
USDA-APHIS
American Embassy
BP 1712 Abidjan
Côte d'Ivoire 01
Fax: (225) 21 32 59

Dr H. Wilps
Forstzoologisches Institut
Universität Freiburg
D-7800 Freiburg
Germany
Fax: (49) 761 203 2496
Tel: (49) 761 203 2496

Dr A. Wodageneh
FAO/BCP Principal Training Officer
IITA Biological Control Programme
Biological Control Centre for Africa
BP 08 0932 Cotonou
Bénin
Fax: (229) 30 14 66
Tel: (229) 30 19 94/35 01 88
Tlx: 5329 Itaben

Dr B. Zelazny
Institute for Biological Pest Control
Biologische Bundesanstalt
Heinrichstrasse 243
D-6100 Darmstadt
Germany
Fax: (49) 6151 42 25 02
Tel: (49) 6151 44061

Dr M. Zweigert
GTZ/BCP Regional Coordinator
IITA Biological Control Programme
Biological Control Centre for Africa
BP 08 0932 Cotonou
Bénin
Fax: (229) 30 14 66
Tel: (229) 30 19 94/36 01 88
Tlx: 5329 Itaben

Author index

Abdalla, A. 97
Auld, B.A. 219
Bahana, J.W. 57
Bani, G. 79
Bateman, R.P. 249, 255
Brader, L. ix
Bradley, C. 296
Brito, J.M. 287
Byaruhanga, E.K. 57
Charnley, A.K. 181
Clarkson, J.M. 191
Coffi, A. 86
Cunningham, G.L. 21
Freres, T. 311
Godonou, I. 133, 237
Goettel, M.S. 122, 230, 296, 356
Greathead, D.J. 4, 105
Henry, J.E. 287
Herren, H.R. 8
Johnson, D.L. 267, 296, 356
Keller, S. 279
Kirkilionis, E. 311
Kitenda, K.R.A. 41
Kooyman, C. 8, 208
Kpindu, D. 133, 255
Krall, S. 44, 311, 337
Langewald, J. 142
Launois-Luong, M.H. 75
Lobo Lima, M.L. 287
Lomer, C.J. 8, 133, 255
Magor, J.I. 64
Maiga, B. 82, 296
Matteson, P.C. 347
Matthews, G.A. 245
Mendonça, A.F. 239
Milner, R.J. 200
Mouhim, A. 38
Nasseh, O. 44, 311, 337
Ndiaye, A.B. 70
Niassy, A. 91
Nkouka, N. 50
Paraïso, A. 8, 133, 255
Peveling, R. 321
Prior, C. 8, 159
Raina, S.K. 54
Roberts, D.W. 230
Schmutterer, H. 142
Shah, P. 208
Smit, J.J. 8, 30
van der Paauw, H. 296
Weyrich. J. 321
Wilps, H. 311, 337
Zelazny, B. 26

Subject index

Acacia spp. 313
Acanthacris ruficornis 91
Acanthodactylus boscianus 324
Acemyia spp. 113
Acorypha glaucopsis 303
Acorypha spp. 91
Acrida bicolor 303
Acridomyia spp. 114
Acrotylus humbertianus 165
acylurea insecticides 181
Adelphocoris lineolatus 170
adipokinetic hormones 337, 339
    see also AKH
Adoryphus couloni 163
Aeneolamia saccharina 165
Aeneolamia varia 165
Aeneolamia sp. 166
Aerobacter aerogenes 115
Aerva javanica 313, 324
Ageneotettix deorum 272
Aiolopus simulatrix 83, 91, 93
AKH 337, 342, 344, 345
    see also adipokinetic hormones
Alcimus sp. 62
alfalfa leafcutter bee 358
Alternaria cassiae 223
Anabrus simplex 24
Anacardium occidentale 91
Anacridium melanorhodon 67, 97
Anacridium wernerellum 313, 315, 316, 318
Anastoechus 109
Anisoptera spp. 62
Anticarsia gemmatalis 187
Antitrogus mussoni 205
Antitrogus parvulus 205
ants 108
aphids 220
Aphis gossypii 235
Apis mellifera 351, 358
    see also honey-bees
APIZYM test system 169
application 234–235, 243
appressorium formation 181
Aristida sp. 324
Aschersonia aleyrodis 186
Ascochyta fabae 174
Asilidae 110
Aspergillus flavus 37, 173
Aspergillus nidulans 125, 191, 192, 193
Aspergillus ochraceus 232
Aspergillus sp. 125
Austracris guttulosa 12, 165, 166
Azadirachta indica 48, 72, 143, 312, 323
    see also neem
azadirachtin 72, 142, 143, 321, 324, 337, 339, 342, 343

B.t. 200
Bacillus cereus 295
Bacillus thuringiensis 71, 115, 167, 200, 223, 224, 231, 364
Bacillus thuringiensis HD1 201

Bacillus thuringiensis var. *israelensis* 201
Bacillus thuringiensis var. *tenebrionis* 201
Bacillus sp. 295
bacteria 10, 15, 28, 29, 47, 67, 72, 109, 115, 134
baculoviruses 10, 247
Beauveria 208, 263, 369, 370
Beauveria as anamorph 174
Beauveria conidia 250
Beauveria conidiophore suspensions 249
Beauveria isolates 18
Beauveria bassiana 11, 24, 49, 122, 125, 125–127, 133, 138, 166, 169, 170, 174, 176, 193, 194, 195, 222, 225, 226, 232, 233, 234, 235, 268, 276, 284, 287, 288–291, 296–309, 311, 312, 314, 317, 318, 319, 321, 323, 324, 325, 327, 329, 330, 331, 332, 333, 334, 335, 357, 359, 363, 365
Beauveria bassiana isolates 137, 140, 162
Beauveria brongniartii 172, 279–285
Beauveria spp. 9, 10, 11, 12, 13, 62, 116, 160, 161, 167, 168, 171, 172, 174, 176, 191, 192, 285
Beauveria spp. isolates 163, 164, 166, 209, 210
bendiocarb 251
benomyl resistance 125, 192
bioassay, field technique 255–261
biological control 24, 41, 42, 43, 44, 61, 70–73, 75, 94–95, 117–118, 163
birds 62, 72, 112, 352
Blaesoxipha filipjevi 113, 117, 133, 135, 137, 138, 139, 140, 155
Blaesoxipha lineata 113
Blaesoxipha spp. 107, 113, 114
Blaps bifurcata mirei 324, 326
Bombyliidae 109
Bombyx mori 176
Boverin 166
Brevicoryne brassicae 319
Brontispa longissima 165
brown necked raven 324

Calliphora vomitoria 184, 185
Calliphoridae 109
Calliptamus italicus 27
Camnula pellucida 127, 272
Carabidae 110
carbaryl 40, 87, 93, 94, 251
cashew 91
cassava 79, 80, 86, 88
Cassia obtusifolia 223
Cataloipus cymbiferus 77, 83, 91, 94, 303, 304
Cataloipus fuscocoeruleipes 83, 87
CAV see crystalline array virus
CDA 11, 18
see also controlled droplet application
Ceracia nomadacris 62, 114
Ceracia spp. 113
Chalcodermus bimaculatus 166
chemical pesticides 118
chlorpyrifos 93, 94, 95, 118, 251
Chortoicetes terminifera 105, 106, 111, 117
Chromolaena odorata 48
chymoelastase 165, 166
Citrullus colocynthis 313, 324
citrus 80
Citrus spp. 80
citrus root weevils 126
clear-winged grasshopper see *Camnula pellucida*
Coccobacillus acridiorum 115
Cochliobolus carbonarum 193
cocoa 80
codling moth virus 364
Coffea spp. 80
coffee 80
coffee berry borer 169
see also *Hypothenemus hampei*
Collego 220
Colorado potato beetle 312
see also *Leptinotarsa decemlineata*
conidia production 298
controlled droplet application 11, 249–254
see also CDA
Coptotermes 205
Coptotermes acinaciformis 205, 206
Coptotermes frenchi 205
Coptotermes spp. 206
Corvus ruficollis 324
Cossus cossus 166
Costelytra zealandica 201
cotton 88
cottonseed oil 319
cream-coloured courser 324
crustaceans 352
Cryptocatantops haemorrhoidalis 83
crystalline array virus 115
Culex pipiens 166
Culicinomyces clavisporus 232
Cunninghamella sp. 111

Curculio caryae 164
Cursoprius cursor 324
cuticle degradation 183–186, 193
cuticle-degrading enzymes 183
Cytherea spp. 109

dark cheeks disease 115
DDT 71
DDVP 251
deltamethrin 40, 251
Dendrolimus punctata 126
desert locust see *Schistocerca gregaria*
destruxins 181, 187, 188, 193
Devine 220
Diabolocatantops axillaris 49, 83, 91, 287, 288, 292, 294, 295, 303
diapause 17, 64, 67
Diaprepes spp. 126
Diatraea saccharalis 166
diazinon 40, 98, 251, 297
dichlorvos 40
Didymella fabae 174
dieldrin 4, 5, 8, 9, 44, 45, 58, 71, 87, 118, 250, 251, 315, 318, 321, 323, 324, 327, 329, 330, 331, 333, 334, 348
diflubenzuron 185
Dimilin 185
Dipel 201
Diuraphis noxia 166
DNA recombinant technology 125
Dociostaurus maroccanus 38, 117

eagles 73, 107
ecdysone 47
see also juvenile hormones
egg parasitoids 111
egg predators 109–110
electrophoretic karyotyping 197
enriched neem oil 311, 312, 314, 316, 317, 318, 319, 339, 341, 343, 345
Entomophaga grylli 10, 14, 15, 24, 27, 116, 117, 122, 125, 133, 134, 135, 137, 175, 211, 231, 232, 268, 276, 357, 366
Entomophaga grylli complex 127–128
Entomophaga spp. 116, 125
Entomophthora spp. 116
entomopox viruses (entomopoxvirus) 10, 27, 115, 118, 287
environmental aspects 44, 89, 276, 347–353
environmental impact & safety 356–360
enzymes 183, 193
Epicauta spp. 110
Eugregarina 114
eugregarines 295
exploration 208–213
Eyprepocnemis plorans ornatipes 133, 135, 139

Fagonia sp. 324
Farinocystis sp. 268
fenitrothion 5, 8, 40, 87, 93, 94, 95, 98, 118, 134, 251, 263, 297
fenvalerate 94
fire ants 126
fish 352
formulation 223–225, 234, 243
fungal spore production 15–16
fungi 15, 28, 29, 47, 106, 109, 116, 122–129, 134, 219–226, 230–235
Fusarium sp. 138

Galleria mellonella 167
gamma HCH 251, 297
see also HCH
genetic recombination 194
Gossypium spp. 88
granulosis virus 364
gregarines 108
gregarization pheromone 153
ground beetles 112
growth regulators 95

HCH 71, 87
see also gamma HCH
Helminthosporium maydis 163
Hieroglyphus 36
Hieroglyphus daganensis 17, 77–78, 83, 86, 92, 94, 303, 304
Hieroglyphus spp. 159–160
Hirsutella thompsonii 232, 233
Hirsutella thompsonii isolates 162
Hirundo obsoleta buchanani 324
honey-bees 347, 351, 358
hormones 71–72, 337
hornbill 107
host death 188–189
host defence mechanisms 186–187
Hypothenemus hampei 166, 169

inoculation 12
insect growth regulators 5, 44, 75, 311, 314, 315
intertropical convergence zone 90
invertebrates 352
isolate variability 203

juvenile hormones 47, 153

kestrel 107
kites 73
Kraussaria 36
Kraussaria angulifera 8, 17, 76, 77, 83, 86, 91, 94, 95, 160, 209, 303, 304
Kraussella amabile 78, 83, 303

lambdacyhalothrin 40, 93, 94, 251
LC_{50} 204
LD_{50} 11, 13, 249, 250, 252
LD_{50}s 251
LD_{90} 252
LD_{99}s 251
Lepidiota consobrina 205
Lepidiota frenchi 205
Lepidiota negatoria 205
Lepidiota noxia 205
Lepidiota squaulata 205
Leptinotarsa decemlineata 125, 312
lizards 112
Locusta migratoria 17, 37, 76, 114, 115, 117, 186
Locusta migratoria migratorioides 36, 71, 251, 267, 275
Locustana pardalina 67
LT_{50} 11, 170

Mahanarva fimbriolata 239
Mahanarva posticata 127, 233, 239–243
maize 86, 88, 193
Malamoeba 260
Malamoeba locustae 15, 54, 55, 114, 295
malathion 4, 5, 8, 40, 87, 88, 93, 94, 251, 297
mammals 112, 352, 357
man 357
Manduca sexta 184, 185, 188, 192, 193
Manihot esculenta 80, 86
see also cassava
marabou 107
mass production 231–233, 240–243
Mastomys natalensis 62
Megachile rotundata 358–359
Melanoplus entomopox virus 287
see also MPV
Melanoplus infantilis 272
Melanoplus packardii 272
Melanoplus sanguinipes 11, 272, 298, 309
Melia volkensii 44, 48
Meloidae 110
Melolontha melolontha 172, 279–285
Melolontha spp. 279
mermithids 108, 114, 133
see also nematodes
Metacemyia calleti 62
Metarhizium 208, 263, 369, 370
Metarhizium conidia 250
Metarhizium isolates 18
Metarhizium anisopliae 11, 116, 122, 125, 127, 163, 166, 167, 168, 173, 176, 181, 182, 183, 184, 185, 186, 188, 191, 192, 193, 195, 196, 201, 202, 222, 223, 225, 232, 233, 239–243, 285, 295
Metarhizium anisopliae ARSEF 324 164, 165
Metarhizium anisopliae FI114 204, 205, 206
Metarhizium anisopliae FI147 204, 205, 206
Metarhizium anisopliae FI153 204, 205, 206
Metarhizium anisopliae FI610 205, 206
Metarhizium anisopliae IIBC 190–574 165
Metarhizium anisopliae IMI 047038 165
Metarhizium anisopliae IMI 152222 165
Metarhizium anisopliae IMI 16877ii 165
Metarhizium anisopliae IMI 298059 165
Metarhizium anisopliae IMI 298061 165
Metarhizium anisopliae ME1 164, 165, 183, 184, 188
Metarhizium anisopliae RS549 187, 188
Metarhizium anisopliae RS1094 188
Metarhizium anisopliae isolates 164, 170, 200–206, 205
Metarhizium anisopliae var. *anisopliae* 168, 169, 170, 173, 195, 203
Metarhizium anisopliae var. *anisopliae* isolates 203
Metarhizium anisopliae var. *majus* 168, 170, 173, 203
Metarhizium flavoviride 11, 15, 18, 37, 125, 127, 168, 249, 255, 260
Metarhizium flavoviride ARSEF 2023 165

Metarhizium flavoviride IMI 324673 165
Metarhizium flavoviride IMI 330189 12, 13, 165, 250, 251, 258
Metarhizium flavoviride isolates 12, 213
Metarhizium flavoviride var. *flavoviride* 168
Metarhizium flavoviride var. *minus* 168
Metarhizium spp. 9, 10, 11, 12, 13, 116, 159, 160, 161, 167, 168, 171, 172, 173, 174, 176, 191, 192
Metarhizium spp. isolates 162, 163, 164, 166, 209, 210
Micro-Ulva sprayer 144
microsporidians 134
migratory locust see *Locusta migratoria*
millet 98
mites 62, 133, 134, 135, 137
molecular markers 195
molecular techniques 191–197
Moroccan locust see *Dociostaurus maroccanus*
mosquitoes 225
MPV 287, 294
multimammate rat 62
Muscidae 114
Mycotal 220
Mylabris spp. 108, 110
Myllocerus elegans 165
Myzus persicae 235, 319

Nasutitermes 205
Nasutitermes exitiosus 166, 205, 206
Nasutitermes spp. 206
neem 48, 72, 143, 312, 327, 330, 331, 332, 333, 334
see also *Azadirachta indica*
neem cake 143
neem oil 88, 142–153, 317, 321, 323, 324, 325, 339, 342, 365
neem products 337, 338, 342
nematodes 10, 15, 62, 114, 117, 133, 134, 135, 140
see also mermithids
Nemestrinidae 113
Neurospora crassa 191
Nilaparvata lugens 127, 170, 171, 194, 210
Nomadacris septemfasciata 57–63, 67, 114, 117, 126, 323
Nomoult 185
Nomuraea rileyi 186, 187, 233
Nomuraea spp. 10
non-target organisms 321–335, 347, 348, 349, 350, 351, 352, 357
Nosema 99, 100, 155
Nosema cuneatum 275, 276
Nosema locustae 10, 24, 49, 71, 77, 95, 118, 226, 231, 263, 267, 268, 269, 270–273, 275, 287, 291–294, 292, 293, 311, 312–313, 314, 317, 319
Nosema spp. 267
nuclear polyhedrosis virus 115

Oedaleus entomopoxvirus 287
see also OPV
Oedaleus nigeriensis 87, 133, 135, 138
Oedaleus senegalensis 4, 8, 17, 36, 37, 49, 64, 67, 76, 77, 83, 87, 90, 95, 105, 106, 109, 159, 287, 288, 292, 293, 294, 295, 303, 323
oil formulations 13
Ommatius variabilis 62
OPV 287, 294
organochlorine insecticides 71
organophosphates 4, 5, 71
Ornithacris 36
Ornithacris cavroisi 12, 165
Ornithacris turbida 91, 93
Ornithacris turbida cavroisi 83
Oryza sativa 86
Ostrinia nubilalis 173
Otiorhynchus sulcatus 126, 189
outbreak areas 59
Oxya chinensis 111
Oxya spp. 111

Paecilomyces canadensis 233
Paecilomyces farinosus 233
Paecilomyces lilacinus 111
Paecilomyces spp. 10, 160
pale crag martin 324
palm oil 337, 342, 343
Panicum turgidum 313
Panolis flammea 247
see also pine caterpillar
Pantorhytes plutus 11, 249
parasitoids 108, 111, 134
pasture 202
Patanga guttulosa 12, 164, 165, 166
Patanga succincta 67
pathogenicity 162

pathogens 10, 44, 111, 134, 137–138, 208–213
PCR see polymerase chain reaction
peanuts 202
pecan weevil 164
Pergularia tomentosa 324
pesticide hazard 348–353
Phenacoccus manihoti 52
pheromones 44, 46, 48, 71–72
Philodicus nigrescens 62
phoresy 111
picornavirus 115
Pimelia sp. 108
Pimelia angulata tschadensis 321, 326, 327, 328, 329, 330, 331, 334, 335
Pimelia senegalensis 94
Pimelia subquadrata chudeaui 326
Pimelia subquadrata tschadensis 324, 325
pine caterpillar 126
see also *Panolis flammea*
pineapple 202
pollinators 347, 352
polymerase chain reaction 196, 200, 203, 206
potatoes 202
PR1 181, 182, 183, 184, 185, 186, 187, 193
pr1 gene 176, 191, 193
PR2 184, 185
PR4 184
Prionotheca coronata coronata 324, 326
propoxpur 87, 94, 98, 134, 251
protease 165
protease *pr1* gene 176
protozoa 10, 28, 29, 47, 114
Pseudeurotium bakeri 174
Pseudomonas aeruginosa 10
Pyrgomorpha cognata 83, 295
pyrrolizidine alkaloids 44, 48, 49

Rastrococcus invadens 52
raven 107
recombination 172–173
red locust see *Nomadacris septemfasciata*
release - risks 171–174
remote sensing 69
reptiles 72, 112, 324
restriction fragment length polymorphisms 195–196
rice 86
rice delphacid 170
see also *Nilaparvata lugens*
Rickettsiella melolonthae 280
rodents 72

Saccharomyces cerevisiae 170, 197
Sarcophaga spp. 113
Sarcophagidae 113
Scapanes australis 165
scarab pests of sugarcane 201, 203–204
Scelio 108
Scelio fulgidus 111
Scelio howardi 62
Scelio pembertoni 111
Scelio spp. 25, 111
Scelionidae 111
Schistocerca cancellata 67
Schistocerca gregaria 4, 8, 11, 12, 13, 15, 17, 27, 36, 38, 39, 44, 45, 46, 49, 54–56, 67, 76, 97, 105, 106, 115, 117, 142–153, 159, 162, 164, 165, 166, 176, 181, 182, 183, 186, 187, 188, 209, 210, 226, 247, 249, 250, 251, 257, 259, 260, 311–320, 321, 323, 324, 335, 337–345, 347
Schistocerca spp. 164
Schizaphis graminum 166
Schouwia purpurea 323, 338
Schouwia thebaica 313, 315, 316, 321, 323, 324, 325, 326, 331, 334, 338
scorpions 112
Segestidea sp. 111
Serratia marcescens 10, 115
Sitona discoideus 210
Sitona spp. 170
Solenopsis spp. 126
solid substrate fermentation 222
sorghum 86, 97
Sorghum sp. 86
Sorosporella sp. 37, 125, 209
southern corn blight 163
sparrow-hawks 73
Spharagemon campestris 272
Sphecidae 112
Sphex aegyptiacus 112
Spodoptera exigua 319
Spodoptera littoralis NPV 115
Stomorhina lunata 106, 109, 118
strain improvement 194
Styphlomerus sp. 95
submerged culture fermentation 220
sugarcane 202
sugarcane spittle bug 127

sumicombi 30 94
summit disease 116, 211
sunscreen 13–14
survey methods 211
Systoechus spp. 106, 108, 109

Tachinidae 113–114
teak 88
Tectona grandis 88
teflubenzuron 185, 315, 316
teleomorphs 173–174
Tenebrionidae 108, 110
termites 201, 202, 204–206
Theobroma cacao 80
thrips 319
tobacco hornworm 124
Tomaspis saccharina 165
Trachyderma hispida 321, 324, 326, 331, 335
Trachyrachys kiowa 272
training 31–36, 69
Tribulus ochroleucus 324
Tribulus spp. 313
Trichoplusia ni 187, 201
Trichopsidea costata 107, 113
Trichopsidea spp. 113
Trogidae 110
trombidiid 137, 138, 139, 140
Trombidiidae 133
Trox procerus 106, 110
Trox suberosus 110
Trox spp. 110
two phase systems 223

ultra-low volume 11
see also ULV
ultra-low volume application 299
ultra-low volume spraying 245–248
ULV 11, 12
ULV formulations 255–261

Vairimorpha sp. 24
Veens Medium 202
Verronia sp. 155
Vertalec 220
Verticillium albo-atrum 194
Verticillium dahliae 194
Verticillium lecanii 163, 186, 194, 220, 232
Verticillium spp. 10, 160
Vieta senegalensis 95
vine weevil 126, 189
virulence 162
viruses 28, 47, 115, 134, 280

wheatear 107
white stork 107
whitefly 220
Wohlfahrtia spp. 113

Xeramoeba oophaga 108, 109

Zacompsa festa 303
Zea mays 86, 193
see also maize
Zonocerus elegans 12, 165, 210
Zonocerus variegatus 14, 15, 48, 52, 72, 76, 77, 79–81, 86, 87, 88, 91, 93, 95, 105, 106, 117, 133–140, 155, 160, 164, 175
Zulia entreriana 166

Handbook to Live Well with Adhesive Arachnoiditis

Second edition

ISBN: 9781955934077
Library of Congress Control Number: 2021912718

Arachnoiditis Research and Education Project
c/o Nancy Kriskovich
14 Hidden River Lane
Bigfork, MT 59911

Ordering Information:

Special discounts are available on quantity purchases by corporations, associations, educators, and others. For details, contact the publisher at the above listed address.

U.S. trade bookstores and wholesalers: Please contact Nancy Kriskovich Tel: (406)249-2002;
or email snkriskovich@gmail.com

All proceeds from the sale of this book will go to the Arachnoiditis Research and Education Project sponsored by the
TENNANT FOUNDATION.
336 ½ S. GLENDORA AVENUE
WEST COVINA, CA 91790-3060
A 501(c)(3) Non-profit Organization

About the Authors

Dr. Forest Tennant Biography

Dr. Forest Tennant has had a long, distinguished career in addiction and pain medicine. He was recently honored with a "Life-Time Achievement Award" by Pain Week and "50 Years of Service" by the journal, "Practical Pain Management" where he served as their medical editor for 12 years. Dr. Tennant began his career in addiction and pain medicine as a US Army medical officer during the Vietnam War Era at which time he helped develop the Army's drug testing, education and treatment programs. After the Vietnam War, he became a Public Health Fellow assigned to the UCLA School of Public Health where he obtained his Masters' and Doctorate in Public Health (MPH, DrPH). Since 1975 to the present day, Dr. Tennant has produced a steady flow of research and publications in addiction and pain medicine. During this time his public notoriety first emerged when he served as an expert witness in the criminal trials of the physicians of Howard Hughes and Elvis Presley. Later he developed the drugs of abuse and anabolic steroid testing programs for the Los Angeles Dodgers and the National Football League. In very recent years Dr. Tennant has chosen to research hormonal testing and treatment of intractable pain and the merging pain problems of adhesive arachnoiditis and genetic collagen disorders. He and his wife Miriam of 52 years reside and work in West Covina, California and Wichita, Kansas.

Ingrid Hollis Biography

Ingrid Hollis began her career as a classically trained artist. This life path was put on hold by the necessity of becoming a family caregiver. This experience, along with a life altering motor vehicle accident in 1996 and the discovery that she has hypermobile Ehlers Danlos syndrome, (hEDS), a genetic collagen disorder that also runs in her family, changed the direction of her life. This knowledge set her on a course to search for answers, medical help and cures.

A great curiosity for research was ignited through this direct experience and fueled the desire to help others in similar situations. She has studied traditional and non-traditional medicine from many remarkable physicians and healers from throughout the world. Her hope has been to glean the wisdom from the many different healing systems and find ways to help and improve the lives of persons and their families who suffer from rare diseases throughout the world. Ingrid resides in Colorado with her retired husband and son. She has two lovely children and two grandchildren to whom her work is dedicated.

She heads the "Publication Team" for the Arachnoiditis Research and Education Project of the Tennant Foundation.

CONTRIBUTORS

A handbook as comprehensive as this could not have been written without the input and advice of many people. We are grateful for the kind assistance of those persons listed here.

Terri Anderson
Lynn Ashcraft
Donna Corley
Lloyd Costello, MD
K. Scott Guess, PharmD, MS Pharm, RPh
Adam Hy, DO
Kate Lamport
Denise Molohon
Kristen Ogden
Caron Pedersen RN, NP, DC
Martin J. Porcelli, DO, MHPE
Rhonda Posey
Gary Snook
Deborah Vallier
Kris Walters

This handbook and the research behind it would never have been written without the pioneering groundwork of Drs. Sarah Smith, Antonio Aldrete, and Charles Burton.

Handbook to Live Well with Adhesive Arachnoiditis

BY

FOREST TENNANT M.D., M.P.H., DR.P.H
with INGRID HOLLIS

Table of Contents

1. MAJOR MESSAGE – BUILD A PERSONAL CARE PROGRAM 17

2. DEALING WITH THE FRIGHT OF AA 18

3. DEFINITIONS YOU MUST KNOW 20

4. HISTORY OF ARACHNOIDITIS 22

5. AA IS INCREASING IN MODERN TIMES 24

6. CAUSES OF ADHESIVE ARACHNOIDITIS 26

7. NATURAL COURSE AND OUTCOME OF ADHESIVE ARACHNOIDITIS 27

8. WHY PREMATURE DEATH OCCURS IN PEOPLE WITH AA 28

9. MAJOR SYMPTOMS AND HARMS OF AA 28

10. CATEGORIES OF SEVERITY 29

11. DIAGNOSIS OF AA 31

12. THE EQUIVOCAL OR INCONCLUSIVE MRI 33

13. MOST COMMON CAUSE OF CONSTANT INCURABLE PAIN IS AA 34

14. I'VE BEEN DIAGNOSED WITH ADHESIVE ARACHNOIDITIS. NOW WHAT? 34

15. TWO STRATEGIES FOR TREATMENT 35

16. MAJOR GOAL OF TREATMENT: STOP PROGRESSION - DON'T GET WORSE 38

17. THE EARLIER THE TREATMENT—THE BETTER THE RESULT 39

18. THREE- COMPONENT MEDICAL TREATMENT 39

19. NEUROINFLAMMATION AND NEURODEGENERATION 42

20. SEVEN FACTS ABOUT NEUROINFLAMMATION (NI) 44

21. PHYSIOLOGIC TREATMENT MEASURES.................................... 46
22. PREVENTIVE MEASURES TO "NOT GET WORSE" 47
23. SPINAL FLUID – RIVER OF HOPE!! 49
24. SPINAL FLUID LEAKAGE AND SEEPAGE 51
25. HOW TO IMPROVE YOUR SPINAL FLUID FLOW 53
26. TREATMENT OF SPINAL FLUID LEAKAGE AND SEEPAGE........... 53
27. STRETCHES TO PREVENT TISSUE SHRINKAGE 55
28. WALKING WITH ARM SWINGS: THE BEST EXERCISE................. 58
29. RETAINED ELECTRICITY – MUST ELIMINATE 58
30. YOU NEED MORE OXYGEN 60
31. A NEW BREAKTHROUGH: ELECTROMAGNETIC ENERGY THERAPY 61
32. THE IMPORTANCE OF SPINE BRACING.................................... 62
33. DO YOU HAVE A GENETIC COLLAGEN DISORDER LIKE EHLERS-DANLOS SYNDROME (EDS)?.. 63
34. COLLAGEN BUILDING PROGRAM FOR PEOPLE WITH AA AND GCD 65
35. INSOMNIA AND SLEEP.. 67
36. HIGH PROTEIN ANTI-INFLAMMATORY DIET 68
37. INVERSION THERAPY.. 70
38. AUTOIMMUNITY WITH AA 70
39. STEM CELLS, MICROSURGERY, AND OTHER NEW PROCEDURES71
40. THERAPEUTIC TRIALS – FIND OUT WHAT WORKS 73
41. HOW TO SAFELY TAKE KETOROLAC AND METHYLPREDNISOLONE 74

42. PAIN CONTROL 75

43. BEST TREATMENT DRUGS FOR AA 76

44. PROTOCOL FOR EMERGENCY TREATMENT OF SUSPECTED AA . 77

45. LOW DOSE NALTREXONE (LDN) FOR ADHESIVE ARACHNOIDITIS (AA) 79

46. DRUGS IN THE 3 MEDICATION COMPONENTS 80

47. PAIN FLARES 82

48. SELF-HELP MEDICATION PROTOCOL 83

49. NEED FOR A COMPOUNDING PHARMACY 85

50. I'M GETTING WORSE, WHAT DO I DO? 86

51. PSYCHOLOGICAL TREATMENT AND SUPPORT 88

52. SUPPORT GROUPS AND PARTNERS 89

53. YOUR FAMILY AND YOUR RELIGION 89

54. WHEN AN ELECTRICAL STIMULATOR OR SPINAL CANAL INFUSION DEVICE ARE NEEDED 90

55. EPIDURAL CORTICOSTEROID INJECTIONS AND SPINAL TAPS 91

56. INFUSIONS OF LIDOCAINE, KETAMINE, AND VITAMIN C 92

57. GENETIC PREDISPOSING SUSCEPTIBILITY TO AA 92

58. NO DOCTOR WILL HELP ME 93

59. THE 21 DAY RULE 94

60. HOW TO DEAL WITH OPIOID RESTRICTIONS 95

61. THREE STRATEGIES TO DEAL WITH OPIOID RESTRICTION 97

62. DEALING WITH THE FEAR OF HORMONES 99

63. HUMAN CHORIONIC GONADOTROPIN (HCG) AND NANDROLONE 101

64. MY MEDICATION PROGRAM HAS QUIT WORKING 103
65. I CAN'T GET A DIAGNOSIS 105
66. WHY CAN'T I GET BETTER? 106
67. AA TREATMENT IS PROTOCOL - NOT EVIDENCE-BASED 107
68. RISK VS BENEFIT AND INFORMED CONSENT 108
69. SUMMARY 111
DISCLAIMER: 112
THE FOE CHART of PHYSIOLOGIC MEASURES 113
REFERENCES 115

INTRODUCTION AND PURPOSE

This handbook has one purpose – to help you live well despite this horrible disease: adhesive arachnoiditis (AA).

We first encountered AA in the 1970's when insoluble dyes (usually "pantopaque") were injected into the spinal canal to help visualize x-rays. Today the causes are different, and AA is increasing in the general population.

AA is a complex neuroinflammatory disease of the spinal canal covering (arachnoid) and the lumbar spinal cord nerve roots (cauda equina). In other words, two different body parts abnormally "glue" together by adhesions. Regardless of cause, AA, once initiated, can be a progressive disease that can result in constant severe pain, paralysis of arms and legs, and impairments of bladder, bowel, and sex organs. Due to the increasing prevalence of AA, the Tennant Foundation has initiated a vigorous and aggressive research project to understand and develop strategies and protocols to control and treat AA. While no absolute cure is known, we have determined that AA is best treated and controlled with a two-fold strategy: (1) medication and (2) physiologic and preventive measures.

We have recently learned that persons with genetic collagen disorders of the Ehlers-Danlos Syndrome and Marfan Syndrome types frequently develop AA. This handbook addresses our efforts to bring treatment to those with this dual disease problem.

Today, few physicians are aware and familiar with the strategies to control AA, which is a major reason this handbook has been written. Although we predict a change in

the future, we have learned that people with AA and their families must currently initiate treatment pretty much on their own. To wait can be a terrible mistake, since AA can swiftly progress and worsen causing deterioration and lead to a miserable, shortened life. This handbook is primarily designed to keep people with AA from getting worse, but there is hope, as most people get better with the measures outlined in this handbook. Plunge in. Even when you find good medical care for AA, you will have to practice measures described in this handbook.

Forest Tennant M.D., Dr. P.H.
Ingrid Hollis

WHY WERE OUR CAST OF CHARACTERS CREATED?

Adhesive arachnoiditis (AA) is an extremely serious disease and not to be taken lightly; however, we have created some characters to emphasize certain points of importance. It is our intent to bring a smile along with getting important points across to the reader.

DR. BEAK

Who is Dr. Beak? A smart old buzzard who received his MD degree from the "Common Sense Medical School." He will give common sense advice.

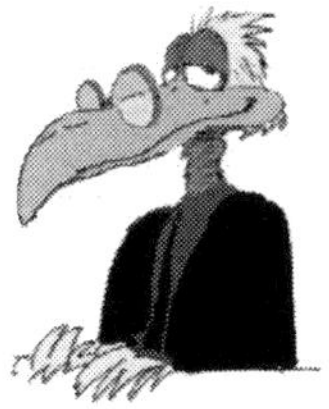

NURSE ROSEY

Who is Nurse Rosey? A pesky, ever present nurse who wrote her nurse's thesis on "How to Shape Up Persons for Their Own Good." She will give you gentle, compassionate, encouragement.

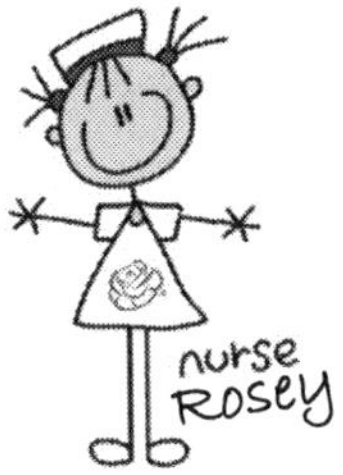

HAPPY SPIDER

How can a spider be happy? Well, it is his web of arachnoid tissue that becomes inflamed with AA. Spiders are meticulous about their web and when you allow his web to be distorted with inflammation, he becomes unhappy. He can be happy when you are following the protocol and his web is no longer inflamed and causing you pain.

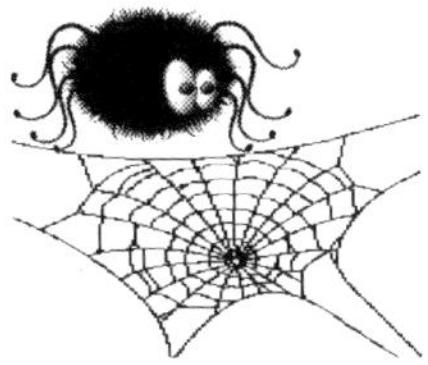

1. MAJOR MESSAGE – BUILD A PERSONAL CARE PROGRAM

Every person who has adhesive arachnoiditis (AA), and obtains this handbook is undoubtedly aware that this disease can result in tragedy, pain, and suffering beyond imagination. A meaningful life can stop on a dime if AA develops and it is not controlled.

Our major message is this: You can build a personal care program that controls this disease and lets you live a quality, meaningful life. It's not, however, easy. You must build a program of medication and physiologic measures. You can't do it all in one day or in a couple of visits to a doctor's office, but it will happen with a little effort and discipline. You must build a program step by step and self-administer and practice your program daily, with a goal of improvement, while constantly enhancing your program.

Here are cautions to know while building your program. Relief of pain is usually the paramount concern of a person with AA. This is understandable but know this: any medication called a pain reliever – prescription or non-prescription – will only provide relief for a limited time period unless you are simultaneously taking medication to suppress neuroinflammation, and medicinal agents to regrow damaged nerve tissue. You must also practice some of the physiologic and preventive measures in this handbook if you want consistent pain relief.

A second caution is this: Modern medicine has done a masterful job in selling a single treatment for a single disease. Media, print, TV, and the internet are constantly trying to sell

the "new" stuff like stem cells, microsurgery, minimally invasive spine surgery, robotic surgery, intravenous infusions, and hyperbaric oxygen chamber treatment among others. While all these may have merit in select clinical situations, there is no substitute for an effective AA care plan which requires medications and specific physiologic measures designed to reduce neuroinflammation, regrow your damaged nerve tissue, and keep you mobile, animated, and living a quality life.

The last caution is to avoid treatments described with buzz words that are usually designed for someone's financial gain or disguised as cost saving measures by insurance carriers and HMO's. Look out for "evidence-based", "patient-centered," and "off-label" cures. Check all the "one-way" or "no-way" words. Don't let propaganda keep you from building an effective treatment program.

2. DEALING WITH THE FRIGHT OF AA

Every person who is informed they have AA is rightfully scared and frightened. To be otherwise would not be human. When one has severe pain, spasms, funny feelings on the skin, an irregular bladder, and blurred vision you will naturally be scared.

What's more, the stories of the past – paralysis, starvation, horrific pain, non-functioning mind and body, and early death were all true at one time, but no more! Our medical protocols for AA aren't totally curative, but because of them, the plight of AA victims in the past doesn't have to occur today.

Follow these steps:

1. Don't let fright paralyze you or cause you not to act. You must take immediate action once you find out you've got AA.

2. Tell someone about your fright – spouse, friend, child, doctor, clergyman – nothing calms fright like sharing it with another person.

3. Understand this new medical fact – modern treatment as outlined in this handbook will almost always keep you from getting much worse – just start. Bottom line – get started with treatment today!

4. First treatment – take a walk – walking is a first-class medicine for AA! Second, go to the health food store and buy one or two non-prescription drugs known to help most people with AA– examples: curcumin, serrapeptase, pregnenolone.

5. Make an appointment with your family doctor (MD, DO, PCP), nurse practitioner (NP), or physician assistant (PA) to discuss treatment strategies.

6. Take out a pencil and paper. Write down every medication, food, exercise, or posture that gives you some comfort. You will be surprised. You already know some things that will help you live a good life!

The best way to rid yourself of fright is to know your challenges and that you have the power to control AA!

3. DEFINITIONS YOU MUST KNOW

Adhesive Arachnoiditis (AA): This condition is present when there are adhesions between the arachnoid layer of the spinal canal covering, and the nerve roots in the cauda equina. Adhesions "glue" the nerve roots to the arachnoid layer, and this can be seen on a magnetic resonance image (MRI). Fundamentally AA is the abnormal "gluing" together of two different body parts, the lumbar nerve roots and spinal canal covering.

Arachnoid: The cover or lining of the spinal canal is scientifically called the "thecal sac" or "meninges." The inner layer is called the "pia mater". It is extremely thin and fragile. The outer layer is the "dura" which is thick and firm. The arachnoid is the middle layer. It contains blood vessels and inflammatory cells and can become inflamed if irritated or damaged.

Arachnoiditis (ARC): Inflammation of the middle layer (arachnoid) of the spinal canal covering (meninges).

Central Nervous System (CNS): CNS is the brain, spinal cord, and cauda equina nerve roots.

Cerebral Spinal Fluid (CSF): Fluid made in the brain that bathes, protects, and nourishes the spinal cord and brain.

Medication Dosage: Milligram is mg. Milliliter is ml.

Nerve Roots: The actual spinal cord runs from the brain down to the top of the lumbar area. Below the spinal cord hangs about 2 dozen string-like structures called nerve roots.

Collectively they are called the cauda equina. The nerve roots can become damaged, inflamed, clump together, and stick or adhere by adhesions to the arachnoid layer of the spinal canal cover. When sticking and adhesions occur, the term AA is applied. If only enlargement, displacement, and clumping of nerve roots is seen on MRI, the term "cauda equina syndrome" is sometimes applied. Symptoms can be similar to AA.

Neuroinflammation (NI): NI is inflammation that occurs inside the CNS. It is the basic cause of AA and must be suppressed to control AA.

Neuroregeneration or Neurogenesis (NR): NR is regrowth of damaged nerve tissue, including nerve roots and supporting cells called glia.

Spinal Canal**:** The spinal canal is fundamentally a pipe that contains 4 components: (1) spinal cord; (2) nerve roots; (3) covering or lining called the meninges; and (4) cerebral spinal fluid. Think of the spinal canal as a closed pipe filled with structures bathed in fluid.

Tarlov Cysts**:** A cyst or outpouching of a spinal nerve root. They are often called "perineural" cysts. Tarlov cysts are frequently associated with ARC/AA.

Three Component Medical Treatment of AA: (1) suppression of neuroinflammation, (2) promotion of neuroregeneration, and (3) pain control.

Troche: Medication in a dissolvable "tablet" or "lozenge" that goes between the tongue and cheek.

<u>Two Strategies for Treatment of AA:</u> (1) medication and (2) physiologic measures.

4. HISTORY OF ARACHNOIDITIS

AA is an old disease first recognized in the mid-1800's (19th century). The causes in that century were primarily the infections of tuberculosis and syphilis. Fortunately, these diseases almost disappeared in the 20th century because antibiotics were discovered that dramatically reduced their prevalence. In the 20th century the major cause of AA was insoluble dyes injected into the spinal canal to enhance x-rays for diagnostic purposes. In 1987, the MRI was invented which lead to the near extinction of AA. In modern times, (the 21st century) AA, has re-emerged due to numerous factors including aging, degenerative spine conditions, obesity, and excessive sitting in front of computers and television screens, invasive spine interventions and surgeries, among other factors.

- The word "arachnoid" refers to a spider's web and the arachnoid membrane was named that because it resembles one.

- The exact year the disease, "arachnoiditis," was named is uncertain, however, the 1873 "Comprehensive Medical Dictionary," published by J.B. Lippincott & Co., included this definition of arachnoiditis: "A faulty term, denoting inflammation of the arachnoid membrane."

- In 1869 the famous neurologist, Dr. Charcot and his colleagues first described a syndrome we now call the

disease, ARC/AA. The causes of the disease were infections, primarily tuberculosis and syphilis.

- Dr. Addison, the physician who discovered adrenal failure, published his findings on 11 autopsied cases in 1855. Two cases had severe pain, atrophied adrenals with calcium deposits, and fluid around the arachnoid layer, which suggested that long-standing, end-stage ARC/AA was a likely cause of pain and adrenal failure.

- The first recorded attempt to treat AA was probably in 1781 when Dr. John Fothergill, a renowned British physician, treated a person with severe back and sciatic pain who had other symptoms compatible with AA. Opioids had failed to relieve this person's pain, but he obtained positive results after treating him with a mercury concoction called calomel.

- Between about 1930 and 1990 pantopaque and other oil-insoluble dyes were infused into the spinal canal for diagnostic (myelogram) purposes. A small percentage of these people developed AA and other neurologic complications.

- MRI's replaced oil-based dyes in the late 1980's, and AA subsequently became a rare, unappreciated disease.

- Beginning around the year 2000, an extended life span, bringing with it increasing rates of chronic painful spinal conditions such as herniated discs and arthritis. This, along with the increasing use of invasive medical interventions and surgeries to treat them, began fueling a rise in the incidence and prevalence of AA that continues to this day.

5. AA IS INCREASING IN MODERN TIMES

- Until recently AA was considered an extremely rare disease. NO MORE. Thanks to the technology of MRI's, AA can be diagnosed in a person with typical history, symptoms, and physical exam.

- While most cases of AA are in the lumbar and sacral spine areas, it can also occur in the cervical (neck) and thoracic (chest) spine. Although there are only a few nerve roots in the cervical and thoracic spine, the arachnoid layer of the spinal canal covering in these spinal areas can become chronically inflamed and produce profound pain and disability. Rarely do adhesions form between the spinal cord and arachnoid lining in the cervical and thoracic areas.

- It now appears that many people who have been labeled with such subjective, non-specific terms like "degenerative spine," "low back pain" or "failed back syndrome" really have AA.

<u>Factors Leading to AA:</u>

- ✓ Sedentary (sitting) lifestyle*
- ✓ Poor posture
- ✓ Non-supportive footwear
- ✓ Bucket seats
- ✓ Risk-taking sports activities
- ✓ Obesity
- ✓ Lack of exercise and walking
- ✓ Risky spinal injections and surgery
- ✓ Longer lifespan and aging

- ✓ Emergency life saving measures following accidents**
- ✓ Increased infant and childhood survival rates due to antibiotics and vaccines***

*Refers to the long hours of sitting in front of television and computers
**Life may be saved but injury left behind
***Immune deficient infants may survive and develop tissue degeneration disorders in adulthood

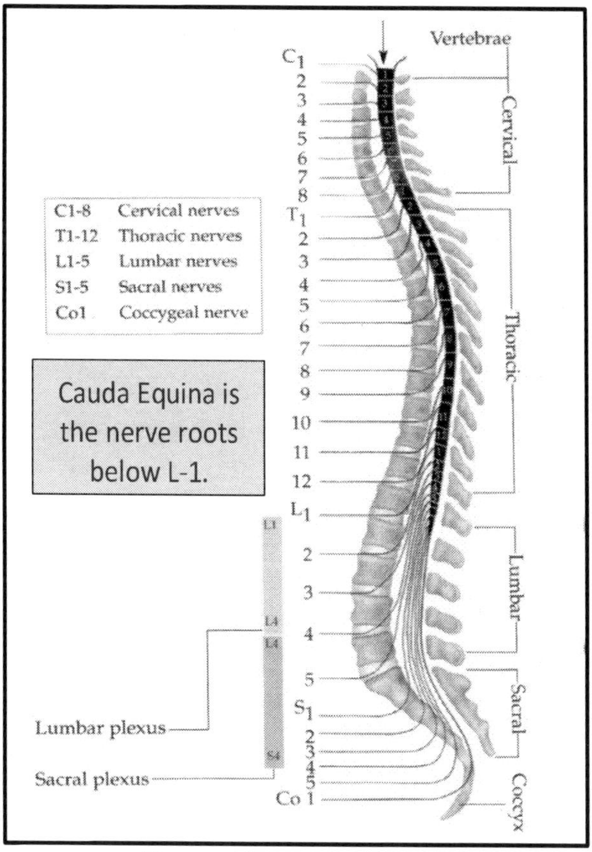

The normal anatomy of the spinal cord and nerve roots

6. CAUSES OF ADHESIVE ARACHNOIDITIS

✓ In the 1800's the common causes of AA were the infections of tuberculosis and syphilis.

✓ In the 1900's the most common cause of AA was oil-based dyes injected into the spinal canal for diagnostic purposes.

✓ In the 2000's the most common causes are chronic spine disorders related to aging, accidents, obesity, bucket seats, lack of exercise, poor posture, and the invasive medical interventions and procedures that are now used to treat common spine disorders.

<u>Listed Here are the Common Causes of AA Today:</u>

<u>Common Spine Disorders</u>

Common spine disorders including chronic herniated discs, stenosis, osteoporosis, and vertebral arthritis that may, over-time, cause nerve roots in the cauda equina to rub or be squeezed together causing friction "sand-paper effect," inflammation, and adhesions.

<u>Genetic Collagen Disorders</u>

The arachnoid and pia mater layers of the spinal covering are thin, soft, and easily damaged because they are composed primarily of very soft and frail tissue compared to other tissues, such as tendons and bone. Genetic collagen disorders that cause tissue degeneration, particularly Ehlers-Danlos and Marfan Syndromes, may cause micro-tears in the arachnoid

layer which lead to inflammation, cysts (Tarlov), and adhesions.

Autoimmune Disease

Many people with AA also have autoimmune diseases such as systemic lupus, psoriatic arthritis, or rheumatoid arthritis. AA may be a direct result from autoimmunity.

Infections

Lyme disease is the most common infection today that may cause AA. Some viruses are also highly suspected to cause AA. Epstein Barr virus is one possibility.

Trauma

A puncture, tear, or traumatic injury to the arachnoid lining from an accident, needle puncture, or chemical irritant may initiate AA. Inflammation and adhesions of the arachnoid lining may later capture, glue and inflame the nerve roots that are close to the traumatic site.

7. NATURAL COURSE AND OUTCOME OF ADHESIVE ARACHNOIDITIS

3 Possible Outcomes of Untreated AA:

- Resolves – a return to the normal uninflamed state (mild or asymptomatic cases)
- Intermittent symptoms, impairments, and pain

- Progressive neurologic symptoms, impairments, and pain (e.g. wheelchair, bed-bound, early death)

AA's natural course and outcome are directly related to neuroinflammation severity. Due to this fact, suppression of neuroinflammation along with neuroregenerative measures is the "baseline" of treatment.

8. WHY PREMATURE DEATH OCCURS IN PEOPLE WITH AA

- Poor mobility
- Obesity, diabetes, hypercholesterolemia
- Endocrine (hormone) suppression
- Immune system impairment - inability to protect against disease from infections and tumors
- Hypertension
- Intestinal digestive defects, gastroparesis, and malabsorption – inability to absorb needed nutrients from food

The Good News: We now know that the natural course and outcome of AA CAN BE greatly changed by treating neuroinflammation and promoting neuroregeneration.

9. MAJOR SYMPTOMS AND HARMS OF AA

Due to nerve entrapment and destruction of nerve roots, these major symptoms may appear: (1) skin sensation of water dripping or bugs crawling, (2) burning feet, (3) can't sit

or stand in one position very long, (4) bladder difficulties, and (5) pain.

Additional symptoms may occur due to AA's complications:

- ✓ Spinal Fluid Flow Obstruction: headache, blurred vision, ringing in ears
- ✓ Spinal Fluid Leakage: back pain, decreased ability to extend arms and legs, difficulty walking
- ✓ Autoimmune Disorder: arthritis, muscle aches, cardiac disorders, seizure, thyroiditis, carpal tunnel
- ✓ Retained Electricity: vibrations, tremors, overheating episodes, sweating, jerking
- ✓ Hormone Suppression; weakness, fatigue, poor pain control, depression, tissue wasting

Key Message: The sooner treatment with anti-neuroinflammatory agents is started, reduction in symptoms and harm can start.

10. CATEGORIES OF SEVERITY

AA has different severities, and we divide the severity into 4 categories: (1) mild; (2) moderate; (3) severe; and (4) catastrophic. Below we list the categories with impairments and functions in each category. If you are in the mild or moderate category, you have an excellent chance of considerable recovery. In fact, you may not even require a prescription drug if you are in the mild category. If you are in the severe or catastrophic categories, you will need a full protocol with the most potent drugs, and you may even need an implanted electrical stimulator or intraspinal opioid pump to get adequate pain relief.

Mild:

- ✓ Full range of motion
- ✓ No back indentation or contracture
- ✓ Normal inflammatory markers
- ✓ No bladder impairment
- ✓ No MRI evidence of spinal fluid leakage or obstruction
- ✓ No hormone abnormalities
- ✓ Can sit and stand in one position for 10 minutes

Moderate:

- ✓ Full range of motion and walks without assistance
- ✓ Mild to zero lower extremity weakness
- ✓ Normal inflammatory markers
- ✓ Some bladder hesitancy, urgency, dripping
- ✓ No MRI or physical evidence of spinal fluid leakage
- ✓ Mild constant pain but no need for sleep medication
- ✓ Can sit and stand in one position for 10 minutes

Severe:

- ✓ Some range of motion impairment and needs assistance (cane or other) to ambulate
- ✓ Weakness in lower extremities with neurologic symptoms (e.g. burning feet, bugs crawling, jerking or other)
- ✓ Elevated inflammatory markers and/or hormone abnormalities
- ✓ Bladder impairment symptoms of hesitancy, urgency, or incontinence
- ✓ MRI and/or physical evidence of chronic spinal fluid leakage and/or flow obstruction
- ✓ Constant pain that impairs sleep
- ✓ Can't sit and stand in one position for 10 minutes

Catastrophic:

- ✓ Requires assistance with activities of daily living (dressing, toiletry, eating, etc.)
- ✓ Significant lower extremity impairment (needs walker, wheelchair, braces)
- ✓ Bladder impairment of hesitancy, urgency, or incontinence
- ✓ Mental deficiencies such as memory loss or reading ability
- ✓ MRI and physical evidence of chronic spinal fluid obstruction and leakage
- ✓ Elevated inflammatory markers and hormone abnormalities
- ✓ Constant pain that impairs sleep
- ✓ Can't sit or stand in one position for 10 minutes

11. DIAGNOSIS OF AA

A final, clinical diagnosis of AA requires typical symptoms, physical findings, and laboratory tests. An MRI is needed to confirm the diagnosis.

Here is a 7-question screen. We have found that if a person answers yes to 4 of the 7, they very likely have AA. The earlier the diagnosis in the course of the disease, the better the results of treatment.

1. In addition to chronic pain, do you ever experience sharp, stabbing pains in your lower back when you twist, turn or bend?
2. Do you ever experience bizarre skin sensations such as crawling insects or water dripping down one or both legs?

3. Do you ever have burning, tingling, or a sensation of walking on broken glass in your feet and/or toes?
4. Does your pain become worse after standing, sitting, and/or walking?
5. Do you have leg weakness and/or pain that radiates down one or both legs?
6. Do you experience any bladder dysfunction such as dribbling, or difficulty when starting or stopping urination?
7. Do you have headaches along with blurred vision?

If you answered yes to four or more of these seven questions, you most likely have AA or some other neuroinflammatory disease of the nerve roots in your lumbar or sacral spine. Your physicians need to be informed of the results of this screening test as you need to obtain both a confirmatory diagnosis, and a treatment plan that is specific for your condition.

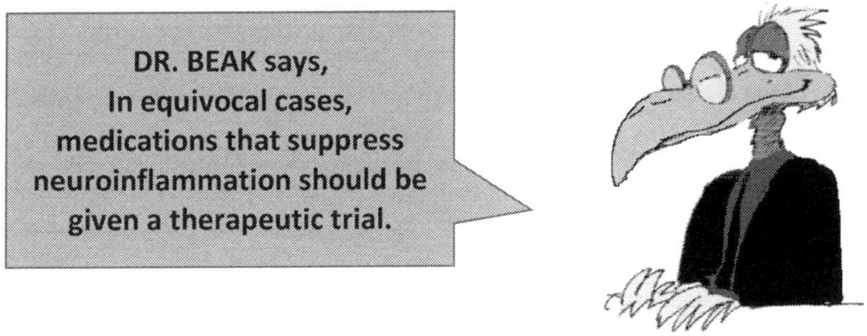

12. THE EQUIVOCAL OR INCONCLUSIVE MRI

AA is usually diagnosed on an axial MRI (foot to head) that shows cauda equina nerve root clumping that is adhered "glued" to the arachnoid lining (meninges) by adhesions. Prior to clumping and adhering to the arachnoid lining, some nerve roots will enlarge (edema), displace, and present an asymmetrical picture. BE CLEARLY ADVISED: In the early phase of the development of AA, or in mild cases, some nerve roots may appear to cling together, enlarge, or displace, but they don't clearly form clumps or "glue" to the arachnoid lining. This can be a major problem in interpretation. "Is there early or mild clumping, or maybe not?"

The lateral (sagittal) MRI views in confirmed cases show such signs as thickened nerve roots, dilated lower spinal canal (thecal sac), spinal fluid flow obstruction, and leakage or seepage. The lateral view, however, is less precise and a diagnosis of AA is not usually possible solely on the lateral view.

What should be done in equivocal or marginal cases? We recommend a blood test for inflammatory markers and therapeutic trials with the potent anti-neuroinflammatory drugs ketorolac and methylprednisolone. If a person's pain and some other symptoms improve with the trial, AA is likely. The 3-component medical treatment for AA should then be instituted, providing the person has a typical history and physical findings of AA.

13. MOST COMMON CAUSE OF CONSTANT INCURABLE PAIN IS AA

It will probably surprise many people in this era of opioid controversy, but a lot of research has recently been done to identify the causes of constant incurable pain and develop treatments for it, which may require opioid medication.

Our studies show that the great majority (over 90%) of persons with constant incurable pain have one of only 6 underlying causes:

- ✓ Adhesive Arachnoiditis (AA)
- ✓ Genetic Collagen Disorders of the Ehlers-Danlos and Marfan Syndrome Types
- ✓ Reflex Sympathetic Dystrophy (RSD) - Chronic Regional Pain Syndrome (CRPS)
- ✓ Post-Stroke
- ✓ Traumatic Brain Injury (TBI)
- ✓ Autoimmune Disorders – Post Viral or Rheumatologic Type

14. I'VE BEEN DIAGNOSED WITH ADHESIVE ARACHNOIDITIS. NOW WHAT?

Don't' panic. AA is now controllable in almost all cases. AA has traditionally been a diagnosis that brought great fear, since nothing could be done. NO MORE! There is now treatment that can allow greater function and pain relief than

ever before! The sooner a treatment protocol is started, the better the potential outcome. It is important to have a “partner” in your care, be it a friend or family member, that can help you understand your disease and help you start a self-care program.

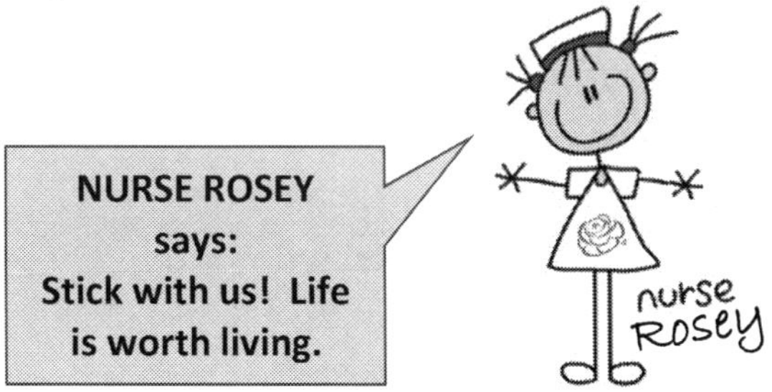

15. TWO STRATEGIES FOR TREATMENT

There are two major strategies of AA treatment: (1) medication to reduce neuroinflammation, promote neuroregeneration, and control pain; and (2) physiologic and preventive measures to enhance spinal fluid flow and prevent shrinkage of nerves, muscles, and collagen-based tissue.

Medication to reduce neuroinflammation, promote neuroregeneration, and control pain.	⟷	**Physiologic and preventive measures to improve spinal fluid flow and prevent tissue shrinkage.**

The nerve roots of the cauda equina and the spinal canal covering (arachnoid and dura in the lower spine) are dependent upon spinal fluid flow to nourish and flush the

spinal canal of toxins including neuroinflammatory waste. Since AA interferes with spinal fluid flow, people with AA must do daily simple physiologic measures to enhance spinal fluid flow such as: walking, arm and leg stretching, deep breathing, water soaking, or paraspinal massage. Other physiologic and preventive measures are to prevent shrinkage and scarring of nerves, muscle and supporting tissues that are either in or surround the spinal canal. For example, if the nerve roots of the cauda equina are not stretched, they may shrink, which leads to bladder and bowel dysfunction, and possible partial leg paralysis. Most people with AA have some spinal fluid seepage into the tissues and muscles that run parallel to the spinal column. If these aren't stretched daily, they may shrink and prevent the arms from doing their normal extension and function. Some specific physiologic measures are designed to help reduce retained electricity which may form heat and inflammation. In summary every person with AA needs an aggressive two-fold strategy of (1) medication; and (2) physiologic and preventive measures. It is our experience that people with AA may procrastinate and put off starting a two-fold strategy in hopes of a "single magic cure" or a physician who will come along and tell them exactly how to improve without the person and family developing their own two-fold strategy.

Here are the purposes and goals of the two-fold strategy:

1. Don't get worse
2. Maintain a quality of life
3. Achieve some permanent recovery

MEDICATION	PHYSIOLOGIC AND PREVENTIVE MEASURES
✓ Suppression of neuroinflammation	✓ Prevent tissue and nerve shrinkage
✓ Regrowth of damaged tissue (neuroregenesis)	✓ Prevent impairment of legs, bladder, bowel (paralysis)
✓ Pain control	✓ Maintain body functions and a "LIFE"

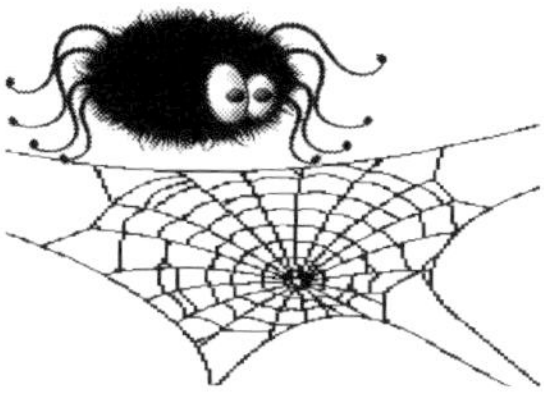

Happy Spider says, "No more paralysis or early death".

NURSE ROSEY says: "Accept it and control it".

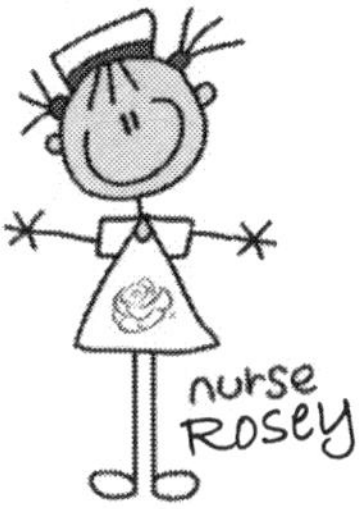

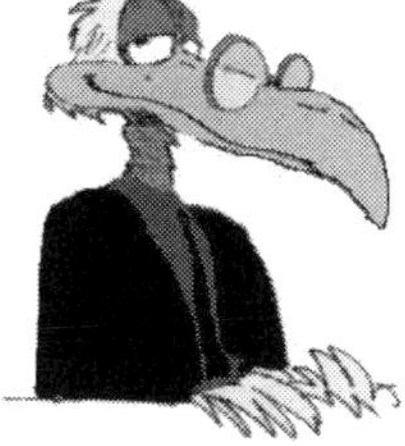

DR. BEAK says, Our 1st goal – "Don't get WORSE".

16. MAJOR GOAL OF TREATMENT: STOP PROGRESSION - DON'T GET WORSE

The major goal of this handbook is to prevent people with AA from getting worse. We caution those who are in the mild or moderate categories against complacency.
Neuroinflammation is the culprit of AA. If you don't constantly take measures to control it, for unknown reasons, it may flare and cause worsening in a short time period. In summary, once you have AA, as documented on an MRI, you must constantly take measures to control neuroinflammation lest you risk sudden and unexpected worsening.

AA is a neuroinflammatory disease of the nerve roots and the spinal canal covering. Once started, the neuroinflammation of AA may take any of these paths:

1. Total recovery or resolution (usually in mild or asymptomatic cases).
2. Cause progressive neurologic damage such as to involve the bladder, intestine, sex organs, or legs.
3. Go into periods of "false" remission, only to episodically flare.

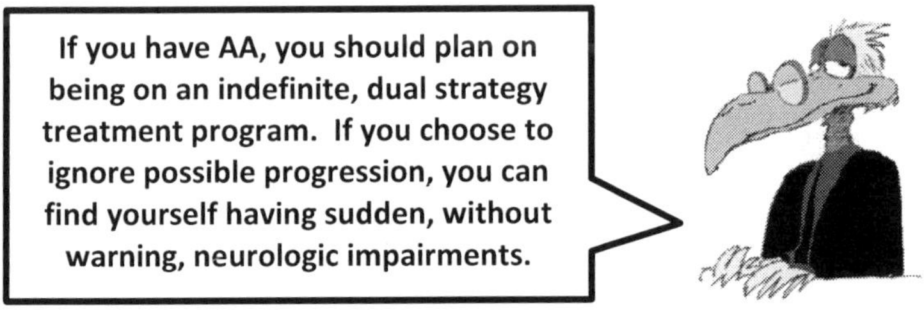

17. THE EARLIER THE TREATMENT—THE BETTER THE RESULT

Our conclusion in evaluating and treating several hundred AA cases is that the earlier treatment is started, the better the result or outcome.

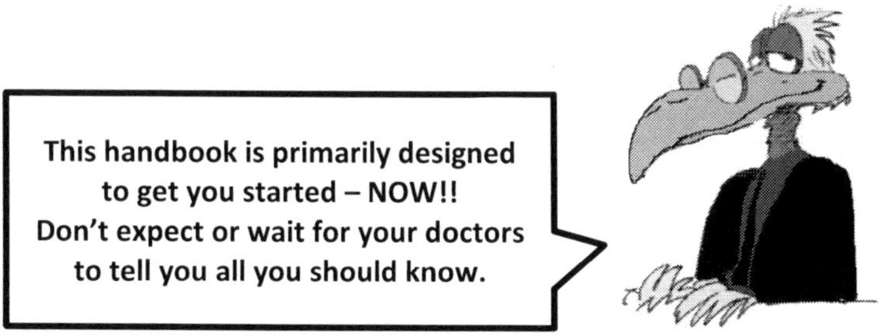

WHY? NI causes adhesions to form between the cauda equina nerve roots and the arachnoid lining of the spinal canal. In the early stage of AA, adhesions and NI can be at least partially resolved. After a time, however, NI and adhesions can cause permanent nerve damage that is not resolvable.

18. THREE- COMPONENT MEDICAL TREATMENT

Our research and experience are clear. Effective medical treatment requires a three-component medication program:

1. Suppression of neuroinflammation;
2. Regrowth of damaged nerve tissue (neuroregeneration)

3. Pain control

The 3-components must be simultaneously administered. Unfortunately, only a limited number of drugs are effective in treating AA. Drugs that help AA must cross the blood-brain barrier, enter the spinal fluid, and bind to action points (called receptors) on specific cells known as glia in the nerve roots of the cauda equina.

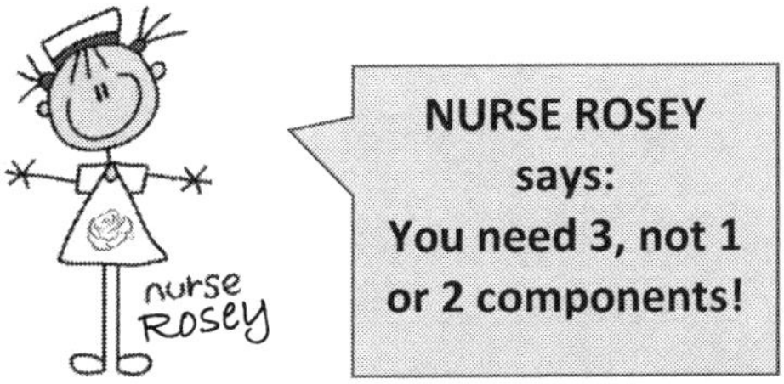

The proper treatment of confirmed cases of AA requires the simultaneous administration of these 3-components:

1. Suppress Neuroinflammation
   Examples: ketorolac, methylprednisolone, acetazolamide
2. Promote Damaged Nerve Regrowth (Neuroregeneration)
   Examples: pregnenolone, human chorionic gonadotropin (HCG), nandrolone
3. Pain Control
   Examples: low dose naltrexone, gabapentin, opioids, clonidine, ketamine

DR. BEAK says:
For relief and recovery, you must simultaneously use all 3-components.

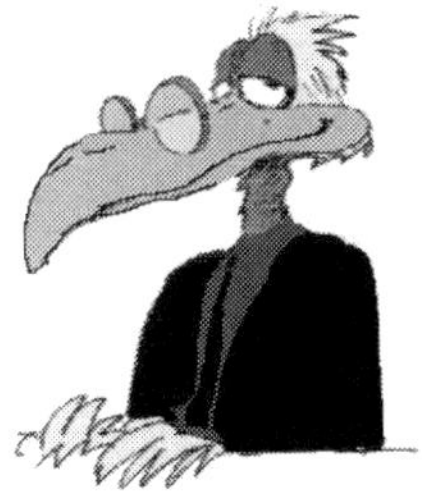

The amount of permanent recovery a person with AA can achieve, in our opinion, is related to the use of the neuroregeneration agents. These are hormones that reduce neuroinflammation and promote neuroregeneration.

Currently most physicians are not yet familiar with the 3-component protocol or treatment. It is no more complex or difficult than the multiple drug protocols necessary to treat such common diseases as asthma, emphysema, diabetes, or depression. The 3-component medical protocol we recommend can and should be done by medical providers in every community.

Out of over a dozen anti-inflammatory drugs on the commercial market, only ketorolac is consistently effective in AA. Sometimes diclofenac and indomethacin seem to help. Out of a dozen corticosteroids on the market, only methylprednisolone (Medrol®) and dexamethasone (Decadron®) are consistently effective. Although the menu of drugs isn't as extensive as we would like, there are enough drugs for a person to get started with AA treatment.

Pain control is what is usual in medical practice today. The drug naltrexone is the preferred pain reliever to start with, but it cannot be given to persons who currently take opioids since it will cause withdrawal symptoms. Many people with AA have constant pain "24/7" as opposed to intermittent "comes

and goes" pain. Severe constant pain will usually require a nerve conduction agent such as gabapentin or topiramate to enhance nerve function.

Undoubtedly, new and better drugs will be identified as the list in this handbook is considered "first generation." Although better drugs are likely in the future, no person with AA should delay starting a 3-component medication program.

Currently, people with AA in the severe and catastrophic categories are typically those who have not had the opportunity to participate in 3-component medical treatment. To move from a severe or catastrophic category to a lesser category is not impossible as we have witnessed many people with AA accomplish this feat. Be advised that almost all have been on a 3-component treatment protocol and have taken the nerve and tissue building hormones: human chorionic gonadotropin and/or nandrolone.

There are some physicians and on-lookers who claim there is no treatment for AA since the United States Food and Drug Administration (FDA) has not labeled a specific drug for AA treatment. Hopefully the future will bring about such labeling, but we seriously doubt that any <u>one</u> drug will do the job since AA is a complex disease.

19. NEUROINFLAMMATION AND NEURODEGENERATION

To treat AA and live a good life, you must clearly understand what these 2 terms mean – "neuroinflammation" and "neurodegeneration". Furthermore, you must know that

these 2 conditions must be treated simultaneously to get improvement.

NEUROINFLAMMATION	**NEURODEGENERATION**
AA can cause microglial cells in the spinal cord and nerve roots to inflame which is called neuroinflammation.	When deterioration and disintegration of nerve tissues is present the tissues become non-functional, and pain, impairment, and bizarre sensations occur. Tissue degeneration leads to autoimmunity
SOME ANTI-NEUROINFLAMMATION DRUGS	**SOME NEUROREGENERATIVE DRUGS**
Ketorolac, methylprednisolone, curcumin, metformin, acetazolamide, pentoxifylline	Nandrolone, human chorionic gonadotropin, dehydroepiandrosterone (DHEA), pregnenolone

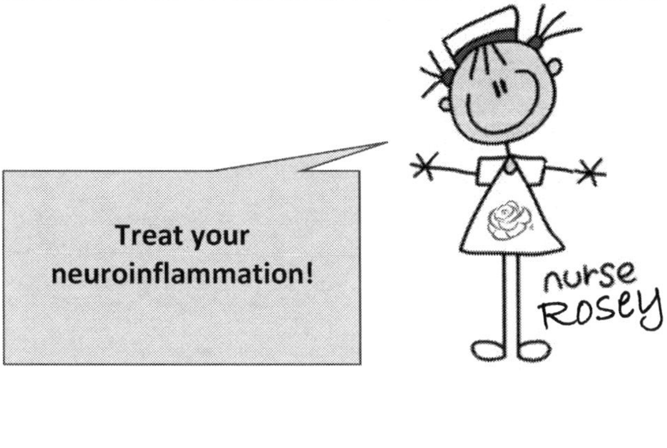

Pain relief drugs such as opioids, gabapentin, and devices such as electrical stimulators provide temporary symptomatic

relief. They do not provide long-term disease reduction which only occurs when anti-neuroinflammatory and neuroregenerative drugs are taken.

ASK YOURSELF: Are you taking drugs to suppress neuroinflammation and promote neuroregeneration? If not, you should start because otherwise you can't expect to control AA, much less achieve some permanent recovery.

20. SEVEN FACTS ABOUT NEUROINFLAMMATION (NI)

Fact 1: The fundamental cause of AA is neuroinflammation. It must be controlled or the person with AA will be in severe pain and will progressively deteriorate.

Fact 2: The term inflammation is a generic term that can apply to any tissue in the body due to any cause. Neuroinflammation is a specific and special type of inflammation caused by nerve cells called microglia, which are found in the spinal cord, brain, and nerve roots of the cauda equina.

Fact 3: Active neuroinflammation causes tissue destruction, adhesions, and fibrosis "scarring." This combination causes clumps or "hard lumps" inside the spinal canal so cerebral spinal fluid (CSF) flow is obstructed "blocked." CSF can also leak through the spinal canal covering into surrounding tissues causing further inflammation and damage. It may also progressively destroy cauda equina nerve root connections to your legs, bladder, sex organs, and bowel.

Fact 4: Neuroinflammation may be active, and will silently, without awareness by the person, destroy nerve tissue.

Fact 5: The drugs that suppress the inflammation of arthritis, allergies, and asthma may not suppress neuroinflammation. Why? To suppress neuroinflammation, a drug must cross the blood-brain barrier and bind or attach to the microglial cell. Consequently, the number of drugs, that suppress neuroinflammation are few.

Fact 6: If you have found that ketorolac (Toradol®), or one of these corticosteroids, methylprednisolone (Medrol®) or dexamethasone (Decadron®), provide pain and symptom relief, you have fundamentally demonstrated that you have active neuroinflammation that needs on-going treatment usually with one of these 2 agents.

Fact 7: Neuroinflammation may lead to autoimmune disorders that can manifest in other areas of the body. Some autoimmune manifestations are arthritis, thyroiditis, muscle pains, fatigue, and carpel tunnel syndrome.

The medical treatment suggested in this handbook cannot be guaranteed as far as outcome. By use of the 3-component medication program few persons in our experience worsen, because it is primarily geared toward suppression of neuroinflammation and promotion of neuroregeneration. Some people with AA have found a "near-cure" with the 3-component program. We are hesitant to use the term "cure" as neuroinflammation may remain asymptomatic and re-emerge later. Once AA is observed on an MRI, treatment must likely be a lifetime endeavor.

21. PHYSIOLOGIC TREATMENT MEASURES

Physiologic measures have 3 major goals:

1. Enhance spinal fluid flow
2. Reduce neuroinflammation,
3. Prevent tissue shrinkage and paralysis.

While it may not be necessary to do every measure, every person with AA should do some of the following every day.

- ✓ Walking with arm swings
- ✓ Water soaking, including foot baths
- ✓ Deep breathing and breath holding
- ✓ Rocking chair or swing
- ✓ Trampoline walking
- ✓ Stretching – side-to-side, arm and leg extension
- ✓ Magnet rubs
- ✓ Copper jewelry
- ✓ Sing or whistle

When our AA research and education project began 10 years ago it was common to see people with AA who had partial paralysis "paraparesis" of the legs and arms. In some cases, the paralysis was so bad that the person had to use a wheelchair or was confined to bed. Many people could not raise their arms or legs to their full extension. Unfortunately, about the only treatment these people ever had was pain medication. Until recently there was no knowledge about spinal fluid flow, leakage and seepage, tissue shrinking, and retained electricity. In recent years as treatment of neuroinflammation and specialized physiologic measures have

become known, we see few new people with AA who have paralysis of the legs and/or a diminution of arm extension.

<u>Here are reasons and some specific physiologic measures:</u>

<u>Increase Spinal Fluid Flow:</u> deep breathing, walking, stand and stretch arms, sing and/or whistle, rock in a rocking chair or swing, walk on a trampoline

<u>Prevention of Tissue Shrinkage and Scarring:</u> walking, side-to-side stretching, extend legs, arms, and feet

<u>Elimination of Inflammation and Electricity:</u> water soaking, foot baths, wearing copper jewelry, magnet rubs, massage

22. PREVENTIVE MEASURES TO "NOT GET WORSE"

The very criteria of an MRI diagnosis of AA means one has nerve clumping with adhesions. This indicates that there is already neuroinflammation and nerve damage <u>INSIDE</u> the spinal canal. When AA is seen on an MRI, goal number one is to "not get worse." Our recommended strategy for treatment of AA is two-fold: (1) medication; (2) physiologic and preventive measures. Here is a list of simple preventive measures for everyday practice to "not get worse."

1. Use bench type chairs/seats (avoid bucket type seats)
2. Posture – sit straight up and walk with head between shoulders.
3. Swing arms when walking

4. Supportive footwear. No thongs, open heel, or high heel shoes. Make sure sandals have heel/ankle straps.
5. Wear a copper bracelet or anklet
6. Deep breath a few times every couple of hours
7. Stretch arms, legs, and hips each day
8. Take walks twice a day
9. Soak in a tub of water. Daily is best. If no tub, jacuzzi, or pool, take a long shower
10. Use an electromagnetic or microcurrent electric device, 3 to 5 times a week (infrared, laser, radio wave)
11. Wear a brace when taking a long automobile or plane ride
12. Don't sit in one position for more than 45 minutes
13. Don't lift over 10-15 pounds
14. Don't exhaust yourself or do activities that cause pain
15. Raise hands above head and hold for a few seconds

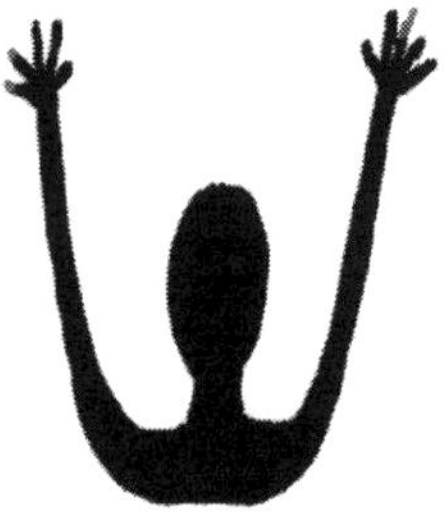

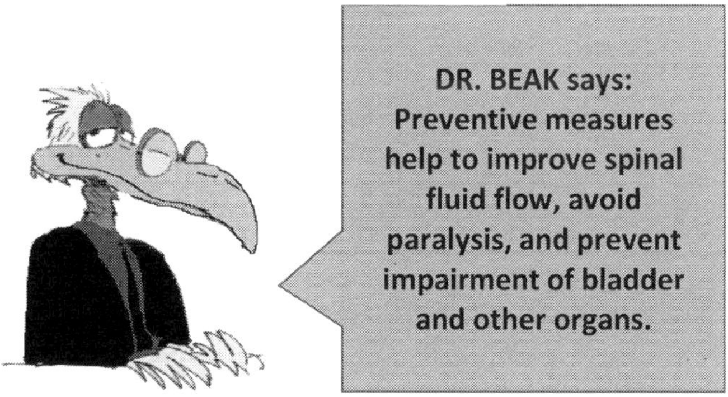

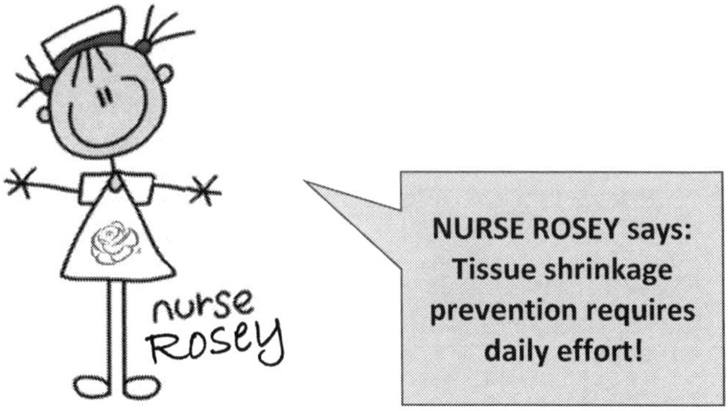

23. SPINAL FLUID – RIVER OF HOPE!!

Optimal function and movement of spinal fluid flow is critical to the relief and recovery of people with AA.

<u>How is it made?</u>

Spinal fluid is made from arterial blood in a structure in the brain called the choroid plexus. Cells with fine structure called cilia and micro-villi strain and produce CSF in the brain. About 125 ml of fluid is produced every 4 to 6 hours for a daily total of about 500 ml.

<u>How does it flow?</u>

Once made, spinal fluid travels like a river around the brain and down the spinal canal. Once it reaches the bottom (lumbar-sacral) area, it flows back up the spinal canal to be filtered by lymph nodes in the neck. Once impurities are removed in the lymph nodes, spinal fluid is pumped into the blood stream to be excreted out of the body by urination. Deep breathing and arm swings helps the spinal fluid flow.

What does spinal fluid do?

1. Carries nutrients and the body's natural healing elements to the brain, spinal cord and cauda equina nerve roots

2. Lubricates and protects the brain, spinal cord, and cauda equina from developing friction, neuroinflammation, and adhesions

3. Carries out toxins (e.g. inflammatory waste)

The clumping of nerve roots and the formation of adhesions cause disruption and obstruction of spinal fluid flow. This is like putting large rocks or a dam in a river – the water flow will slow down, back up, or reroute around the blockage.

When blockage occurs inside the spinal canal symptoms of headache, blurred vision, nausea, dizziness, mental confusion, loss of memory, ringing in ears, loss of balance, dysphoria (opposite of euphoria), vertigo and fatigue may occur.

One medication that often reduces the symptoms of spinal fluid flow obstruction is acetazolamide, given 50 to 500 mg a day. Our suggestion is to start at about 50 mg a day and work up the dosage to 250 mg a day over 2 weeks. Stop if it's not helping. Continue and even raise the dosage if acetazolamide helps. This drug also reduces neuroinflammation. Every person with AA should consider it.

The "rusty" seeping "pipe"

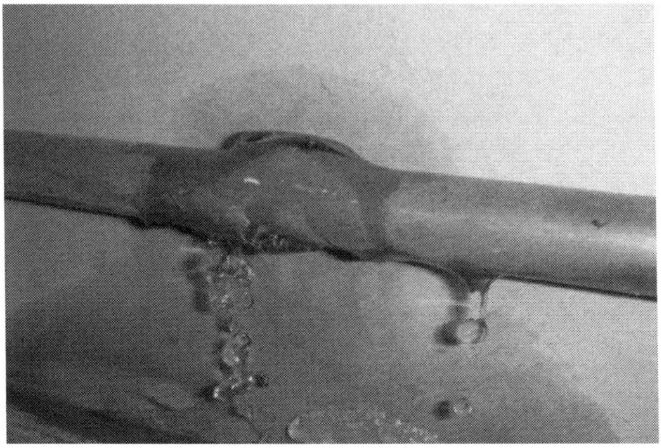

24. SPINAL FLUID LEAKAGE AND SEEPAGE

We have learned from MRI reviews and physical examinations most people with AA chronically leak or "seep" spinal fluid into the tissues between the lumbar spine area and skin over the area. The process resembles a pipe that rusts and chronically leaks or "seeps" fluids out of the pipe. Unfortunately, the formation of inflammation between the nerve roots and arachnoid lining may cause microleaks through the outer spinal canal covering.

The Problem

Spinal fluid is toxic to muscle, subcutaneous fat, and skin which is why spinal fluid is in a closed canal away from non-CNS tissue. The exposure of spinal fluid to the general circulation may also cause an autoimmune disorder.

Spinal fluid that leaks into the tissues between the spinal column and skin over the lumbar spine area is toxic to these

tissues. It will cause inflammation, scarring, and shrinkage of muscles, fascia, nerves and skin.

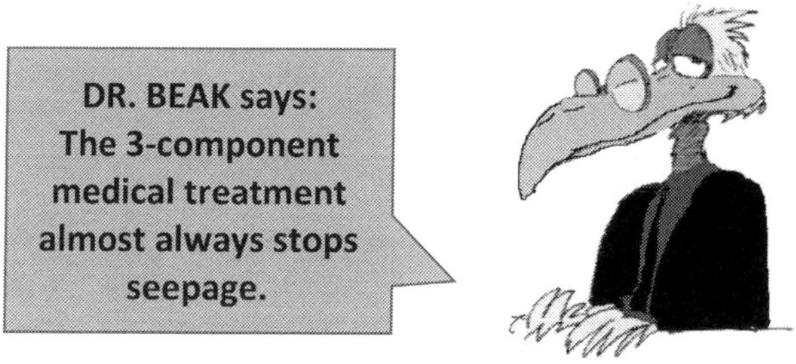

Symptoms and Complications

Pain and indentation of the skin along the spine may occur from leaking spinal fluid. A major complication is that muscles and nerves that run along the spinal column may shrink and decrease one's ability to fully extend the arms and legs.

Diagnosis

Active "seepage" is suspected if there is pain upon pressing on the skin and tissues over the lumbar spine. If a topical skin anesthetic such as lidocaine relieves pain, seepage is likely. Seepage evidence can be seen on MRI.

Over-time, these complications from spinal fluid seepage may occur:

1. Shrinkage of paraspinal muscles to the point that you can't fully extend your arms or legs.
2. Pain over the spine – worse when pressure is applied.
3. Abnormal, off-balance leaning – asymmetry of back muscles.
4. Indentation (caving in) of tissues over the spine.

25. HOW TO IMPROVE YOUR SPINAL FLUID FLOW

All people with AA will have some disruption or blockage of spinal fluid flow. Good spinal fluid flow is necessary to wash away waste products and bring nutrition and healing power to the inflamed site.

Here are simple physiologic measures to enhance spinal fluid flow. We recommend daily use of at least some of them.

- ✓ Rock in a rocking chair or swing
- ✓ Walk on a trampoline
- ✓ Use vibrator or massager over spine (Back scratchers and scrubbers are good)
- ✓ Soak or wade in water or use foot baths
- ✓ Walk and swing your arms "Power Walking"
- ✓ Rock back and forth on your feet
- ✓ Rub your spine with copper and/or a magnet
- ✓ Nod your head up and down
- ✓ Scrub your back with a brush
- ✓ Deep breathing (diaphragm) with stomach

26. TREATMENT OF SPINAL FLUID LEAKAGE AND SEEPAGE

If seepage is present it can almost always be seen on your MRI. Above all else, you need to be on a 3-component medical treatment program for AA:

1. Suppression of neuroinflammation
2. Promotion of neuroregenesis
3. Pain control

Here are some other measures used to stop spinal fluid leakage and seepage:

- Add an anti-inflammatory or neuroregenerative agent to the current treatment program
- Massage into the lumbar area a topical cream which contains a corticosteroid like prednisone.
- Inject a corticoid and/or homeopathic agent into the tissue around (not in) the spinal column.

SPECIAL NOTES

1. We believe spinal fluid leaks regularly stop with the anti-neuroinflammatory and neuroregeneration agents suggested in this handbook.

2. We do not recommend blood patches since they are for acute, and not the chronic leakage present in people with AA.

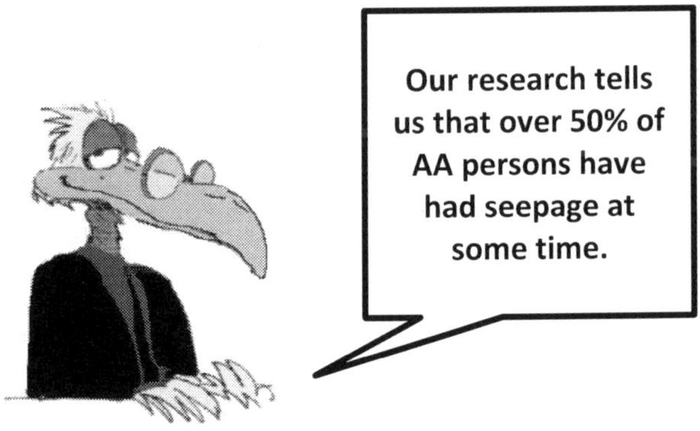

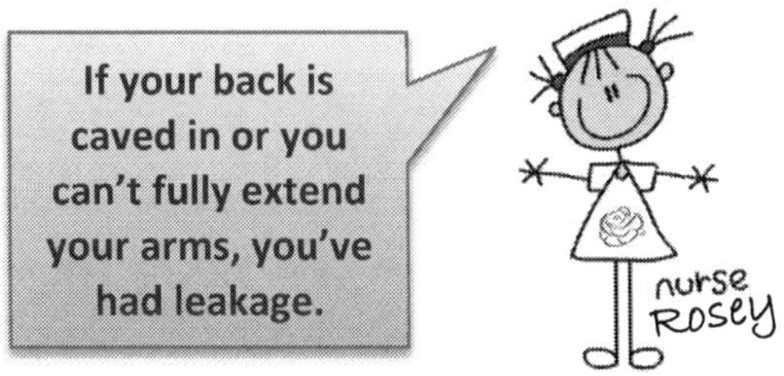

27. STRETCHES TO PREVENT TISSUE SHRINKAGE

Stretching Principals

1. Stretch to a point you feel tugging or pulling but not pain
2. Standing is best to stretch but sitting or lying down is OK
3. Stretch your arms and legs into positions that let you know you are tugging or pulling on your lumbar area

It is the shrinking, scarring, and shortening of nerves, muscle, and tendons that cause severe neurologic impairments such as partial paralysis "paraparesis." The nerve roots of the cauda equina are the first section of long nerves "e.g. sciatic nerve" that reach into your legs, feet, bladder, intestine, stomach, rectum/anus, and sex organs.

Muscles and tendons that attach to the vertebrae and joints can also shrink, particularly with chronic spinal fluid seepage.

Here are simple stretching exercises to prevent tissue shrinkage.

1 – Reach for the sky. Spread your fingers, raise both arms straight up. Hold for 5 to 10 seconds. Raise only as high as you can without causing pain.

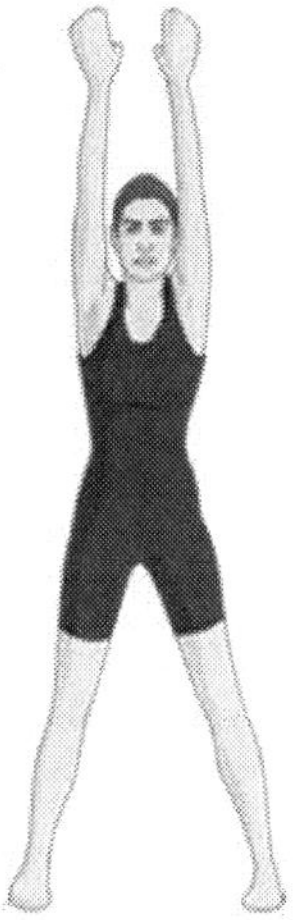

2 – Side to side bends. Stand with hands on head. Lean right for 5 to 10 seconds, then left for 5 to 10 seconds. Bend only right and left to feel a "tug" or "pressure" in your lower back, but not pain.

NURSE ROSEY says: These exercises help spinal fluid flow and prevent tissue shrinkage.

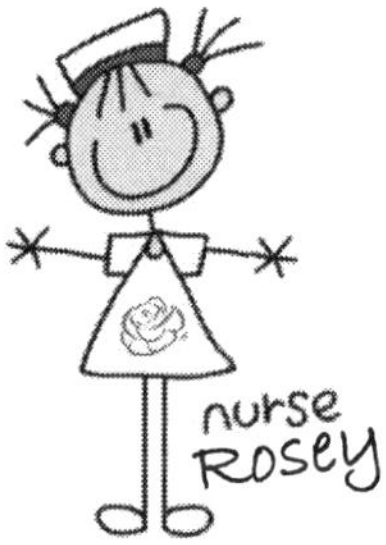

Other Helpful Stretching Exercises

Full-Body Stretch Laying Down: Lay down on a flat surface (if physically possible) and do a full-body stretch with arms over head. Count to 10.

Sit and Stretch Arms: Stretch your arms above your head and spread your fingers. Count to 10. Can do while sitting in a car or plane.

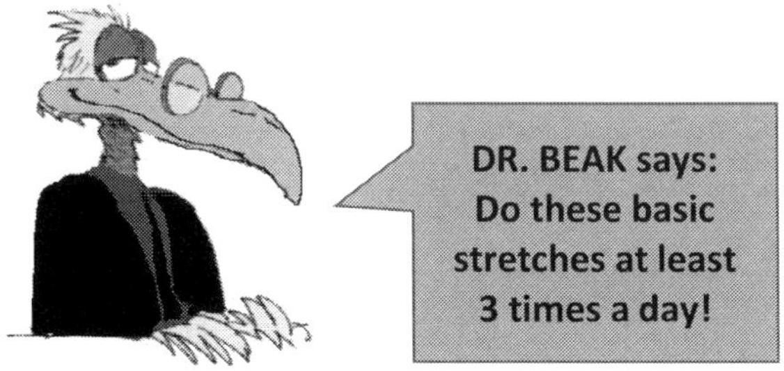

Leg Raise While Laying Down: Raise each leg until you feel tugging in your back. Count to 10.

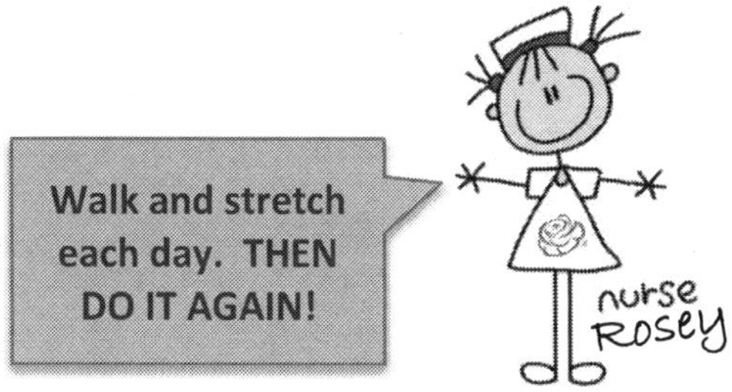

Leg Raise While Standing: Stabilize yourself next to a table or wall. Raise your leg and flex your foot. Count to 10.

Knee Pull While Laying Down: Pull one knee back until you feel tugging in your back. Count to 10. Repeat with the other knee.

28. WALKING WITH ARM SWINGS: THE BEST EXERCISE

A person with AA **must take walks every day** to move spinal fluid and prevent shrinking of nerves and muscles. Walk with toes pointed straight ahead. Swing your arms during part of your walk. Lift your head so that your ears are directly over your shoulders. Breathe deeply. Quit at the first feeling of fatigue. Don't overdo or push too hard.

People with AA should wear supportive, tie shoes such as tennis shoes unless tie shoes cause pain. There are also some shoes that have copper or magnets in the soles. These are excellent to help control pain.

Bare foot is often better for people with AA than the modern-day practice of wearing thongs, sandals, flip flops, or slip-ons. Non-supportive footwear is a risk in 2 ways: (1) falls; (2) prevents walking with correct posture.

One slip, slide, or fall can set a person with AA back to square one, or worse. A fall may tear adhesions, which may cause severe pain and when the injured tissue heals, can cause scar tissue to form with more permanent, nerve entrapments and impairments!

29. RETAINED ELECTRICITY – MUST ELIMINATE

Nerves function and control our body's organs and structures by transmitting electricity. With AA, nerve roots are clumped

with adhesions and scarring so electricity won't pass easily up or down the nerve root. Consequently, electricity is retained and accumulates.

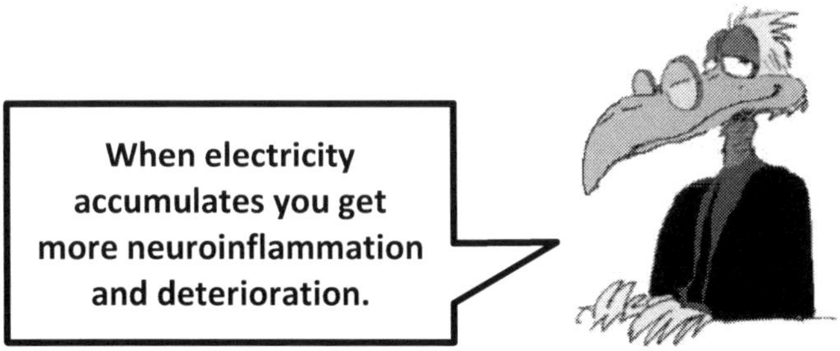

When electricity accumulates, it causes increased neuroinflammation and it may suddenly release itself in dysfunctional bursts. That is why a person with AA gets:

- ✓ Shooting and burning episodes of pain
- ✓ Leg jerks and tremors

Abnormal electricity retention and release also contributes to such symptoms as burning feet and funny sensations on skin such as "bugs crawling" and "water dripping."

Here are physiologic measures to eliminate electricity. Do some daily:

- ✓ Rub your spine with copper or a magnet 2 to 3 times a day
- ✓ Wear a copper anklet or bracelet
- ✓ Use magnets in your shoes or mattress
- ✓ Wear lots of jewelry, particularly copper
- ✓ Hold doorknobs or other metal a second longer
- ✓ Soak in water and foot baths (Epsom salts help)
- ✓ Pet your dog or cat (any animal's fur will do.)
- ✓ Walk barefoot on carpet, or outside on your lawn

30. YOU NEED MORE OXYGEN

Oxygen is necessary for healing, nerve function, and medication effectiveness. Without enough, you may progressively deteriorate.

Symptoms of Low Oxygen:

- fatigue and lethargy
- slow or forgetful thinking
- depression and feeling of hopelessness
- tired, but can't sleep
- pain medication works poorly
- deep sighing

How Do I Get Oxygen?

Oxygen is breathed in through your lungs and enters your blood stream to be carried throughout your body. Whether your pain site is in the spine, brain, joints, or muscles, you must have oxygen for pain relief and healing. The more oxygen, the better.

How Do I Get More Oxygen?

Your base oxygen intake and carrying capacity is what is in your blood when you are quietly sitting or lying down. Anytime you become active you breathe a little harder and deeper and your heart pumps a little faster, so you carry more oxygen in your blood. The healing and pain relief formula is simply to stay more active than what you are when you sit or lay down. Just increasing your breathing and heart rate will increase oxygen at your pain site.

1. Stay active! Walk every day.
2. Breathe as deeply as you can with your stomach (diaphragm) and hold it for a few seconds. Do it while sitting or standing. Do it in a car, church, or at home. Do this at least 10 times a day.

31. A NEW BREAKTHROUGH: ELECTROMAGNETIC ENERGY THERAPY

A new therapy that is gaining more and more supporters and advocates is electromagnetic energy (EME) therapy. We highly recommend it as we believe EME enhances the standard treatments of medicinal agents and physiologic measures.

Human beings are alive and functioning because cells metabolize and communicate with each other by electromagnetic energy (EME). EME is biologically ½ magnetism and ½ electricity, and the devices administer it in waves. Devices that "pulse" or administer the energy in "waves" are most effective.

EME Devices: There are 3 medical devices that administer EME in various wave lengths and frequency to obtain a clinical effect:

1. Radio waves that are deep, long waves of slow frequency (Provant®)
2. Infrared has shallow warm waves
3. Laser has deep, short, and hot waves of high frequency

Difference with Other Devices

- ✓ TENS and electrical stimulators provide pure electricity which may provide temporary pain relief. Microcurrents are particularly effective for pain relief
- ✓ Acupuncture –moves retained electricity, unblocks and opens energy channels to enhance healing

Benefits of EME

EME reduces inflammation, edema, and retained electricity; These devices have been shown to have considerable healing power unless the tissue is scarred and non-functional.

We believe EME devices are helpful to heal spinal fluid leakage and even promote neuroregeneration in some cases. At this point in time we recommend a one-month trial of EME to see if a positive clinical effect can be obtained. To date, about 2/3 of people with AA report a positive benefit in pain reduction and functional improvement. We also recommend electric devices. In summary, all people with AA should be on the 3-componant medication program accompanied by physiologic measures. Once in place, all people with AA should explore the use of EME and electrical devices.

32. THE IMPORTANCE OF SPINE BRACING

People with AA must be very cautious and careful while lifting, bending over, or walking in an unfamiliar area. If you attempt to lift something that weighs more than about 10-15 pounds, you run the risk of tearing adhesions or scars in and around your lower spinal canal. When you bend over, raise up slowly

because a jerk or rapid movement can cause a tear or rip. If this happens, severe pain follows, and the damaged area may end up being worse than ever.

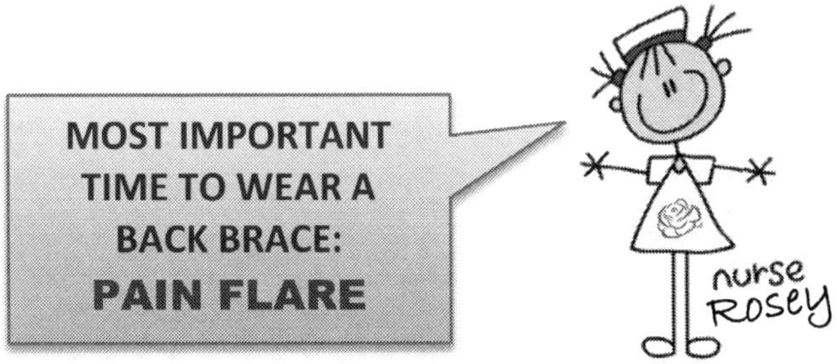

People with AA need to wear a brace to protect their damaged area in these circumstances.

Worst Situation: Riding in a car or plane that has bucket seats.

Danger Situation: Walking in unfamiliar areas such as a shopping center, grocery store, or social event.

33. DO YOU HAVE A GENETIC COLLAGEN DISORDER LIKE EHLERS-DANLOS SYNDROME (EDS)?

AA occurs frequently in persons who have a genetic collagen disorder of which Ehlers-Danlos Syndrome (EDS) and Marfan Syndrome are the most common. These genetic disorders have a built-in gene that prevents soft (non-bone) tissues from being formed properly. As a person grows into childhood and adulthood this gene defect causes tissue to be formed with faulty collagen, and tissues, progressively deteriorate, degenerate, and form micro-tears throughout the body.

Tissues most affected are those that are known as "connective" in that they support and connect such organs as the intestine, joints, skin, blood vessels, and spinal cord to bones and fibrous tissue. Fundamentally, the disorder causes tissue to stretch, loosen, and collapse due to the dissolution of collagen. Unfortunately, the spinal canal has many soft connective tissues like the pia mater and arachnoid. They may collapse and cause an array of spinal conditions such as Chiari malformations, Tarlov Cysts, tethered cord, syringomyelia, and AA.

<u>Test yourself with these questions to see if you may have a genetic collagen disorder.</u>

1. Has anyone in your family had Ehlers-Danlos Syndrome, Marfan Syndrome, or a ruptured organ or aneurysm?

2. Have you developed a sudden, without warning or trauma, a loss or impairment of a neurologic function such as being able to lift, flexing your arms and legs, urination, or had a ruptured organ or aneurysm?

3. Do you have soft, sensitive gums or, have you had multiple teeth totally deteriorate or fall out?

4. Have you developed a sudden, constant pain in one, or multiple places in your body without warning or trauma?

5. Do you have fallen arches, or extra flexibility of your hands or feet?

6. Can you now (or could you ever) do a forward bend and place your hands flat on the floor without bending your knees?

7. Can you now (or could you ever) bend your thumb to touch your forearm?

8. As a child did you amuse your friends by contorting your body into strange shapes or could you do the splits?

9. As a child or teenager did your shoulder or kneecap dislocate on more than one occasion?

10. Do you consider yourself double-jointed?

11. Does your skin easily break, tear, crack, or bruise?

If you answered yes to 4 or more of these questions, your physician should evaluate you for the presence of a genetic collagen disorder of which the best known are called "Ehlers-Danlos and Marfan Syndromes."

34. COLLAGEN BUILDING PROGRAM FOR PEOPLE WITH AA AND GCD

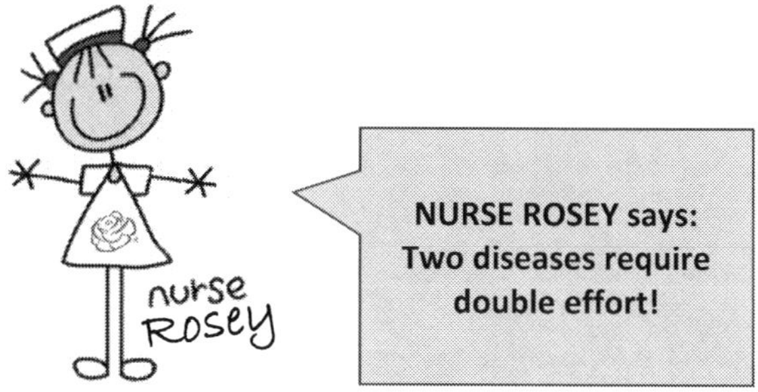

People with genetic collagen disorders (GCD), of which Ehlers-Danlos Syndrome
(EDS), and Marfan Syndromes are the best known, frequently develop AA and other neurologic complications such as Tarlov Cysts, Chiari malformations/herniations, tethered cord, and syringomyelia among others.

> Our research and experience are clear. When you have the dual diseases of AA and GCD, you must be treated with the 3-component medical protocol - **PLUS** – You must take measures to build collagen, **BOTH INSIDE AND OUTSIDE** of the CNS.

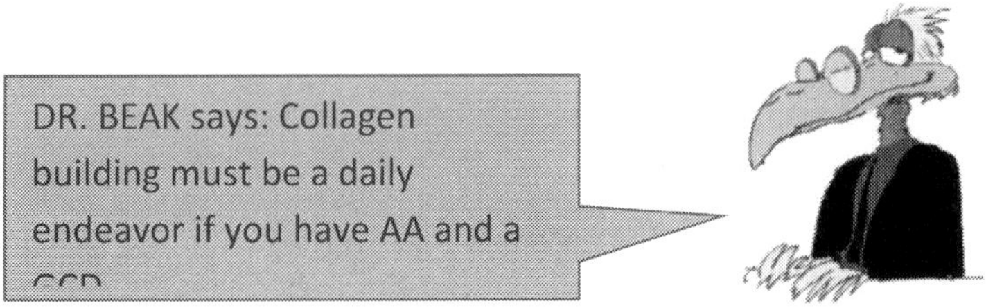

<u>RATIONALE:</u> Persons with GCD's are genetically programmed at birth to build faulty collagen which causes tissue to dissolve and break down easily in their "connective" tissues that hold organs in place. Some persons start to dissolve tissues in childhood and others in adulthood. Tissues in the spine, eye, gums, and brain such as the pia mater and arachnoid are made of collagen. A person with AA and a GCD must constantly attempt to build collagen to combat its dissolution.

<u>Here are our Collagen Building Measures for Dual Diseases</u>

DIET & DIETARY SUPPLEMENTS	EXERCISES	NON-PRESCRIPTION HORMONES	PRESCRIPTION HORMONES
High Protein Diet DIETARY SUPPLEMENTS Collagen (gummies, powder, liquid), Bone Broth, Vitamin B_{12}, Vitamin C, Magnesium	Light Weightlifting Walking Mild Stretching	Colostrum Gonadal Extract (Orchex®, or other) Deer Antler Velvet	Human Chorionic Gonadotropin: 250-500 units, 3 times a week and/or Nandrolone Troche: 25mg, 1 a day on 3-5 days a week or injection, 25-50mg, once a week

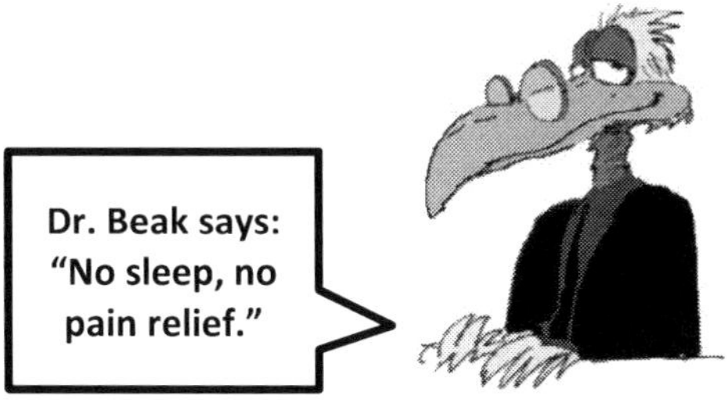

35. INSOMNIA AND SLEEP

A regular sleep pattern enhances the hormone and immunologic systems that are necessary for healing and neuroregeneration. Here are some guidelines:

- ✓ Be in bed between 10:00 and 11:30 PM
- ✓ Perform your last stretches and take your medications 30 to 60 minutes before bedtime

- ✓ Keep your pain medications beside your bed. Take additional dosages during the night, if necessary
- ✓ Take your first morning pain relief medications so you can be out of bed between 6:00 and 8:00 AM
- ✓ Goal is 4 to 8 sleeping hours each night. Do not expect more than four hours of consecutive sleep
- ✓ If a sleep aid is needed, we recommend clonidine, gabapentin, melatonin, valerian root, or temazepam

36. HIGH PROTEIN ANTI-INFLAMMATORY DIET

Our recommended diet is principally based on the physiological fact that amino acids and collagen build tissue. It is designed to help reduce neuroinflammation and promote healing.

Although much has been written and proclaimed about various diets for pain control, hard evidence that they really contribute is lacking. Our experience, however, is that people with AA who follow a high protein, anti-inflammatory diet, do better than the average person.

<u>THE DIET</u>

<u>Protein Food:</u> red meat, pork, poultry, fish, eggs, soy, dairy products, cottage cheese. If you can't or won't eat any of these, you must obtain protein powder drinks and/or protein bars.

<u>Collagen/Amino Acid Preparations:</u> To help build tissue take collagen or amino acid preparations every day. Collagen

gummies, capsules, liquid powder, amino acid capsules, liquid, powders. (See label for instructions.)

<u>Vegetables and Fruits:</u> Some vegetables and fruits have anti-inflammatory properties. Eat one or more of these each day.

Carrot	Celery	Avocado	Tomatoes
Broccoli	Onion	Dark Leafy Greens	Cucumbers
Radish	Berries	Apple	Citrus fruits
	Beets		

<u>Drinks:</u> (Only use dietary sugars if weight is a problem): Coffee, Tea, Dietary Drinks, Water, Low alcohol content drinks are acceptable.

<u>Banned to Control Weight</u>: milk, regular sodas, fruit juice, bread, pastries, pancakes, waffles, donuts

<u>Highly Restricted</u> (eat these very sparingly): potatoes, corn, cakes/pies, pasta/pizza, ice cream, whipping cream

<u>Gluten Restriction:</u> bread, pasta, rolls, noodles (For some, avoiding gluten helps digestion)

<u>Dietary Supplements:</u> Pick some for weekly use
Co-Enzyme Q-10
Omega 3 Fish Oil
Vitamins: C, D, B_{12}, B_6
Minerals: Calcium and Magnesium
Probiotic

37. INVERSION THERAPY

Inversion therapy (IT) is a form of super-stretching. It is usually done on a commercial stretcher. Some people with AA hang upside down as a therapy. The purpose of IT is to stretch out nerves, muscles, and tendons that have shrunk or are about to shrink. This is especially a problem with persons who have had spinal fluid leakage. It must be done gently and for only a short time (e.g. 3 to 5 minutes) to begin. Later, stretch time can be extended. Only some people with AA seem to benefit from IT. Those persons who can't fully extend their arms or legs are the best candidates. We only recommend IT for persons who are on a 3-component medication program. IT is an ancillary measure and not a primary treatment.

CAUTION: Only stretch to the point of pressure. NEVER cause pain because pain means you may be tearing tissue that may later scar, shrink, and produce even more pain.

DANGER: Not to be done by people with AA who have heart disease or GCD.

38. AUTOIMMUNITY WITH AA

It is known that neither spinal fluid nor spinal cord tissue should get outside the spinal canal. Why? They are toxic to the general circulation and may cause an autoimmune disorder if too much spinal fluid or tissue gets out. In AA, leakage or seepage of fluid into the tissues surrounding the spinal canal is a potential autoimmune trigger. So are tissue fragments from neuroinflammation that reach the general

circulation through the normal spinal fluid cleansing mechanism in the brain and lymph nodes in the neck.

The presence of an autoimmune disorder becomes known to the person and medical practitioner when the person with AA begins to develop aches and pains in joints and muscles which are anatomically far away from the lumbar spine. Some common autoimmune manifestations that may occur are Hashimoto's thyroiditis, carpal tunnel (and other nerve entrapments), temporal mandibular joint disease, and migraines. Food smell and medication sensitivities can develop. The most ominous sign of an out-of-control autoimmune disorder is tissue wasting, loss of appetite, weight loss, and susceptibility to infections. This "wasting" state calls for tissue building hormones such as testosterone, human chorionic gonadotropin (HCG), or nandrolone.

39. STEM CELLS, MICROSURGERY, AND OTHER NEW PROCEDURES

People with AA may be consistently bombarded with offers to try experimental or expensive procedures. While we are aware of anecdotal, positive results with some of these treatments, we are also aware of reports of no effect or even worsening of AA. We believe all people with AA must initially be treated with a medical program consisting of 3 components:

1. Suppression of neuroinflammation
2. Regrowth of damaged nerves (neuroregeneration)
3. Pain control

Once a person with AA is on a 3-component medical treatment, a trial of stem cells, microsurgery, or other expensive or high-risk techniques are options if the person knows the risk.

Before any person with AA attempts a medical treatment outside the 3 basic medical components of treatment, discuss it with your family, other people with AA, and your primary medical practitioner.

There is not a day that goes by that we don't get asked, "What do you think about this or that new treatment?" The most common inquiries today involve stem cells. Here is our current view.

Stem Cells: An exciting development. Many techniques are being used under this broad title. In addition to cells, some non-cellular substrates that mimic or activate your own stem cells (e.g. laminins, amniotic fluid) are being tried. To date we have received mixed (some good, some worthless) reports on effectiveness, but none have reported any harm from any of the various stem cell therapies. Also, we have not received enough positive reports to **highly** recommend the treatment.

Any person with AA who tries a stem cell treatment is on their own for expense, risk, and benefit as experience with stem cells is still very meager.

Microsurgery: Not recommended at this time.

40. THERAPEUTIC TRIALS – FIND OUT WHAT WORKS

No two people with AA will likely have the same precise medical program. You must find your own "suit of clothes." We recommend a trial of 10 to 20 days of most medications as this is a long enough period to find out if a medication will work. Essentially every medication in the 3-component medical protocol can be given a 10 to 20-day trial. After that time, you will know if the drug causes side-effects or has a positive effect on pain, function, energy, or well-being.

Therapeutic trials with ketorolac, methylprednisolone (Medrol®), or dexamethasone (Decadron®) are highly recommended as they indicate whether neuroinflammation is at a high or low level. If you do a trial with one of these drugs and you feel much better, continue it on a low, intermittent dosage on 2 to 3 days a week. If a drug produces no positive effects after 10-20 days, there is no reason to continue it.

Common questions we get are: (1) Do I have AA? (2) If I have it, what do I do now? and (3) Why has my pain control stopped working? A therapeutic trial is used to find answers to these questions. If you relate to one of the above 3 questions, you are a candidate for therapeutic trials with ketorolac (Toradol®) and methylprednisolone (Medrol®).

We have found that ketorolac (Toradol®) and methylprednisolone (Medrol®) to be the most consistent agents to control neuroinflammation and treat AA. Unfortunately, many doctors and people with AA have erroneously been led to believe that these two drugs are too dangerous to use. Any party who believes this should re-

evaluate their opinion due to new research and clinical experience.

RISK vs BENEFIT
The risk vs benefit of developing serious complications of untreated AA is greater than the risk of Toradol® and Medrol® if these 2 drugs are used as we suggest.

41. HOW TO SAFELY TAKE KETOROLAC AND METHYLPREDNISOLONE

Ketorolac Trial: Take an injection or troche of 30 to 60 mg on 2 consecutive days.

Safety Measures with Ketorolac (Toradol®)

a. Never use oral ketorolac (Toradol®)
b. Use ketorolac (Toradol®) as a compounded troche or as a commercially manufactured injection. Inject into buttocks.
c. Take blood urea nitrogen (BUN) and creatinine blood tests every 6 to 12 weeks if the person is high risk for kidney disease. High risk persons have diabetes, one kidney, or are over 70 years of age.

Methylprednisolone Trial: Take a 6-Day Dose Pak (Medrol® is the Trade Name)

Both ketorolac (Toradol®) (30 to 60 mg) and methylprednisolone (Medrol®) (2 to 4 mg) should only be

taken maximally on 2 to 3 days a week. On this basis the risk is limited. The key to safety is to skip days between dosages.

42. PAIN CONTROL

BE CLEARLY ADVISED. New research clearly shows that there are three types of pain you must treat, if you have constant "24/7" pain. This table lists the 3 types of pain, cause, and some treatment agents:

1. **NEUROINFLAMMATORY PAIN**	Due to inflammation in your cauda equina nerve roots and in the arachnoid lining of the spinal canal
Common treatment agents: ketorolac, Medrol®, acetazolamide, metformin, curcumin, indomethacin, low dose naltrexone (LDN), oxytocin, ketamine, opioids	
2. **NEUROPATHIC PAIN**	Due to nerve tissue (neurons, nerve roots, spinal cord) that has been damaged but is not inflamed
Common treatment agents: gabapentin, topiramate, clonazepam, carisoprodol, clonidine, diazepam	
3. **CENTRAL ELECTRICAL "Descending" PAIN**	Pain that is centralized and sends out aberrant electricity
Common treatment agents: Adderal®, methylphenidate, phentermine, modafinil, tizanidine	

43. BEST TREATMENT DRUGS FOR AA

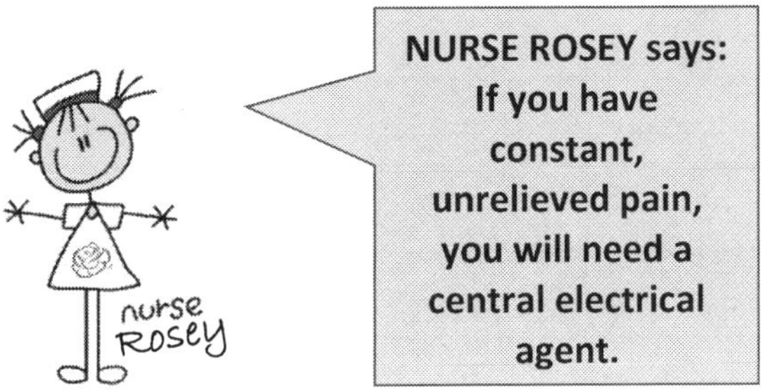

Our research has found 7 drugs to be the most consistently effective in controlling AA. They are listed here. Other drugs help many individuals, but these shown here have been consistently effective in about 70-80% of people with AA. You would be well-advised to show this list to your medical providers.

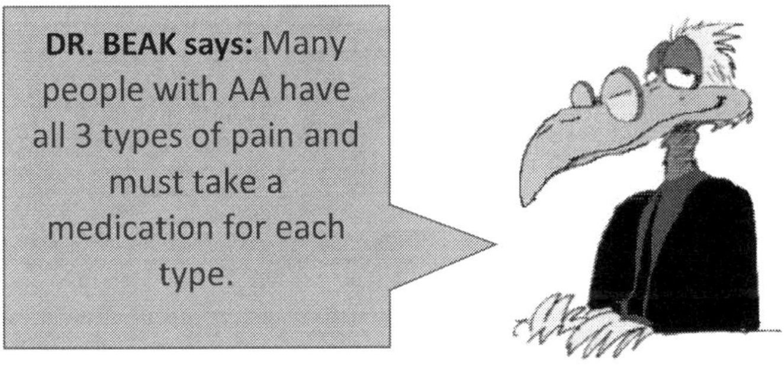

Most consistent drugs to date:

NEUROINFLAMMATION SUPPRESSORS
Low Dose Naltrexone
Ketorolac
Methylprednisolone
Dexamethasone
Acetazolamide
NERVE REGROWTH AGENTS “NEUROREGENERATION”
Human Chorionic Gonadotropin
Nandrolone

44. PROTOCOL FOR EMERGENCY TREATMENT OF SUSPECTED AA

Indication: A person who has these SYMPTOMS within about 60 days after an epidural injection, spinal tap, or spine surgery.
Lumbar pain, plus 2 of these symptoms:

1. Burning/painful feet
2. Bladder hesitancy/difficult to empty, can’t hold urine
3. Can’t sit or stand in one place over 10 minutes
4. Headache
5. Blurred vision
6. Leg pains

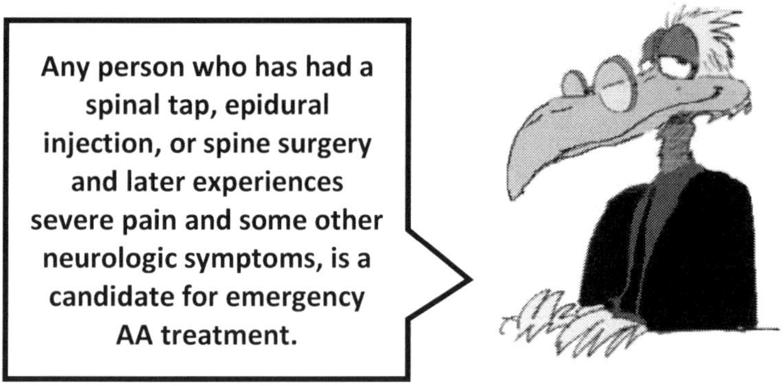

Treatment:

1. 6-day methylprednisolone, (Medrol®) dose pack
2. Ketorolac (Toradol®) – 30 – 60 mg injection, daily for 2 or 3 days

Interpretation

If the person's pain and some other symptoms improve during the treatment, a diagnosis of early AA, cauda equina inflammation, or other CNS neuroinflammatory process has essentially been established. If during, or at the end, of emergency treatment clinical improvement is apparent, we recommend the use of the 3-component medical protocol. If no improvement occurs, the logical conclusion is that pain and other symptoms are primarily non-inflammatory.

45. LOW DOSE NALTREXONE (LDN) FOR ADHESIVE ARACHNOIDITIS (AA)

About 75% of people with AA who have taken LDN have done well with it. Some people with AA in the mild and moderate categories even appear to be achieving almost a full recovery. Some are able to go about their pre-AA daily activities without much pain or impairment of body functions.

Why Does LDN Work?

Neuroinflammation is a major cause of pain. LDN is a potent neuroinflammation suppressor. LDN also activates the nervous system's pain centers that provide pain relief. You get two AA fighting actions with one drug.

Dosage

Dosage of LDN ranges from 0.5 to 5.0 mg a day. Most persons start at 0.5 or 1.0 mg and work up. Persons usually take LDN on 5 to 7 days a week. A compounding pharmacy can make LDN capsules, usually for a low monthly cost.

IMPORTANT TREATMENT LIMITATION
Persons on DAILY opioid drugs CANNOT take LDN, because it will cause withdrawal symptoms.

<u>Adding LDN to Your Current Treatment Protocol</u>

You can add LDN to your current protocol if you are not on opioids. (Some people on low dose opioids can also take LDN.) LDN can be taken with other anti-neuroinflammatory and neuroregeneration drugs including ketorolac, methylprednisolone, and all other non-opioid agents recommended in the 3-component protocol.

<u>Suggestion:</u> All people with AA NOT ON HIGH DOSE OPIOIDS should give LDN a 2 to 4-week trial. You will know in this time frame whether it is helping you. A few people can have increased pain or have other side effects with LDN and cannot take it.

46. DRUGS IN THE 3 MEDICATION COMPONENTS

Only a few drugs effectively suppress neuroinflammation, promote neuroregenesis (nerve regrowth), and control the pain of AA. Why? To be effective a drug must cross the blood brain barrier, enter the spinal fluid, and attach to receptors on cauda equina nerve roots and glial cells. Shown in the following table are drugs reported to us by people with AA to be effective.

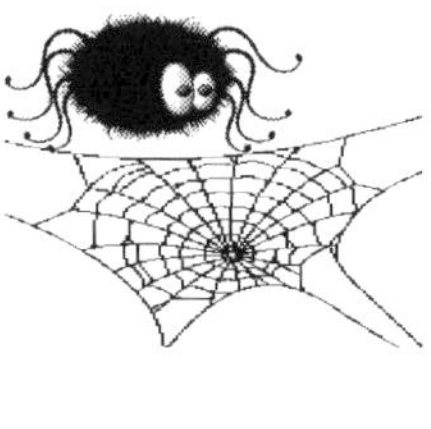

Happy Spider says: Non-Prescription drugs will boost your regular prescriptions drugs.

NURSE ROSEY says: Don't rely on only 1 or 2 components. You need 3!

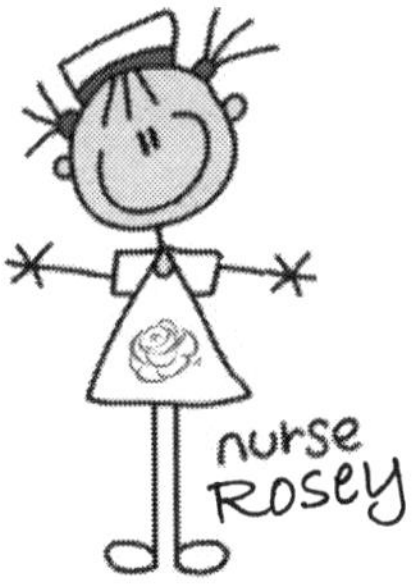

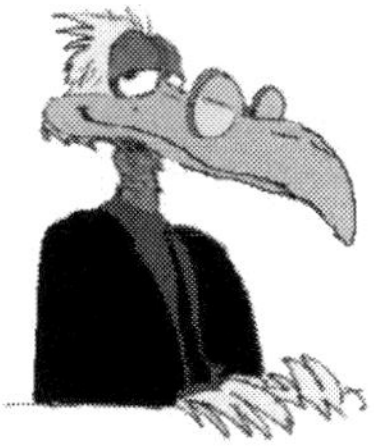

DR. BEAK says: To not get WORSE, you will need drugs from all 3 components.

COMPONENT NO 1	COMPONENT NO 2	COMPONENT NO 3
SUPRESSION OF NEUROINFLAMMATION	NEUROREGENERATION (RE-GROWTH OF DAMAGED NERVES)	PAIN CONTROL
Prescription drugs	**Prescription drugs**	**Prescription drugs**
methylprednisolone (Medrol®), ketorolac, dexamethasone, metformin, acetazolamide, minocycline, indomethacin	human chorionic gonadotropin, nandrolone, testosterone, medroxyprogesterone	**General Agents:** naltrexone, oxytocin, ketamine, opioids
		Nerve Damage: gabapentin, clonidine, topiramate, diazepam, carisoprodol, clonazepam, duloxetine, pregabalin

		Central/Electrical Agents: amphetamine salts (Adderall®), methylphenidate (Ritalin®), phentermine, modafinil, tizanidine
Non-Prescription Drugs	**Non-Prescription Drugs**	**Non-Prescription Drugs**
curcumin/turmeric, serrapeptase, adrenal extract	gonadal extract (Orchex®), deer antler velvet, colostrum, pregnenolone, DHEA	palmitoylethanolamide (PEA), cannabinoid oils (CBD), kratom, corydalis, valerian

47. PAIN FLARES

Every person with AA needs to be prepared for a pain flare. Don't kid yourself into thinking it won't happen. Most people with AA encounter an occasional, disabling flare. It's a little demoralizing, but flares occur without explanation. Don't blame yourself or the treatment that keeps you stable 90% of the time.

There are several options for flare treatment. We list some here as flare medication should be in your home ready to be used as soon as you know a flare is coming.

Here are some choices, but you may discover something better:

1. Ketorolac (Toradol®) injection 30-60 mg for 2 days with or without methylprednisolone (Medrol®) 20-30 mg
2. 6-Day methylprednisolone (Medrol® Dose Pak)
3. Suppository of hydromorphone 3 mg.
4. Suppositories of diazepam (Valium®) 5 to 10mg.

5. Patch of lidocaine, diclofenac or other.

48. SELF-HELP MEDICATION PROTOCOL

AA is a progressive neuroinflammatory disease. EVERY DAY that you delay treatment puts you at greater risk for increased pain, suffering, paralysis, bladder dysfunction, bed-bound state, and early demise. Too many people with AA are looking and waiting for a doctor to treat them. While waiting you must get started with treatment yourself.

Take at least one (two is usually better) of the non-prescription drugs listed in each component. These are available in health food stores or on the internet. Follow the dosage on the label except for pregnenolone and DHEA. The dosage for these hormones is listed here:

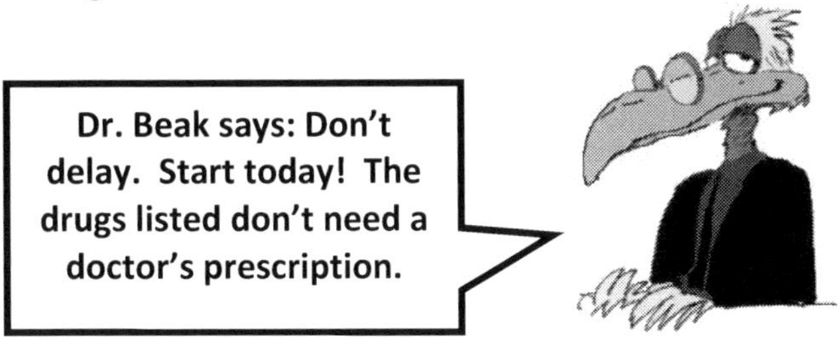

UPPRESSION OF NEUROINFLAMMATION	PROMOTION OF NEUROREGENERATION	CONTROL OF PAIN
Curcumin/Turmeric Serrapeptase Bovine Adrenal Extract	Pregnenolone and/or DHEA *Start pregnenolone or DHEA at 50 mg a day and increase slowly as tolerated up to 200 to 400 mg a day.* Colostrum Collagen Preparations *(Gummies, Capsules, Liquid)* Gonadal Extract (Orchex®) Deer Antler Velvet	CBD Oil Kratom Palmitoylethanolamide (PEA) Corydalis

Start Today! The drugs listed here do not need a doctor's prescription. You can take non-prescription drugs with prescription drugs. Don't delay!

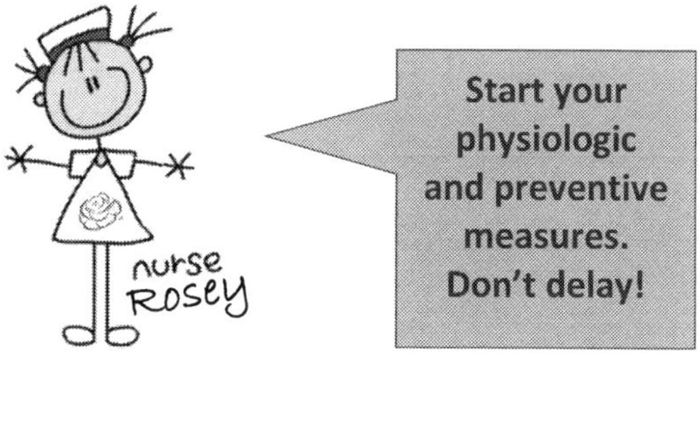

49. NEED FOR A COMPOUNDING PHARMACY

Compared to hypertension and asthma, AA is a "rare" disease. Because of this proper treatment will require some unusual medications. "Unusual" means a medication that isn't commercially available in most drug stores.

Listed here are compounded medications which are now regularly used by AA persons:

1. Ketorolac: 15, 30, or 60 mg – troche
2. Oxytocin: 40 or 80 units – troche or sublingual tablet
3. Ketamine: 25 or 50 mg per ml sublingual liquid or troche
4. Nandrolone: 25 to 50 mg troche, or injection
5. Human Chorionic Gonadotropin (HCG): 250 to 500 units - troche, sublingual tablet, or injection
6. Low Dose Naltrexone (LDN): .5 to 2 mg capsule
7. Diazepam (Valium®) suppositories 5-10mg

Every person with AA should take this list to their local compound pharmacy and determine their cost and capability to make the above compounded medications.

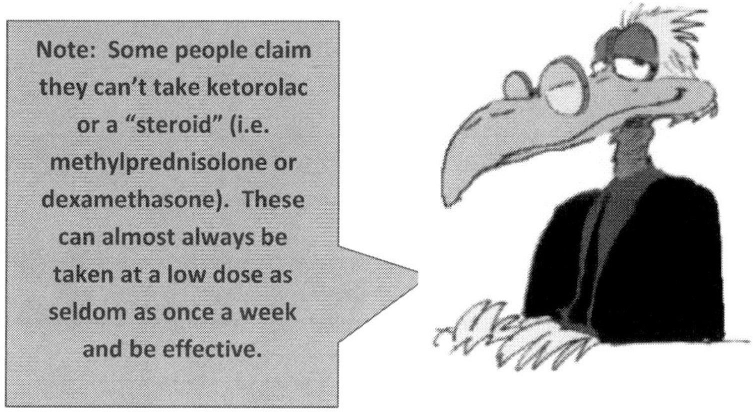

50. I'M GETTING WORSE, WHAT DO I DO?

In our experience almost every person with AA who is progressively getting worse is only using symptomatic drugs for pain relief and not taking the drugs that suppress neuroinflammation or regenerate damaged nerves. Keep this key point always in mind. AA is a neuroinflammatory disease of the lumbar-sacral nerve roots and arachnoid covering of the spinal canal which may progressively destroy additional tissue. Worsening simply means you are neither suppressing neuroinflammation nor regrowing damaged nerve tissue.

Follow These Steps:

1. Review the drugs that are in each of the 3 treatment components: (1) neuroinflammation suppression; (2) neuroregeneration; and (3) pain control. If you are not taking at least 1 drug in each component, you can expect to get worse.
2. Review the physiologic measures in this handbook which involves, spinal fluid flow, oxygen level,

electricity retention, and tissue shrinkage prevention. Are you walking and doing other physiologic measures each day? How are your hormone levels? Have your medical practitioner do a blood test for these hormones and replenish any that are low: cortisol, DHEA, estradiol, pregnenolone, progesterone, testosterone.

3. We have found only 7 drugs to be consistently effective in controlling AA: ketorolac (Toradol®), methylprednisolone (Medrol®), dexamethasone, acetazolamide, low dose naltrexone (LDN), human chorionic gonadotropin (HCG), and nandrolone. If you are not taking at least 2 of these 7, we believe you may get worse. Find out which ones your medical practitioner will prescribe.
4. If you feel your pain is worse, review the agents for pain control in this handbook. If you have constant pain, you may need a central electrical agent such as amphetamine salts (Adderal®). If you can only get a limited supply of opioids, take one or two of these non-prescription pain relievers: palmitoylethanolamide (PEA), cannabinoid oil (CBD), kratom, corydalis. Take them simultaneously with your opioid and/or between opioid dosages.

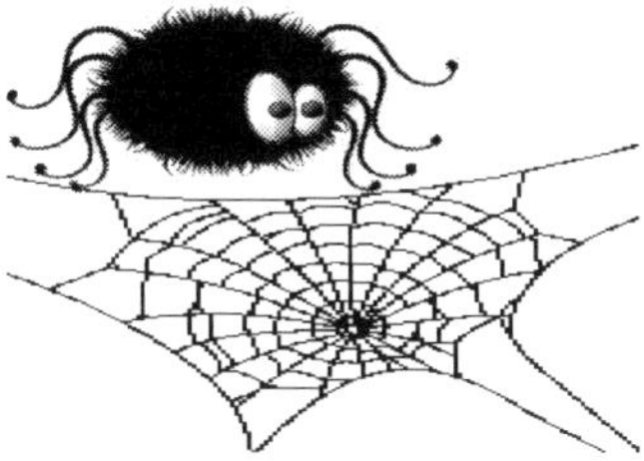

Happy Spider says:
If your doctor won't
help, look for a new one!

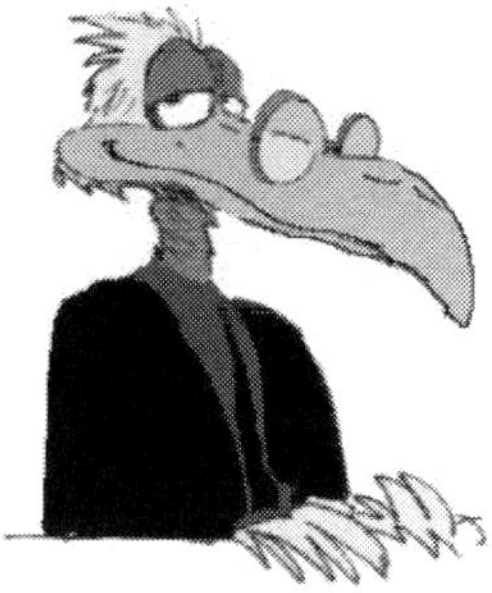

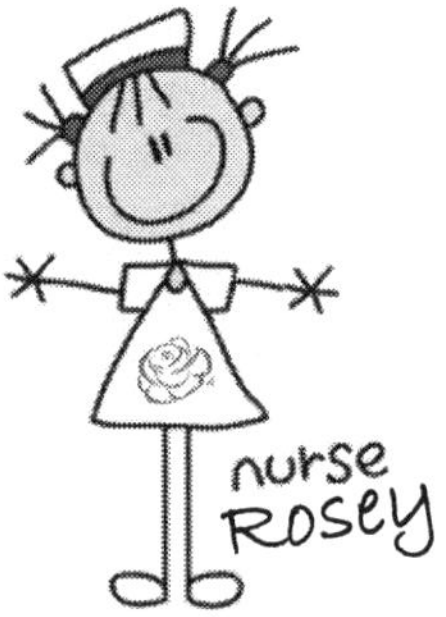

51. PSYCHOLOGICAL TREATMENT AND SUPPORT

AA is a frightening disease as it carries a high risk of severe disability, pain, misery, and a shortened life. It can also produce depression and loss of mental capacity.

Today there are psychologists who specialize in pain matters. They can often help you find comfort and peace. Mainly, they may be able to help you put together a game plan on how you are going to accomplish your therapeutic goals and simultaneously cope and maintain the other aspects of your

life. Don't settle for any old therapist. Seek out only those that understand AA and constant, incurable pain.

52. SUPPORT GROUPS AND PARTNERS

Every person with AA needs to have a partner or buddy who has AA. It may take a while but find at least one other person with AA with whom you can share your goals, fears, and hopes. Today, thanks to computer technology, you can find social media group members who have AA. Your partner or buddy may be someone you find online. Our caution about groups and partners is negativism. Find people and groups who are positive about life and AA treatment potential.

53. YOUR FAMILY AND YOUR RELIGION

Too many people with AA feel ashamed and isolated. They even feel they are somehow to be blamed or even cursed by the devil. Get rid of these false beliefs. If you're lucky enough to have a loving spouse, share all. Next best is a family member you love and trust. People close to you need to know you have a serious disease of the spinal cord. This is as important as your physicians and medical help.

We highly recommend you have a clergyman with whom you can discuss your case. Whatever your religion and beliefs, please become better acquainted with your spiritual advisor. This handbook's goal is to give you the best guidance we can give. Be clearly advised; We have seen that deep religious and spiritual beliefs sometimes bring about healing, comfort, and well-being beyond our medical treatments and expectations.

54. WHEN AN ELECTRICAL STIMULATOR OR SPINAL CANAL INFUSION DEVICE ARE NEEDED

The physiologic measures and 3-component medical treatment described in this handbook have been developed over the past 10 years. Thanks to this research and development, fewer and fewer people with AA are ending up in the severe and catastrophic categories. People with AA who have had their disease over 5 years and who have not had the benefits of either physiologic measures or the 3-component medical treatment may have so much nerve root adhesion, entrapment, damage, and scarring that pain cannot be relieved by the use of the medicinal agents described in this handbook. Another disabling factor in long-term, untreated people with AA is the additional pain caused by autoimmunity. In these situations, a trial with an implanted electrical stimulator and/or spinal canal (intrathecal) infusion device is warranted.

People with AA who possibly might need high dose opioid therapy may need to have it administered by injection, sublingual formulation, or by infusion directly into the spinal canal. A special implanted device is necessary to administer opioids directly into the spinal fluid. Those devices are often called "intrathecal pumps."

It is critical to understand that implanted electrical stimulators and high dose opioids are only symptomatic pain relievers that enhance physiologic functions and ease of movement for activities of daily living. With meaningful pain control people experience a better quality of life. They do not stop or slow

the progression of AA. It is, therefore, critical that the medical components of neuroinflammation suppression and neuroregeneration be simultaneously administered with an implanted electrical stimulator and/or high dose opioid therapy given by injection, sublingual formulations, or intraspinal administration. The physiologic and preventive measures described in this handbook should also be continued.

55. EPIDURAL CORTICOSTEROID INJECTIONS AND SPINAL TAPS

Once a person has developed AA, an injection of any sort that goes into the epidural space or the spinal canal is not recommended except in lifesaving situations. The reason here is more intuitive than based on any scientific data. Here is our logic. AA is a neuroinflammatory disease of the nerve roots in the cauda equina and the arachnoid covering of the spinal canal. Since neuroinflammation is present, it seems logical that any chemical intrusion or trauma might aggravate or cause more neuroinflammation. It is also now known that there are micro-conduits between the epidural space and the interior of the spinal canal. This is how chemicals injected into the epidural space may enter the spinal fluid.

If a person who has AA wants to try an epidural corticosteroid injection, our recommendation is that the person, family, and physician be aware and acknowledge that there is an unknown risk as to whether AA may worsen with the procedure.

Spinal taps also carry a risk to the person with AA, since the needle must penetrate the arachnoid lining. In our opinion, they should only be done in the case of a life-threatening emergency in people with AA.

56. INFUSIONS OF LIDOCAINE, KETAMINE, AND VITAMIN C

As this handbook is being written, we are receiving more and more positive feedback on intravenous infusions of lidocaine, Vitamin C, and ketamine. They don't work for every person, but they are often providing about 1 to 3 months of comfort and reduced pain in many people with AA. The best news is that reports of side-effects are minimal. In other words, the benefits seem to outweigh the risks. Although the future may change our mind, we currently recommend these infusions to AA persons who are already on a 3-component medical program along with physiologic and preventive measures. Also, our research and education project are encouraging medical providers to provide intravenous infusions as positive ancillary measures to people with AA.

57. GENETIC PREDISPOSING SUSCEPTIBILITY TO AA

There is now the belief among some medical practitioners and that some people are more susceptible to developing AA after an epidural injection, spinal tap, or trauma including surgery. Certainly, people with a genetic collagen disorder are susceptible and should consider avoiding any and all trauma in

and around the spinal canal such as an epidural injection and surgery. People who have an autoimmune disorder such as psoriasis or systemic lupus erythematosus may also be susceptible. This is an area of research and people with these conditions should be aware that they may have a genetic susceptibility to AA.

58. NO DOCTOR WILL HELP ME

Keep looking. Don't forget that almost every community has nurse practitioners (NP) and/or physician assistants (PA) who can prescribe medications. Oftentimes the NP's and PA's are more interested in assisting those with long-term illnesses, such as, AA than many MD's.

We are much better off today relative to physician access than we were 2 years ago. There is more and more awareness that AA is in every community and that it must be treated.

While looking for medical help, start the self-help medical protocol and physiologic measures provided in this handbook. It is intentionally designed with all non-prescription medications. It may even suffice for some mild cases. The self-help protocol may go a long way toward slowing or stopping the disease of AA until you can obtain more potent prescription drugs.

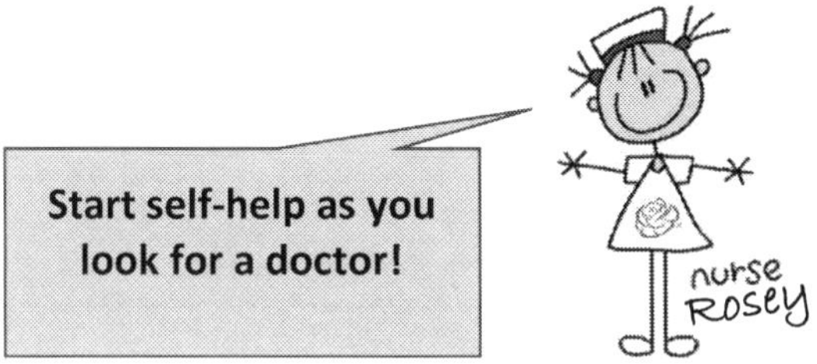

When you go to a doctor, bring written materials about AA and documentation that you have AA. Tell him or her that you have most of the 4 cardinal symptoms: (1) pain that improves when reclining or positional change; (2) bladder impairment; (3) feeling of water or bugs on your legs; and (4) burning feet. Know ahead of time what your insurance will pay for and where you can obtain supplies. Know which compounding pharmacy can make any supplies that are not carried by a standard pharmacy. Ask other people with AA about which doctor to seek out. Be prepared to travel some distance to a knowledgeable doctor. Be prepared to tell a medical practitioner which drugs you want to try and that you know the risks and benefit of treatment.

59. THE 21 DAY RULE

Each person with AA must develop their own medication program with the help of their medical provider. We strongly advise a 3-component medication approach as described in this handbook. We present several agents in each component that we believe to be effective in some people with AA. You will have to try different medications to build an effective program. Which ones you end up with depend on multiple factors including allergy, side-effects, and cost.

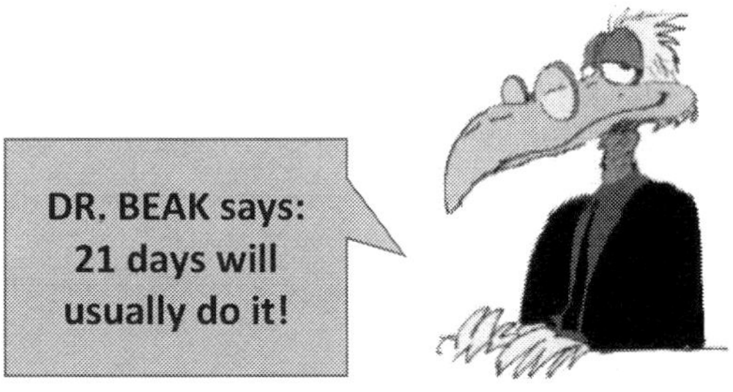

As you try different medications and dosages, we recommend the 21-day rule. Take any new medication for 21 days. If you can't tell an improvement in pain control, energy, motivation, comfort, or mental ability, stop the medication. Don't keep taking a medication that you are unsure about, because one medication may render another one to be ineffective.

When you stop a medication, sometimes you feel worse and realize the medication was helping. In this case just restart the medication with the knowledge of your medical provider.

60. HOW TO DEAL WITH OPIOID RESTRICTIONS

Opioid prescribing restrictions and poor availability of opioids is now standard. Each state is slightly different. There is a maximal amount of daily opioid medication recommended by the United States Centers for Disease Control and Prevention (CDC). They recommend a daily 90 mg limit called a morphine milligram equivalence (MME). Physicians can prescribe higher levels if they justify the need. However, physicians must limit their opioid prescribing to comply with their state and local restrictions. Some physicians are also restricted by their malpractice carrier or employer. The federal government and state pharmacy boards are progressively limiting supplies in pharmacies. Some veteran's hospitals have essentially banned opioids.

From a practical standpoint, we recommend that every person with AA pick a strategy to find relief with zero or limited amounts of opioids. A federal 90 mg morphine equivalence table is given here to provide a rough idea as to the maximal

amount of daily opioid that can be prescribed in most locations.

MAXIMAL DAILY OPIOID DOSAGES ALLOWED	
Approx. Oral Doses a Day	**OPIOID (Oral or Patch)**
8-9	Morphine – 10 mg
3-4	Methadone – 10 mg
8-9	Hydrocodone/APAP – 10/325 mg (Vicodin®, Norco®)
3	Morphine – 30 mg
6	Oxycodone/APAP – 10/325 mg (Percocet®)
5	Hydromorphone – 4 mg (Dilaudid®)
2-3	Hydromorphone – 8 mg (Dilaudid®)
6	Oxycodone Plain – 10 mg
2-3	Oxycodone Plain – 20 mg
2	Oxycodone Plain – 30 mg
16-20	Codeine 30 mg
8-10	Codeine 60 mg
16-18	Tramadol 50 mg
8-9	Tramadol 100 mg
1	Fentanyl Patch – 25 mcg per hour
1	Fentanyl Patch – 50 mcg per hour is 120 mg of morphine equivalence
	OPIOID INJECTIONS
2-4	Hydromorphone 50 mg/ml, .05 to .1 ml (2.5 to 5 mg)
3-4	Fentanyl 1000 mcg/ml, 0.1 ml (100 mcg) sub cu per injection
8-9	Morphine 10 mg per injection
3-4	Meperidine (Demerol®) 50-100 mg per injection
• **This table is based on recommendations of the Federal Centers for Medicare and Medicaid.**	
• **If a person wishes, they can take 2 opioids, each at half the maximal number a day which is listed above.**	

61. THREE STRATEGIES TO DEAL WITH OPIOID RESTRICTION

Here are 3 strategies to deal with the limited availability of opioids. If you are unable to get the amounts of opioids you would like, review these 3 strategies and select one.

Strategy No. 1 – Comprehensive, Symptomatic Pain Relief

Take one or more pain reliever from each of the 6 categories listed here. Many people on prescription opioids prescribed by their doctor don't use a comprehensive pain control program and rely solely on opioids.

1. Opioid – hydrocodone, oxycodone, morphine, hydromorphone, tapentadol
2. Non-opioid Pain Relievers – ketamine, oxytocin, corydalis, CBD oil, PEA, kratom, valerian
3. Neuropathic (injured nerve) – gabapentin, topiramate, carisoprodol, diazepam
4. Electrical/Central/Descending – amphetamine, methylphenidate, phentermine, modafinil, tizanidine
5. Bedtime Aid/Pain Reliever – clonidine, gabapentin
6. Topical/Skin – Lidocaine patch or gel

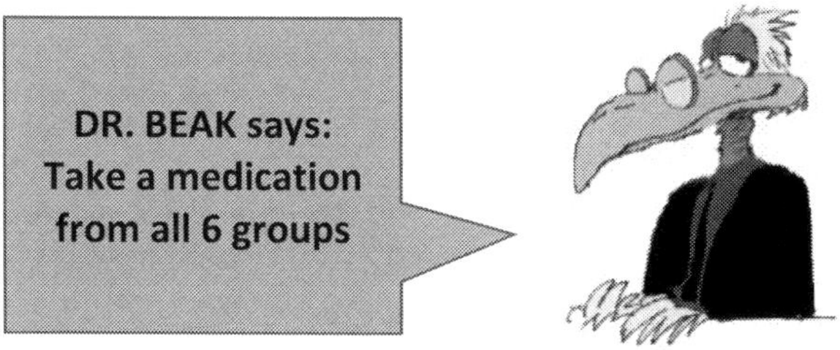

Strategy No. 2 – Potentiate or "Boost" Opioid Effectiveness for Maximal Pain Relief

Take agents that boost opioid power. Take your opioid on a regular, same time each day basis, such as every 4 to 6 hours. Take a potentiator or booster simultaneously with your opioid and between opioid dosages. Example: Take hydrocodone with corydalis. One or two hours later, take another dose of corydalis.

Potentiator or boosting agents: corydalis, CBD products, kratom, palmitoylethanolamide (PEA), ketamine, oxytocin

Strategy No. 3 – Treat Underlying Cause of Pain (AA)

We have found that the most effective way to reduce opioid dosage is to vigorously treat AA with a 3-component medication program plus physiologic measures.

Anti-Neuroinflammatory Agents - Examples

1. Ketorolac (Toradol®) – 2 to 3 days a week
2. Methylprednisolone (Medrol®) or dexamethasone – 3 days a week
3. Acetazolamide – 5 days a week

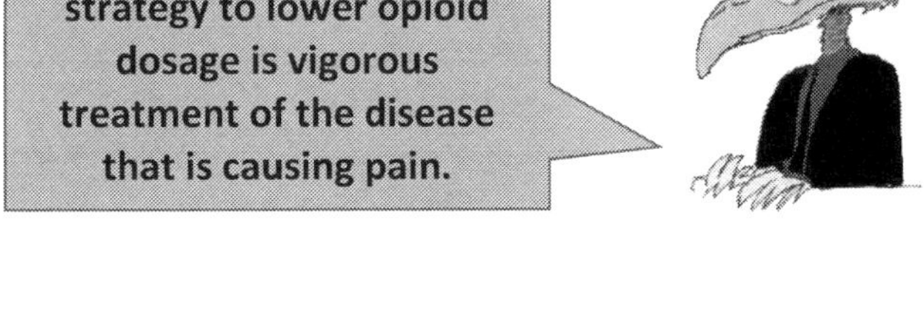

Neuroregenerative Agents - Examples

1. Pregnenolone and/or DHEA 200 to 300 mg 2-3 times a week
2. Nandrolone troche– 25 mg on 3 to 5 days a week
3. Human Chorionic Gonadotropin (HCG) – 500 units on 3 days a week

For all 3 strategies, replenish any of these hormones that are deficient in the blood: pregnenolone, DHEA, testosterone.

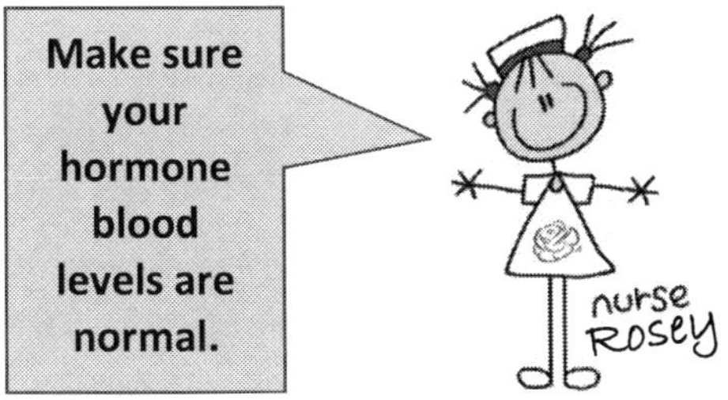

SPECIAL NOTE: Parts of all 3 strategies may be more effective than one alone.

62. DEALING WITH THE FEAR OF HORMONES

The American public and the average doctor has become unduly afraid of hormones. This has been brought about by incessant, negative propaganda about their possible complications. Vested financial interests have grossly overblown the cases of estrogen or testosterone

administration that caused breast, uterine, or testicular cancer. The term “steroid” has become a synonymous term with cortisone, when it is the chemical structure that is the basis of almost all hormones that are made by the body.

Those of us who constantly work with hormones know precisely why vested pharmacologic interests have done their best to keep people and practitioners away from hormones. They simply are very effective in both prevention and treatment of many medical conditions. We consider the use of some hormones, or their synthetic derivatives, to be essential in the treatment of AA.

Be advised. The frightening reports about cancer, bone degeneration (osteoporosis), and impotence with hormones were all based on persons who took high dosages of a hormone on a regular, daily basis. No wonder complications occurred. Check it out. Hormones for AA including corticoids are taken in low or modest dosages on only some days each week or month. Hormone complications are best avoided by using them on a low dosage intermittent basis.

We describe here some of the hormones you will need, in our experience, to slow or stop progression of your disease and find some relief and recovery. First, some cortisone derivatives are the most potent suppressors of neuroinflammation. The most effective are methylprednisolone (Medrol®) and dexamethasone (Decadron®). People with AA can take a low oral dosage of either hormone on 2 or 3 days a week. Some people take an injection of methylprednisolone (Medrol®) 1 to 4 times a month (e.g. weekly). A Medrol® six-day dosage package is a good flare or emergency treatment.

A recent research discovery has found that the spinal cord and brain make some specific hormones which are called neurosteroids. Their function is to protect nerve cells from inflammation and regrow damaged cells (neuroregeneration). These hormones include pregnenolone, DHEA, progesterone, and estradiol. Although these neurosteroids are in an early stage of clinical use, we find them to be useful for people with AA. We recommend a blood test to see if any are depleted and need replenishment. Each can be given as a 21-day trial.

There are now some hormone products that people with AA can obtain without a prescription. In case you can't find a doctor, who will prescribe hormones, you should obtain one or more of the non-prescription hormonal agents. These include adrenal and gonadal extracts, colostrum, and deer antler velvet. Neither pregnenolone nor DHEA require a prescription. The dosage is 200 to 300 mg taken at one time on 3 to 5 days a week.

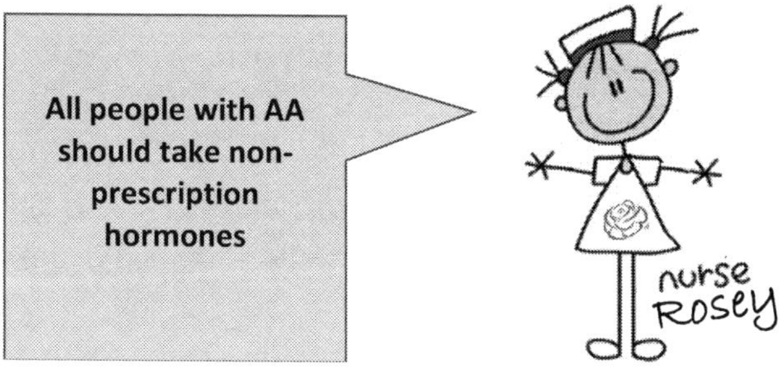

63. HUMAN CHORIONIC GONADOTROPIN (HCG) AND NANDROLONE

These 2 hormonal agents are proving to be essential for some people with AA. HCG is the hormone whose natural function is to grow brain, spinal cord, skin, nails, and hair "ectoderm"

tissue in the embryo. In the adult, its function is to maintain hormone levels of thyroid, progesterone, estradiol, and testosterone and regrow any damaged nerve tissue. Studies in laboratory animals show it can regenerate spinal cord tissue. Unfortunately, HCG has some prohibitive expense and availability for people with AA. Except for persons in the mild category, we recommend it as an injection, sublingual solution, or troche. Dosage is 250 to 500 units taken 2 to 5 times a week. We have observed some remarkable results including the elimination of paralysis and the reduction of pain great enough that opioids were no longer needed. Once people with AA have stabilized on some anti-neuroinflammation and pain control medication, we recommend a 3-month trial of HCG. Side-effects are rare but may include acne and hair loss. If this occurs the dosage should be lowered. HCG can be stopped for a period and alternated with another hormone. We are aware of people with AA who have taken HCG for over 5 years and continue to recover. All people with AA are highly encouraged to locate a supplier and work with family, insurance carrier, or other party to finance a 3-month trial.

Nandrolone is a synthetic testosterone derivative approved by the US Food and Drug Administration (FDA) for regeneration of tissue in wasting states caused by a severe disease. AA qualifies. It will regenerate nerve, muscle, and other soft (non-bone) tissue. Although available as an expensive injectable compound, it can be made into a relatively inexpensive troche by compounding pharmacies. The starting troche dosage is 25 mg given on 3 to 5 days a week. Nandrolone has pain-relief properties.

We consider nandrolone almost essential for persons with the dual disease problem of a genetic collagen disorder (Ehlers-

Danlos/Marfan types) and AA. All people with AA except those in the mild category should have, in our opinion, a 21-day trail of nandrolone. It works much faster than HCG, so persons usually feel a benefit within the first week.

HCG and nandrolone can be taken together. We have used both hormones in cases of AA with multiple spinal cord complications like Chiari herniations, syringomyelia, and Tarlov cysts. These two hormones can also be alternated. For example, one month of nandrolone and then rotate to HCG.

People with AA must realize that the use of these hormones is considered "revolutionary" in the minds of most physicians. They represent a departure from mainstream medical practice. Our position is this: AA is a progressive, devastating disease unless treated. Genetic collagen disorders progressively dissolve collagen and render tissue painful and dysfunctional. As this handbook is being written (2019) we are becoming increasingly more adamant that these two hormones should become a "backbone" of treatment for the dual disease problem of AA and the genetic collagen disorders such as EDS. The benefit of the 2 hormones far outweigh the risks of AA and GCD.

64. MY MEDICATION PROGRAM HAS QUIT WORKING

When your medication program suddenly stops working, it is usually due to a lack of neuroinflammation control. Always remember that AA is a neuroinflammatory disease of the cauda equina nerve roots and the arachnoid covering of the spinal canal.

In our experience people with AA who complain of sudden lack of effectiveness of their medical protocol are usually not taking ketorolac (Toradol®) and methylprednisolone (Medrol®) or its close relative, dexamethasone. Due to our clinical experience, we believe that at least a single dosage of ketorolac (Toradol®) and methylprednisolone (Medrol®) are necessary every 7 to 10 days unless the person with AA is in the "mild" category. Even then, occasional dosages of ketorolac (Toradol ®) and methylprednisolone (Medrol®) are well-advised. These 2 drugs have emerged to be the backbone of AA treatment. Always keep in mind that neuroinflammation may be silently clumping and destroying your nerve roots. Consequently, you may suddenly, without warning, take a "turn for the worse."

Another reason your medication program may stop working is the development of a hormone deficiency of pregnenolone, progesterone, cortisol, estradiol, or testosterone. A blood test is a wise move to determine if you have a deficiency. If so, replenishment of one or more hormones is necessary, as adequate hormone levels are necessary to make inflammatory and pain control drugs maximally effective.

Naturally, you will want to review the 3-medication components and physiologic measures presented in this handbook. Perhaps you need to change some drugs. Make sure you are taking agents from all 3- components and doing physiologic measures each day.

65. I CAN'T GET A DIAGNOSIS

Unfortunately, there is far too much reliance on the MRI to make the diagnosis of AA. A diagnosis of AA is rather clear cut. There is usually an initiating disease or event such as an accident or genetic disease. There are major symptoms: (1) pain decreases on reclining or with positional change; (2) feeling of water or bugs on the legs; (3) urinary difficulty; and (4) burning ankles or feet. Physical exam usually shows some neurologic deficit in the legs or feet. The MRI confirms what the history and physical indicate.

Although it is changing, some communities and physicians still don't want to accept AA as a diagnosis or disease. They still remember the days of malpractice claims and blame over AA. They still believe that AA is only caused by physician error which today is rarely the case. Some radiologists just haven't seen it often enough to diagnose it. Another problem is that some MRI's don't show classic nerve root clumping and adhesions. This problem may be technical. An MRI is a series of photographs, and a small area of AA can be missed.

Please heed this advice. If you are sure that you have AA or it was diagnosed by physicians other than your primary doctors, let your doctors know this. If your doctors deny you have AA, simply ask them "What do I have?" and "What is the treatment you recommend?" We are aware that physicians in communities everywhere are beginning to diagnose and treat AA. Too many people now have AA to keep sweeping the diagnosis under the rug. Keep looking for a knowledgeable and willing doctor. They are "cropping up."

66. WHY CAN'T I GET BETTER?

There are usually one or two reasons why you may not get better. One is that you have had AA for a long time before any known treatment was available, and second, you simply have severe nerve damage that won't resolve or repair. The problem is that AA is a neuroinflammatory disease of the cauda equina nerve roots and arachnoid covering. Unfortunately, neuroinflammation can destroy nerve tissue to the point of scarring and permanent non-function. Pain relief and retention of some neurologic function may be the best you can do, but we highly recommend you attempt to get better, no matter how much damage or neurologic impairment you have.

Most people with AA don't get better because they don't have a good 2 strategy treatment: (1) specific physiologic measures; and (2) 3-component medical program. To get better a person with AA must clearly understand the difference between "symptomatic" or "comfort" measures and "curative" or "improvement" measures.

<u>Here Are Some Examples of Curative or Improvement Measures and Drugs:</u>

<u>Physiologic Measures</u>

- ✓ Walking
- ✓ Water Soaking
- ✓ Stretching

<u>Improvement Medications</u>

- ✓ Ketorolac (Toradol®)
- ✓ Methylprednisolone (Medrol®)

- ✓ Human chorionic gonadotropin (HCG)
- ✓ Nandrolone

Many people with AA make this mistake. They get to feeling better with their new treatment, so they are satisfied. Don't do this as our culprit, neuroinflammation, may be lurking and doing silent damage. Push yourself to do more physiologic measures. For example, walk a little farther or stretch a little more. Keep up a vigorous hormone therapy program as these are the body's natural agents that suppress neuroinflammation and stimulate regrowth of damaged nerves.

67. AA TREATMENT IS PROTOCOL - NOT EVIDENCE-BASED

There is a great "fight" and controversy in today's medical practice. Some parties demand that any treatment, including drugs and other measures, be "evidence-based". The meaning here is that there must be double-blind, random, controlled studies or some other statistical parameter showing "evidence" before a treatment should be used. Naturally, the parties pushing for "evidence" are those paying the bills. They don't want to pay for anything that is not "evidence-based." In other words, "one size fits all", and there should be no payment or financing for any other treatment. Unfortunately, the cost and effort to do these types of studies is so prohibitive that only a small percentage of drugs and medical therapies can ever be tested under statistical control.

"Evidence -based" is not, however, the way medicine has always been practiced. Certainly, there will be more

"evidence" in the future, but traditional medical practice will, for the foreseeable future, continue to be protocol-based. Be clearly advised; another name for protocol is "old-fashioned common-sense medicine." All it means is that we have a basket of therapies. The medical provider is to pick one or two. Try them. If they work – terrific! If they don't, try another one. The idea is to take several measures, and through trial and error come up with a satisfactory treatment plan. AA is a complex neuroinflammatory disease of multiple causes and symptoms. No two persons will end up with precisely the same treatment program. Just like people with cardiac, pulmonary, or diabetic disorders, "one size won't fit all." Remember this. If someone tells you that you need "evidence-based" treatment, stay with the drugs and therapies that you and your practitioner know work. Your comfort and well-being are the "best evidence."

68. RISK VS BENEFIT AND INFORMED CONSENT

You cannot find any relief or recovery with AA unless you are willing to take some risks. All the medications, including those that are non-prescription, have risks, better known as side-effects and complications. Even the physiologic measures have risks. For example, you might overstretch or walk too far and tear apart an adhesion.

Here is the basic fact. All the best treatment agents identified to date for AA have risks. The best drugs and their best-known complications or side- effects are listed here:

1. Ketorolac (Toradol®) – kidney damage

2. Methylprednisolone (Medrol®) and Dexamethasone – osteoporosis, weight gain, hyperglycemia
3. Acetazolamide – dizziness, nausea, dysphoria (opposite of euphoria)
4. Human Chorionic Gonadotropin (HCG) – acne, hair loss
5. Pregnenolone – acne, hair loss
6. Nandrolone – acne, hair loss
7. Naltrexone – increase in pain, dysphoria (opposite of euphoria)

Simply put, we don't believe you can find much long-term relief, much less recovery, unless you are taking at least a couple of the drugs listed above. You must accept their risks to get their benefit. AA is a progressive neuroinflammatory disease of cauda equina nerve roots. Unless controlled, it has serious sequelae with an autoimmune component and shortened life span. There is no more miserable disease or one that ruins a quality of life more drastically. What's important is that you inform your medical providers that you know the risks and are willing to accept them. This is known as "informed consent."

The best way, and it is our firm recommendation, to prevent complications is to take AA drugs on only 3 to 5 days a week or even monthly. Complications occur most often with daily use of a drug.

Ketorolac (Toradol®) is a special case, and we make special note of it here as it is the most consistent drug for treatment of the neuroinflammation of AA. For over 2 decades it is known and labeled by the US Food and Drug Administration (FDA) that it cannot be taken for over five days in a row. We firmly agree. Some ill-informed persons in the medical field, especially some pharmacists, believe this means 5 days in a

lifetime. This is not the case. We recommend that the maximal dosage be 3 days a week and that days must be skipped between dosages. If one is over 70 years old, we recommend that a kidney blood test for damage be done at least every 3 to 6 months.

We normally like to see the corticosteroids methylprednisolone (Medrol®) and dexamethasone, only be taken on 2 to 3 days a week in a low, oral dosage. Some people with AA find they can't function and experience unbearable pain without a higher dosage taken almost daily. There are obviously greater risks with higher dosages taken more frequently. Simply put, you may have to take more risk. Many people with AA and their physicians are learning that a periodic (e.g. 7-10 days interval) injection of about 10 to 20 milligrams of methylprednisolone (Medrol®) may be more effective than oral dosages and have less risk.

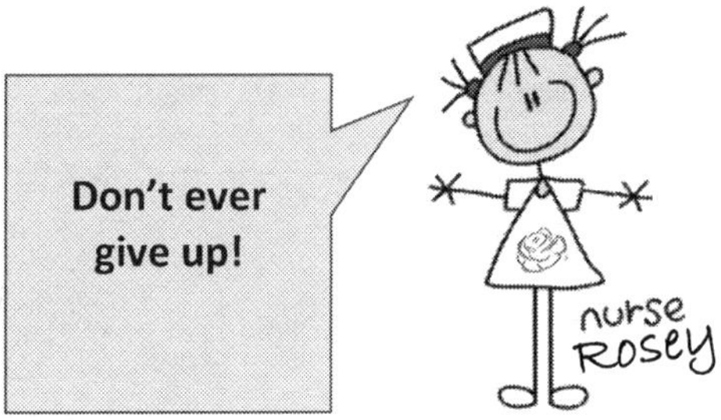

The take home message is this. AA, like cancer, is a devastating disease, and the drugs that treat it have risks that a person must accept to get their benefits and improve.

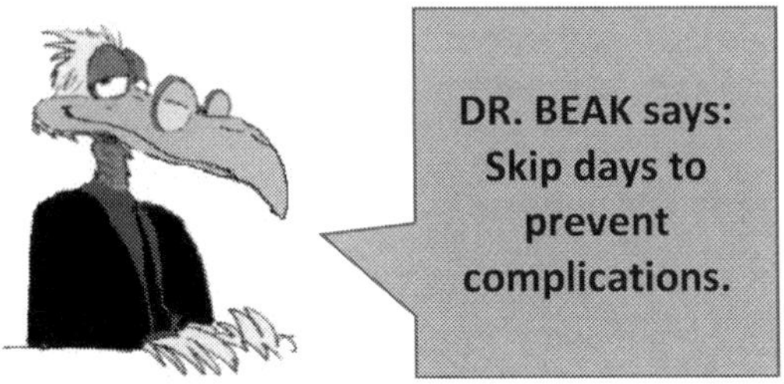

69. SUMMARY

The treatment strategy outlined in this handbook is two-fold: (1) medication and (2) physiologic and preventive measures. Medication administration has 3-components: (1) suppression of neuroinflammation; (2) regrowth of damaged nerves (neuroregeneration); and (3) pain control. The first goal of treatment is to "not get worse!"

Once a person is on a 3-componant medical protocol with accompanying physiologic and preventative measures, we highly recommend electromagnetic energy therapy, intravenous infusions, and other potential experimental measures such as stem cells. There are four categories of AA severity; mild, moderate, severe, and catastrophic. Some people with AA who are in the severe or catastrophic categories will require the implantation of an electric stimulator or opioid infusion pump for symptomatic pain relief.

Medical providers are just starting to understand and treat AA. Some uninformed providers still deny and reject it as a disease, but they will change in the future because AA is increasing in the population. In the meantime, every person with AA and their family needs to start self-help treatment

with the help of the measures and suggestions in this handbook.

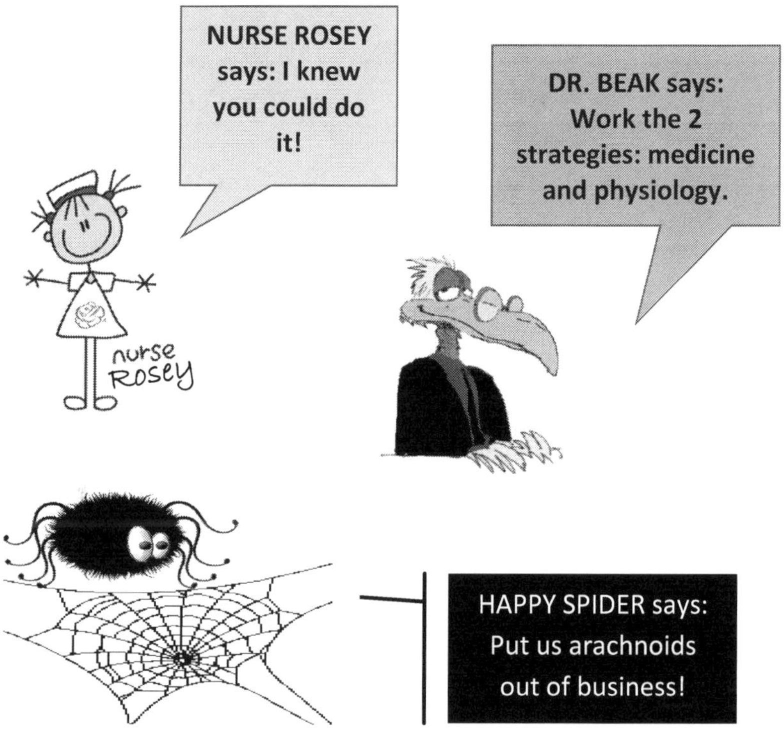

DISCLAIMER: No content in this handbook can be considered a medical order or advice. All materials and recommendations of the authors are based on experience and research. No guarantees or assurances can be derived from this handbook. All medical advice must come from a licensed medical practitioner who has examined and evaluated a person who is their patient.

THE FOE CHART of PHYSIOLOGIC MEASURES	
F-	Flow of Spinal Fluid - "Power Walking"
O-	Oxygen Intake- "Deep Breathing"
E-	Electricity Elimination- "Water Soak"
S-	Seepage and Shrinkage- "Stretch and Extend Arms and Legs"

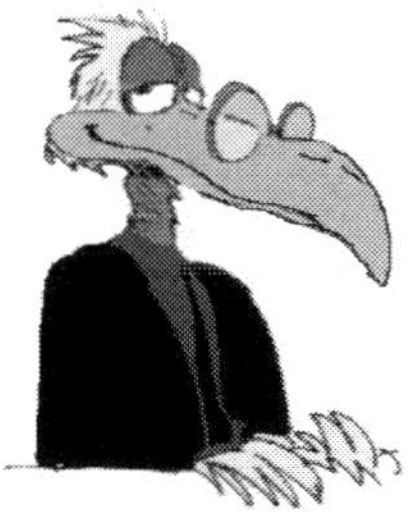

Neuroinflammation and adhesions are our **FOES**

THINK FOES

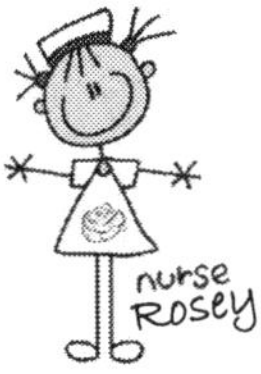

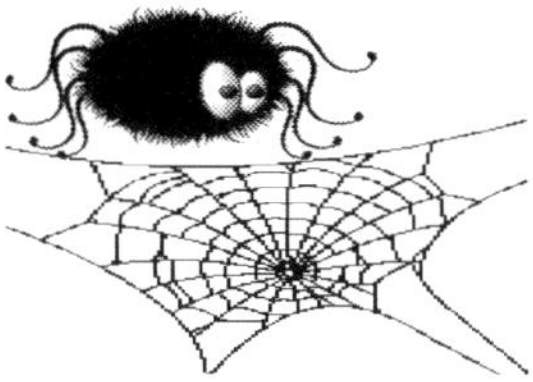

Simple measures will send me packing

REFERENCES

HISTORY

1. Thomas J. Arachnitis and Arachnoiditis. *Comprehensive Medical Dictionary.* Philadelphia, J.B. Lippincott & Co. 1873; p57.
2. Aldrete JA. History and evaluation of arachnoiditis: the evidence revealed. Insurgentes Centro 51-A. Col San Rafael, Mexico 2010; p3-14.
3. Horsley VAH. Chronic spinal meningitis: its differential diagnosis and surgical treatment. Br J Med 1909; 1:513-517.
4. Charcot JM, Joffrey A. Deax cas d'atrophic musculaire progressive avec lesions de a substance gris et des faisceaux anterolateraux de la moelle spinaire. Arch de Physiologic 1869; 2:354-358.
5. Addison T. The constitutional and local effects of disease of the supra-renal capsules. London: Samuel Highley;1855.
6. Elliott J. Of the cure of sciatica in a complete collection of the medical and philosophical works of John Fothergill. Pater-Nofter-Row, London;1781: p355-363.
7. Meningitis, Cerebral, Spinal, and Tubercular in Merck's 1899 Manual of the Materia Medica: A Ready Reference Pocket Book for the Practicing Physician. Merck & Co. New York, 1899; p146.
8. Harvey SC. Meningeal adhesions and their significance. Interstate Post Grad Med, North America Prac 1926;2:27-31.

DIAGNOSIS

9. Quiles M, Marchiselo PJ, Tsairis P. Lumbar adhesive arachnoiditis: etiologic and pathologic aspects. Spine 1978; 3:45-50.
10. Burton C. Lumbosacral arachnoiditis. Spine 1978; 3:24-30.
11. Jackson A, Isherwood I. Does degenerative disease of the lumbar spine cause arachnoiditis? A magnetic resonance study and review of the literature. Brit J Radiology 1994; 67:840-847.
12. Aldrete JA. Suspecting and diagnosing arachnoiditis. Pract Pain Mgt 2006;16(5):74-87.
13. Tennant F. Arachnoiditis: clinical description. Pract Pain Mgt 2016;14(7):63-69.
14. Tennant F. Erythrocyte sedimentation rate and C-reactive protein: old but useful biomarkers for pain treatment. Pract Pain Mgt. 2013;13(2):61-65.
15. Tennant F. Arachnoiditis: diagnosis and treatment. *Pract Pain Mgt* 2016; 16(5):74-87.

16. Tennant FS. Hormone abnormalities in severe chronic pain persons who fail standard treatment. Postgrad Med 2015;127(1):1-4.

TREATMENT

17. O'Callgan JP, SriranT, Miller DB. Defining "neuroinflammation". Ann NY Acad Sci 2008; 1139:318-330.
18. Tsuda M. Microglia in the spinal cord and neuropathic pain. J Diabetes Investig 2016;7(1):17-26.
19. Loggia MI, Chunde DB, Oluwaseum A, et al. Evidence for brain glial activation in chronic pain persons. Brain 2015; 138:604-615.
20. Mika J. Modulation of microglia can attenuate neuropathic pain symptoms and enhance morphine effectiveness. Pharmacol Rep 2008; 60:297-300.
21. Bilello J, Tennant F. Patterns of chronic inflammation in extensively treated persons with arachnoiditis and chronic intractable pain. Postgrad Med 2016;92(17):1-5.
22. Compagnone NA, Mellon SH. Neurosteroids: biosynthesis and function of these novel neuromodulators. Front Neuroendocrinol 2000; 21:1-56.
23. Jones KJ. Gonadal steroids and neuronal regeneration: a therapeutic role. Adv Neurol 1993; 59:227-240.
24. Joels M, DeKloet E. Control of neuronal excitability by corticosteroid hormones. Trends Neurosci 1992; 15:25-30.
25. Guth L, Zhang Z, Roberts E. Key role for pregnenolone in combination therapy that promotes recovery after spinal cord injury. Proc Natl Acad Sci 1994; 91:12308-12312.
26. Kilts JD, Tupler LA, Keefe FJ, et al. Neurosteroids and self-reported pain in veterans who served in the military after September 11,2001. Pain Med 2010; 10:1469-1476.
27. He J, Evans CO, Hoffman SW, et al. Progesterone and allopregnanolone reduce inflammatory cytokines after traumatic brain injury. Exp Neuro 2004; 189:404-412.
28. Patil AA. The effect of human chorionic gonadotropin (HCG) on restoration of the spinal cord: A preliminary report. Int Surg 1990;75(1):54-57.
29. Inyang K, Szabo-Pardi T, Price T. Treatment of chronic pain: long-term effects of metformin on chronic neuropathic pain and microglial activation. Poster presented at Annual Meeting of the American Pain Society, May 11-14, 2016; Austin, TX Poster 309.

30. Aldrete JA. Epidural injections of indomethacin for post-laminectomy syndrome: a preliminary report. Anesth Anal 2003;96(2):463-468.
31. Nakano M, Matsui H, Miaki K, et al. Post-laminectomy adhesion of the cauda equina: inhibitory effects of anti-inflammatory drugs on cauda equina adhesion in rats. Spine 1998;23(3):298-304.
32. Tawfik VL, Nutile-McMenemy N, Lacroix-Fralish MI, et al. Efficacy of propentofylline, a glial modulating agent, on existing mechanical allodynia following peripheral nerve injury. Brain Behav Immun 2007; 21:238-246.
33. Tikka TM, Kaistinaha JE. Minocycline provides neuroprotection against n-methyl-d-asparate neurotoxicity by inhibiting microglia. J Immunol 66:7527=7533.
34. Mika J. Modulation of microglia can attenuate neuropathic pain symptoms and enhance morphine effectiveness. Pharmacol Rep 2008; 60:297-300.
35. Radhakrishnan R, Sluka KA. Acetazolamide, a carbonic anhydrase inhibitor, reverses inflammation-induced thermal hyperalgesia in rats. J Pharmacol Exp Ther 2005; 313:921-927.
36. Harvey JW, Otterson M, Yun H, et al. Acetazolamide reduces referred postoperative pain after laparoscopic surgery with carbon dioxide insufflation. Anesthesiology 2003; 99:924-928.)
37. Liu J, Feng X, Yu M, et al. Pentoxifylline attenuates the development of hyperalgesia in a rat model of neuropathic pain. Neurosci Lett 2007; 412:268-272.
38. Vale ML, Benevides VM, Sachs D, et al. Antihyperalgesic effect of pentoxifylline on experimental inflammatory pain. Br J Pharmacol 2004; 143:833-844.
39. Asiedu M, Ossipov MHG, Kaila K, et al. Acetazolamide and midazolam act synergistically to inhibit neuropathic pain. Pain 2010;148(2):302-308.
40. Pi R, Wenning L, Nelson TK, et al. Minocycline prevents glutamate-induced apoptosis of cerebellar granule neurons by differential regulation of p38 and akt pathways. J Neurochem 2004; 91:1219-1230.
41. Tikka T, Usenius T, Tenhunon M, et al. Tetracycline derivatives and ceftriaxone, a cephalospaorin antibiotic, protect neurons against apoptosis induced by ionizing radiation. J Neurochem 2001; 78:1409-1414.
42. Pabreja K, Dua K, Sharma S, et al. Minocycline attenuates the development of diabetic neuropathic pain: possible anti-inflammatory and antioxidant mechanism. Eur J Pharmacol 2011;661(1-3):15-21.

43. Liu J, Li W, Zhu J, et al. The effect of pentoxifylline on existing hypersensitivity in a rat model of neuropathy. Anaesth Analog 2008; 106:650-653.
44. Singh R, Sen I, Wig J, et al. An acetazolamide based multimodal analgesic approach versus conventional pain management in persons undergoing laparoscopic living donor. Indian J Anaesth 2009;53(4):434-441.
45. George C, Lefain JL, Delonion S. Case report: resolution of symptomatic epidural fibrosis following treatment with combined pentoxifylline-tocopherol. Br J Radiol 2004; 77:885-887.
46. Delanian S, Porcher R, Balla-Mekias S, et al. Randomized placebo-controlled trial of combined pentoxifylline and tocopherol for regression of superficial radiation-induced fibrosis. J Clin Oncol 2003; 21:2545-2550.
47. Lefaix JL, Delanizan S, Vozenin MC, et al. Striking regression of subcutaneous fibrosis induced by high doses of gamma rays using a combination of pentoxifylline and alpha tocopherol: an experimental study. Int J Radiat Oncol Biol Phys 1999; 43:839-847.
48. Compagnone NA, Mellon SH. Neurosteroids: biosynthesis and function of these novel neuromodulators. Front Neuroendocrinol 2000; 21:1-56
49. Mensah-Nyagan A.G., Meyer L., Schaeffer V., et al. Evidence for a key role of steroids in the modulation of pain. Psychoneuroendocrinology, Volume 34, Issue SUPPL. 1, 2009, S169-S177.
50. Reddy DS. Neurosteroids: endogenous role in the human brain and therapeutic potentials. Prog Brain Res 2010; 186:13-137.
51. Dawson-Basoa M, Gintzler AR. Estrogen and progesterone activate spinal kappa-opiate receptor analgesic mechanisms. Pain 1996;64: 608-615.
52. Ceccon M, Runbaugh G, Vincini S. Distinct effect of pregnenolone sulfate on NMDA receptor subtypes. Neuropharm 2001; 40:491-500.
53. Frye CA, Duncan JE. Progesterone metabolites, effective at the GABA(A) receptor complex, attenuate pain sensitivity in rats. Brain Res 1994; 643:194-23.
54. Garcia-Estrada J, Luquin S, Fernandez AM, et al. Dehydroepiandrosterone, pregnenolone, and sex steroids down-regulate reactive astroglia in the male rat brain after a penetrating brain injury. Intern J Develop Neuro 1999;17(2):145-151.
55. Evrard HC, Balthazart J. Rapid regulation of pain by estrogens synthesized in spinal dorsal horn neurons. J Neurosci 2004; 24:7225-7229.

56. Webster KM, Wright DK, Sun M, et al. Progesterone treatment reduces neuroinflammation, oxidative stress and brain damage and improves long-term outcomes in a rat model of repeated mild traumatic brain injury. J Neuroinflammation 2015 Dec 18;12-238.
57. Chang DM, Chu SJ, Chen HC, et al. Dehydroepiandrosterone suppresses interleukin 10 synthesis in women with systemic lupus erythematosus. Ann Rheum Dis 2004; 63:1623-1620.
58. McEwen BS, de Kloet ER, Rostene W. Adrenal steroid receptors and action in the central nervous system. Physio Rev 1986; 66:1121-1188.
59. Joels M, DeKloet E. Control of neuronal excitability by corticosteroid hormones. Trends Neurosci 1992; 15:25-30.
60. Bohn MC, O'Banion NK, Young DA, et al. In vitro studies of glucocorticoid effects on neurons and astrocytes. Amer NY Acad Sci 1994; 746:243-258.
61. Roglio I, Bianchi R, Gotti S, et al. Neuroprotective effects of dehydroprogesterone and progesterone in an experimental model of nerve crush injury. Neurosci 2008 Aug 26;155(3):673-685.
62. Djeball M, Guo Q, Pertus EH, et al. The neurosteroids progesterone and allopregnanolone reduce cell death, gliosis, and functional deficits after traumatic brain injury in rats. J Neurotrauma 2005; 22:106-118.
63. Morlin R, Young J, Corpechot C, et al. Neurosteroids: pregnenolone in human sciatic nerves. Proc Natl Acad Sci 1992; 98:6790-793.
64. Akwa Y, Young J, Kabbadj K, et al. Neurosteroids: biosynthesis, metabolism and function of pregnenolone and dehydroepiandrosterone in the brain. J Steroid Biochem Molec Biol 1991:40(1-3):71-81.
65. Jones KJ. Gonadal steroids and neuronal regeneration: a therapeutic role. Adv Neurol 1993; 59:227-240.
66. Fednekar J and Mulgacnker V. Role of testosterone on pain threshold in rats. Indian J Physci Pharmacol 1995; 39:423-24.
67. Hau M, Dominguez OA, Evrard HC. Testosterone reduces responsiveness to nociceptive stimuli in a wild bird. Horm Behav 2004; 46:165-170.
68. Aloisi AM, Ceccarelli I, Fiorenzani P, et al. Testosterone affects pain-related responses differently in male and female rats. Neurosci Lett. 2004; 361:262-264.
69. Matura S, Okashi M, Chen HC, et al. Physiochemical and Immunological Characterization of an HCG-Like Substance from human pituitary glands. Nature 1980; 286: 740-741.
70. Lei ZM, Rao CV. Neural actions of luteinizing hormone and human chorionic gonadotropin. Seminar Reprod Med 2001; 19:103-109.

71. Lei ZM, Rao CV, Kornyei JL, et al. Novel expression of human chorionic gonadotropin/luteinizing hormone receptor gene in brain. Endocrin 1993; 132:2262-2270.
72. Tennant F. Human chorionic gonadotropin in pain treatment. Prac Pain Mgt 2009; 9:44-46.
73. Vielkind U, Walencewicz A, Levine JM, et al. Type II glucocorticoid receptors are expressed in oligodendrocytes and astrocytes. J Neurosci Res 1990;27(3):360-323.
74. Kiefer r, Kreutzberg GW. Effects of dexamethasone on microglial activation in vitro: selective downregulation of major histocompatibility complex class II expression in regenerating facial nucleus. J Neuroimmunol 1991;34(2-3):99-108.
75. Chao CC, Hu S, Close K, et al. Cytokine release from microglia: differential inhibition by pentoxifylline and dexamethasone. J Infect Dis 1992;166(4):842-853.
76. Tanaka J, Fujita H, Mostsudo S, et al. Glucocorticoid and mineral corticoid receptors in microglial cells: the two receptors mediate differentiation effects of corticosteroids. Glia 1997; 20:23-37.
77. Rash JA, Aguirre-Camancho A, Campbell TS. Oxytocin and pain: a systemic review and synthesis of findings. Clin J Pain 2014;30(5):453-462.
78. Paloyells Y, Krahe C, Mahazos S, et al. The analgesic effect of oxytocin in humans: a double-blind placebo controlled cross-over study using easer-evoked potentials. J Neuroendocrinol 2016;28(4):10,111.
79. Tennant F, Pedersen C. Sublingual oxytocin and ketamine for pain relief. Poster Presented at PainWeek. September 5-9, 2017. Las Vegas, Nevada.
80. Gold J, High HA, Li Y, et al. Safety and efficacy of nandrolone decanoate for treatment of wasting in persons with HIV infection. AIDS 1996 Jun;10(7):745-52.
81. Sattler FR, Jaque SV, Schroeder ET, et al. Effects of pharmacological doses of nandrolone decanoate and progressive resistance training in immunodeficient persons infected with human immunodeficiency virus. J Clin Endocrinol Metab 1999 Apr;84(4):1268-76.
82. Hassager C, Jensen LT, Podenphant J, et al. Collagen synthesis in post-menopausal women during therapy with anabolic steroids or female sex hormones. Metabolism 1990 Nov;39(11):1167-9.

SPINAL FLUID

83. Damkier HH, Brown PD, Praetorius J. Cerebrospinal fluid secretion by the choroid plexus. Physiol Rev 2013;93(4):1847-92.

84. Kiiski H, Aanismaa R, Tenhunen J, et al. Healthy human CSF promotes glial differentiation of hESC-derived neural cells while retaining spontaneous activity in existing neuronal networks. Biology Open 2013;2(6):605-612.
85. Whendon JM, Glassey D. Cerebrospinal fluid stasis and its clinical significance. Altern Ther Health Med 2009;15(3):54-60.
86. Weller RO, Djuanda E, Yow H, et al. Lymphatic drainage of the brain and the pathophysiology of neurological disease. Acta Neuropathol 2009; 117:1-14.
87. Csarr HF, Harling-Berg CJ, Knopf PM. Drainage of brain extracellular fluid into blood and deep cervical lymph and its immunological significance. Brain Path 1992; 2:259-296.
88. Laman JD, Weller RO. Drainage of cells and soluble antigen from the CNS to regional lymph nodes. J Neuroimmune Pharmacol 2013; 8:840-856.
89. Rydovik B, Holm S, Brown MD, et al. Diffusion from the cerebrospinal fluid as a nutritional pathway for spinal nerve roots. Acta Physiol Scand 1990; 138:247-248.

GENETIC COLLAGEN DISORDERS

90. Henderson FC, Austin C, Benzel E, et al. Neurological and spinal manifestations of the Ehlers-Danlos Syndromes. Amer J Men Gen 2017;175C:195-211.
91. Castori M, Voermann NC. Neurological manifestations of "Ehlers-Danlos Syndromes. Iran J of Neurol 2014; 13:190-208.
92. Sevesto S, Merli P, Ruggier M, et al. Ehlers-Danlos Syndrome and neurological features: a review. Childs Neuro Syst 2011; 27:365-371.
93. Schievink WI, Gordon OK, Tourje J, et al. Connective tissue disorders with spontaneous spinal cerebrospinal fluid leaks and intracranial hypotension: a prospective study. Neurosurgery 2004;54(1):65-71.

AUTOIMMUNITY

94. Wang L, Wang FS, Gershwin ME. Human autoimmune disease: a comprehensive update. J Intern Med 2015; 278:369-395.
95. Zweiman B, Levinson AI. Immunologic aspects of neurological and neuromuscular diseases. JAMA 1992;268(20):2918-2922.
96. Meisel C, Schwab JM, Prass K, et al., Dirnage U. Central nervous system injury-induced immune deficiency syndrome. Nat Rev Neurosci 2005;6(10):775-786.
97. Javidi E, Magnus T. Autoimmunity after ischemic stroke and brain injury. Fron in Immunol 2019; 10:1-12.

98. Tennant F. The physiologic effects of pain on the endocrine system. Pain Ther. 2013 Dec;2(2):75-86.

RISKS

99. Epstein NE. The risks of epidural and transforminal steroid injections in the spine: commentary and a comprehensive review of the literature. Surg Neurol 2013;4(supe2):574-593.

100. Eisenberg E, Goldman R, Shclag-Eisenberg D, et al. Adhesive arachnoiditis following lumbar epidural steroid injections: a report of two cases and review of literature. J Pain Research 2019; 12:513-518.

101. Nelson DA. Dangers from methylprednisolone acetate therapy by intraspinal injection. Arch Neurol 1988;45(7):804-806.

102. Kitson MC, Kostopanagiotau G, Alimeric K, et al. Histopathological alterations after single epidural injection of rapivacaine, methylprednisolone acetate, or contrast material in swine. Cardiovasc Interven Radiol 2011;34(6):1288-1295.

Read Other books by Forest Tennant

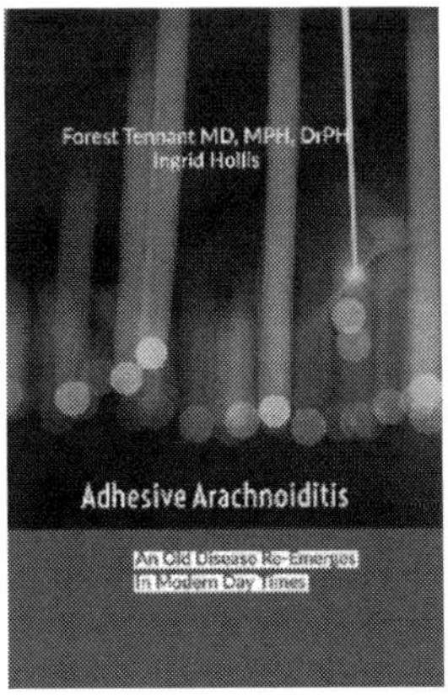

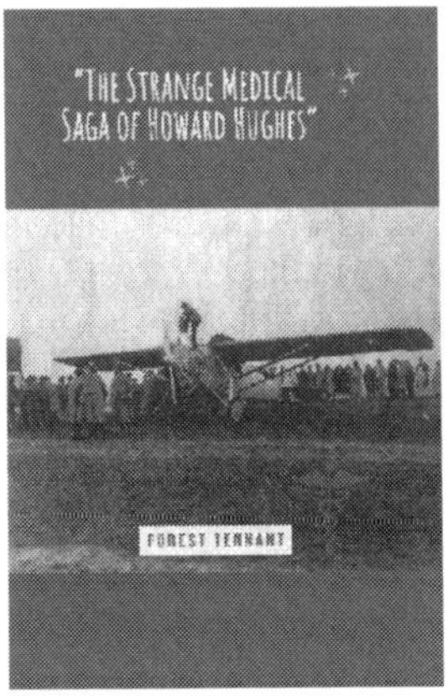

Coming Soon

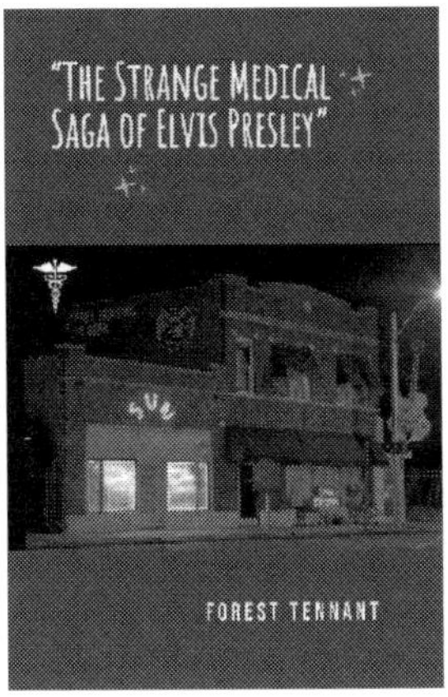

Available on Amazon

Made in the USA
Monee, IL
12 November 2026

7e24e6d4-d678-4c08-8082-b31f47449e92R01

Canon Law Society of America

Proceedings of the Eighty-First Annual Convention

Atlantic City, New Jersey
October 14-17, 2019

Canon Law Society of America

ISBN 978-1-932208-54-2
ISSN 0277-9889
SAN 237-6296

Unless otherwise noted, all canons quoted are from the *Code of Canon Law, Latin-English Edition* (Washington, DC: Canon Law Society of America, 2012) and the *Code of Canons of the Eastern Churches, Latin-English Edition* (Washington, DC: Canon Law Society of America, 2002).

Printed in the United States of America.

Canon Law Society of America
415 Michigan Avenue NE, Suite 101
Washington, DC 20017-4502

Table of Contents

Foreword vii

Keynote Address

What's All This about Missionary Discipleship? It is enough for the disciple that he becomes like the teacher (Mt 10:25)
The Most Reverend Andrew H. Cozzens, STD 1

Major Addresses

Impelling Obligation: Forming Intentional Discipleship in the New Missiondom
Ms. Sherry Weddell 15

Can We Open the Door Wider under Current Law?
The Most Reverend Mark O'Connell, JCD 28

Seminars

Opportunities in Canon Law for Interecclesial Ministry
The Reverend Jobe Abbass, OFM Conv., JCD 41

Cor Orans: Implementing New Papal Norms for Nuns
Sr. Nancy Ann Bauer, OSB, JCD 60

Canonical Norms Regarding Place of Marriage: Both a Challenge and an Opportunity
The Reverend Sean Bransfield, JCL 78

Ten Years Later: The Special Faculties Granted to the Congregation for the Clergy, 2009-2019
The Very Reverend Georges de Laire, JCL 102

Qui propter nos homines et propter nostram salutem: Justice and Mercy in the Distribution of the Salvific Goods of the Church
The Very Reverend Peter A. Faulk, JCL 112

Proceed with Caution: Canon 1071 and Licit Assistance at Marriage
The Reverend David Fulton, JCD 128

The Separation of Spouses: Old Law, New Questions
Mr. Vincent Gardiner, JCL 160

The Permanent Diaconate: A Holy Order in Search of (Canonical) Reality
Deacon Matthew Glover, JD, JCL 192

Custom as an Expression of the Canonical Creativity of a Community of the Faithful
Dr. Wojciech Kowal, OMI, JCD 217

From Tripoli (1976) to Abu Dhabi (2019): How Catholic-Muslim Relations Have Evolved
The Reverend Elias Mallon, SA, STL, PhD 234

Conducting a Diocesan Synod in Service of Missionary Discipleship
The Most Reverend Thomas John Paprocki, JD, JCD 247

Officers' Reports

President
Dr. Zabrina Decker 268

Treasurer
Sister Nancy Reynolds, SP 271
Independent Auditor Report
Linton Shafer Warfield & Garret, P.A. 274
Supplementary Information 286
Fiscal Year 2019-2020 Budget 287

Staff Reports

Executive Coordinator
Mrs. Donna Miller 294

General Secretary
Ms. Colleen Crawford 298

Committee Reports

Constitutional Standing Committees
Nominations 301
Resolutions 303
Resource and Asset Management 304
Professional Responsibility 305

On-Going Committees

Church Governance 307
Clergy 307
Consecrated Life and Apostolic Life 313
Convention Planning 308
Eastern Churches 312
Laity 316
Publications Advisory Board 317
Research and Development 320
Sacramental Law 322

Varia

Business Meeting Minutes
Mr. Timothy M. Olson 324

Homily, Convention Liturgy
The Reverend John P. Donovan 331

Role of Law Award Citation
Dr. Zabrina Decker 334

Role of Law Award Response
The Reverend Patrick Lagges 335

Note, re Tribunal Statistics 2018 338

Board of Governors and Administrative Staff 339

Convention Contributors 340

List of Participants 341

Foreword

The Canon Law Society of America is pleased to publish the *Proceedings of the Eighty-First Annual Convention*, which convened in Atlantic City, New Jersey, from October 14 through October 17, 2019, at the Bally's Atlantic City Hotel.

The convention *Proceedings* have been published for almost fifty years, thus providing a significant volume of presentations and reports.

We are grateful to the presenters who submitted their texts for this publication. The texts have been edited to be in conformity with the most recent CLSA style sheet, publication guidelines, and previous editions of *CLSA Proceedings*. Included in this edition are minutes of the Society's annual business meeting, varia, and a list of the participants at the Atlantic City convention.

Special thanks are extended to Ms. Susan Mulheron and Monsignor John Foster, both of whom spent many hours assisting with the editing of this edition of *Proceedings*, in preparation for publication.

The CLSA, established as a professional association on November 12, 1939, presently has more than 1,100 members who minister in more than thirty-five countries. Interested persons may apply for membership via the CLSA website or by contacting the administrative office. We offer Active, Associate and Student memberships to qualified persons.

Additional copies of this 2019 volume of *Proceedings* may be purchased from the online bookstore at www.clsa.org.

Donna Miller, JD, JCL
Executive Coordinator
Canon Law Society of America
415 Michigan Avenue NE, Suite 101
Washington, DC 20017-4502
(202) 832-2350

Keynote Address

What's All This about Missionary Discipleship? It is enough for the disciple that he become like the Teacher (Mt 10:25)

The Most Reverend Andrew H. Cozzens, STD

I recently was at an ecumenical dialogue with a group of evangelical Protestants and we were sharing about our ministry and what we are focusing our efforts upon. I was surprised to hear them speak about the word "discipleship" and the fact that they were really working on making disciples not just churchgoers. They articulated the same struggle that we are seeing in the Catholic Church today. They are seeing many of their people giving into the pressures of modern culture and falling away because they were Christian in name only, and not committed disciples. We noted together all those passages in scripture where Jesus speaks about discipleship and how important this is becoming in today's world. They could see what many Catholics see: the Church needs committed disciples who are deeply rooted in their relationship with Jesus, not only so that they can stand against the secular streams in our culture, but also so they can become the evangelists Jesus called his disciples to be.

You all know that this is not new thinking in the Catholic Church. Before Pope Francis' clarion call for all Catholics to be missionary disciples, we had the landmark encyclical of St. Paul VI on Evangelization in the Modern World, where he pointed out that the Church is a community of evangelizing disciples.[1] In the United States, at least since Sherry Weddell's now famous book *Forming Intentional Disciples*,[2] "discipleship" has become the way to speak about someone who is a committed Catholic. When we speak about being a disciple, we mean someone who is seeking to follow Jesus with their whole life and wants to invite others to follow him as well. In this talk, I want to explore the meaning of discipleship, and especially how this relates to the cross. I hope to give you some practical help for your own discipleship as you serve the Church in difficult times as canon lawyers.

---

1 See Paul VI, apostolic exhortation *Evangelii Nuntiandi* 15, December 8, 1975: *AAS* 68 (1976) 13-15.

2 See Sherry Weddell, *Forming Intentional Disciples* (Huntington, IN: Our Sunday Visitor, 2012).

We know that discipleship itself is a concept that pre-dates even Jesus, although he gives it a unique meaning. In the first century Jewish world in which Jesus lived, there were other rabbis who had disciples. The word disciple (in Greek, *mathetes*) means student or learner. Rabbis would invite a person to join their school and learn from their example. It was a kind of apprenticeship where one began to live in the company of the rabbi and learn his whole way of life. The goal of discipleship was imitation. It was to imitate the master's way of life.

It is in the New Testament, however, that the concept of discipleship takes on a unique meaning. In the Gospels, followers of Jesus are not called Christians, they are called disciples. The picture we get of a disciple is someone who begins by being fascinated by Jesus. They begin by observing and listening, but eventually they encounter him and they are changed by that encounter. Consider, for example, Andrew and John, who were first disciples of St. John the Baptist, and through John they began to follow Jesus. This following led to an encounter. Jesus turned and looked at them and asked, "What are you looking for?" Andrew and John responded by asking, "'Rabbi, where are you staying?' [Jesus] said to them, 'Come, and you will see.' So, they went and saw where he was staying, and they stayed with him that day. It was about four in the afternoon."[3]

Why do we have this detail of *four in the afternoon*? In commenting on this passage, Pope Francis suggests that this was such a life-changing moment for St. John that he remembered and recounted the exact moment it happened.[4] What was so life changing about the encounter? As Andrew and John spend the day with Jesus, they begin to realize that he is someone they cannot live without and soon they are willing to stake their whole lives on this Jesus. As they spend time with him, they began to discover that he speaks to the deepest desires of their hearts. They see that he is unlike any other man.

If you are familiar with Fr. Luigi Giusanni of the Communion and Liberation Movement, he calls this the "exceptionality" of Jesus, which corresponds to the deepest needs of the human heart. He says, "There are deep needs that give a goal to living, to reasoning and to moving. When something corresponds to the criteria by which everything is judged and lived, when it corresponds to the criteria by which life is lived, should be lived . . . when it corresponds to the deepest needs of the heart . . . when it brings to fruition what life has been awaiting then it's exceptional."[5] He then argues that this exceptionality of Jesus, what made him so different from everyone else and at the same time so attractive, was a sign of

---

3 John 1:38-39.

4 See Francis, General Audience, August 30, 2017, http://www.vatican.va/content/francesco/en/audiences/2017/documents/papa-francesco_20170830_udienza-generale.html (accessed on 2 Mar. 2020).

5 Luigi Giussani, *Is It Possible to Live This Way? An Unusual Approach to Christian Existence, Volume 1: Faith* (McGill-Queen's University Press, 2008) 31.

his divinity. The encounters with Jesus take on different forms in scripture. Some involve people who are healed, like Bartimaeus. Others are forgiven, like Mary Magdalene. But the result is the same. Through their encounter with Jesus, each realizes who Jesus is and that they cannot live without him. Each then seeks to become his disciple.

The early Church captured the uniqueness of being a disciple with a phrase: "Jesus is Lord." The disciple of Jesus recognizes him as Lord and submits his or her life to his Lordship. A disciple is willing to surrender everything within to Jesus. Only this Lordship of Jesus can explain the incredible and shocking demands that he speaks about regarding his disciples: "Whoever loves father or mother more than me is not worthy of me, and whoever loves son or daughter more than me is not worthy of me."[6] Or even more shocking:

> If any man would come after me, let him deny himself and take up his cross and follow me. For whoever would save his life will lose it; and whoever loses his life for my sake and the gospel's will save it. For what does it profit a man, to gain the whole world and forfeit his life? For what can a man give in return for his life? For whoever is ashamed of me and of my words in this adulterous and sinful generation, of him will the Son of man also be ashamed, when he comes in the glory of his Father with the holy angels.[7]

Let's all admit that we find these radical notions of discipleship uncomfortable at times. If we take Jesus at his word, discipleship is a way of life that will demand all of our hearts. Of course, there are different stages on the journey of discipleship. In the beginning, when we are fascinated, we don't always realize what we are getting into. Even in scripture we see that some followed Jesus for a time, but when the cost of discipleship got to be too much, they fell away. We think of John, chapter 6, for example. Here we see the difference between true disciples and false disciples. When some leave because they don't understand the Bread of Life discourse of Jesus, what is his reaction? He turns to his closest disciples, the twelve, and he says to them, "Do you also want to leave?"[8] Simon Peter gives the answer of the true disciple: "Master, to whom shall we go? You have the words of eternal life. We have come to believe and are convinced that you are the Holy One of God."[9] There is a great mystery here. I am sure that you all, like me, have had close friends decide not to be disciples anymore, walking away from their vocation or from the Lord. What is clear is that the Lord usually tries his disciples, that is, he puts them in situations that are meant to purify them, to help them grow deeper in their discipleship. Yet sometimes, in these trials,

---

6 Mt. 10:37.

7 Mk. 8:34-38.

8 Jn. 6:68.

9 Jn. 6:69.

people walk away and stop being disciples, as is evidenced in the parable of the sower and the seed.[10]

I love the way C.S. Lewis describes this journey into deeper discipleship in one of his sermons, "A Slip of the Tongue," which he preached at evening prayer in January of 1956. He says that one morning when he was praying, he accidentally misread the collect for the fourth Sunday after Trinity. Instead of praying "that I might so pass through things temporal that I finally lost not the things eternal," he accidentally prayed, "so to pass through things eternal that I finally lost not the things temporal." In other words, he prayed that he would not get so caught up in following Jesus that he would have to let go of the things he likes so much on this earth. He said he did not think that all such slips of the tongue were significant, but he feared that this one was. He worried that a part of him actually feared the total self-gift that real discipleship demanded. When we are honest, we can relate to this fear.

In this sermon, Lewis beautifully expresses what you and I know is a real human temptation: we want to follow Jesus, we want to be his disciples, but we want to do this within reason, being careful not to get carried away. Lewis captures this natural human fear so well:

> This is my endlessly recurrent temptation: to go down to that Sea (I think St. John of the Cross called God a sea) and there neither dive nor swim nor float, but only dabble and splash, careful not to get out of my depth and holding on to the lifeline which connects me with my things temporal. It is different from the temptations that met us at the beginning of the Christian life. Then we fought against admitting the claims of the eternal at all. And when we had fought, and been beaten, and surrendered, we supposed that all would be fairly plain sailing. This temptation comes later. It is addressed to those who have already admitted the claim in principle and are even making some sort of effort to meet it. Our temptation is too look eagerly for the minimum that will be accepted. We are in fact very like honest but reluctant taxpayers. We approve of an income tax in principle. We make our returns truthfully. But we dread a rise in the tax. We are very careful to pay no more than is necessary. And we hope – we very ardently hope – that after we have paid it there will still be enough left to live on. . . . There is no parallel to paying taxes and living on the remainder. For it is not so much of our time and so much of our attention that God demands; it is not even all our time and all our attention; it is ourselves. . . . For He has, in the last resort, nothing to give us but Himself; and He can give that only insofar

10 Cf. Mk. 4:1-9; Mt. 13:3-9.

as our self-affirming will retires and makes room for Him in our souls.[11]

To put it into Biblical terms, a Christian disciple does not enter into a contract with God, such that if he fulfills the minimum of the commandments and the precepts of the Church, or at least goes to confession when he fails, then God will give him eternal life. Rather, a Christian disciple enters into a covenantal, life-long relationship with Jesus Christ. This covenant is a gift of self. Christ gives himself to us and he asks us to surrender our entire selves to him as our Lord. This means following him on the path that he set for us. As Jesus himself said, "A disciple is not above his teacher, nor a servant above his master; it is enough for the disciple to be like his teacher, and the servant like his master."[12]

It is actually here, on the role of the cross in the life of the disciple, that I want to focus the rest of my thoughts for you all this evening. In consulting and praying about what I might share with you about discipleship, it seemed to me it would be good to reflect with you as canon lawyers on the role of the cross in Christian discipleship. This is because your vocation at this time in the history of the Church involves you in her suffering. Having lived through the real depths of the current crisis in the Church in my own Archdiocese of St. Paul and Minneapolis, I know how much canon lawyers are involved in this crisis. Also, I know how often you get to see the wounded side of the Church, especially in her clerics—her deacons, her priests and her bishops.

I remember listening to a bishop friend of mine speak about becoming a bishop. He said that rather than being raised up in the Church, he felt like, on becoming a bishop, he was taken deeper into the Church, and deeper within he could see more of her wounds and weakness. Anyone who has had to deal closely with the failures of our Church knows how painful this is to see and experience, and how much it weighs on us, especially when it is part of our daily experience. We can be tempted to doubt God's work in the Church, or even to give up. Certainly, we face the temptation of losing our joy. Pope Francis has challenged us to be missionary disciples who evangelize others by our joy. How is this possible in the midst of the difficulties and sufferings of serving a Church that has been compromised by scandal? How do I live my discipleship when it brings me to the cross?

I want to turn here to the example of St. Paul, whose teaching in this regard I find to be a great help. In St. Paul's second letter to the Corinthians, he speaks about the difficulties and struggles in his life, as he reflects on his (and our) human frailties. He begins in chapter four, where he is reflecting on the incredible gift it is to serve in ministry in the Church. When he gets to verse seven, he says:

---

11 C.S. Lewis, "A Slip of the Tongue," *The Weight of Glory and Other Addresses* (San Francisco: Harper, 1980) 187-190.

12 Mt. 10:24-25.

"We hold this treasure in earthen vessels, that the surpassing power may be of God and not from us."[13] He is speaking not primarily about the weaknesses of all those who minister, but about himself. He continues:

> We are afflicted in every way, but not constrained; perplexed, but not driven to despair; persecuted, but not abandoned; struck down, but not destroyed; always carrying about in the body the dying of Jesus, so that the life of Jesus may also be manifested in our body. For we who live are constantly being given up to death for the sake of Jesus, so that the life of Jesus may be manifested in our mortal flesh. So death is at work in us, but life in you.[14]

Do you see what St. Paul is saying here? He acknowledges the painful suffering that his ministry has involved him in, but then he notes two things about it. First, he notes that although it has been painful it has not destroyed him. He is afflicted but not ultimately constrained. He is perplexed, but he does not end in despair. He is persecuted, but not abandoned, struck down but not destroyed. It is as if he begins to recognize in himself in the midst of his ministry that there is another force within him, something which prevents him from being destroyed. Of course, he recognizes that this force is the very life of Jesus in him. Second, he recognizes that his own suffering is not only his suffering. Rather, his suffering is Jesus living his Paschal Mystery in him. This is so real for him that he can say that Jesus is dying in his body and Jesus is rising in his body: "We who live are constantly being given up to death for Jesus' sake, so that the life of Jesus may be manifested in our mortal flesh."[15] Third and most important, Paul's participation in Jesus' own death and suffering on the cross is producing life for those whom he loves: "Death is at work in us, but life in you."[16] This is very important to be able to see in the midst of my own suffering. Can I learn to see that in a very real way, my suffering can contribute spiritually to the *salus animarum*?

St. Paul has certainly experienced the cross in his life, but he comes to see it as a gift that allows him to participate in the redemptive love of Jesus. His suffering is Jesus living his Paschal Mystery in him, and this is fruitful for God's people. In fact, this understanding allowed St. Paul to find joy in the cross. He expresses this joy in many places, but perhaps nowhere more clearly than in his letter to the Colossians, where he says, "Now I rejoice in my sufferings for your sake, and in my flesh I am filling up what is lacking in the afflictions of Christ on behalf of his body, which is the church."[17]

---

13 2 Cor. 4:7.

14 2 Cor. 4:8-12.

15 2 Cor. 4:11.

16 2 Cor. 4:12.

17 Col. 1:24.

At this point, I find that personally I can get discouraged. I understand that true discipleship involves the cross, but how can I possibly do this? How can I practically learn to find joy in my sufferings? Pope Francis spoke about this struggle to find joy in our pastoral service in *Evangelii gaudium*. He spoke about the evil of *acedia*, a spiritual ailment that was often spoken of by the desert fathers. St. Thomas Aquinas calls it "sadness about a spiritual good."[18] Pope Francis says,

> The problem is not always an excess of activity, but rather activity undertaken badly, without adequate motivation, without a spirituality which would permeate it and make it pleasurable. As a result, work becomes more tiring than necessary, even leading at times to illness. Far from a content and happy tiredness, this is a tense, burdensome, dissatisfying and, in the end, unbearable fatigue. This pastoral acedia can be caused by a number of things. Some fall into it because they throw themselves into unrealistic projects and are not satisfied simply to do what they reasonably can. Others, because they lack the patience to allow processes to mature; they want everything to fall from heaven. Others, because they are attached to a few projects or vain dreams of success. Others, because they have lost real contact with people and so depersonalize their work that they are more concerned with the road map than with the journey itself. Others fall into acedia because they are unable to wait; they want to dominate the rhythm of life. Today's obsession with immediate results makes it hard for pastoral workers to tolerate anything that smacks of disagreement, possible failure, criticism, the cross.[19]

I might add that some fall into *acedia* because they are asked to deal with very difficult things. I remember at one point in the midst of our own crisis in St. Paul and Minneapolis I was reading the Gospel of Matthew where Jesus says, "Come to me, all you who labor and are burdened, and I will give you rest. Take my yoke upon you and learn from me; for I am gentle and lowly in heart, and you will find rest for your souls. For my yoke is easy, and my burden is light."[20] I remember that moment in prayer well. I thought to myself, I believe that Jesus wants me to experience this lightness, but I do not experience it. Right now, I do not experience the burden he is asking me to carry as light. I knew at this moment that my spiritual life was in trouble. If you are experiencing something similar,

---

18 Aquinas, *Summa Theologica* II-II.35.2, corp.

19 Francis, apostolic exhortation *Evangelii gaudium* 82, November 24, 2013: *AAS* 105 (2013) 1054; English translation at http://www.vatican.va/content/francesco/en/apost_exhortations/documents/papa-francesco_esortazione-ap_20131124_evangelii-gaudium.html (accessed on 2 Mar. 2020).

20 Mt. 11:28-30.

I recommend a great book on the subject of *acedia* called *The Noonday Devil.*[21] Every now and then I find the Lord sends me the right book just at the time I need it, and this book really helped me in a difficult moment in my ministry.

So, what do we need to do when we experience that our work or something in our service of the Lord gets this heavy? What do we need to do if we experience sadness about serving the Lord, which should make us joyful? I do not pretend that this is easy. Suffering and the cross bring us to the deepest and most mysterious aspects of Christian discipleship. But I would like to share with you a way of praying that I have learned that has helped me, at times, to be able to find God's love and peace in the midst of difficult circumstances. It is a practical tool that I learned from the Institute for Priestly Formation. You might be familiar with this Institute, which we call IPF, based out of Omaha, Nebraska. IPF is dedicated to helping seminarians and priests grow in a deep spiritual life. If you want to learn more about this after my lecture, you can get a book on their website called *The Parish as the School of Prayer.*[22]

Here are the four steps of prayer: Acknowledge, Relate, Receive and Respond. I want to talk about each of them. They are really four steps to surrender and to allowing God to be with me in my trials. It is really the heart of the spiritual life of a disciple.

The first step is to acknowledge. Whenever I am having some struggle, the first thing I have to do is to admit that it is a struggle. This is already something important. It is having a necessary self-awareness. Many times, something is bothering me but I never actually acknowledge it. I am feeling lonely, angry or discouraged, but instead of dealing with the pain, I distract myself so I don't have to face it. Sometimes there is a fear of acknowledging, because I don't want to give the thing too much power. I think it is better to ignore it. I have some problem or something which is bothering me and I don't have any solution to it, so I just try not to think about it. My own experience is that this usually makes it worse. Unless I face the pain that I have and acknowledge that it is real, I cannot begin to see it the way God sees it. It just remains an annoyance, or a pain, or a place of desolation. Or worse, it can become a subtle place of despair in my life, a place where I don't believe God is good or God wants to work.

The second step after acknowledging is relating the situation to God. What this means is that I have to bring this situation, this painful reality, into my relationship with God. Relating is very practical. I have to tell God about it. I acknowledge to God what I am feeling: "Lord, this is really difficult for me."

21 See Dom Jean-Charles Nault, O.S.B., *The Noonday Devil: Acedia, the Unnamed Evil of Our Times* (San Francisco: Ignatius Press, 2015).

22 See *The Parish as a School of Prayer* (Omaha, Nebraska: Institute of Priestly Formation) https://saintjoe.com/products/the-parish-as-a-school-of-prayer-foundations-for-the-new-evangelization (accessed on 30 Mar. 2020).

"Lord, I feel alone." "I feel overwhelmed, where are you, Lord?" "I'm really angry about this Lord, how could you let this happen!" It is important to really pour out what I'm feeling. One of the reasons relating can be difficult is because I judge myself first for my feelings. I am bothered by something, but I think that I should not be bothered by it. I think, if I were a holy person then this wouldn't bother me. The reality is that it does not help to pretend that I am not bothered. The only way that God can actually speak his truth to me, is if I honestly acknowledge what I really feel. If I really am hurting, I need to pour it out to him.

It is good to remember that this pouring out of one's heart to God in prayer is scriptural and also something we see the saints doing. Do you remember how Hannah poured out her heart to God in the first book of Samuel, expressing such pain that he had left her barren? The prophet Eli even thought she was drunk. Hannah said, "No, my lord, I am a woman sorely troubled; I have drunk neither wine nor strong drink, but I have been pouring out my soul before the Lord."[23] The Lord heard her prayer and gave her a son. Or we can remember the words of Psalm 22, which the Lord himself made his prayer on the cross: "My God, my God, why have you abandoned me?"[24] Have you ever read the letters of St. Teresa of Calcutta in her darkness? She cries out to her spiritual director: "Heaven means nothing to me—to me it looks like an empty place . . . ."[25] This pouring out of my feelings, relating my feelings to God, is not complaining simply for the sake of complaining, or stewing. The goal is to supernaturalize the trial. I have to relate the situation to God with faith. As I am pouring out what I really feel, I am also saying, "God I know that you are good. I know that you are with me. Show me how you are working in this situation." I am trying to see the situation as God sees it, not just to be stuck in myself.

I see this pouring out sometimes like opening the wound and letting the puss out. Often times it is in pouring out what I feel that I discover just how much something is bothering me. I also am able to see what the real pain or difficulty is. Sometimes the thing that is bothering me is only the surface. This allows God to speak to the real issue. It allows God's truth to penetrate to the depth of my wound, so that it can begin to heal.

What happens as I pour out my complaint to God is that eventually I can receive from God a new way of seeing things. Receiving is God's part of the action, and I cannot control it. But I can have faith that he will do it! God desires to give me his peace. He wants to let me see how he sees. God is always good, in every situation, and if I have faith, he can show me how he is good. There are two

23 1 Sam. 1:15.

24 Mt. 27:46.

25 José Tolentino Mendonça, *Our Father Who Art on Earth: The Our Father for Believers and Unbelievers* (Adelaide: ATF Press, 2014) 57.

important scripture verses from St. Paul that are helpful in understanding this. The first is Romans 8:28: "For we know that God makes all things work for good for those who love him and are called according to his purpose." Sometimes in prayer I want to say, "Really, St. Paul? All things? Even my own sins? Even the sins of priests and bishops? Even bankruptcy as an Archdiocese? God can use these things for good?" Yes, God's word is true—all things. A second passage I find helpful is 2 Corinthians 1:3-8: "Blessed be the God and Father of our Lord Jesus Christ, the Father of mercies and God of all comfort, who comforts us in all our affliction, so that we may be able to comfort those who are in any affliction, with the comfort with which we ourselves are comforted by God." Again, we are invited to the faith that God wants to console us in all the afflictions we face in our lives. Do we believe this? Do we come to prayer believing it?

What does receiving look like? It could be a word that touches my heart, or a phrase from scripture that stands out to me. It could be just a sense of peace that comes over me in Adoration or at Mass that lets me know it is going to be okay, and that God is with me. This receiving is very important. It is the key to the whole spiritual life. It is the peace that Jesus promises even in the greatest trials.[26] It is the way I can receive joy in the midst of my sufferings. It is the key to being a joyful disciple even in the midst of suffering.

When I receive this way of seeing from Jesus, then I can respond differently. I can respond with Jesus, and sometimes I can actually experience peace even in the midst of the difficulty. Sometimes I can even experience the joy that St. Paul talks about.

I hope you can see how different this process is from just grinning and bearing it, or white knuckling it. In this process, when I receive from God how to see my struggle, when I receive that he is with me, Jesus' words in Matthew chapter 11 become true for me: "Take my yoke upon you, and learn from me; for I am gentle and lowly in heart, and you will find rest for your souls. For my yoke is easy, and my burden is light."

Let me share with you a couple of examples of this process of surrender to make this concrete. The greatest example comes from Jesus himself in the Agony in the Garden. I don't know about you, but I find the way the Lord prays in his agony to be astounding. What actually happens when the Lord comes face to face with his cross? He does not pretend it will all be okay. He doesn't say, "Father, I know you will be with me. I can do this. This is what I was born for." No, in fact he cries. He pours out his heart, he sweats blood and he says, "Father, if it be your will let this cup pass from me."[27] According to Cardinal Ratzinger, this is the place we can see the two natures of Christ most clearly, his divine nature

26 Cf. Jn. 14:27.

27 Mk. 14:36.

and his human nature. We can actually see the freedom of the human will of Christ which submits to his divine will. Cardinal Ratzinger explains: "Indeed it is as if we were actually looking in on the inner life of the Word-made-man. It is revealed to us in the sentence which remains the measure and model of all real prayer: 'Not what I will, but what thou wilt' (Mk 14:36). Jesus' human will assimilates itself to the will of the Son. In doing this, he receives the Son's identity, i.e., the complete subordination of the I to the Thou, the self-giving and self-expropriation of the I to the Thou."[28] Christ's human nature trembles before the cross. He acknowledges and relates the pain of his human heart. He relates with absolute trust in the Father—not my will but yours be done. And his human soul receives peace from his divinity.

Did you ever notice the difference in Christ from the moment when he is in agony in the Garden of Gethsemane to the next moment when they come to arrest him? One moment he is in agony and the next he is in perfect peace of soul. What happened? Without presuming to understand the hypostatic union, I would argue that his humanity surrendered and received from his divine nature.

Another scriptural example is found in St. Paul. It is found in 2 Corinthians, chapter 12, after St. Paul recounts a powerful mystical experience in which he was "caught up into Paradise and heard ineffable things, which no one may utter."[29] St. Paul goes on to speak about a thorn he was given in his flesh. He never says what this thorn was, and it doesn't really matter for our point. It was some painful thing in his life—another person, a physical ailment, a heavy problem or a moral weakness—which he begged the Lord to take away. He says, "Three times I begged the Lord about this, that it might leave me."[30] What is he doing here? He is acknowledging and relating. He is pouring out his pain to the Lord. I don't imagine that this was all within the context of one time of prayer. I imagine that over a period of weeks or months St. Paul found himself on his knees crying out to the Lord, "Please take this thorn from me!" And then St. Paul receives this: "He said to me, 'My grace is sufficient for you, for power is made perfect in weakness.'"[31] When he receives this, it changes everything for St. Paul. He sees that God is with him, and that God is allowing this thorn. It gives him peace, even joy. What was a thorn becomes a gift.

And how does St. Paul respond in this grace? He says, "I will rather boast most gladly of my weaknesses, in order that the power of Christ may dwell with me. Therefore, I am content with weaknesses, insults, hardships, persecutions

---

28 Joseph Cardinal Ratzinger, *Behold the Pierced One* (San Francisco: Ignatius Press, 1986) 41.

29 2 Cor. 12: 4.

30 2 Cor. 12: 8.

31 2 Cor. 12: 9.

and constraints, for the sake of Christ; for when I am weak, then I am strong."[32] He is able to respond with great joy and peace even though the thorn has not gone away, because relating the thorn to God in prayer, he is able to see it the way God sees it. The weakness becomes a cause for boasting.

As we speak about learning to carry the cross with Jesus, and even doing so with joy, we begin to see how important prayer is to the process. A true disciple must have a life of prayer, because he must have a relationship with God where he can surrender and come to see the way God sees. I love the way Pope Benedict stated this early in his papacy, "[P]rayer is not an accessory or 'optional', but a question of life or death. In fact, only those who pray, in other words, who entrust themselves to God with filial love, can enter eternal life, which is God himself."[33] Why is prayer essential? Because when the cross comes, if I don't entrust myself to God through prayer, through relating it to him and receiving his way of seeing, then I will grow bitter or sad and may even begin to fall away from being a disciple. Certainly, I won't be a disciple who is completely surrendered and joyful, but rather one who becomes bitter.

The *Catechism of the Catholic Church* also states it quite strongly: "*Prayer is a vital necessity*. Proof from the contrary is no less convincing; if we do not allow the Spirit to lead us, we fall back into the slavery of sin. How can the Holy Spirit be our life if our heart is far from him?"[34] As I grow in prayer and relate the struggles of my life to God, I begin to learn to surrender and am able to be led by the Holy Spirit. This is the very heart of being a disciple. Jesus Christ becomes more and more my "Lord." My heart grows in union with him and I am led by him.

The other thing that happens as I surrender to the cross which the Lord invites me to carry with him is that I begin to see that the cross is fruitful. We begin to see through faith what we saw in St. Paul above. Our suffering is Jesus living his Paschal Mystery in us and therefore, although death is at work in us, it is bringing life to the Church. I love the way that Pope Francis speaks about this fruitfulness of the cross in missionary discipleship in *Evangelii gaudium*. He says,

> Because we do not always see these seeds growing, we need an interior certainty, a conviction that God is able to act in every situation, even amid apparent setbacks: "We have this treasure in earthen vessels" (2 Cor 4:7). This certainty is often called "a sense of mystery." It involves

---

32 2 Cor. 12: 9-10.

33 Benedict XVI, Angelus, Mar. 4, 2007, available at http://www.vatican.va/content/benedict-xvi/en/angelus/2007/documents/hf_ben-xvi_ang_20070304.html (accessed on 2 Mar. 2020).

34 *Catechism of the Catholic Church* 2744, 2nd ed. (Washington, DC: United States Catholic Conference, 2000) 658.

> knowing with certitude that all those who entrust themselves to God in love will bear good fruit (cf. Jn 15: 5). This fruitfulness is often invisible, elusive and unquantifiable. We can know quite well that our lives will be fruitful, without claiming to know how, or where, or when. We may be sure that none of our acts of love will be lost, nor any of our acts of sincere concern for others. No single act of love for God will be lost, no generous effort is meaningless, no painful endurance is wasted. All of these encircle our world like a vital force. . . . It may be that the Lord uses our sacrifices to shower blessings in another part of the world which we will never visit. The Holy Spirit works as he wills, when he wills and where he wills; we entrust ourselves without pretending to see striking results.[35]

When I see my sufferings the way Christ sees them, I can trust that they are bearing fruit as he desires.

What is missionary discipleship? It is the surrender of my life completely to the Lord. It is learning to say a deeper and deeper yes to him, even to his cross. Let me just share with you one final example of a man I met who showed me what true missionary discipleship is. Through the Missionaries of Charity, I was able to meet a man named Fernand, who lives near their home in Ghent, Belgium. When I lived in Rome, I was privileged to go to Ghent to give a couple of retreats for Mother Teresa's sisters. Fernand was a paralyzed man, who was only able to move his head. He could speak without any problem, but the rest of his body was paralyzed, except that he had the strength to squeeze his right hand enough to press a button that opened the front door of his house when someone came to visit. Fernand wanted to be a priest, but just a few months before he was to enter the seminary he came down with this strange paralysis, a disease that has left him in bed for more than fifty years.

The sisters took me to his room where I celebrated Mass for him. He said to me after Mass that he knows he has done more good on that bed than he would have as a priest. He said, "This bed is my altar, here is where I offer my sacrifice." He was perhaps the most joyful man I have ever met. In fact, the sisters told me that when they are having a bad day they go and see Fernand, because they always feel cheered up by being in his presence. He is actually the reason that the Missionaries of Charity are in Ghent, Belgium. When Mother Teresa went to Ghent to give a talk, they asked her to send some of her sisters. She responded, "You don't have poor people here." They said, "Come meet Fernand." Mother Teresa spent a couple of hours talking with Fernand through a translator. At one point in the conversation, the translator, a co-worker of Mother Teresa, said, "Fernand, you have no crucifix in your room." Mother got upset with her and said, "Don't you get it? He is the crucifix." In fact, Fernand keeps a crucifix on

---

35 *Evangelii gaudium*, n. 279.

his chest between his arms, so he remembers why he is in that bed.

When I would visit him he would speak about his work of praying and offering his suffering for the world, which brought him great joy. You can imagine that this was not Fernand's first reaction when he was paralyzed over 50 years ago. Rather, there must have been many a lonely night in that bed as he related and received from the Lord the meaning of his suffering. In the end, he was able to accept his vocation with great joy. The last time I visited him in 2008, he said something that has stuck with me ever since. He said, "Fr. Andrew, I am just a man with all my weakness, but I am burning with love." In that moment I felt like I was before the burning bush – the fire that burned but was not consumed. I felt like I was before the burning heart of Christ – a man who had so surrendered to Christ that his own heart burned with the same fire. "I'm just a man with all my weakness, but I am burning with love." As I prayed with that line, I so wanted to be able to say it myself. Isn't this what happens to us as we relate our suffering to the Lord? Isn't this how we are transformed as we grow in prayer and learn to see our crosses with joy?

My prayer is that we too one day will be able to say, "I am just a man, just a woman, with all my weakness, but I am burning with love." This is the heart of a missionary disciple.

Major Address

Impelling Obligation: Forming Intentional Discipleship in the New Missiondom

Ms. Sherry Weddell

I entered the Church as a young evangelical with an unusual background. I had been studying to become a missionary in the Middle East. My BA was in Near Eastern History and Arabic and then I studied Islamics and cross-cultural studies at one of the foremost evangelical graduate schools of missions. When I became Catholic and tried to explain what I had been preparing to do, Catholics just looked at me in speechless surprise. They thought the whole idea was beyond extraordinary, even though missionary work in Muslim contexts was a full-blown movement in the world I came from.

So I was thrilled to come across this particular canon as a new Catholic:

> Since, like all the Christian faithful, lay persons are designated by God for the apostolate through baptism and confirmation, they are bound by the general obligation and possess the right as individuals, or joined in associations, to work so that the divine message of salvation is made known and accepted by all persons everywhere in the world. This obligation is even more compelling in those circumstances in which only through them can people hear the gospel and know Christ.[1]

I was *so* excited to realize that, even though most Catholics did not seem to understand, canon law recognized my baptismal right to evangelize the world! It was a true epiphany to discover that the law of the Church had such a strong missionary orientation.

Welcome to Missiondom

The implications of this particular canon are crucial for us because we do not live in Christendom any more. Geo-political Christendom has slowly but largely disappeared over the course of the last several generations in the West. And the informal cultural consensus that lingered in parts of the United States, like Flannery O'Connor's Christ-haunted south, is also quickly disappearing.

1 C. 225 §1; all English translations of canons in *Code of Canon Law, Latin-English Edition: New English Translation* (Washington, DC: Canon Law Society of America, 2012).

This has shocked many Catholics because the assumption that Christendom and the West were one and the same was something that many held on to as an essential part of what it *means* to be Catholic. The Catholic Church was the spiritual center, the heart of western Europe, for over 1,000 years, and that kind of history creates a sense of self that lingers long after the reality on the ground has changed. A lingering corollary belief is that since we *should* be living in Christendom, the Catholic faith *should be supported and reinforced by the larger culture*.

Today we find ourselves in a very different situation, one that I call "Missiondom." Missiondom is the new western reality where faith and religious identity are not supported by the larger culture and not primarily inherited but chosen (or *not* chosen). For instance, one-half of American Millennials who were raised Catholic—and are now in their mid-twenties through late thirties—have already jettisoned their Catholic identity.[2]

The next generation, often called "Gen Z," are the new emerging adults. Many have no imaginative category for a Christian cultural norm at all and were not raised in a believing Christian family or any religious context. One-third of Gen Z are already completely secular. They don't believe in God, they never pray, and they never attend religious services. They do not consider themselves to be either religious or spiritual.[3] *If* members of the Gen Z generation remain Catholic as adults or become Catholic, it will be because they have chosen to do so. In Missiondom, a living Catholic faith is usually the fruit of a *voluntary* personal journey.

This cultural shift is not temporary. It is essential that we understand that we are heading into an era of *enduring* Missiondom. Christian cultural hegemony as we knew it in historic Christendom can never be re-established as long as something like the internet exists and most people are a ten-second Google search away from access to every religious or spiritual idea on the planet. None of us or our children or grandchildren will see that kind of Christendom again and the Church will need to find new ways to respond to the challenges of our new cultural reality.

In my book, *Forming Intentional Disciples*, I describe three concurrent journeys that all Catholics are called to make and that are at the heart of our dilemma.

---

2 See Pew Research Center, "America's Changing Religious Landscape," May 12, 2015, 41, https://www.pewforum.org/2015/05/12/americas-changing-religious-landscape/ (accessed on 9 Jan. 2020).

3 See, e.g., Jean M. Twenge, *iGen: Why Today's Super-Connected Kids Are Growing Up Less Rebellious, More Tolerant, Less Happy—and Completely Unprepared for Adulthood—and What That Means for the Rest of Us* (New York: Atria Books, 2017).

1. The *personal interior journey of a lived relationship with Christ* resulting in intentional discipleship.

2. The *journey of active practice* evidenced by receiving the sacraments, attending Mass, and participating in the life and mission of the Christian community.

3. The *ecclesial journey into the Church* through reception of the sacraments of initiation.[4]

In Christendom, we presumed that normal Christian development would begin with the sacraments of initiation such as the baptism of infants (journey 3), who would gradually pick up a living faith from their parents and families as they grew older (journey 2); a faith which would be reinforced by the larger culture. In practice, the first journey of the living relationship with Christ, conversion, and personal discipleship was assumed to not be absolutely necessary for ordinary Catholics and really only for those called to priesthood and religious life or very exceptional lay people. As long as you retained your religious identity, attended Mass with some regularity, went to confession occasionally, and didn't do anything dramatically bad, you were a reasonably good Catholic.

But in a highly secularized setting like ours, post-modern culture eats through a merely notional faith or inherited cultural identity like acid. If our understanding or experience of being Catholic is merely institutional, impersonal, and obligation-driven, many 21st century people, especially those under 40, will simply walk away. Without the first journey of personal conversion, most Millennial and Gen Z Catholics won't practice the faith, and those who don't practice will not bother to baptize their children. The decline in infant baptism in the United States has already begun; the baptism of infants and children under the age of seven dropped 38% between 2000 and 2017.[5]

Three Stages of Adult Christian Development

We use a very simple schema to describe adult Christian development, which we have found enormously useful, and which is rooted in the Church's Tradition. We speak of three basic stages: Seeker, Disciple, and Apostle or Missionary Discipleship.

Seeker refers to what the *Catechism* calls the "first and fundamental

---

4 See Sherry A. Weddell, *Forming Intentional Disciples: The Path to Knowing and Following Jesus* (Huntington, IN: Our Sunday Visitor, 2012) 54.

5 See Center for the Applied Research in the Apostolate, "Baptisms of Infants in Previous Years," *Frequently Requested Church Statistics*, https://cara.georgetown.edu/frequently-requested-church-statistics/ (accessed on 9 Jan. 2020).

conversion."[6] This is the initial spiritual journey—perhaps starting as far back as "I don't believe in any kind of God" or "I'm an agnostic"—leading to and culminating at the point where a person begins to follow Jesus Christ as his disciple in the midst of his Church.

The second stage, which we call *Disciple* and which the *Catechism* describes as the "second conversion,"[7] is the lifelong journey of transformation as we follow Jesus as disciples. The second journey is an experience of gradual but ever deeper level of conversion that shapes us into a person who is ready to be sent by Jesus on mission into the world.

Which brings us to the *Apostle stage,* or what Pope Francis calls a *Missionary Disciple.* Christian adulthood or Christian maturity is another way to think of "missionary disciple." A missionary disciple is not just someone seeking to *follow* Christ. He or she has now become someone with a strong sense of personal mission whom Jesus is sending out as his emissary to others. A Christian who has reached the Apostle level of spiritual development is not only capable of taking responsibility for their own relationship with God but they have become a man or woman for others who can help draw them closer to Christ. This is the developmental stage at which personal vocations are discerned and deliberately lived and where great fruit, the sort of fruit that changes history, is born.

At the Catherine of Siena Institute, we have worked with 170,000 Catholics in over 1,000 parishes in 200+ dioceses all over the world. For 22 years, we have been listening to Catholics tell us stories of their relationship with God and of being used by God. And we have come to realize that a majority of Catholics are not yet disciples, much less *missionary* disciples. They retain a Catholic identity; they may even be active in the parish in addition to attending Mass. But that does not necessarily mean that they have a personal faith or a personal relationship with God.

Last year, one of my collaborators and I did interviews with 25 highly engaged Catholics—leaders in their parish. Half of them told us that even though they were raised Catholic and attended Mass regularly as a child and had even received First Communion, they thought of God as a distant authority figure when they were children. This childhood God was a rule-enforcer who did not love them or their families, a God with whom they had no relationship, and whose primary purpose was to punish people who didn't obey the rules.

Stunningly, half of these "practicing" Catholics also told us that they had not known who Jesus Christ was as children. They had heard the name but Jesus was

---

6 *Catechism of the Catholic Church* 1427, 2nd ed. (Washington, DC: United States Catholic Conference, 2000) 359.

7 Ibid., n. 1428.

just a mysterious figure, a good man that Catholics respected or revered although what Jesus has done to deserve reverence was not at all clear. As children, they had not believed that Jesus was God. Most of the 25 had left the Church early, often as soon as they graduated from high school. They were gone for years or even decades, and then each one had slowly made the journey back. But there was nothing automatic about it.

We have discovered that you can be raised in the Church and attend Mass every week, but still not believe in or trust the personal God become incarnate in Jesus Christ that the Catholic Church proclaims. Forty years ago, St. John Paul II wrote about the same phenomenon when he observed that many Catholic children are "still without any explicit personal attachment to Jesus Christ; they only have the capacity to believe placed within them by Baptism and the presence of the Holy Spirit."[8]

When people do develop that explicit personal attachment to Christ and begin the journey of discipleship, their priorities change. Disciples will want to worship. They want to learn how to pray. They want to serve because they really care about the Church. They give. When a parish seriously evangelizes, giving goes up. Evangelizing leaders tell us, "We have the highest per capita giving in the diocese."

Disciples are also intensely curious spiritually. They are eager to study the Church's teaching and will fill every class you offer at the parish and diocesan level. Disciples clamor to discern God's call. They want to know, "Now that my relationship with God is coming alive, what does this mean? What does God want of me?" None of this is motivated by mere obligation. It flows out of a living and growing relationship with God.

Catechesis really comes into its own when people are on the verge of becoming disciples or in their early days as disciples. Now catechesis answers questions they are actually asking. This is the stage where people start to develop the basic habits of discipleship: prayer, discernment, obedience, etc. This is where spiritual mentoring becomes very important. This is the stage at which people begin to have the strength to go public with their faith even in hostile or indifferent environments. And this is the point where the charisms, which all the baptized receive when they receive the Holy Spirit in baptism, begin to manifest.

We have been told many times that charisms started to manifest a year or two after someone has gone through a major conversion and with a charism comes a call. The emergence, recognition, and discernment of one's charisms is part of what sparks a larger sense of responsibility for the Church and her mission.

8 John Paul II, apostolic exhortation *Catechesi Tradendae* 19, October 16, 1979: *AAS* 71 (1979) 1293; English translation from Weddell, *Forming Intentional Disciples*, text accompanying footnote 15.

People tell us, "Discerning my charisms has changed everything." It has changed how they understand themselves, how they understand the Church, how they relate to God, and how they relate to other people in their lives and to the world.

Fruit bearing now becomes a way of life. This is the time when Catholics begin to discern and live personal vocations of all kinds: ordained, religious, and lay. Mature missionary disciples undertake amazing and creative works of charity and social justice, vocations that sometimes may affect the lives of millions.

My best rough estimate at this point is that only about one percent of baptized Catholics have reached the Missionary Disciple stage of spiritual development. Our vocational problem is a developmental problem. Most of our people are not yet consciously seeking to follow Jesus as his disciple in the midst of his Church. They are not being helped to mature to the point where they really begin living and functioning as Missionary Disciples.

The issue of spiritual adulthood is crucial. What we desperately need now are millions of Catholics who are spiritual adults not just in name but in living reality. We need people who are true Missionary Disciples and Apostles whom Christ can send into thousands of different mission fields. Our problem is that most of our people are simply not yet there spiritually. In practice, we have come to accept religious "activity" or "identity" without personal faith and Missionary Discipleship as *normal*. The challenge before us is: how can we intentionally help Catholics grow into spiritual adults and Missionary Disciples?

One parish that we have worked with for years has helped a number of merely notional, non-practicing, or "former" Catholics not only come back to the Church but become full blown spiritual adults. One such story took place just after 9/11 when many Americans showed up at church again looking for some kind of hope. One young man who had left his parish at age sixteen and been away for 20 years suddenly showed up at Mass at his childhood parish looking for something he could not put into language. He stood in the back and was moved to hear the youth minister say, "Raise your hand if you want to get to heaven and if you want to bring a teen with you." He hesitantly raised his hand and the youth minister saw him and talked to him after Mass. That was the beginning. He got involved with youth ministry, and the youth minister spent many hours mentoring him, teaching him how to pray, etc. Now that young man is a priest.

The Evangelizing Tasks of the Church

Canon 787 has something really important to say to our situation in Missiondom: "By the witness of their life and word, missionaries are to establish a sincere dialogue with those who do not believe in Christ so that, in a manner adapted to their own temperament and culture, avenues are opened enabling

them to understand the message of the gospel."

There are three tasks the Church teaches that we need to tackle in order to accompany people on the journey to discipleship: Pre-Evangelization, Initial Proclamation of Jesus Christ, and Catechesis. Since the late sixteenth and early seventeenth centuries, the Catholic retention strategy has been: (a) sacramental initiation and (b) childhood catechesis. But that catechesis occurred in a world that was still dominantly Christian. Indeed, we never thought about pre-evangelization in the United States because the only missionaries who had to worry about that sort of thing were bound for Asia or Africa to evangelize non-Christians who lived *outside* Christendom. But Americans lived *inside* Christendom and therefore all we needed to offer was catechesis. We assumed that because we were still living in an overwhelmingly Christian setting, pre-evangelization and an introductory knowledge of Jesus' story would "just happen" within our already Christian and practicing families and in the larger culture *if* we catechized our people properly. Even today, Catholic leaders are still prone to leap directly into Catechesis. We are comfortable with it, we understand it, we have a lot of model and structures set up to support, and we tend to presume the catechesis automatically includes pre-evangelization and the initial proclamation as well.

Now we live in a very different world where we cannot presume that even practicing cradle Catholics believe in a personal God who loves them or know why Jesus is important. These first two tasks—pre-evangelization and initial proclamation of Jesus—cannot be taken for granted at all in a situation where the majority of Catholic families do not practice and the culture no longer transmits basic Christian knowledge and values. They are absolutely critical in our setting, and yet they are the evangelistic tasks with which we are the least familiar and comfortable and for which we have the fewest structures and tools.

What canon 787 is describing is pre-evangelization, which addresses the concerns of people in the very beginning of the journey to initial conversion.

Pre-evangelization

The first task of pre-evangelization is establishing trust. Spiritual trust requires that a person has some kind of positive association with Christianity or Christ or the Church. Trust is not the same as personal faith. They may not believe any part of the faith themselves but they have a good relationship with a believing Catholic. Their Catholic friend serves as a kind of living bridge to the Christian faith and the Church.

Someone without any positive association with Christianity—who does not have a living bridge of trust already in place—is almost certainly not going to walk spontaneously through the door of one of our parishes. Fifty-five percent of Americans who still retain a Catholic identity seldom or never attend Mass.

Many non-practicing or former Catholics no longer trust us for various reasons. There may have been a bridge of trust in place in the past but that trust was broken. Until the bridge of trust is rebuilt, people will not move closer to or return to Jesus Christ and his Church.

On the other hand, people who have a bridge of trust in place are spiritually and emotionally *near* and much more accessible. They are much more likely to show up in our parishes to attend Mass or, if invited by a friend, to a social gathering or an evangelizing group experience like the Alpha course.[9] About 45% of Catholics are *active*, meaning they attend Mass at least once a month. In our experience, if someone is active, you will find that a bridge of trust is already in place. In terms of their spiritual development, about 90% of U.S. Catholics are either at distrust or at trust. A small minority of practicing Catholics have grown beyond spiritual trust into early curiosity and are often some of our highly engaged members.

Pre-evangelization is the first and most fundamental evangelical task in our secularized setting. Unfortunately, it is a task for which Catholics have little or no training, skills, vision, or structures in place. Most of our parishes and parish leaders still function as though we are living in a Christian rather than missionary setting. We are going to have to start thinking like true missionaries and seek new ways of going outside the parish to former Catholics and skeptics who will never come to us. We need evangelizers who pro-actively build bridges of trust and walk with non-believers and skeptics while they are still outside and before they will feel comfortable walking through our doors. We need to form "far" evangelizers.

At the Catherine of Siena Institute, we train such evangelizers and call them "Ananiases." Ananiases are evangelizing spiritual companions who can recognize the work of the Holy Spirit in another's life, can recognize when people are going through spiritual change or are seeking, and come alongside to help. An Ananias leaves the Christian community to meet spiritual wanderers where they are right now and to help foster a transforming encounter with Jesus Christ that will create a bridge to the Church itself. *We, as parish leaders and as entire parish communities, need to intentionally foster, form, and support such evangelizers*. These evangelizing companions function as an arm of the Church to reach families, circles of friends, neighborhoods, businesses, professions, schools, and the larger world.

Initial Proclamation of Jesus Christ

---

9 "Alpha is an 11-week course that creates a space, online or in person, where people are excited to bring their friends for a conversation about faith, life and God." See https://www.alpha.org/about/ (accessed on 28 Apr. 2020).

The second task of the Church—the initial proclamation of Jesus Christ—helps people become more curious and open to the possibility of personal and spiritual change and helps them grapple more profoundly with who Jesus is and how to respond to him. This second task is also very crucial and is also one for which we have relatively few structures. Catholics have just started to grapple seriously with how to tell Jesus' "Great Story" in compelling and accessible ways in our parishes and campus ministries, schools, and families in the last five years. The conversation is beginning to change tremendously. But in practice, the majority of our people still have not heard and cannot articulate who Jesus is, what he has done for us, why it matters, and, therefore, are not yet ready to grapple with the challenge, "How will you respond to Jesus's call to follow him in the midst of his Church?"

Ananias Training

To help foster a growing cohort of evangelizing bridge-builders, the Catherine of Siena Institute offers what we call Ananias Training. Our goal is to form hundreds and thousands of ordinary Catholics and give them an evangelizing skill set that can be used inside *and* outside the parish so that they can accompany others on the path of discipleship. Our goal is to train laity to recognize the people who are on spiritual journeys; to understand and recognize the stages of conversion (the developmental stages that 21st century people typically go through on their way to discipleship); and to learn how to hold what we call "threshold conversations" (of which more in a moment).

In addition, we train our Ananiases to really grapple in depth with the kerygma, the basic gospel proclamation. The goal is that they will grasp it so deeply that it will permeate their sharing with other people. We teach them how to share their own story of their encounter with God and how that has changed their life, and how to share Jesus' story. We want to enable as many believing Catholics as possible to acquire the basic skills and awareness necessary to be evangelizing bridge-builders on the spiritual frontier.

One of those skills is having threshold conversations, where, after building trust, we can ask to hear the story of another's lived relationship with God to this point in their life, whatever it has been: good, bad, indifferent, or non-existent. Such conversations are very simple and can be done formally in the course of ministry or informally in a pub. I've had threshold conversations on airplanes with total strangers. You can have these conversations with self-proclaimed *atheists*, Buddhists or *Nones*. People may tell you that they are a "practicing Catholic," a "skeptic," an "agnostic" or say, "I don't use the word 'God.'"

People in the 21st century often don't use religious labels in definitive, dictionary ways. What they often mean by a religious label is, "This is how I am identifying myself right now." In our culture, that could change tomorrow

or a year from now, or it may never change. Someone may self-identify as a Catholic, and you literally do not know what that means in practice anymore. I have met Catholics who were really functional atheists. We have learned to never just accept a religious label at face value. Always ask what they *mean*. Always ask for the *story* behind the label.

That's why our motto is, "Never accept a religious *label* in the place of a *story*." So if somebody says to me, "I was raised a Catholic, but now I'm an agnostic," I typically reply along the lines of, "Really? That is fascinating. When you say *agnostic*, what does that mean for you? How did you get there?" Then we're off and running: we're into the *story*. Threshold conversations are a great example of *listening evangelism*.

What is fascinating is that recent studies have found that good spiritual conversations create greater spiritual openness in both Christians and non-Christians! Indeed, the more *positive* conversations people have about faith, the more open they become to additional faith conversations. We have seen people move through whole developmental stages just by telling their story to someone who really listened. Even a single conversation in the course of an entire year can move someone into greater spiritual openness. Five or more positive conversations about faith can double someone's spiritual openness. So good conversations are really critical. It is crucial that we remember what non-believers consider to be a *good* faith conversation is one in which the Christian listened without judgment and left the other free to come to their own conclusion.

Remember that *many people don't know what their journey is because they've never tried to put it into words before*. That is why it is so vital at the beginning to let people tell their story and listen hard to understand. Our purpose at this moment is not to fix them, catechize them, do apologetics or correct all their loopy ideas about Catholics and the Catholic Church (you can do that later but that's not the job of *this* moment). The purpose of the threshold conversation is for the listener to *understand the other's journey from their perspective* and to give the speaker the chance to describe, not just what happened objectively, but the emotional and spiritual impact on them. People tell us over and over, "No one ever asked me that question before and no one ever listened."

As canon lawyers, you encounter so many Catholics at moments of personal struggle and crisis, at moments when they may feel as though their faith in God and in the Church has been crushed or even shattered. At that moment you can be both a canonist and a witness to God's abiding presence and love, a sign of hope. When we really listen, people's emotional and spiritual defenses drop dramatically and they become much more open to the possibility of something new and good. You can help strengthen or help rebuild their trust in God and the Church and rouse fresh hope and spiritual curiosity by both the questions you ask and the way you listen to them.

One last passage that I find especially compelling comes from the introduction to the *Code*:

> [T]he Code is in no way intended as a substitute for faith, grace, charisms and especially charity in the life of the Church and of the faithful. On the contrary, its purpose is rather to create such an order in the ecclesial society that, while assigning the primacy to love, grace and charisms, it at the same time renders their organic development easier in the life of both the ecclesial society and the individual persons who belong to it.[10]

To put it very simply, canon law is a kind of ecclesial trellis whose purpose is to support the branches of the true Vine so they bear abundant fruit for the world.

Similarly, Pope St. John Paul II puts it this way in *Pastores dabo vobis* 40:

> Indeed, God with his call reaches the call of each individual, and the Spirit, who abides deep within each disciple (cf. 1 Jn. 3:24), gives himself to each Christian with different charisms and special signs. Each one, therefore, must be helped to embrace the gift entrusted to him as a completely unique person, and to hear the words which the Spirit of God personally addresses to him.[11]

This is why priests are called to recognize, uncover with faith, acknowledge with joy, foster with diligence, appreciate, judge and discern, coordinate and put to good use, and have "heartfelt esteem" for the charisms of all the baptized.[12] In the Church's understanding, there are three basic categories of charisms: hierarchical charisms, founding charisms (given those who found religious orders or lay movements), and the gifts that I am addressing here, the charisms given to individuals.

These individual charisms are given to each and every baptized person, not for his or her sake but for the sake of others. This is why Saint Thomas Aquinas

---

10 John Paul II, apostolic constitution *Sacrae disciplinae leges*, January 25, 1983: *AAS* 75/2 (1983) xi; English translation in *Code of Canon Law, Latin-English Edition: New English Translation,* xxix-xxx.

11 John Paul II, apostolic exhortation *Pastores dabo vobis* 40, March 25, 1992: *AAS* 84 (1992) 657; English translation at http://www.vatican.va/content/john-paul-ii/en/apost_exhortations/documents/hf_jp-ii_exh_25031992_pastores-dabo-vobis.html (accessed on 2 Mar. 2020).

12 Second Vatican Council, dogmatic constitution *Lumen gentium*, November 21, 1964: *AAS* 57 (1965) 5, n. 30; Second Vatican Council, decree *Presbyterorum ordinis* 9, December 7, 1965: *AAS* 58 (1966) 991; *Pastores dabo vobis* 40, 74; John Paul II, apostolic exhortation *Christifideles laici* 32, December 30, 1988: *AAS* 81 (1989) 393.

calls them "gratuitous graces." Charisms are given to us not for our own salvation but to enable us to cooperate with God's redemptive purposes for our neighbor. These gifts are ways that we are supernaturally empowered to become channels of God's love, mercy, beauty, truth, provision, and healing for others.

The Church says that all the baptized have a "right and duty" to use their charisms.[13] She also says that the charisms call us to be "active and co-responsible" and that they enable each person to make a totally unique contribution to the mission, life, and ministry of the Church.[14] Finally, the Church tells us that discernment is always necessary for discovering one's charisms.[15]

I don't have time to describe the whole discernment process, but I will end with this on the impact discernment can have.

One of the parishes we worked with for a long time began offering evangelization retreats and the Called & Gifted discernment workshop.[16] As a result, people's lives started changing in very dramatic ways. One was a woman named Ellen. I happened to be visiting the parish and sat down to lunch next to Ellen (whom I had never met) and she turned to me and exclaimed, "Boy, do I have to talk to you!"

She told me that a couple of years earlier she had gone through the evangelization retreat. She had been a sort of ordinary, essentially passive show-up-once-a-week Catholic. But when she came out of that retreat, she was on fire. She said she had had a dream in which she saw the words "WORKS OF MERCY" carved into stone. She asked herself, "What does that mean?" Then she went through the Called & Gifted workshop, and she scored high in the charism of Mercy when she took the inventory that is part of the process.

She said, "It's that *Mercy* word again! God is trying to tell me something." She said her first step was to volunteer for her parish Saint Vincent De Paul Society, which made perfect sense. But by the time I talked to her, two years later, she was negotiating with state and local officials to start the first day shelter for the homeless in the entire state of Idaho. And that was only the beginning!

After that, she helped found the local Catholic Worker movement. Then she set up two homes, one for homeless women and the other for homeless men.

---

13 Second Vatican Council, decree *Apostolicam actuositatem* 3, November 18, 1965: *AAS* 58 (1966) 837.

14 *Christifideles laici* 20, 21.

15 Ibid., 24.

16 "The Called & Gifted™ Discernment Process . . . is designed to help Christians discern the presence of charisms in their lives." See https://siena.org/called-gifted (accessed on 28 Apr. 2020).

Finally, she earned her master's degree in Addiction Studies and become a licensed social worker. She had two questions for me:

1. How do I find a spiritual director who understands what has happened to me?
2. How do I explain this to my husband?

Ellen's parish was the catalyst for her spiritual development, but the whole community was transformed in turn by watching her go through this maturation process as a mature missionary disciple. Lay leaders had been holding a three-day evangelizing retreat for parishioners for the past nineteen years. They estimated that at least a quarter of their adults were full-blown intentional disciples, many of whom had been away from the Church for decades and then had come back as a result of going through this retreat. Forty percent of all adults in their parish were involved in parish ministries of some kind, and almost all of them had gone through the retreat. At Ellen's parish, both their Mass attendance and their giving went up. They had, in fact, the highest per capita giving in the diocese.

Witnessing Ellen's journey named a larger call for the whole parish community, which then set out to have as big an impact as possible on their part of the city. I don't have time to tell you all the extraordinary things that happened as a result. They got involved in working with drug addicts, feeding the homeless, refugee resettlement, "No One Dies Alone,"[17] healing prayer and a host of other ministries. Parishioners went around the country bringing the evangelization retreat to other parishes at their own expense and another group took the Called & Gifted discernment process out to remote mountain and desert towns in their diocese.

The obvious question is, "Which came first: The chicken or the egg?" The parish changed the lives of Ellen and other individuals by offering the evangelization retreats. But the conversion of individuals and the fruit those disciples bore changed many other people's lives within and outside the parish. Their conversion also changed the cultural and spiritual norm of the whole parish community itself. It created a parish culture where becoming Christian adults and bearing the abundant fruit of a missionary disciple did not seem weird or only for an exceptional few but was considered absolutely normal for ordinary Catholics and the whole community.

---

17 See, e.g., https://www.peacehealth.org/sacred-heart-medical-center/noda/start-your-own-program (accessed on 9 Jan. 2020).

Major Address

Can We Open the Door Wider under Current Law?

The Most Reverend Mark O'Connell, JCD

Please allow me to recognize two things as I begin this talk. First, I am fully aware that the third major address is the one where many bags are packed and in the back of the room and that almost all of you have some place to get to right after this morning's schedule. So, I fully understand that some of you will be getting up to leave and catch a flight or an Uber, and I promise not to take it personally. Should you want me to take it personally, you should perhaps stamp your feet and slam the door on the way out, and I'll get the message. In our divided world and Church these days, I am bound to offend some of you. Second, I had an interesting experience writing this speech after three years of being an auxiliary bishop and therefore no longer a part of the day-to-day canon law world. For fifteen years I was doing canon law work every day, and I gained a lot of experience. But for the past three years I still have participated, but it is not daily, and I find myself a bit out of practice.

There is an interesting balance here that fits into the premise of this talk; this is not just idle speculation. I used to be one the ones who wanted to get my opinion into the mix of opinions, but I am on the other side of this now. As an auxiliary bishop, what I want more now is to get a variety of people's opinions to help inform me. But where is the variety of opinions? Of course, it exists in this room. But how do we as the Canon Law Society of America get the availability of a variety of canonical opinions to the private side-meetings that truly run our Church? Articles and synods and councils and staff members all are important; but when there is a crisis in your diocese how many of you are truly in the decision-making room?

Let me demonstrate. I will ask three series of questions here and will ask for a show of hands if you are comfortable. Please be honest with yourselves and not nice to whoever is your bishop. In other words, I am asking you to answer strictly and not generously.

Dear members of the Canon Law Society of America, when your diocesan bishop confronts a situation where a priest has acted scandalously and the bishop has to make a decision as to the priest's canonical status, does he consult with you directly, face to face, such that you feel that you have helped him make up

his mind? If you feel you have that level of decision-influencing clout, please raise your hand.

Let's move to tribunal work because many of you specialize in that area. [*Aside* - is that a good thing for a diocese to have canon lawyers who only do marriage cases and are not part of the other canonical decisions?] Let's have those whose jobs are principally marriage tribunal related please raise your hand. Now please keep your hand raised only if your bishop has ever consulted you directly and included you in his decision making of anything canonical. Now let me be clear, I am not asking if the judicial vicar consulted you about something for the bishop, I am asking if your bishop heard your opinion unfiltered and made a decision based on it.

Final series of questions: first, please raise your hand if you have been involved in meetings where your bishop or even your vicar general brings together a small group to discuss a difficult problem. I assume a lot of you have been to this type of meeting; there is a problem of some sort and they gather a team for crisis management and you are someone who gets invited to that type of meeting along with the PR people and the money people and the lawyers that are inevitably in the room. Now here is something that I notice repeatedly: at the end of the meeting, two to three people are usually asked to stay behind. If you feel that you are usually dismissed after your opinion is given, whereas two or three others stay behind, please lower your hand.

Let me conclude this section with the "why" of this talk I am giving. Real decision influencing authority is to be in the room when the decision is made and to have been consulted such that you are certain that you have been heard. But in so many dioceses the ones left in the room at the end of the day are priests and *not* lay people and *not* women. Notice, I am in no way here taking away the bishop's authority to make these kinds of decisions and to lead. I am just pointing out that real consultation on critical issues—including the scandalous things that the bishop wants few to know—should involve lay people and, in particular, lay women. But the Code of Canon Law doesn't require this type of consultation, and I would argue there is nothing wrong with that *per se*; instead, our bishops and priests need to consciously open the door.

That's my premise. Now let me take you back to the eye of the storm in 2002 when the scandal first surfaced in the Archdiocese of Boston and a tsunami of accusations crashed onto our unsuspecting shores. On January 6, 2002, the Feast of the Epiphany, I was a brand-new canon lawyer in the Archdiocese of Boston with the title Assistant to the Moderator of the Curia for Canonical Affairs. It was my job to be the delegate for dispensations and answer canonical questions and every now and then give a canonical opinion when the Archbishop or the Vicar General asked for one. Later that winter I would defend my doctorate, so I was very new. That was the day (as most of you know) that the first article about an

abusing priest appeared in the major newspaper, to be followed by day after day revelations, which spread throughout the country and the universal Church. As the intensity grew behind the walls of the chancery we were scrambling to come up with, among other things, a canonical process to handle the cases. But, as you know, there wasn't one, for two reasons: first, because almost every case was past canonical prescription,[1] and second, because the law before it was reformed urged vigorously for these things to be settled outside of court. One only has to read canon 2214 §2 of the 1917 Code of Canon Law to see an example of the mindset.[2] Because of this there were few-to-no records of complete canonical processes as they had not taken place, and there was no place to look for canonical precedents as to how to handle violations of canon 1395 of the 1983 Code after prescription had passed; yet the People of God and the archbishop demanded one. Since our more senior canon lawyers were compromised in various ways it fell to the more junior canon lawyers on staff to figure this all out as best we could. I was part of it, as were three other relatively inexperienced canon lawyers (three of us priests and a laywoman). We did our best.

In the middle of that whole thing, the People of God understandably became more and more angry, and they demanded a hearing in the whole sordid mess. A few groups were formed in the midst of all this, and one of these was "The Voice of the Faithful." They came for discussions, and Cardinal Law assigned his vicar general/moderator of the curia to the task of meeting with them. He brought with him his Assistant for Canonical Affairs, and that would be me.

---

1 1983 *CIC* c. 1362 §1, 3° plus special derogations, April 25, 1994, and extension April 26, 1999.

2 1917 *CIC* c. 2214 §2:

> She shall always have before her eyes the advice of the Coun. of Tr., sess. 13, *on ref.*, chap 1: "Let Bishops and other Ordinaries bear in mind that they are pastors and not prosecutors and that they ought so to preside over those subject to them so as not to lord it over them, but to love them as children and brethren and to strive by exhortation and admonition to deter them from what is unlawful, that they may not be obliged, should [their subjects] transgress, to coerce them by due punishments. In regard to those, however, who should happen to sin through frailty, that command of the Apostle is to be observed, [namely] that they reprove, entreat, and rebuke them in all kindness and patience, since benevolence toward those to be corrected often effects more than severity, exhortation more than threat, and charity more than force. But if on account of the gravity of the offense there is need of the rod, then is rigor to be tempered with gentleness, judgment with mercy, and severity with clemency, that discipline, so salutary and necessary for the people, may be preserved without harshness and they who are chastised may be corrected, or, if they are unwilling to repent, that others may, by the wholesome example of their punishment, be deterred from vices."

The 1917 Pio-Benedictine Code of Canon Law in English Translation, cur. Edward N. Peters (San Francisco: Ignatius Press, 2001) 701-702.

They came to the meeting with righteous anger and armed with the level of canon law that all lay people have access to, which is the index of our CLSA *New Commentary on the Code of Canon Law*;[3] they wanted to assert their authority as members of the Church in accord with c. 212 §§2-3.[4] They asked, where do the people of God have the power to step in and stop the presumed outrageous activity of the hierarchy? They wanted to take over the purse strings of the Archdiocese/Archbishop, and they sought direction on how to do that. They wanted to lecture the culprits, and they focused on the two of us. It was eye-opening at the same time as it was canonically unsophisticated; it caused me to be in protection mode at the same time as I related to their outrage. It, and subsequent meetings, were a whirlwind, and I am still sorting it all out to this day.

The reason I bring it up here is not to tell the whole story of those meetings and that time, as much as I would like to set the record straight from what was published. It is to point out the deficiency of the Code of Canon Law for moral outrage to be expressed by the People of God. Depending on the reaction of the bishop, it often pushes the People to mass media, social media, hit-or-miss accusations and shaming as their most powerful options. For what exists in the code is easily rendered ineffective if a bishop chooses that route.

- The diocesan pastoral council[5] exists, but it is a suggestion in the code[6] and has none of the "consult or consent" power that the presbyteral council or the college of consultors has.[7]

---

3 *New Commentary on the Code of Canon Law,* ed. John Beal et al. (Mahwah, NJ: Paulist Press, 2000).

4 1983 *CIC* c. 212:

> §2 The Christian faithful are free to make known to the pastors of the Church their needs, especially spiritual ones, and their desires.
> §3 According to the knowledge, competence, and prestige which they possess, they have the right and even at times the duty to manifest to the sacred pastors their opinion on matters which pertain to the good of the Church and to make their opinion known to the rest of the Christian faithful, without prejudice to the integrity of faith and morals, with reverence toward their pastors, and attentive to common advantage of the dignity of persons.

English translation of canons is from *Code of Canon Law, Latin-English Edition: New English Translation* (Washington, DC: Canon Law Society of America, 2012) unless otherwise indicated.

5 See 1983 *CIC* cc. 511-514.

6 See 1983 *CIC* c. 511: "In every diocese and to the extent that pastoral circumstances suggest it, a pastoral council is to be constituted which under the authority of the bishop investigates, considers, and proposes practical conclusions about those things which pertain to pastoral works in the diocese."

7 Although the diocesan pastoral council has a "consultative vote," according to 1983 *CIC* c. 514, there are no corresponding canons where this consultation is required by the law.

- The diocesan finance council has some real authority to stop major actions, but its membership is at the whim of the diocesan bishop and there is no requirement that it be representational.[8]
- Ultimately, no one can judge a bishop except the Apostolic See.[9]
- Those who work for the diocesan curia have some access[10] but are bound to secrecy[11] and easily removed.
- Lay institutes exist, but they depend completely on the approval of their statutes to gain any recognition. *De facto* lay institutes only really have a voice if the bishop chooses to listen.
- Appeals over the bishop's head need a specific grievance.

In the end, the code is easily used to shut the doors to the complaints of the people; but at the same time, it *can* be used much more effectively if a diocesan bishop is unafraid to open the doors. Naturally, a diocesan bishop should not obstruct or prohibit real, meaningful, decision-making consultations with those who are truly qualified from the People of God. Indeed, in my experience, many bishops are very open with those they trust. However, I think the modern bishop should consciously set up and find ways to encourage consultation with lay people. It is critical to our Church that the bishop be especially conscious to open the doors to women's voices only because in my experience these voices are underrepresented given that all clerics are men.

Future codes of canon law will hopefully be more open to real, visible and meaningful decision-making capacity among lay people without reducing the theological standing of the bishop. But the Code of Canon Law is adaptable now, as is, to create real avenues of meaningful decision-making capacity for lay men and women. Or, it is adaptable to discourage the truly meaningful decision-making capacity from lay men and women and to be very clerical. It is up to the bishop. I admit that I speak to you as an auxiliary bishop, a position also too easily marginalized. But as a bishop, I ask: *what are we afraid of?*

---

8 1983 *CIC* c. 492 §1: "In every diocese a finance council is to be established, over which the diocesan bishop himself or his delegate presides and which consists of at least three members of the Christian faithful truly expert in financial affairs and civil law, outstanding in integrity, and appointed by the bishop."

9 1983 *CIC* c. 1405.

10 See 1983 *CIC* c. 228:

> §1 Lay persons who are found suitable are qualified to be admitted by the sacred pastors to those ecclesiastical offices and functions which they are able to exercise according to the precepts of the law.
>
> §2. Lay persons who excel in necessary knowledge, prudence, and integrity are qualified to assist the pastors of the Church as experts and advisors, even in councils according to the norm of law.

11 See 1983 *CIC* c. 471: "All those who are admitted to offices in the curia must: . . . 2° observe secrecy within the limits and according to the manner determined by law or by the bishop."

With that premise and my own experience, I reread the Code of Canon Law, and here forthwith I simply list and comment on canons that can be held up in this same light. It is not an exhaustive study, and it does not dwell on already heavily utilized canons that impart important responsibility upon lay people such as the offices of chancellor,[12] finance officer,[13] or judge in the tribunal.[14] It hopefully will begin a conversation and not attempt to limit it in any way.

Of course, the foremost canon when discussing the inclusion of lay people in real meaningful decision-making capacities is c. 129 §2.[15] Many of you have weighed in on the issue of what the limitations of the word "cooperate" (*cooperari*) are, but my focus is on its potential. The code contradicts itself, for example with cc. 1421 and 494 spoken of earlier as compared to c. 274 §1 which limits most offices to clerics,[16] but rather than be discouraged by the pessimism of strict interpretation, can we be encouraged by the inclusion of cc. 129 §2, 1421 and 494 and others into the code without seeking to attack the theological basis of c. 274 §1? Like the other canons mentioned in this paper, these canons can be used to slam doors or to open them.

A bishop considering these canons, I submit, should not feel threatened that his "power of jurisdiction" is slipping away but should be pushed to hear the counsel of all the People of God and not just those who exercise the power of orders. The definition of "cooperate" is easily stated as "to work jointly toward the same end," and its synonyms include "join up," "join together," "join forces," and "come together."[17] Besides the obvious limiting, it is an invitation to exactly what I feel must happen—that the doors to real meaningful consultation have to be consciously opened by bishops. Unless this cooperation by the laity is consistent and visible to the People of God, such that they see that lay men and women are relied upon by their bishops, the bishops' credibility will be lesser. The power of jurisdiction given to the apostles by Christ led to the real, visible leadership in the early Church of Phoebe, Priscilla and Aquila, Andronicus and Junia and many others.[18] Now that was cooperation!

---

12 1983 *CIC* cc. 482-483.

13 1983 *CIC* c. 494.

14 1983 *CIC* c. 1421, as modified by *Mitis Iudex Dominus Iesus.*

15 1983 *CIC* c. 129 §2: "Lay members of the Christian Faithful can cooperate in the exercise of this same power according to the norm of law."

16 1983 *CIC* c. 274 §1: "Only clerics can obtain offices for whose exercise the power of orders or the power of ecclesiastical governance is required."

17 *Oxford English Dictionary* (Oxford: Oxford University Press, 2004): "To work together, act in conjunction with another person or thing, to an end or purpose."

18 See, for example, Romans, chapter 16.

Let's look at canon 212 quoted earlier,[19] with the duty of the Christian faithful to let their opinion on matters which pertain to the good of the Church be known. What institution of your diocese consciously does this besides the pastors of local parishes (which I do not question as it is an important part of being a pastor)?[20] The strongest authority lay people possess is, in my opinion, the right to appeal a decision of a bishop that affects them, especially if the ecclesiastical authority did not consult them prior to acting.[21] Canons 1732–1739 lay out the proper way of appeal (known as having "recourse"), and when used properly it is effective.

My personal experience with the recourse process, however, shows it to be an inconsistent and at times overly adversarial procedure. It begins benignly enough where the one offended is to contact the author of the decree to attempt to find an equitable solution to the problem.[22] The code encourages this conversation and offers a handy idea for the conference of bishops to establish norms for each diocese to have a stable office to handle these complaints or each diocese can do so on their own in accord with canon 1733 §2.[23] But pause here, because the United States Conference of Catholic Bishops (USCCB) has not issued this complementary norm. Moreover, how many dioceses in the country that you know have indeed established a stable office of this type? There are some, for sure, but I would submit that they are few and far between. Not only would this facilitate better redress for grievances between the People of God and the bishop, but what a perfect spot for lay people to cooperate in the power of governance!

To conclude the section on canonical recourse, however, I note that the process can indeed be effective with the able assistance of a motivated canon lawyer on one's side. But it is far from "user-friendly." This, as I stated, is the layperson's strongest authority. But how does the angry lay person or group truly manifest their opinion to bishops that are comfortable on the other side of the door? I do not know the answer to that question, and it is not the premise of this paper—the premise is that bishop's need to consciously open the door, and canons 212 and 1733 are ways to facilitate this.

---

19 See footnote 4.

20 See c. 529.

21 See c. 50.

22 See 1983 *CIC* c. 1733 §1: "Whenever a person considers himself or herself aggrieved by a decree, it is particularly desirable that the person and the author of the decree avoid any contention and take care to seek an equitable solution by common counsel, possibly using the mediation and effort of wise persons to avoid or settle the controversy in a suitable way."

23 See 1983 *CIC* c. 1733 §2: "The conference of bishops can determine that each diocese establish in a stable manner an office or council whose function is to seek and suggest equitable solutions according to the norms determined by the conference. If the conference has not ordered this, however, the bishop can establish a council or office of this kind."

Canon 229,[24] regarding the right of lay people to acquire knowledge appropriate to their capacity which includes the sacred sciences taught at ecclesiastical universities, leads me to observe from my premise that this is a key way that bishops can open the door to future cooperation. I wonder how many of you here today who are not priests worked in financial partnership to obtain your canon law degree? If I asked the same question of the priests in the room, I would wager that most of them were sent by their bishop or superior for their degree and that many of the priests, like me, had that degree paid for. How many lay people have been intrigued with the canonical field only to confront their own financial and family situations and let that dream go? I commend every one of you here who somehow figured out a way to get it done and I admire your incredible dedication to your calling. It is not a guarantee, but obtaining an ecclesiastical decree is a very real way of having true, meaningful, decision-making authority in the Church. The Church is greatly blessed by those who have climbed that mountain. But, as with everything else in the Catholic Church, if it is not literally a priority such that it actually appears in the budget; it probably is not going to happen, well-meaning intentions or not.

I wonder how many of you have ever filled out one of those forms from the Nuncio when a person is being vetted for the office of bishop. The envelopes have appeared in my mailbox over the years due mostly to my former title of Judicial Vicar. They contain a series of detailed questions about a potential candidate and are clearly labeled as "Pontifical Secret." The last question asked on the form is for recommendations as to who else the Holy See could consult who knows the candidate. Canon 377 §3 speaks of the papal legate's inquiry among the bishops, suffragan bishops, conference of bishops, and those on the College of Consultors and Cathedral Chapter (all clerics), and then it states "if he judges it expedient, [the papal legate] is also to seek individually and in secret the opinion of others

---

24 See 1983 *CIC* c. 229:

§1 Lay persons are bound by the obligation and possess the right to acquire knowledge of Christian doctrine appropriate to the capacity and condition of each in order for them to be able to live according to this doctrine, announce it themselves, defend it if necessary, and take their part in exercising the apostolate.
§2 They also possess the right to acquire that fuller knowledge of the sacred sciences which are taught in ecclesiastical universities and faculties or in institutes of religious sciences, by attending classes there and pursuing academic degrees.
§3 If the prescripts regarding the requisite suitability have been observed, they are also qualified to receive from legitimate ecclesiastical authority a mandate to teach the sacred sciences.

from the secular and non-secular clergy and from laity outstanding in wisdom."[25] Let me appeal then directly to you in the room who are bishops and clerics, it is imperative that you and I use that final question to suggest qualified lay people for the Nuncio to ask. It is too easy for a bishop to be selected without the Holy See ever directly hearing from a member of the laity or any woman whatsoever. It is a small example of what it means to consciously open the door.

Canon 458 speaks of the office of the general secretary of the bishops' conference. Here in the United States, the USCCB statutes allow for a non-bishop cleric to be the General Secretary, and I have no issue with the current office holder. But just think of the good fruit if this office was filled instead by a layperson. There is nothing in the law that prevents it, and it is without a doubt an extremely influential position in the Church hierarchy. What if, when the leadership of the USCCB were to go to meet with the Pope in the future, instead of having three men sit with the Pope to discuss the Church in the United States, instead, it was two bishops and a lay woman. What would just the picture of that say to the women of our Church, let alone what would that add to the conversation? What a huge door that would open!

This paper has already mentioned the diocesan pastoral council as described by canons 511 to 514. I have already pointed out that it is an option of the bishop to the extent that pastoral circumstances suggest it.[26] Let us go by the premise that clearly it should be in every diocese, what should a bishop do with it? Should not the bishop have it mirror the requirement of the Presbyteral Council that "the diocesan bishop is to hear it in affairs of greater importance?"[27] I know that many diocesan bishops utilize this counsel this way already, but opening the doors and allowing lay people to truly have a voice would mean that they all should do this consciously.

---

25 1983 *CIC* c. 377 §3:

> Unless it is legitimately established otherwise, whenever a diocesan or coadjutor bishop must be appointed, as regards what is called the ternus to be proposed to the Apostolic See, the pontifical legate is to seek individually and to communicate to the Apostolic See together with his own opinion the suggestions of the metropolitan and suffragans of the province to which the diocese to be provided for belongs or with which it is joined in some grouping, and the suggestions of the president of the conference of bishops. The pontifical legate, moreover, is to hear some members of the college of consultors and cathedral chapter and, if he judges it expedient, is also to seek individually and in secret the opinion of others from both the secular and non-secular clergy and from laity outstanding in wisdom.

26 See footnote 6.

27 1983 *CIC* c. 500 §2: "The presbyteral council possesses only a consultative vote; the diocesan bishop is to hear it in affairs of greater importance but needs its consent only in cases expressly defined by law."

Some dioceses do have lay leadership of parishes in the United States, as allowed by canon 517 §2. But I wonder at the interpretation of the canonical standard; namely, who defines the words "because of a lack of priests?"[28] It would seem to me that this gets strictly interpreted by diocesan bishops to speak literally of the actual number of priests and the large geographic area in which they minister. But what makes this interpretation need be so strict? What if the interpretation was more than the mere number of priests and spoke to the number of qualified priests? I ask the question: which person would you rather have in charge of the non-sacramental pastoral and financial administration of your family's parish: a priest who has no competence in pastoring, yet counts as a number, or a qualified deacon or lay person truly trained for the job? Put that way, I think it is a no-brainer; yet clergy personnel departments across the country are crossing their fingers and sending incompetent priests back into parishes.

Canons 759 and 766 are obvious canons for a paper such as this one. Canon 759 calls for all the Christian faithful to cooperate in the exercise of the ministry of the word with the bishops and presbyters.[29] Canon 766 lays out when and under what limited circumstances lay people can preach.[30] The USCCB complementary norms spell out the specifications in the United States for lay preaching. I am not challenging these norms (you may, of course), but this paper does not take objection to what is already established; rather, it pushes where the law can legitimately be pushed. To that end, bishops and priests should concentrate on c. 759 and create as many opportunities as possible for lay men and women to witness to the gospel message apart from the celebration of Mass. They also should take the time to attend and benefit from our laypeople's teaching.

There are so many places where bishops and priests are the keynote speakers that do not have to be so. Missions, sacramentals, conventions, retreats, days of reflection, all sorts of ways that already happen in abundance in our Church but merely being conscious of this need would create many more opportunities. Speaking of which, why is the definition of "catechists" as found in c. 785 so narrowly interpreted to traditional missions? Can we contemplate expanding that

---

28 1983 *CIC* c. 517 §2: "If, because of a lack of priests, the diocesan bishop has decided that participation in the exercise of the pastoral care of a parish is to be entrusted to a deacon, to another person who is not a priest, or to a community of persons, he is to appoint some priest who, provided with the powers and faculties of a pastor, is to direct the pastoral care."

29 See 1983 *CIC* c. 759: "By virtue of baptism and confirmation, lay members of the Christian faithful are witnesses of the gospel message by word and the example of a Christian life; they can also be called upon to cooperate with the bishop and presbyters in the exercise of the ministry of the word."

30 See 1983 *CIC* c. 766: "Lay persons can be permitted to preach in a church or oratory, if necessity requires it in certain circumstances or it seems advantageous in particular cases, according to the prescripts of the conference of bishops and without prejudice to can. 767 §1."

definition of what constitutes "missionary work?"[31]

The rest of the code proved to me to be less primed for opening the doors wider to lay people, but I think a major section of the law to concentrate on are the canons on the formation of priests. How many of you here believe that the traditional system for the formation of priests is the best we can do to form future leaders of lay people and parishes? Does anyone really believe that our seminary systems as they function in general now are exactly what is needed to form priests ready for ministry? Personally, I think the priests and lay people currently dedicated to this important work are doing the best they can, but the current system is designed to create a routine of prayer, life and ministry that does not echo in any way the life of a diocesan priest; it does not enough expose seminarians to lay people. One can completely excel in every way as a seminarian and completely fail in the first year as a parish-level priest; more frequently than some would like to admit, new priests in fact do fail at an alarming rate. Living chastely as a celibate is far more clear-cut behind the walls of the seminary than it is in the almost completely unsupervised atmosphere of the parish.

Who is more qualified to judge the effectiveness of a homilist's style to connect with lay people than lay people? In no way does this mean that we sacrifice theological training for priests and proper biblical exegesis, but there is room and need for both. I would submit that canon 1025, where the bishop is to decide the usefulness of the potential priest to the church before ordaining,[32] could be better determined with a more lay-involved system, and canon 1028, which speaks to proper instruction by the seminary about those things the People of God truly need,[33] would be changed significantly if lay people were advising how to train them. A more lay-involved system of seminary training would help the rector truly fulfill canon 1051, 1° in describing the candidate's "genuine piety, good morals, and aptitude to exercise the ministry."[34] I conclude it is more tradition than canon law that prevents a responsible bishop from opening the doors and the windows and destroying the "no trespassing" signs that close up the seminaries.

---

31 1983 *CIC* c. 785 §1: "Catechists are to be used in carrying out missionary work; catechists are lay members of the Christian faithful, duly instructed and outstanding in Christian life, who devote themselves to setting forth the teaching of the gospel and to organizing liturgies and works of charity under the direction of a missionary."

32 See 1983 *CIC* c. 1025 §2: "Furthermore, it is required that he is considered in the judgment of the same legitimate superior as useful for the ministry of the Church."

33 See 1983 *CIC* c. 1028: "The diocesan bishop or the competent superior is to take care that before candidates are promoted to any order, they are instructed properly about those things which belong to the order and its obligations."

34 1983 *CIC* c. 1051, 1°: "There is to be a testimonial of the rector of the seminary or house of formation about the qualities required to receive the order, that is, about the sound doctrine of the candidate, his genuine piety, good morals, and aptitude to exercise the minitry, as well as, after a properly executed inquiry, about his state of physical and psychic health."

With respect to the sacramental canons, my eye did not linger on too many canons in my study. But one thing that seems painfully obvious to me is that we as a whole do not do a good job with the post-marriage help to new couples envisioned by canon 1063, 4°.[35] There is no celibate-never-married cleric who is fully qualified by holy orders to fulfill this mandate. This is an ideal task for lay people to be leaders. Yet how many dioceses and parishes have a real program for the newly married? Even though it is a real need and a natural fit for lay people, how our clerical Church functions is that bishops and priests must consciously get the ball rolling for it to truly happen.

Canon 1168 seems rather open to the premise of this paper in that the administration of sacramentals by lay people is left to the judgment of the local ordinary, as long as the chosen lay people possess the appropriate qualities for "some sacramentals."[36] I mean, there are so many questions here to explore: which sacramentals? What are the appropriate qualities? Why is this all up to the local bishop and not in the hands of pastors? I am not a liturgist, and the liturgist I consulted for this paper told me he was intrigued with the canon, but that he didn't know what to do with it. Therefore, I shall merely highlight and move on.

As I said, the utilization of lay judges of canon 1421 and lay finance officers of canon 494 seems to be no secret and widely used in dioceses. Here lay people are functioning well in roles traditionally occupied by a priest. Other functions in the Church are still mandated to be fulfilled by clerics, but permission can be sought for a qualified lay person to serve instead. I believe it is worth asking, for example, for the use of a lay person as promoters of justice in criminal trials, which indult is granted regularly by the Congregation for the Doctrine of the Faith. Moreover, the use of lay experts assisting in investigations—even for bishops—is allowed in *Vos estis lux mundi*, Article 13.[37] I would submit that beyond the obvious "review boards," anything a bishop can do to add qualified lay people to the criminal process is worth doing for the sake of credibility of the criminal process, which credibility the People of God may find to be lacking.

Doing anything suggested by this paper involves a conscious decision—as has been repeated—to open the door to more involvement of lay people. Clericalism starts with:

---

35 See 1983 *CIC* c. 1063, 4°: "[This assistance must be offered especially by] help offered to those who are married, so that faithfully preserving and protecting the conjugal covenant, they daily come to lead holier and fuller lives in their family."

36 1983 *CIC* c. 1168: "The minister of sacramentals is a cleric who has been provided with the requisite power. According to the norm of the liturgical books and to the judgment of the local ordinary lay persons who possess the appropriate qualities can also administer some sacramentals."

37 See Francis, apostolic letter *Vos estis lux mundi,* May 7, 2019, *L'Osservatore Romano* 159 (2019) n. 106.

- those from whom a bishop or a pastor invites feedback;
- those from whom the bishop or pastor seeks advice;
- those who are allowed into the critical decision-making meetings;
- those who can see all the facts of a situation (and not just advise on side issues), and
- those whom the bishop and the pastor nominate to speak.

In turn lay people offer a very different and critical perspective. For example, it occurs that when a priest is accused of a violation (that perhaps does not rise to "abuse of a minor" but is still unseemly), a bishop or priest can choose to give another bishop or priest a break because their standard can too easily be "the people do not have to know." In contrast, a lay person's first reaction is more likely to be, "I don't want this priest ministering to my family!" Whereas a bishop or priest might think something is already inclusive of all involved, I submit the layperson's idea of "inclusive" can be widely differing. And finally, whereas a bishop and a priest may think that something is sufficiently sensitive to women, they are necessarily not fully qualified for the judgment.

Let us clerics, and in particular bishops, consciously open the doors wider where the code already allows; what are we afraid of?

Seminar

Opportunities in Canon Law for Interecclesial Ministry

The Reverend Jobe Abbass, OFM Conv., JCD

Regarding the possibilities for interecclesial ministry in canon law, this paper will examine the question from the perspective of the norms contained in the 1990 *Codex Canonum Ecclesiarum Orientalium* (*CCEO*). The examination will be made both by treating Eastern canons that apparently allow for ministry among the various Churches *sui iuris* and, then, by considering *CCEO* norms that are seemingly more restrictive in terms of interecclesial ministry especially with reference to the Latin Church. In what ultimately comes down to a question of canonical interpretation, this study does not intend to provide any definitive answers. Nor can it do so since that is the competence of the Legislator or those to whom he has entrusted the power to interpret laws authentically (*CCEO* c. 1498 §1). However, in an area of canonical interpretation that has continued to develop over time, the study must first focus on the appropriate meaning to be given to *CCEO* canon 1.[1] It states: "The canons of this Code concern all and only the Eastern Catholic Churches, unless, with regard to relations with the Latin Church, it is expressly (*expresse*) established otherwise."[2]

When Pope John Paul II promulgated the Eastern code almost thirty years ago, the intent and scope of canon 1 were already quite clear. According to the precise wording of the canon, the Legislator's intention was to apply the Eastern code only to the Eastern Catholic Churches and not to the Eastern Orthodox Churches. This was also the intent of the expert draftsmen within the *Pontificia Commissio Codici Iuris Canonici Orientalis Recognoscendo* (*PCCICOR*) who wanted to avoid extending, even indirectly, the application of the Eastern code

---

1 For a detailed commentary on *CCEO* c. 1, see J. Abbass, "The Eastern Code and Latin Church," in *A Practical Commentary to the Code of Canons of the Eastern Churches*, ed. John D. Faris et al. (Montréal: Wilson & Lafleur, 2019) [hereafter *A Practical Commentary*] I:1-50.

2 In this study, English translations for the *CCEO* canons are taken from *Code of Canons of the Eastern Churches, Latin-English Edition* (Washington, DC, Canon Law Society of America, 2001). Unless otherwise indicated, other foreign language translations are the author's.

to the Orthodox.[3] However, from the very first canon, the Legislator was equally clear in establishing an interrelationship of the Eastern and Latin codes. In fact, on October 25, 1990, a week after promulgating the Eastern code, the pope presented the Eastern code to the twenty-eighth General Congregation of the Synod of Bishops and declared: "In presenting to this Assembly, so representative of the universal Church, the code which governs the common discipline of all the Eastern Catholic Churches, I regard it as part of one *Corpus Iuris Canonici....*"[4] Despite this language that already recognized the Eastern code in relationship to a larger body of canon law, including the Latin code and *Pastor bonus*, some canonists initially felt that the interrelationship of the Eastern and Latin codes did not amount to much except for the nine canons in which the Eastern code explicitly names the Latin Church. Indeed, several canonists argued over the years that the rule expressed in Eastern canon 1 was peremptory and intended to exclude the Latin Church unless it was explicitly established.[5] Other canonists maintained that the interrelationship of the codes was broader and that the Legislator expressly established it, either explicitly or implicitly, for example, through the use of the expression "Church *sui iuris*" or even by reason of the nature of the matter (*ex natura rei*).[6]

It was not until December 8, 2011, that the Pontifical Council for Legislative Texts published an official Explanatory Note regarding the meaning of Eastern canon 1 and the Eastern code's application in relation to the Latin Church. After recognizing "that the express (*expresse*) mention of the Latin Church in

---

3 For the pertinent observations made regarding canon 1 and the experts' replies, see *Nuntia* 22 (1986) 13 (c. 1). For further detail concerning the legislative history to *CCEO* c. 1, see J. Abbass, "*CCEO* Canon 1 and Absolving Eastern Catholics in the Latin Church," *Studia canonica* 46 (2012) 79-83.

4 John Paul II, allocution, "In aula Synodi episcoporum habita: de novo Codice Canonum Ecclesiarum Orientalium," October 25, 1990: *AAS* 83 (1991) 490.

5 See Marco Brogi, "Licenza presunta della Santa Sede per il cambiamento di Chiesa *sui iuris*," *Revista Española de Derecho Canonico* 50 (1993) 645; Peter Erdö, "Questioni interrituali (interecclesiali) del diritto dei sacramenti (battesimo e cresima)," *Periodica de re canonica* 84 (1996) 317-318; and Pablo Gefaell, "Impegno della Congregazione per le Chiese orientali a favore delle comunità orientali in diaspora," in *Nuove terre e nuove Chiese: Le comunità di fedeli orientali in diaspora,* ed. Luis Okulik (Venice: Marcianum Press, 2008) 137-138.

6 See Dimitri Salachas, "Problematiche interrituali nei due codici orientale e latino," *Apollinaris* 75 (1994) 641-648; Carl G. Fürst, "Interdipendenza del diritto canonico latino ed orientale," in *Il Diritto Canonico Orientale nell'ordinamento ecclesiale,* ed. Kuriakose Bharanikulangara (Vatican City: Libreria Editrice Vaticana, 1995) 21-24 and 28-30; Jobe Abbass, "The Interrelationship of the Latin and Eastern Codes," *The Jurist* 58 (1998) 12-20; René Metz, "Preliminary Canons," in *A Guide to the Eastern Code: A Commentary on the Code of Canons of the Eastern Churches,* ed. George Nedungatt (Rome: Pontifical Oriental Institute, 2002) [hereafter *A Guide*] 72; and Lorenzo Lorusso, "L'ambito d'applicazione del Codice dei Canoni delle Chiese Orientali: Commento sistematico al can. 1 del CCEO," *Angelicum* 82 (2005) 471-472.

the (*CCEO*) canons can occur both in an 'explicit' and an 'implicit' way," the Pontifical Council declared:

> According to this distinction, that appears reasonably confirmed by the normative provisions of *CCEO*, besides the canons in which the Latin Church is "explicitly" named, there are also other canons of the same code in which it is included "implicitly," if one takes into account the text and context of the norm, as *CCEO* canon 1499 requires. It is therefore necessary to begin with the expressions contained in the norm to be interpreted and with the context in which it is found to determine if the Latin Church is implicitly included in it or not. This is the case, for example, of the norms of the Eastern Code that concern juridical relations with the various Churches of the one Catholic Church.
>
> Consequently, one must hold that the Latin Church is implicitly included by analogy each time that CCEO explicitly uses the term "Church *sui iuris*" in the context of interecclesial relations. We say "by analogy" keeping in mind that the characteristics of the Latin Church, though not coinciding completely with those of the Church *sui iuris* described in canons 27 and 28 §1 of CCEO, are nevertheless, in this regard, substantially similar.[7]

By this official interpretation, the Explanatory Note allows for a more extensive application of the Eastern code to the Latin Church, at least with regard to those Eastern canons in which the expression "Church *sui iuris*" is employed in the context of interecclesial relations. Indeed, in referring to the other canons of the same (Eastern) Code in which it (the Latin Church) is included implicitly, the note does not limit them to only those canons that contain the expression "Church *sui iuris*" but could include those norms that apply also to the Latin Church by reason of the nature of the matter (*ex natura rei*) in interecclesial contexts involving various Churches *sui iuris*. These findings have implications for the Latin Church going forward as canonical studies continue the ongoing definition of the interrelationship of the Eastern and Latin codes. However, the Explanatory Note did not open the door to a broader and unchecked application of the Eastern code to the Latin Church.[8] Following the publication of the Explanatory Note, for example, this writer examined the Eastern code's use of the expression "Church

---

7 Pontifical Council for Legislative Texts, "Explanatory Note Regarding CCEO Canon 1," December 8, 2011, *Communicationes* 43 (2011) 316. The manner of the Roman See's intervention here is noteworthy. There was evidently no need for an authentic interpretation since the significance of *CCEO* canon 1 was clear; the Holy See simply had to explain its meaning. For more detail, see Jobe Abbass, "The Explanatory Note regarding *CCEO* Canon 1: A Commentary," *Studia canonica* 46 (2012) 293-318.

8 Cf. Giacomo Incitti, "Quale concordanza tra i Codici? Ancora su un progetto di *Lex Ecclesiae Fundamentalis*," in *La costante sollecitudine per la concordanza tra i Codici (Quaderni di Ius Missionale)*, 13 (Rome: Urbaniana University Press, 2018) 48.

sui iuris" 243 times and found that certainly more than one-half could not intend to regard the Latin Church. In some cases, the Eastern norms are addressed only to the Eastern Churches by definition or context; others refer solely to Eastern liturgical norms or the particular law of each Eastern Church *sui iuris*; in still other cases, the Eastern canons simply cannot apply to the Latin Church which already has parallel Latin norms governing the same matter. Nevertheless, there were found to be many Eastern norms that potentially regard the Latin Church *ex natura rei* in the context of ascription/transfer between Churches, interritual celebration of the sacraments and interecclesial collaboration generally.[9]

In a subsequent and important legislative development regarding the interrelationship of the Eastern and Latin codes, Pope Francis published his *motu proprio, De concordia inter Codices* on September 15, 2016.[10] In the Preamble to the *motu proprio*, Pope Francis explained that his solicitude for harmonizing the codes is motivated by two specific reasons: 1) to seek an equilibrium between safeguarding the law proper to the Eastern minority with the canonical tradition of the Latin majority, especially in the West, and 2) to better define relations with the faithful of the non-Catholic Churches particularly regarding Catholic ministers' celebration of the sacraments of baptism and marriage for non-Catholic faithful. These pastoral considerations constitute the key and backdrop against which the articles of the *motu proprio* are to be interpreted.

Despite the pope's intent to harmonize the codes, all eleven articles of the *motu proprio* considered, His Holiness essentially sets limits on the application of the Eastern code to the Latin Church in three ways.[11] First, by adding norms to the Latin code (cc. 112 §3; 868 §3 and 1116 §3) to mirror those already found in the Eastern code (cc. 36; 681 §5 and 833 §§1-2), Pope Francis implies, in effect, that these Eastern norms could not have been considered, beforehand, to be applicable to the Latin Church. Secondly, by not adding other unique Eastern canons (for example, cc. 588; 701, 899; 1102 §1) to the Latin code, the Legislator has effectively indicated that these Eastern norms, common to all the Eastern Catholic Churches, are still not universal Latin norms. Thirdly, while Pope Francis observes that the codes often have common or parallel norms, which should have "an appropriate degree of harmony," he nevertheless acknowledges that the codes have "their own peculiarities which make them mutually independent." Consequently, parallel norms of the codes (for example,

---

9 For a detailed analysis, see: Jobe Abbass, *The Eastern Code (Canon 1) and Its Application to the Latin Church* (Bangalore: Dharmaram Publications, 2014) [hereafter *The Eastern Code (Canon 1)*].

10 For the text see Pope Francis, motu proprio *De concordia inter Codices*, September 15, 2016: *AAS* 108 (2016) 602; or see *Communicationes* 48 (2016) 326. For an unofficial English translation and a commentary on the *motu proprio*, see Jobe Abbass, "*De concordia inter Codices*: A Commentary," *Studia canonica* 50 (2016) 323-345.

11 For a detailed study, see Jobe Abbass, "Setting Limits on the Application of the Eastern Code to the Latin Church," *Studia canonica* 51 (2017) 25-54.

CCEO c. 193 §1/*CIC* c. 383 §§1-2; *CCEO* c. 828 §1/*CIC* c. 1108 §1; *CCEO* c. 826/*CIC* c. 1102) that remain mutually different in some significant respect result in a certain disharmony between the codes.[12] Unique differences in *CCEO* norms cannot oblige the Latin Church just as differences found in *CIC* norms cannot bind the Eastern Catholic Churches. Given that the Eastern and Latin codes are separate and distinct juridical systems, any parallel matter may be regulated in a different manner and the norms of one code simply cannot be imposed on the other.

Given these significant markers in the ongoing development of canonical knowledge regarding the interrelationship of the codes of the Catholic Church, this study can begin to examine the possibilities for interecclesial ministries from the vantage point of the norms of the Eastern code. In light of the 2011 official Explanatory Note and the 2016 *motu proprio*, *De concordia inter Codices,* part one will look at three cases (*CCEO* cc. 678 §1; 916 §4 and 1068 §1) in which it can reasonably be argued that the Eastern norms do foresee the possibility of ministry for both Easterners and Latins. On the other hand, taking into account the 2011 Explanatory Note together with the possible implications of the 2016 *motu proprio*, part two will deal with three other cases (*CCEO* cc. 1102 §1; 247 §4 and 899) in which the Eastern norms may not, in the final analysis, allow for interecclesial ministry for both Easterners and Latins. Again, any definitive answer in these cases must remain the competence of the Legislator or those to whom he has entrusted the power to interpret laws authentically.

1. Eastern Norms that Foresee the Possibility of Interecclesial Ministry

1.1. Baptism Administered by a Priest of Another Church *sui iuris* (*CCEO* c. 678 §1)

Unique to the Eastern code, *CCEO* canon 678 §1 establishes that, while permission is required to baptize in the territory of another, a pastor cannot deny such permission to a priest of another Church *sui iuris* in which the person to be baptized is to be ascribed. The norm states:

In the territory of another it is not licit for anyone to administer baptism

12 For more detail, see Jobe Abbass, "*De concordia inter Codices:* Towards a Harmonization of the Eastern and Latin Codes," *Iustitia* 8 (2017) 15-48. In the Preamble, the Holy Father specifically deals with the parallel norms (*CCEO* c. 193 §1/*CIC* c. 383 §§1-2) regarding a bishop's duty of care towards faithful from another Church *sui iuris. CCEO* c. 193 §1 clearly establishes that a bishop has the grave obligation of providing everything (*gravi obligatione tenetur omnia providendi*) so that these faithful observe their own rite in all its respects wherever they are. Clearly, the *motu proprio* does not go this far with respect to Latin bishops entrusted with the care of Easterners. In not imposing on them the more serious obligation in *CCEO* c. 193 §1, the pope states that "the competent ecclesiastical authority is to take care most earnestly that appropriate means are provided (*congrua media apparentur*) them to be able to fulfill this obligation."

> without the required permission; this permission cannot be denied by a pastor of a different Church *sui iuris* to a priest of the Church *sui iuris* in which the person to be baptized is to be ascribed.[13]

Within *PCCICOR*, the *Coetus de sacramentis* based their first draft of this norm on the initial text that had been proposed in 1958 but was never promulgated.[14] Concerning the rationale behind the norm, then Chorbishop Moussa Daoud, reporting for the group, stated:

> The right to baptize is limited by a double requirement: the territory and the rite. The proper pastor and hierarch can only baptize within the limits of their territory, even if they baptize persons of their own rite; and, within their territory, if they wish to baptize persons belonging to other Particular Churches, they need permission.
>
> But there are territories where there is no proper pastor of such a Particular Church. Who then has the right to baptize the persons before them belonging to that Particular Church?
>
> In order to foster the rite, two dispositions are foreseen by the new canon:
>
> 1) The pastor of the territory, who is of another rite (*diversi ritus*) from that of the person to be baptized, cannot refuse a priest, who would be present and of the same rite of the person being baptized, the permission for him to administer the baptism.
>
> 2) The local hierarch is urged to designate for the faithful, who do not have a proper pastor in the territory, a priest who is of the same rite as them to administer baptism to their children.
>
> But the words "*diversi ritus*" ("of a different rite") caught the attention of the group. Do they also include the Latin rite? The old base-text found it necessary to add "*latini quoque*" ("also Latin") and "*latino non excepto*" ("Latin not excluded"). Our group, imbued with ideas of equality among the rites and wishing to avoid all discrimination, states with a note attached to the text of the new canon 4 that these words include the Latin rite itself, and they dispense us from having to add each time "*latini quoque*" ("also Latin").[15]

Already substantially the same as the promulgated norm, provisional canon 4

---

13 *CCEO* c. 678 §1.

14 See *Nuntia* 4 (1977) 45 (c. 9 §§1-2).

15 *Nuntia* 4 (1977) 21 (c. 4).

§1 stated: "In the territory of another, it is not licit to administer baptism without the required permission; this permission cannot be denied by the pastor of a different rite to a priest who is present and who is of the same rite as the person to be baptized;" the norm subsequently became canon 13 §1 of the 1980 *Schema canonum de culto divino et praesertim de sacramentis* (1980 Schema).[16] In the *Praenotanda* to the 1980 Schema, the *Coetus de sacramentis* clearly reiterated: "In can. 13, we substantially retained what was already proposed in 1958, namely, the obligation of pastors of whatever rite, the Latin by no means excluded, not to deny a Catholic priest the faculty of administering baptism to those who are of the same rite. . . ."[17] During the *denua recognitio* of the 1980 Schema, no observations were made to change canon 13 §1.[18] The *Coetus de coordinatione* slightly modified the formulation before it became *SCICO* (*Schema Codicis Iuris Canonici Orientalis)* canon 675 §1, which was identical to the promulgated norm.[19]

The use of the expression "Church *sui iuris*" twice in *CCEO* canon 678 §1 clearly implies the Latin Church. To deal first with the second use of the expression, in relation to the words "priest of the Church *sui iuris* in which the person to be baptized is to be ascribed," it implicitly involves the Latin Church in a passive sense. That is to say, regarding the administration of baptism, an Eastern pastor cannot deny permission to a priest of another Church *sui iuris*, including the Latin Church, to which the person to be baptized is to be ascribed. In the context of interecclesial relations, this interpretation logically follows the indications of the 2011 Explanatory Note, which held that the Latin Church is implicitly included by analogy when the Eastern norm explicitly uses the expression "Church *sui iuris*."

Now, given that Latin Catholic parishes are found almost everywhere in the world, the circumstance may be rare that a Latin priest approaches an Eastern Catholic pastor for permission to celebrate the baptism of a person to be ascribed to the Latin Church. Nevertheless, let us take the example of the Latin Catholic husband and wife who work for the American embassy in Asmara, Eritrea and who, like all Catholics there, are entrusted to the care of an Eritrean Catholic pastor. They have invited their cousin, a Latin Catholic priest from Washington, to visit and celebrate the baptism of their first child. Since the child would be ascribed to the Latin Church,[20] it seems clear, based on the 2011 Explanatory Note, that the Eastern pastor could not deny this Latin priest the permission to administer his cousin's baptism.

---

16 *Nuntia* 10 (1980) 20 (c. 13 §1).

17 *Nuntia* 10 (1980) 5.

18 See *Nuntia* 15 (1982) 15 (c. 13 §1).

19 See *Nuntia* 24-25 (1987) 127 (c. 675 §1).

20 See *CIC* c. 111 §1, which begins: "Through the reception of baptism, the child of parents who belong to the Latin Church is enrolled in it."

Now, it can also be argued that the first use of the expression "Church *sui iuris,*" in the words "pastor of a different Church *sui iuris,*" implicitly obliges the Latin Church in an active sense. That is to say, in these cases regarding baptism, Eastern as well as Latin pastors cannot deny permission to a priest of another Church *sui iuris* in which the person to be baptized is to be ascribed. The problem is that *CCEO* canon 678 §1 is a norm unique to the Eastern code and apparently only addressed to pastors of the different Eastern Catholic Churches *sui iuris*. Because the Eastern and Latin codes are separate and distinct, the characteristic norms of one code cannot simply be imposed on the other. Moreover, since the pastorally motivated *motu proprio*, *De concordia inter Codices*, did not add Eastern canon 678 §1, or a similar norm, to the Latin code, it could be argued that Latin pastors are simply not governed by *CCEO* canon 678 §1. In addition, Pope Francis insisted that, despite the pastoral intent of the *motu proprio* to effect "an appropriate degree of harmony" between the Eastern and Latin codes, he nevertheless acknowledged that the codes would still have "their own peculiarities which make them mutually independent."

Nevertheless, it seems clear from the detailed legislative history concerning Eastern canon 678 §1 that the Eastern draftsmen intended it to oblige Latin as well as Eastern pastors. While the Eastern and Latin codes are separate and distinct, they are still interrelated (*CCEO* c. 1). The 2011 Explanatory Note allows for the explicit use of the expression "Church *sui iuris*" in interecclesial relations to imply also the Latin Church. Then, even as Pope Francis' *motu proprio De concordia inter Codices* meant to harmonize the codes in some areas, that harmonization was limited and certainly did not intend to harmonize the codes in every respect. Therefore, as this writer has argued in the past,[21] it still seems more reasonable to argue that the first use of the expression "Church *sui iuris*" in Eastern canon 678 §1 also implicitly obliges Latins in an active sense. That is to say, Eastern as well as Latin pastors are not to refuse the permission for administering baptism to a priest of any other Church *sui iuris*, either Eastern or Latin, in which the person to be baptized is to be ascribed.

Let us take a practical example. An Eritrean Eastern Catholic couple works for the Eritrean embassy in Washington and is entrusted to the care of a Latin pastor in the capital. They have invited their cousin, an Eritrean priest studying canon law at the Catholic University of America, to administer baptism to their first child. Upon the basis of *CCEO* canon 678 §1, when the Eritrean priest asks the Latin pastor for the required permission to baptize the child, the Latin pastor cannot deny him that.

---

21 See Jobe Abbass, "The Interrelationship of the Latin and Eastern Codes," *The Jurist* 58 (1998) 15-16; Abbass "CCEO and Code in Comparison," in *A Guide,* 888; Abbass, *The Eastern Code (Canon 1),* 200-202; and Abbass, "The Eastern Code and Latin Church," in *A Practical Commentary*, I:25-26.

1.2. Designating a Pastor from Another Church *sui iuris* (*CCEO* c. 916 §4)

If, in a country or region, the hierarchy of an Eastern Catholic Church *sui iuris* has been established but groups of that Church's faithful remain isolated and without a proper pastor, the eparchial bishop for those faithful is to designate a pastor for them from another Church *sui iuris*. In Canada and the United States, for example, where Eastern Catholic bishops are responsible for vast territories, this is often the case. The applicable norm, *CCEO* canon 916 §4, which is unique to the Eastern code, basically repeats the previous norm in *Cleri sanctitati* (*CS*) canon 22 §2.[22] Eastern canon 916 §4 states:

> If there is no pastor for the Christian faithful of a certain Church *sui iuris*, the eparchial bishop for those same faithful is to designate the pastor of another Church *sui iuris*, who is to assume their care as their proper pastor, with the consent, however, of the eparchial bishop of the pastor to be designated.[23]

Within *PCCICOR*, the draft of this norm, which followed *CS* canon 22 §2 almost literally, first appeared as canon 6 §4 of the 1981 *Schema canonum de normis generalibus et de bonis Ecclesiae temporalibus*.[24] During the *denua recognitio*, no observations or changes were made regarding the norm.[25] After becoming *SCICO* canon 912 §4,[26] only one small redactional change was made before promulgation.[27]

CCEO canon 916 §4, which is addressed to and binds Eastern bishops, does not apply to Latin bishops in any active sense. The norm undoubtedly finds no parallel in the Latin code since the matter it regulates, the lack of a proper pastor, is a rare occurrence in the Latin Church. However, the Eastern norm does regard the Latin Church in a passive sense for two reasons. First, as the 2011 Explanatory Note held, the Latin Church is implied by the use of the expression "Church *sui iuris*" in this context of interecclesial relations.[28] Secondly, consistent with a long line of Eastern norms that urge interecclesial cooperation and communion,

---

22 *CS* c. 22 §2 stated: "If a pastor is lacking for the faithful of a certain rite, their hierarch is to designate a pastor of another rite who is to take care of them, after the same hierarch will have received the consent of the hierarch of the pastor being designated." Pius XII, apostolic letter, *Cleri sanctitati* 22, June 2, 1957: *AAS* 49 (1957) 433-603.

23 *CCEO* 926 §4.

24 See *Nuntia* 13 (1981) 14 (c. 6 §4).

25 See *Nuntia* 18 (1984) 9-11 (c. 6 §4).

26 See *Nuntia* 24-25 (1987) 164 (c. 912 §4).

27 For this change, see *Nuntia* 27 (1988) 77 (c. 912 §4).

28 See also John Huels, "The Proper Hierarch and Pastor," in *A Practical Commentary*, II:1716.

Eastern canon 916 §4 also implies the Latin Church *ex natura rei.*[29] Now, as in the past, wherever Eastern Catholic faithful are without a pastor, their eparchial bishop is to designate for them a pastor from another Church *sui iuris,* even the Latin Church. While pastors of many other Eastern Catholic Churches *sui iuris* may be present, they might not be as available as the more numerous Latin pastors. In any event, as Eastern canon 916 §4 stipulates, whichever pastor is designated must have the consent of his diocesan (eparchial) bishop.

Let us give a practical example of the application of *CCEO* canon 916 §4. Suppose that there is no pastor for a community of Melkite faithful living in Parma, Ohio. Since an eparchy for the Melkite Church has been erected in the United States at Newton, Massachusetts, its eparchial bishop could designate a pastor from any one of several Churches *sui iuris* present there: Ruthenian, Ukrainian and Latin. While the Melkite Church comes from the same Byzantine (Greek) tradition as the Ruthenian and Ukrainian Churches, the Melkite bishop is still free to designate as their pastor a priest of the Latin Church. The consent of his diocesan bishop, the bishop of Cleveland, would be required according to the Eastern norm. If the Latin priest has not had any liturgical training in the celebration of the sacraments according to the Melkite rite, that formation will evidently be necessary. Towards the same end, the Latin priest will also require an indult of biritualism which cannot be granted by either bishop. Instead, the Melkite bishop will need to apply for the indult to the Apostolic See of Rome since, according to *Orientalium Ecclesiarum* (*OE*) n. 4, this See alone is the supreme arbiter over the individual Churches *sui iuris*.

1.3. Interecclesial Tribunals (*CCEO* c. 1068 §1)

In order to assist, in a particular way, those eparchies which lack trained tribunal personnel, *CCEO* canon 1068 §1 encourages eparchial bishops of various Churches *sui iuris* to establish a common tribunal. This Eastern norm updates the previous, similar prescript in canon 39 §1 of *Sollicitudinem nostram* (*SN*).[30] Unique to the Eastern code, *CCEO* canon 1068 §1 states: "The eparchial bishops of various Churches *sui iuris* exercising their power within the same territory can agree among themselves to establish a common tribunal, which is to adjudicate either contentious or penal cases of the Christian faithful subject to any one of these eparchial bishops."

Within *PCCICOR*, a first draft of this norm appeared as canon 13 §1 of the

29 See Jobe Abbass, "Interecclesial Structures in the Eastern Code," *CLSA Proceedings* 77 (2015) 60-88.

30 *SN* c. 39 §1 stated: "Local hierarchs having jurisdiction in the same territory within the patriarchate can agree among themselves to establish a common tribunal which is to adjudicate cases, whether contentious or criminal, of the faithful of whichever rite subject to any one of these local hierarchs." Pope Piux XII, motu proprio *Sollicitudinem nostram* 39, January 6, 1950: *AAS* 42 (1950) 14.

1977 provisional canons on procedure.[31] Although some consultors advanced good reasons for arguing that these common tribunals be imposed, the *Coetus de processibus* decided that the matter would remain optional. However, to offer some direction in those situations where it is difficult to find qualified tribunal personnel, the *Coetus* added a norm (now *CCEO* c. 1068 §2), which states: "If suitable judges and other tribunal officers are lacking, the eparchial bishops are to take care that a common tribunal is constituted." Underlining a worry evidenced in *PCCICOR*, the *Coetus* stated: "The exhortation on this point is not a strict obligation. And that, again, is to safeguard the *status sui juris* of each Eastern Church."[32] Canon 13 §1 subsequently entered the 1982 *Schema canonum de tutela iurium seu processibus* (1982 Schema).[33] During the *denua recognitio* of the 1982 Schema, the norm was only revised to reflect the precise terminology adopted for the future Eastern code.[34] As *SCICO* canon 1083 §1,[35] the norm was almost identical to *CCEO* canon 1068 §1.

In areas where resources are scarce and trained tribunal personnel are lacking, *CCEO* canon 1068 §1 proposes a common, interecclesial tribunal as a wise, concrete solution. This is one of a great many Eastern norms that promote a unity of action through the collaborative efforts of eparchial bishops of various Churches who exercise their power in the same territory.[36] The repeated formula in these norms, "*Episcopi eparchiales diversarum Ecclesiarum sui iuris in eodem territorio potestatem suam exercentes*" (eparchial bishops of various Churches *sui iuris* exercising their power within the same territory) strongly suggests that, with the expression "Church *sui iuris*," the Legislator meant, *ex natura rei*, to signal the active participation of all the bishops, including the Latin bishops, in these collaborative structures.[37] The 2011 Explanatory Note also seems to support such a finding in the specific case of *CCEO* canon 1068 §1. The norm

---

31 See *Nuntia* 5 (1977) 17 (c. 13 §1). Canon 13 §1 stated: "Local hierarchs having jurisdiction in the same territory can agree among themselves to establish a common tribunal which is to adjudicate cases, whether contentious or penal, of faithful of whichever rite subject to any one of these local hierarchs."

32 *Nuntia* 5 (1977) 17 (c. 13 §1).

33 See *Nuntia* 14 (1982) 22 (c. 13 §1).

34 See *Nuntia* 21 (1985) 43 (c. 13 §1). The words local hierarchs, jurisdiction, and rite were changed, respectively, to eparchial bishops, power and Church *sui iuris*.

35 See *Nuntia* 24-25 (1987) 194 (c. 1083 §1). Only the word *iisdem* was subsequently changed to *eisdem;* see *Nuntia* 27 (1988) 63 (c. 1083 §1).

36 See Jobe Abbass, "The Eastern Code at the Service of Interecclesial Communion," *CLSA Proceedings* 68 (2006) 60-88 and 65-86; see also Abbass, *The Eastern Code (Canon 1)*, 220-247.

37 In fact, among these Eastern norms, one does explicitly name the Latin Church (c. 322 §1); one had explicitly named the Latin Church within *PCCICOR* but before promulgation (c. 84 §1); from the discussions within *PCCICOR*, two others clearly implied the Latin Church (cc. 1013 §2 and 1405 §3) and one other even included consultation with Orthodox bishops present in a territory (c. 720 §3).

undoubtedly regards interecclesial relations and, by the expression "Church *sui iuris*," it surely implies the active involvement of any Latin bishops in the territory also because of the nature of the matter.

According to Eastern canon 1068 §1, the eparchial bishops involved can reach an agreement among themselves to establish a common tribunal and no mention is made at this stage of any intervention by the Holy See. However, regarding the approval of statutes and the erection of the common tribunal, the unique *CCEO* canon 1070 states: "Any authority that erects a tribunal is to take care that the tribunal has its own statutes approved by the same authority, in which must be determined the manner of appointing judges and other officers, the duration of their function, their remuneration and all the other matters required by law." Given the involvement of bishops from different Churches *sui iuris*, the authority mentioned in canon 1070 is undoubtedly the Holy See (Apostolic Signatura) since, as mentioned earlier, it alone is the supreme arbiter among the Churches (*OE* n.4). What is important, though, for the purposes of this paper is that, in the statutes the bishops propose for approval, the appointment of judges and other tribunal officials needs to be detailed. Therein lies the possibility for numerous interecclesial ministries as judges, officials and other personnel from the various Churches *sui iuris* to collaborate in the operation of the common tribunal.

2. Eastern Norms That May Not Foresee the Possibility of Interecclesial Ministry

2.1. Tribunal Personnel from Another Church *sui iuris* (*CCEO* c. 1102 §1)

Another unique Eastern norm, *CCEO* canon 1102 §1, provides for the recruitment of judges and other personnel of ecclesiastical tribunals from one's own or even another Church *sui iuris*. It provides:

> Judges and other officers of the tribunals may be chosen from any eparchy, religious institute or society of common life in the manner of religious, of one's own or even of another Church *sui iuris*, with the written consent, however, of their own eparchial bishop or major superior.[38]

As the reported proceedings of *PCCICOR* indicate, the *Coetus de processibus* presented the first draft of this norm while revising the former Eastern canon in *SN* canon 71. The proposed formulation stated: "Judges and other ministers of the tribunals can be taken from any eparchy, monastery or institute of the same or a different rite, provided the written consent of proper hierarch is given."[39]

---

38 *CCEO* c. 1102 §1.

39 *Nuntia* 5 (1977) 26-27 (c. 40 §1). *SN* canon 71 stated: "Judges and ministers mentioned in can. 38 seqq., can also be taken from persons of another rite."

That formulation became canon 44 §1 of the 1982 Schema.[40] Thereafter, no observations were reported in *Nuntia* regarding the norm and it only underwent terminological or other minor changes before promulgation.[41]

Regarding the interpretation of *CCEO* canon 1102 §1, the norm is addressed to Eastern Catholic bishops. There is no corresponding *CIC* norm for Latin bishops and they cannot simply adopt it as their own. While this Eastern norm therefore does not regard the Latin Church in an active sense, it does involve the Latin Church, in a passive sense, in the context of the recurring theme of interecclesial cooperation that characterizes the Eastern legislation. Thus, for example, an Eastern Catholic bishop can choose judges and other tribunal personnel from any eparchy of his own Church *sui iuris* or even from an eparchy of another Church *sui iuris*. Given the 2011 Explanatory Note, since the implicit meaning of the expression "Church *sui iuris*" can also include the Latin Church, an Eastern bishop could appoint judges and tribunal personnel from an eparchy of his own Church or from an eparchy (diocese) of another Eastern Church or even the Latin Church. The Eastern bishop can also hire his tribunal personnel from among the religious or the members of societies of common life of his own Church or another Eastern Catholic Church *sui iuris*. However, in the case of the Latin Church, the same Eastern bishop can hire religious or members of societies of apostolic life mentioned in *CIC* canon 731 §2, since the latter are to be equated with Eastern societies of common life, as defined in *CCEO* canon 554 §1.[42] In whichever case, the Eastern bishop will need the written consent of the relevant eparchial (diocesan) bishop or major superior.

Although this writer still argues for the interpretation of *CCEO* canon 1102 §1 outlined above, the *motu proprio*, *De concordia inter Codices*, has raised a number of issues that question the sureness of that interpretation. While the *motu proprio* added several norms to the Latin code to mirror those already found in the Eastern code, it did not add other unique Eastern norms, like *CCEO* canon 1102 §1. Did this mean to imply that Eastern canon 1102 §1 is strictly Eastern and does not apply to the Latin Church either in an active or passive sense? Even though the expression "Church *sui iuris*" appears in the norm, it may be one instance in which the Latin Church is not implied, notwithstanding the 2011 Explanatory Note. Indeed, *CCEO* canon 1102 §1 could intend that Eastern bishops necessarily hire tribunal judges and officers who are experts, not in Latin canon law, but rather in the common law (*CCEO*) and traditions of their own

---

40 See *Nuntia* 14 (1982) 29 (c. 44 §1).

41 See *Nuntia* 21 (1985) 46 (c. 44); *Nuntia* 24-25 (1987) 200 (c. 1117 §1); *Nuntia* 27 (1988) 85 (c. 1117 §1) and *Nuntia* 31 (1990) 38 (c. 1117 §1).

42 For the comparison between Eastern societies of common life in the manner of religious (*CCEO* c. 554 §1) and Latin societies of apostolic life, whose members assume the evangelical counsel with some bond (*CIC* c. 731 §2), see Jobe Abbass, *The Consecrated Life: A Comparative Commentary of the Eastern and Latin Codes* (Ottawa: Saint Paul University, 2008) 419-425.

Eastern Catholic Churches. Moreover, the norm speaks of eparchies and institutes of consecrated life characteristic of the same Eastern Churches. If, in the final analysis, *CCEO* canon 1102 §1 only implies hiring tribunal personnel from the same or another of the Eastern Catholic Churches *sui iuris*, then there would be fewer possibilities for interecclesial ministry, at least in relation to the Latin Church. In any event, as canonical knowledge regarding the interrelationship of the two codes of the Catholic Church continues to grow, more guidelines and rules for interpretation from the Legislator or the Pontifical Council for Legislative Texts will be extremely helpful.

2.2. Eparchy's Protosyncellus/Syncelli from another Church *sui iuris* (*CCEO* c. 247 §4)

For the most part, both the Eastern (c. 247) and Latin (cc. 477 §1 and 478) codes prescribe comparatively similar norms regarding the appointment of the protosyncellus (vicar general) and the syncelli (episcopal vicars). Essentially, candidates must be celibate priests, who are not less than thirty years of age, and have a doctorate, licence or expertise in canon law or theology. Uniquely, however, the Eastern code adds that the eparchial bishop can take on personnel for these offices from another Church *sui iuris*. *CCEO* canon 247 §4 states: "The eparchial bishop can also take the protosyncellus or syncelli from another eparchy, or from another Church *sui iuris*, however, with the consent of their eparchial bishop."

When the *Coetus de S. Hierarchia* presented the draft of this canon in 1979, there was no mention of the possibility of hiring someone from another Church *sui iuris*. The proposed canon simply stated: "The bishop can take the protosyncellus and syncellus from another eparchy."[43] The same norm appeared as canon 219 §3 of the 1984 *Schema canonum de constitutione hierarchica Ecclesiarum orientalium* (1984 Schema).[44] Although no observations were made regarding the norm during the *denua recognitio* of the 1984 Schema, the expert study group *ex officio* made the change allowing for these officials to come from another Church *sui iuris*. The experts stated: "In §3, however, it was specified *ex officio* that, if an eparchial bishop wanted to appoint as his own protosyncellus or syncellus a priest of another eparchy, he must have *consensum eius Episcopi eparchialis* (his eparchial bishop's consent) for this and, in addition, it was specified that such a priest can be ascribed to *altera Ecclesia sui iuris* (another Church *sui iuris*)."[45] Because the study group added another paragraph to the canon, canon 219 §3 became canon 219 §4, which read: "The eparchial bishop can also take the protosyncellus and syncellus from another eparchy, even if from another Church

---

43 *Nuntia* 9 (1979) 42 (c. 60 §3).

44 See *Nuntia* 19 (1984) 70 (c. 219 §3).

45 Ibid.

sui iuris, however, with the consent of his eparchial bishop."[46] After the identical norm became *SCICO* canon 245 §4,[47] the ending was reformulated once to read as it does in *CCEO* canon 247 §4.[48]

Because *CCEO* canon 247 §4 is unique to the Eastern code and the canons regulating Eastern bishops, it simply cannot be added to the Latin code and the norms governing Latin bishops. A Latin bishop follows *CIC* canons 477 §1 and 478 with regard to the appointment of a vicar general and his episcopal vicar(s). Therefore, Eastern canon 247 §4 does not apply to bishops of the Latin Church in an active sense. However, Eastern canon 247 §4 does involve the Latin Church in a passive sense. In applying *CCEO* canon 247 §4, an Eastern bishop may well decide to appoint his protosyncellus or syncellus not from another eparchy of his Church but, rather, from another Eastern Catholic Church *sui iuris* or, to be implied here, even the Latin Church. This inclusive interpretation is consonant with the Eastern code's characteristic theme of interecclesial collaboration and it is consistent with the 2011 Explanatory Note.

While the interpretation outlined above is still valid for this writer, the same reservations made regarding *CCEO* canon 1102 §1 also apply with respect to *CCEO* canon 247 §4. Certainly, in promulgating *De concordia inter Codices,* the Legislator did not intend to harmonize the Eastern and Latin codes entirely. Nevertheless, *CCEO* canon 247 §4 has not been mirrored in the Latin code. The Legislator may always have intended norms such as Eastern canons 1102 §1 and 247 §4 to be strictly Eastern for a reason. Perhaps a doctorate, license or expertise in Latin canon law (see *CIC* c. 478 §1) would not suffice for the office of protosyncellus or syncellus in an Eastern Catholic Church, distinguished by its different traditions and, above all, by a separate and distinct code. Despite the 2011 Explanatory Note, perhaps the expression "Church *sui iuris*" never meant to imply the Latin Church even in a passive sense here.

2.3. Exercise of Orders by Eastern Clerics Received into Full Communion (*CCEO* c. 899)

Regarding the question of baptized non-Catholics coming into full communion with the Catholic Church, title XVII of the Eastern code is entirely unique. Among its six canons (896-901), *CCEO* canon 899 deals with the exercise of orders by Eastern clerics entering into full communion with the Catholic Church. It states:

> A cleric of an Eastern non-Catholic Church entering into full communion with the Catholic Church can exercise his sacred order in accord with

46 *Nuntia* 23 (1986) 58 (c. 219 §§3-4).

47 See *Nuntia* 24-25 (1987) 46 (c. 245 §4).

48 See *Nuntia* 27 (1988) 43 (c. 245 §4).

> the norms established by the competent authority; a bishop, however, cannot validly exercise the power of governance except with the assent of the Roman Pontiff, head of the college of bishops.[49]

With specific respect to clerics, the canon essentially repeats its source found in *OE* n. 25. It states:

> Nothing more than what a simple profession of the Catholic faith requires should be asked of people of separated Eastern Churches coming into the unity of the Catholic Church under the influence of the grace of the Holy Spirit. And since the valid priesthood has been preserved among them, Eastern clerics joining the Catholic Church may exercise their own orders in accordance with the norms established by the competent authority.[50]

While this canon is addressed to authorities of the Eastern Catholic Churches, the question of receiving Eastern clerics and having them exercise their priestly ministry has also come up in the Latin Church. Suppose that a Latin bishop in the United States has received a Russian Orthodox priest into the Catholic Church and wishes to have him exercise his priestly ministry in his Latin diocese. Can the Latin bishop invoke *CCEO* canon 899? Since the Eastern canon is unique to the Eastern code and concerns all and only the Eastern Catholic Churches (*CCEO* c. 1), *CCEO* canon 899 cannot simply be applied by Latin authorities. The expression "Church *sui iuris*" is not found in this Eastern norm and therefore cannot be used to imply the Latin Church by way of the 2011 Explanatory Note. The *motu proprio, De concordia inter Codices,* does not even broach the topic of title XVII of the Eastern code, not to mention the more particular *CCEO* canon 899.

However, *OE* n. 25, which is the canon's source, while principally concerning the Eastern Catholic Churches, is part of a conciliar decree of the entire Catholic Church and one could argue that it could be applied in this case. Still, even if we were to overcome the lack of a codical norm in this manner, we run into another problem. When the Russian Orthodox priest was received into the Catholic Church, he was ascribed by law to the Russian Catholic Church. That is because *CCEO* canon 35 stipulates that non-Catholics coming into full communion with the See of Rome are to be ascribed to the Church *sui iuris* of the same rite to which they belong. This Eastern norm literally repeats the conciliar prescript in

---

49 *CCEO* c. 899.

50 Second Vatican Council, decree *Orientalium Ecclesiarum* 25, November 21, 1964: *AAS* 57 (1965) 83-84.

OE n. 4,[51] which again applies in the Latin Church even though it has not been incorporated into the Latin code. Unique to the Eastern code, *CCEO* canon 35 states:

> Baptized non-Catholics coming into full communion with the Catholic Church are to retain and practice their own rite and are to observe it everywhere in the world as much as humanly possible. Thus, they are to be ascribed to the Church *sui iuris* of the same rite with due regard for the right of approaching the Apostolic See in special cases of persons, communities or regions.[52]

One might argue that the Russian priest should be able to choose to be ascribed to the Latin Church since *CCEO* canon 35 does not mention validity. In fact, within *PCCICOR*, the expert study group entrusted with the *denua recognitio* of this canon responded to a proposal that the norm be prescribed for validity. The experts replied: "Although it is agreed that the canon is *ad liceitatem*, that is nevertheless not specified in order to adhere more to the conciliar text . . . ."[53] The fact is that neither *CCEO* canon 35, nor *OE* n. 4 that it repeats, is purely exhortative but, rather, prescriptive.[54] Moreover, this is also the interpretation and practice currently followed by the Congregation for Eastern Churches in these matters.[55] Therefore, to transfer to the Latin Church, the Russian priest would need to apply to the Roman See in accord with *CCEO* canon 32 §1, which states: "No one can validly transfer to another Church *sui iuris* without the consent of the Apostolic See." According to *CCEO* canon 32 §2, the Holy See's consent would be presumed if there were both a Latin bishop and a Russian Catholic bishop in the same territory who consented in writing to the transfer.[56] However, since there is no Russian Catholic hierarchy in the United States, this

---

51 *OE* 4 states: "Each and every Catholic as well as baptized members of any non-Catholic Church should keep (*retineant*), follow (*colant*) and as far as possible observe (*observent*) their own rite everywhere in the world, without prejudice to the right of recourse to the Apostolic See in cases of persons, communities or regions." *Orientalium Ecclesiarum* 4, 77; English translation in *Decrees of the Ecumenical Councils,* ed. Norman Tanner (London and Washington: Sheed & Ward and Gregorian University Press, 1990) 2: 901.

52 *CCEO* c. 35.

53 *Nuntia* 22 (1986) 31 (c. 14).

54 See also George Nedungatt, "Churches *sui iuris* and Rites," in *A Guide*, 125, note 60.

55 See also Francesco Catozzella, "Le modifiche in materia di forma canonica del matrimonio introdotte dal *Motu proprio De concordia inter Codices*, 'Stato, Chiese e pluralismo confessionale, Rivista telematica'" (February 20, 2017) n. 6, 16-17, https://riviste.unimi.it/index.php/statoechiese/article/view/8107 (accessed on 2 Mar. 2020).

56 See *CCEO* canon 32 §2: "In the case of Christian faithful of an eparchy of a certain Church *sui iuris* who petition to transfer to another Church *sui iuris* which has its own eparchy in the same territory, this consent of the Apostolic See is presumed, provided that the eparchial bishops of both eparchies consent to the transfer in writing."

option would not be available.

In the case of a Russian Orthodox priest who is received into the Catholic Church, there are certainly possibilities for interecclesial ministry. If he had been received by a Russian Catholic bishop, he could exercise his orders in that Church or even in another Eastern Catholic Church in accord with *CCEO* canon 899. It is also possible to exercise his orders in the Latin Church but not by way of Eastern canon 899. It is not a Latin canon and nothing suggests that it implicitly addresses Latin bishops. Nor can it be argued that either the 2011 Explanatory Note or the 2016 *motu proprio, De concordia inter Codices*, has somehow made *CCEO* canon 899 a Latin norm. Outside the codes, there is *OE* n. 25, which the Latin bishop could rely on in this case. However, in accord with *CCEO* canon 35, the Russian priest must first apply to the Roman Apostolic See to transfer to the Latin Church. Then, as far as exercising his sacred orders in the Latin Church, according to *OE* n. 25, the "competent authority" mentioned there would again be the Roman See as it, alone, is supreme arbiter among the Churches.

Conclusion

From the perspective of the 1990 *Codex Canonum Ecclesiarum Orientalium,* many concrete opportunities for interecclesial ministry are present in the Eastern canonical norms. However, the frequency of these possibilities will vary depending on one's expansive or restrictive interpretation of *CCEO* canon 1, by which the Legislator initially established the interrelationship of the Eastern and Latin codes. A more expansive interpretation of Eastern canon 1, based on the 2011 Explanatory Note, might envisage more opportunities for interecclesial ministry as the two codes and their unique canons are seen to be interrelated and applicable in the entire Catholic Church. On the other hand, a more restrictive interpretation of *CCEO* canon 1, based on the apparent limits set by *De concordia inter Codices* on the interrelationship of the codes, might well see fewer opportunities for interecclesial ministry as the two codes are seen as totally separate and distinct juridical systems.

Part one of this paper examined Eastern norms (*CCEO* cc. 678 §1; 916 §4; 1068 §1) which undoubtedly offer the possibility of interecclesial ministry for Easterners as well as Latins. A priest of any Church *sui iuris*, including the Latin Church, can administer baptism to a person who is to be ascribed to his Church and that person's pastor, of any Church *sui iuris*, even the Latin Church, cannot deny the priest that permission (c. 678 §1). An Eastern bishop can designate a priest from another Church *sui iuris*, also the Latin Church, as pastor for his faithful who find themselves in an area without a proper pastor (c. 916 §4). Eparchial bishops, as well as diocesan bishops, who exercise their power in the same territory can agree to establish a common ecclesiastical tribunal (c. 1068 §1). The interpretations which afford these interecclesial ministries are consistent with the wider interpretation given *CCEO* canon 1 by the Holy See's

2011 official Explanatory Note.

Part two looked closely at other Eastern norms (*CCEO* cc. 1102 §1; 247 §4; 899) which may not ultimately offer the same opportunities for interecclesial ministry. It was argued, for example, that Eastern bishops can hire tribunal personnel from other Churches *sui iuris*, including the Latin Church (c. 1102 §1). However, if it is eventually decided that, since this is a unique *CCEO* norm, Eastern bishops are limited to hiring those who are versed in Eastern canon law and traditions, then there would be fewer opportunities for Latins to carry out interecclesial ministry. In the same way, an Eastern bishop may be able to appoint his protosyncellus or syncellus from another Church *sui iuris,* even from the Latin Church (c. 247 §4). However, this unique Eastern norm might also limit the bishop to appointing only other Easterners who are experts in Eastern canon law and traditions. Finally, *CCEO* canon 899 and the entire title XVII are unique to the Eastern code. While Eastern Catholic bishops can receive Eastern Orthodox clerics into the Catholic Church and have them exercise sacred orders in accord with canon 899, it is not a canon upon which Latin bishops can rely. This is not only because the priest must be received into the Church as Eastern Catholic, but also because the competent authority in any case involving different Churches would be the See of Rome, as supreme arbiter among the Churches. These more restrictive interpretations follow from the limits that effectively were set by *De concordia inter Codices* on the interpretation of Eastern canon 1 and the interrelationship of the codes.

In sum, we have felt a certain unsureness in the interpretation of these canons regarding the interrelationship of the codes and the norms associated with opportunities or possibilities for interecclesial ministry. As canonical knowledge in this area continues to grow, more guidelines and rules for interpretation from the Legislator or the Pontifical Council for Legislative Texts will prove to be an indispensable help.

Seminar

Cor Orans: Implementing New Papal Norms for Nuns

Sister Nancy Bauer, OSB, JCD

Introduction

If there is a community of contemplative nuns in your diocese, or you provide canonical counsel for such a community, or you simply know a few nuns, you are aware that the instruction *Cor orans* is a force to be reckoned with.[1] *Cor orans* was issued by the Congregation for Institutes of Consecrated Life and Societies of Apostolic Life (CICLSAL) on April 1, 2018, and, since then, monasteries of nuns have been hard at work, first trying to understand its intricacies and then trying to implement it. You could say that *Cor orans* is to monasteries of nuns what *Mitis Iudex* has been to tribunals. But before I delve into the instruction, I will review the steps along the yellow brick road that got us to the land of *Cor orans*.[2]

Not much had changed in church law regarding contemplative monasteries of nuns from the Middle Ages up until 1950 when Pope Pius XII issued his apostolic constitution *Sponsa Christi*. Pius recognized that, for too many monasteries, centuries of increasingly strict papal enclosure had resulted in an unhealthy isolation and near destitution.[3] In *Sponsa Christi*, he provided for two levels of papal enclosure: major papal enclosure for nuns wholly engaged in the contemplative life and minor papal enclosure for nuns who needed to acquire revenue by engaging at least minimally in works external to the monastery.[4] Pius also "highly recommended" that monasteries of nuns form or join federations,

---

1 See Congregation for Institutes of Consecrated Life and Societies of Apostolic Life [hereafter CICLSAL], instruction *Cor orans*, April 1, 2018: *AAS* (2018) 814-864, English translation at http://www.vatican.va/roman_curia/congregations/ccscrlife/documents/rc_con_ccscrlife_doc_20180401_cor-orans_en.html (accessed on 30 Mar. 2020).

2 For a more in-depth review of the lead-up to *Vultum Dei quaerere* and thus *Cor orans*, see Nancy Bauer, "*Vultum Dei Quaerere*: New Norms for Nuns," *The Jurist* 76 (2016) 379-414.

3 See Pope Pius XII, apostolic constitution *Sponsa Christi*, November 21, 1950: *AAS* 43 (1950) [hereafter *SpC*] 10-11; English translation in *CLD* 3: 227-228.

4 See *SpC* 12-13; *CLD* 3: 229-230.

but he did not require them to do so.[5]

Vatican II conciliar and postconciliar documents that addressed women's contemplative life focused primarily on enclosure. Major and minor papal enclosure were replaced by papal and constitutional enclosure.[6] The Sacred Congregation for Religious and for Secular Institutes issued the first postconciliar revision of papal enclosure in its 1969 instruction *Venite seorsum*.[7] The 1983 Code of Canon Law contains a few canons specific to nuns, including canon 667 §§3-4 on cloister.[8] However, the life of contemplative nuns had not been addressed in a comprehensive way after *Sponsa Christi* until sixty-six years later—five decades after the close of Vatican II—when, in 2016, Pope Francis issued a new apostolic constitution on women's contemplative life *Vultum Dei quaerere*, which contains new papal legislation for nuns.[9] *Cor orans* is the implementing instruction for *Vultum Dei quaerere*.

The new norms for nuns are in continuity with the evolution begun in *Sponsa Christi*, but also emerge from more recent realities. There are about 4,000 monasteries of contemplative nuns around the world, with a total membership (in 2014) of about 39,000, with 23,000 of those in Europe.[10] In a ten-year period beginning in the mid-1990s, there was a decline of about 10,000 nuns.[11] Some monasteries that have been in continuous existence for centuries now have only

5 *SpC* 18, Art. VII §2, 2°: "Monasteriorum Foederationes quamvis regula generali non praecipiantur, tamen a Sede Apostolica valde commendantur." *CLD* 3: 237.

6 See Second Vatican Council, decree *Perfectae caritatis* 16, October 28, 1967: *AAS* 58 (1966) 710; English translation: *Vatican Council II: Constitutions, Decrees, Declarations*, ed. Austin Flannery (Northport, NY: Costello Publishing Company, 1996) 397.

7 See Sacred Congregation for Religious and for Secular Institutes, instruction *Venite seorsum,* August 15, 1969: *AAS* 61 (1969) 674-690.

8 See *Codex Iuris Canonici auctoritate Ioannis Pauli PP. II promulgatus* (Vatican City: Libreria Editrice Vaticana, 1983). English translation of canons of this code are from *Code of Canon Law, Latin-English Edition: New English Translation* (Washington, DC: Canon Law Society of America, 2012). Canon 667 requires cloister for all religious institutes, whether female or male, but prescribes various levels of enclosure for various kinds of institutes. Canon 667 §3 prescribes papal enclosure for monasteries of nuns that are ordered entirely to contemplation and constitutional enclosure for other monasteries of nuns. Other canons specific to nuns (*moniales*) are cc. 609 §2, 614, 616 §4, 630 §3, and 686 §2. Canon 686 §2 on exclaustration of nuns is derogated by *Cor orans*.

9 See Pope Francis, apostolic constitution *Vultum Dei quaerere*, June 29, 2016: AAS 108 (2016) [hereafter *VDq*] 835-861; English translaton at http://w2.vatican.va/content/dam/francesco/pdf/apost_constitutions/documents/papa-francesco_costituzione-ap_20160629_vultum-dei-quaerere_en.pdf (accessed on 30 Mar. 2020).

10 See Carol Glatz, "Pope issues rules to help contemplative women be beacons for world," Catholic News Service, July 22, 2016. Available at https://cnstopstories.com/2016/07/22/pope-issues-rules-to-help-contemplative-women-be-beacons-for-world/ (accessed on 19 Jan. 2020).

11 Ibid.

a few members, as few as three or four.

Several other developments provide the immediate impetus for provisions that appear in *Vultum Dei quaerere* and *Cor orans*. At the conclusion of the 1994 Synod of Bishops on consecrated life, synod members, in their final dispositions, called for equality between contemplative women and contemplative men; specifically, they recommended that nuns have the same freedom and flexibility regarding cloister that monks have always had.[12] The subsequent 1999 instruction *Verbi Sponsa* maintains papal enclosure for contemplative women, but inches closer to equality by giving major superiors of nuns greater authority in granting short absences from cloister.[13] In November 2008, CICLSAL, in its plenary assembly, focused on "The Monastic Life and Its Meaning in the Church and in the World Today," with particular emphasis on female monasticism.[14] Speakers addressed issues and challenges in women's contemplative life, including the decline in vocations and the progressive aging of nuns in Europe and North America, with the consequent lack of nuns qualified to serve as superiors and formators, financial difficulties, and impoverished liturgical prayer.

In 2014, CICLSAL sent a letter and questionnaire to monasteries of nuns around the world asking for comments on the topics of autonomy, formation, and the evangelical meaning of the wholly contemplative life in the Church.[15] In February 2016, the Year of Consecrated Life closed with a theological symposium which included sessions on women's contemplative life. [16] Speakers addressed the distinction between the juridical autonomy of monasteries and "real autonomy of life," the tendency of monasteries to recruit candidates from distant countries to avoid suppression, and the growing trend of monasteries resorting to postulation or appointing administrators because of a lack of members capable of being superiors. There was also a recommendation that all monasteries of nuns be required to join a federation.

In light of these developments, Pope Francis issued *Vultum Dei quaerere* in which he identifies twelve "matters calling for discernment and renewed norms:" formation, prayer, the Word of God, the sacraments of Eucharist and

12 See Johnson Michael Kallidukil, *The Canonical Significance of the Synod of Bishops of 1994 on Consecrated Life from the Lineamenta to the Vita consecrata* (Frankfurt am Main: P. Lang, 2003) 256.

13 See CICLSAL, instruction *Verbi sponsa* norm 17, May 13, 1999 (Vatican: Libreria Editrice Vaticana, 1999), in *CLD* 14: 579.

14 See Vatican Information Service, "Monasteries: Oases of Ascetic Life," in *Vatican Information Service Bulletin*, November 20, 2008, http://visnews-en.blogspot.com/2008/11/monasteries-oases-of-ascetic-life.html (accessed on 19 Jan. 2020).

15 See CICLSAL, letter to "Dear Reverend Mothers and Sisters," April 29, 2014, Prot. 28513/2014 (unpublished).

16 The presentations of the symposium are available at https://www.vitanostra-nuovaciteaux.it/o-pepe-le-federazioni-dei-monasteri/ (accessed on 19 Jan. 2020).

Reconciliation, community life, autonomy, federations, cloister, work, silence, communications media, and asceticism.[17] In the concluding section, he issues new papal law regarding these twelve matters. For example, he requires every monastery of nuns to belong to a federation,[18] extends the duration of initial formation,[19] and invites each community to choose the form of cloister it wishes to observe.[20]

The implementing instruction *Cor orans* does not address every one of the twelve matters identified by Pope Francis. Following a brief introduction and "General Norms," *Cor orans* addresses five of those matters—autonomy; federation; separation from the world, which includes both social communications and cloister; and formation. The instruction ends with final dispositions and a conclusion. The conclusion lists canons of the code that are derogated by the new norms and one article of *Verbi Sponsa* that is abrogated. *Cor orans* was approved *in forma specifica* by Pope Francis.[21]

Introduction and General Norms

The introduction to *Cor orans* recognizes the gift of women's contemplative life within the Church.

> Praying heart, guardian of gratuity, wealth of apostolic fruitfulness and of a mysterious and multiform holiness is the feminine contemplative life in the Church. The contemplative life of nuns, rooted in the silence of the cloister, from its beginnings through a mysterious apostolic fruitfulness enriches the Church of Christ with fruits of grace and mercy.[22]

The introduction recalls that Pope Pius XII, in *Sponsa Christi*, recognized the autonomy of monasteries of nuns, advocated federations to overcome isolation and facilitate collaboration, and accommodated cloister to newer times.[23] Finally, the introduction notes that Pope Francis mandated the instruction to help monasteries of the Latin Church apply *Vultum Dei quaerere*.[24]

The General Norms (*CO* 1-14) provide important definitions of terms as they will be used in the instruction. The first four general norms answer the question:

17 *VDq* 12.

18 *VDq* 9 §1.

19 *VDq* 15.

20 *VDq* 10 §1.

21 *CO* Conclusion.

22 *CO* Introduction.

23 Ibid.

24 Ibid.

"Who is a nun?" Canonically, there has always been a distinction between nuns and sisters, although what constitutes the distinction has changed from time to time. In the 1917 Code of Canon Law, nuns (*moniales*) were defined as women religious in solemn vows and sisters (*sorores*) as women religious in simple vows.[25] The 1983 code, in the section on religious, does not distinguish between solemn and simple vows. Rather, all religious profess the evangelical counsels of poverty, chastity, and obedience by public vow.[26] The term "*sorores*" does not appear in these canons. Instead, the inclusive term "*sodales*" or "members" is used to refer to all religious, male and female.[27] Although a few canons, such as canon 667 §§3-4, refer explicitly to "*moniales*," the 1983 code does not define the term. In *Cor orans*, a nun is defined as a woman religious who leads a wholly contemplative life, more specifically, a "canonical contemplative life," which is "the external profession of religious discipline that, whether through the exercises of piety, prayer, and mortification, or through the occupations which the nuns must attend to, is so ordered to interior contemplation that their whole life and all actions can easily and must efficaciously be imbued by the desire for it."[28] The term "nun" does not exclude engagement in works external to the cloister.[29] For example, some monasteries operate schools or retreat centers, but the primary occupation and preoccupation of the members is interior contemplation.

Because *Vultum Dei quaerere* requires all monasteries to be federated unless dispensed by the Holy See, the definitions of a federation and equivalent entities are important for interpreting the instruction. Three kinds of affiliation among monasteries are identified as "structures of communion." They are federations, associations, and conferences. A federation of monasteries is "a structure of communion among some autonomous monasteries of the same Institute erected by the Holy See that approves the Statutes, so that in sharing the same charism, the federated monasteries overcome isolation and promote regular observance and contemplative life."[30] An association of monasteries is "a structure of communion between several autonomous monasteries of the same Institute erected by the Holy See so that, in sharing the same charism, the associated monasteries collaborate among themselves according to the Statutes approved by the Holy See."[31] A conference of monasteries is "a structure of communion among autonomous monasteries belonging to diverse Institutes and present in the same region, erected by the Holy See that approves the Statutes, with the aim of promoting contemplative life and of favoring collaboration among the

---

25 See *Codex Iuris Canonici Pii X Pontificis Maximi iussu digestus Benedicti Papae XV auctoritate promulgatus* (Rome: Typis Polyglottis Vaticanis, 1917) c. 488, 7°.

26 See 1983 *CIC* c. 607 §2.

27 See, for example, cc. 607 §2, 610, 619, 622, 623, etc.

28 *CO* 4.

29 *CO* 2.

30 *CO* 7.

31 *CO* 8.

monasteries in particular geographic or linguistic contexts."[32] It is hard to detect anything significant that distinguishes a federation from an association. Both are composed of monasteries of the same institute, while a conference is composed of monasteries of different institutes or perhaps monasteries that are truly one of a kind. What is important to note is that whatever *Cor orans* says about a federation applies equally to an association and a conference and the requirement to belong to a federation is fulfilled by membership in any one of these three structures of communion.[33] In other words, what is prescribed in *Cor orans* regarding the structure of a federation and the role of the federal president and other officers also applies to an association and conference.

The General Norms also mention a monastic congregation, which is a "structure of governance," rather than a "structure of communion."[34] This indicates that the president of a monastic congregation, who is a major superior, has a greater level of jurisdiction in relation to the member monasteries than presidents of structures of communion, who are not major superiors. It is clear from the context that *Cor orans* is referring here to a congregation of women's monasteries. Membership in such a congregation fulfills the requirement of federating and whatever pertains to a federation in *Cor orans* pertains to a monastic congregation, with the necessary adaptations.[35]

Chapter 1. The Autonomous Monastery (*CO* 15-85)

The first chapter of *Cor orans* identifies the juridical elements of an autonomous monastery, the distinction between juridical autonomy and real autonomy of life, how a new monastery is established, options for a monastery that is struggling to maintain real autonomy, ecclesial vigilance of a monastery, and the relationship between a monastery of nuns and the diocesan bishop.

The chapter begins by defining a monastery *sui iuris* as "a religious house which enjoys legal autonomy: its Superior is a Major Superior, its community is permanently established for the number and quality of the members; by law it is the place of the novitiate and of formation, is considered a public juridical person, and its assets are ecclesiastical goods."[36] In other words, a monastery that enjoys legal or juridical autonomy elects its own superior who is, in law, a major superior; she has all the authority she needs to direct the members in the pursuit of their vocation according to the proper law and charism of the monastery. By contrast, *Cor orans* will later say explicitly that the federal president is not a

32 *CO* 9.

33 *CO* 13.

34 *CO* 12.

35 *CO* 14.

36 *CO* 15.

major superior.[37] A monastery with legal autonomy also enjoys a sense of stability or permanence. The members can reasonably expect to live out their vocations in *that* monastery until death. Some even profess a vow of stability.[38] However, permanence or stability does not mean that a monastery cannot lose its legal autonomy—a situation addressed further along in chapter 1.

An autonomous monastery has its own novitiate and formation. The superior of the monastery has the right to admit new members and to see that they are formed in the ways of the monastery, that is, in the living tradition of the community. Candidates cannot be imposed on the monastery by any external authority and, as long as they are qualified by universal and proper law, external authority is not qualified to prevent admission of specific candidates. An autonomous monastery is a public juridic person which acquires, possesses, administers, and disposes of its own temporal goods. The temporal goods belong to the monastery itself, even if the monastery is federated. Finally, legal autonomy means the community has internal autonomy; it has its own way of life in accord with its charism. Like all religious institutes, monasteries of contemplative nuns enjoy a "just autonomy of life, especially of governance."[39]

Pope Francis, in *Vultum Dei quaerere*, recognizes the importance of autonomy for monasteries of contemplative nuns: "Autonomy favors the stability of life and internal unity of each community, ensuring the best conditions for contemplation."[40] Likewise, *Cor orans* affirms that autonomy promotes stability of life and internal unity and it preserves the character and identity of a monastery.[41] It provides the "best conditions for the life of the nuns according to the spirit and character of the institute to which they belong."[42]

However, autonomy is not absolute. It means that there will be no unnecessary intervention in the life of the community but, like all religious institutes, monasteries of nuns are subject to ecclesiastical authority. Furthermore, *Vultum Dei quaerere* and *Cor orans* distinguish between juridical or legal autonomy and real or authentic autonomy of life.[43] In order to acquire juridical autonomy, a new foundation must demonstrate that it has achieved real autonomy which is

---

37 *CO* 110.

38 Religious who observe the Rule of Benedict, such as Benedictines and Cistercians, profess stability, fidelity to the monastic way of life, and obedience. See Benedict of Nursia, *Regula Sancti Benedicti* 58.17, in *RB 1980: The Rule of St. Benedict in Latin and English*, ed. Timothy Fry et al. (Collegeville, MN: Liturgical Press, 1981) 269.

39 1983 *CIC* c. 586 §1: "Singulis institutis iusta autonomia vitae, praesertim regiminis."

40 *VDq* 28.

41 See *CO* 16.

42 *CO* 17.

43 See, for example, *VDq* 8 §1: "Juridical autonomy needs to be matched by a genuine autonomy of life."

"the ability to manage the life of the monastery in all its dimensions."[44] These dimensions are vocational, formational, governmental, relational, liturgical, financial, etc.[45] In other words, the monastery must be vital and viable which means it has sufficient vocations and potential vocations, members capable of leadership, a family spirit, the ability to carry out liturgical functions in a solemn and dignified manner, financial stability, and a proper physical plant.[46] *Cor orans* will also say that a monastery *sui iuris* must maintain real autonomy in order to retain its legal autonomy.[47]

A new foundation, or dependent house, can be initiated by an existing autonomous monastery or by a federation.[48] When a monastery or federation considers the possibility of initiating a foundation, it must proceed prudently, choosing a location where there is a potential for vocations, financial stability, sacramental life, and separation from the world.[49] In the beginning, the founding monastery or federation must send a minimum of five nuns, at least three of them in perpetual vows.[50] Establishing a dependent house also requires the prior written consent of the diocesan bishop where the house will be located and authorization of the Holy See.[51] Other requirements are prescribed in *Cor orans.*[52]

In order for the foundation to obtain legal autonomy, it must have grown in membership and stability. Specifically, there must be eight nuns in perpetual profession, as long as most of them are not elderly.[53] Among those eight or more nuns, there must be members capable of serving as superior, formator, and financial administrator.[54] The community must have achieved financial independence and vital community life and it must have suitable facilities.[55] These criteria should be accomplished within fifteen years or the Holy See will assess whether there is a "well-founded hope" that the dependent house will acquire "real autonomy."[56] If not, it will be suppressed.[57]

---

44 *CO* 18.

45 Ibid.

46 *VDq* 8 §1.

47 *CO* 43.

48 *CO* 20.

49 *CO* 24-28.

50 *CO* 29.

51 Ibid.

52 *CO* 20-38.

53 *CO* 39 a.

54 *CO* 39 b.

55 *CO* 39 c-d.

56 *CO* 38.

57 Ibid.

In order for a monastery *sui iuris* to retain legal autonomy, it must maintain real autonomy. If the number of members in perpetual profession declines to five, the monastery loses its right to elect its own superior and an "administrator superior" is appointed.[58] The Holy See, having been informed of the situation by the federal president, establishes an *ad hoc* commission to assess the monastery's viability.[59] *Cor orans* provides three options when a monastery's real autonomy is deemed precarious or non-existent: 1) affiliation; 2) transfer; and 3) suppression. With affiliation or entrustment, the monastery's juridical autonomy is suspended and it becomes dependent on another monastery or on the federation itself.[60] The major superior of the affiliating monastery or the federal president becomes the major superior of the affiliated monastery, while the affiliated monastery has a local superior.[61] The affiliated monastery may accept candidates, but they have their novitiate and formation in the affiliating monastery.[62] During the period of affiliation, the struggling monastery is assessed as to whether its apparent lack of viability is only temporary and reversible, or whether it is irreversible.[63] If it proves to be irreversible, the monastery is suppressed.[64]

In the case of transfer, a monastery retains its juridical autonomy and its own major superior and membership, but it changes its geographic location.[65] In some cases, a new location may provide the opportunity to regain authentic autonomy of life. In other cases, a monastic community may transfer with the intention of "coming to completion" in a place that is more conducive to a declining and aging membership.[66]

In some cases, when a monastery has lost real autonomy, the Holy See will establish an *ad hoc* commission to determine whether suppression is warranted. The commission will consider the following criteria: the number of nuns and

---

58 *CO* 45.

59 Ibid.

60 *CO* 57.

61 *CO* 58-59.

62 *CO* 60-61.

63 *CO* 55.

64 Ibid.

65 *CO* 65.

66 For example, in February 2018, the members of a Franciscan Poor Clare community, most of whom were elderly, moved from their monastery in Bloomington, Minnesota, in the Archdiocese of St. Paul-Minneapolis, to a wing of the motherhouse of the Sisters of St. Francis in Rochester, Minnesota, in the Diocese of Winona-Rochester. The Poor Clares maintain their own way of life but join the Franciscan Sisters for daily Eucharist. Matthew Davis, "Bloomington Poor Clares moving to Rochester after 63 years in archdiocese," *The Catholic Spirit*, December 1, 2017, http://thecatholicspirit.com/news/local-news/bloomington-poor-clares-moving-rochester-63-years-archdiocese/ (accessed on 19 Jan. 2020).

their ages and capacity for governance and formation, a lack of candidates for a number of years, and a lack of vitality in living and transmitting the charism in dynamic fidelity.[67] A specific number of nuns is not identified, nor is the number of years during which there have been no candidates. All of these criteria must be considered together. In some circumstances, a relatively small membership can sustain authentic autonomy of life.

The final sections of chapter 1 of *Cor orans* address ecclesial vigilance of monasteries and the relationship between monasteries and diocesan bishops. Ecclesial vigilance is described as "the service of supervision."[68] Each female monastery is entrusted to the vigilance of a single ecclesial authority.[69] In the case of a female monastic congregation, the "congregated monasteries" are under the vigilance of the president whose scope of supervision is defined in the constitutions.[70] Female monasteries that are juridically associated with the male branch of the same institute, or "juridically associated monasteries," are under the vigilance of the religious ordinary whose scope of supervision is also defined in the constitutions.[71] Monasteries *sui iuris* as they are described in canon 615 are entrusted to the vigilance of the diocesan bishop.[72] His functions in relation to the entrusted monastery are given in the Code of Canon Law and repeated in *Cor orans*. Specifically, he presides at the election of the major superior; conducts regular visitations; examines the annual financial report; in derogation of canon 638 §4, gives his written consent for particular administrative acts, *if established by its proper law*; confirms an indult of departure of a member in temporary profession; and issues a decree of dismissal.[73]

However, all monasteries, including those that are congregated and juridically associated, are subject to the diocesan bishop in some matters. An exhaustive list of these matters is given in *Cor orans*. They include (1) the public exercise of divine worship, care of souls, and the apostolate; (2) the bishop's ability to provide solutions when he discovers abuses in monastic life that the major superior fails to address; (3) the requirement of the bishop's written consent to establish a monastery in his diocese; (4) the intervention of the bishop to appoint a chaplain and approve ordinary confessors; (5) the intervention of the bishop through

---

67 *CO* 70.

68 *CO* 75.

69 *CO* 76.

70 *CO* 75.1.

71 *CO* 75.2.

72 *CO* 75.3. According to canon 615, the diocesan bishop has special vigilance of "an autonomous monastery which does not have another major superior besides its own moderator and is not associated to another institute of religious in such a way that the superior of the latter possesses true power over such a monastery as determined by the constitutions."

73 *CO* 81 a-f.

expression of his opinion regarding the possible suppression of a monastery; (6) the bishop's care of an exclaustrated nun residing in the diocese; and (7) the bishop's faculty allowing him to enter the cloister and to allow others to enter, with the consent of the major superior.[74] These are the "only possible forms of intervention by the diocesan Bishop" to safeguard the rights and duties of the president of a congregation or the religious ordinary of associated monasteries.[75]

Chapter 2: The Federation of Monasteries (*CO* 86-155)

The chapter on autonomy is followed immediately by a chapter on the federation of monasteries. Autonomy and federation are two sides of the same coin. Even as Pope Francis advocates autonomy as the best condition for contemplation, he says autonomy "ought not to mean independence or isolation"[76] and he legislates that every monastery of nuns must be federated, unless dispensed from this obligation by the Holy See.[77] Note that the requirement to be federated is fulfilled by membership in a federation, association, or conference and what is said about a federation in *Cor orans* applies equally to associations and conferences.

Federations are erected, suspended, united, and suppressed by the Holy See and are of pontifical right.[78] They are public juridic persons capable of acquiring, possessing, managing and alienating temporal goods.[79] The temporal goods of a federation are separate from those of each member monastery. A federation does not own or control in any way the temporal goods of the individual monasteries.

About half of the world's monasteries of nuns were already federated before promulgation of *Vultum Dei quarere*, which means that about half were not.[80] Since *Cor orans* was issued, a number of monasteries have requested dispensation from the obligation of federating and a dispensation has been granted in certain circumstances. Monasteries of nuns that belong to a monastic congregation that includes male and female monasteries have been dispensed, but only on condition that essential requirements of *Cor orans* be incorporated into the constitutions.

---

74 *CO* 83 a-g.

75 *CO* 84.

76 *VDq* 28.

77 *VDq* 9 §1.

78 *CO* 88, 90.

79 *CO* 97.

80 At the May 15, 2018, press conference introducing *Cor orans*, Cistercian Father Sebastiano Paciolla, undersecretary of the Congregation for Institutes of Consecrated Life and Societies of Apostolic Life, said that, despite Pius XII's recommendation, almost half of women's monasteries of nuns had not yet joined a federation. See Carol Glatz, "Vatican issues new rules for communities of contemplative nuns," Catholic News Service, May 15, 2018, https://www.globalsistersreport.org/news/trends/vatican-issues-new-rules-communities-contemplative-nuns-53791 (accessed on 17 Mar. 2020).

The Order of Cistercians of the Strict Observance (Trappistines and Trappists) petitioned CICLSAL for an exemption of the order's nuns from the obligation of federating. The exemption was granted because of the unique "legal link" of the female monasteries with the order as a whole.[81] Specifically, "the Abbots and Abbesses form a single chapter . . . the Abbesses are members of the General Assembly with an active vote in the election of the Abbot General and an active and passive vote in the election of the members of the General Council."[82] The Benedictine Congregation of Solesmes also requested an exemption for its female member monasteries. The response from CICLSAL noted: "In principle, it seems possible and even justified that monasteries belonging to a monastic congregation are dispensed from the obligation of Federation required by the Apostolic Constitution to the extent that this congregation is actually an organ of communion and government and that its constitutions incorporate the new provisions."[83] The dicastery added that exemption depends on incorporation of the new norms regarded as "essential" into the constitutions of the monastic congregation, including the new norms on papal enclosure, the development of the responsibility of the nuns and the new faculties granted to major superiors, the participation of a nun as co-visitator, the provisions on initial and permanent formation, and the support and communion among monasteries.[84] The Order of Cistercians (O.Cist.) received a similar response to its request for dispensation.[85] Specifically, the dicastery noted that the new norms of *Vultum Dei quaerere* and *Cor orans* must be incorporated into the proper law of the order, the constitutions of the congregations, and the statutes of foundations, especially the new norms regarding papal enclosure, the criteria of vital autonomy for foundations, the development of responsibility of nuns and the new faculties granted to major superiors, the inclusion of a nun as co-visitator for canonical visitations, the prescriptions on initial and ongoing formation, and the support and communion among monasteries.[86] On the other hand, there have been reports that some stand-alone monasteries, that is, monasteries that are not affiliated with any others, have requested dispensations from the obligation of federating and they have been denied. Other monasteries that had not been federated are seeking to join existing structures of communion or are initiating new federations, associations, or conferences.

81 CICLSAL, Letter to Abbot General, April 1, 2019, Prot. N. C. 79-1, available at https://www.ocso.org/2019/04/17/civcsva/ (accessed on 3 Mar. 2020).

82 Ibid.

83 CICLSAL, Letter from José Rodríguez Carballo, O.F.M., to Révérend Père, March 5, 2019, Prot. n. 385/2019 (unpublished).

84 Ibid.

85 CICLSAL, Letter from João Braz Card. de Aviz to Révérend Père, May 3, 2019, Prot. n. C 109/2019 (unpublished).

86 Ibid.

According to *Cor orans*, the officers of a federation include a president and four councilors, elected for six-year terms by the federal assembly, which is comparable to the general chapter of other religious institutes.[87] Each federation also has a financial administrator elected by the federal assembly, a federal secretary selected by the president, and a federal formator, appointed by the president with the consent of the federal council.[88] One of the functions of the federation is to assist the member monasteries with formation, especially with formation of formators and of those who will serve as superiors in the member monasteries.[89]

An "ordinary federal assembly" is held every six years at which the president and councilors are elected and the major business of the federation is addressed.[90] The "intermediate federal assembly" is convened every three years to assess progress on whatever was decided in the ordinary assembly.[91] An "extraordinary federal assembly" is called when there is a need.[92]

Cor orans assigns significant functions to the federal president, even though she is not a major superior. For example, she serves as "co-visitator" in the canonical visitation of each member monastery, accompanying the regular visitator, who is the diocesan bishop for "entrusted" monasteries and the religious ordinary for "juridically associated monasteries."[93] The federal president also visits a monastery when a need arises.[94] *Cor orans* does not specify what kind of "need" would warrant this kind of visit, but it could be a financial difficulty or another crisis such that a monastery would benefit from the intervention or input of the president. The federal president can also visit on an informal basis, but only when agreed on by the superior of the monastery.[95] In the canonical visitation, the president exercises vigilance in relation to specific matters, such as how the community is observing the twelve items specified by Pope Francis in *Vultum Dei quaerere*, initial and ongoing formation, and the viability of the monastery.[96] She submits a report to CICLSAL after each canonical visitation.[97]

---

87 *CO* 110, 123.

88 *CO* 142 (financial administrator), 144 (federal secretary), 148 (federal formator).

89 *CO* 118-119.

90 *CO* 135, 141 a-j.

91 *CO* 136.

92 *CO* 137.

93 *CO* 111.

94 *CO* 113.

95 *CO* 114.

96 *CO* 116-117.

97 *CO* 115.

Each federation has a "religious assistant" who is a priest appointed by CICLSAL.[98] The federation, through the president, has the opportunity to recommend the names of three priests to serve in this capacity.[99] The religious assistant represents the Holy See to the federation, not to the individual monasteries.[100] He is not a major superior; his role is to assist the president and council, especially regarding formation at the federal level and financial matters.[101] The religious assistant submits to the Holy See a brief annual report on the progress of the federation.[102]

Chapter 3: Separation from the World (*CO* 156-218)

In chapter 3 on "Separation from the World," *Cor orans* addresses social communications and cloister. Some degree or form of separation from the world is characteristic of all religious institutes[103]; all institutes have some form of cloister[104]; and all are called to "discretion" in the use of social communications.[105] Regarding the use of the various forms of social communications within monasteries of nuns, *Cor orans* calls for sobriety and discretion, but it is for the conventual chapter of each monastery to establish guidelines suitable to their own way life.[106]

The instruction introduces significant changes regarding cloister. Since *Sponsa Christi* in 1950, there have been two levels of cloister available for nuns: at first, major and minor; since Vatican II, papal and constitutional. *Cor orans* provides a third option called "monastic cloister." Papal enclosure is for those who lead a wholly contemplative life; it excludes the possibility of engagement in the external apostolate and usually nuns under papal enclosure do not participate in diocesan or other church events outside the cloister.[107] The major superior can permit a nun to leave the cloister for ordinary situations, such as, for health care, participation in initial and ongoing formation meetings organized by the federation or by another monastery, the exercise of civil rights, and to provide for other needs of the monastery which cannot be provided for in another way.[108] Constitutional cloister, as the name implies, is cloister defined in the constitutions of the monastery and is for nuns who are dedicated to the contemplative life but

98 *CO* 150.

99 *CO* 154.

100 *CO* 149.

101 *CO* 151.

102 *CO* 155.

103 1983 *CIC*, c. 607 §3.

104 1983 *CIC*, c. 667.

105 1983 *CIC*, c. 666.

106 *CO* 170.

107 *CO* 184, 188 a-c.

108 *CO* 200.

who also engage in some work of the apostolate or charity that draws them out of the cloister proper.[109] Monastic enclosure is a form of constitutional enclosure, but allows for greater engagement in hospitality, that is, in receiving guests into the monastery.[110] According to *Vultum Dei quaerere*, each monastery is to discern the form of cloister it wishes to embrace.[111] Note that it is for the nuns themselves to choose one of the three forms of cloister and for the Holy See to approve the choice. It is not for the diocesan bishop or regular superior to impose a form of enclosure on a monastery. The nuns' choice should be based on the charism and tradition of the monastery, but also on reality, that is, on the real ability to observe the kind of cloister selected, especially if the choice is papal enclosure which requires specific architectural accommodations.

While some monasteries will remain under papal enclosure, with *Cor orans*, Pope Francis derogates from canon 667 §4 and abrogates *Verbi Sponsa* n. 17.2.[112] The major superiors of all monasteries of nuns, including those under papal enclosure, can now grant dispensations from cloister on their own, with no permission needed from a diocesan bishop or religious ordinary.[113] If it is an absence of more than fifteen days, the major superior needs the consent of her council.[114] For a longer absence, up to one year, she needs the consent of her council and she must hear, that is, consult, the diocesan bishop or religious ordinary, but she does not need the consent of the bishop or ordinary.[115] Also, in derogation from canon 686 §2, the major superior, with consent of her council, can grant exclaustration for up to one year after hearing the diocesan bishop or religious ordinary.[116] The federal president, having obtained the consent of the federal council and the opinion of the diocesan bishop or religious ordinary, can extend the exclaustration for another two years.[117]

---

109 *CO* 205.

110 *CO* 210.

111 *VDq* 10 §1.

112 *CO* 174, 176. According to c. 667 §4, the diocesan bishop has the faculty of permitting nuns to leave the enclosure for a truly necessary period of time. *Verbi sponsa* n. 17 §2 says: "For other just and grave reasons the Superior, with the consent of her Council or the conventual Chapter, and in accordance with the norms contained in the Constitutions, can authorize a departure for whatever time is needed, not however beyond one week. If the stay outside the monastery has to be further extended, up to three months, the Superior will seek the authorization_of the Diocesan Bishop, or the regular Superior if there is one. Should the absence exceed three months, other than in cases of health care, permission must be obtained from the Holy See."

113 *CO* 174.

114 *CO* 175.

115 *CO* 176.

116 *CO* 177. According to c. 686 §2, only the Holy See can grant an indult of exclaustration for nuns.

117 *CO* 178-179.

Chapter 4: Formation (*CO* 219-289)

The final chapter of the instruction addresses formation, both initial and ongoing. Formation in contemplative life, as in all forms of religious life, consists above all in identifying with Christ, which means formation lasts a lifetime.[118] It is a continual process of growth and conversion that involves the whole person and includes development of the human, Christian, and monastic dimensions of the candidates and nuns, radically living the Gospel, "so that one's life becomes a prophecy."[119]

One of the most controversial provisions of *Vultum Dei quaerere* is the new requirement regarding the duration of initial formation for nuns: a minimum of nine years and a maximum of twelve.[120] Nine years is longer than the minimum duration of initial formation prescribed for validity by the Code of Canon Law and twelve years exceeds the maximum permitted by the code.[121] Therefore, the length of formation for nuns is now longer than for all other religious, whether women or men. The required stages also differ. According to the code, life in the institute begins with the novitiate, which is followed by a period of temporary profession.[122] While canon 597 §2 calls for "suitable preparation" before admittance into an institute, the code does not require any particular form or duration of preparation. It is for each institute to prescribe how candidates are prepared for the novitiate. *Cor orans*, on the other hand, identifies four stages of initial formation and a minimum and maximum length for each. The first stage, the aspirancy, is a period of mutual discernment on the part of the inquirer and the community and a time of getting to know each other.[123] This stage involves "a series of contacts and times of community experience, even prolonged."[124] The minimum period of the aspirancy is twelve months and the maximum is two years.[125] The postulancy, which also must be a minimum of twelve months and a maximum of two years, is when the candidate begins to live in the monastery

---

118 *CO* 222.

119 *CO* 224.

120 *VDq* 15.

121 The 1983 Code of Canon Law requires, for validity, a minimum of twelve months in the novitiate (c. 648 §1), with some exceptions that could lessen that period to eleven months (c. 649), and a maximum of thirty months (cc. 648 §3, 653 §2). The minimum period in first profession is three years (c. 655), with the possibility of shortening that by up to three months (c. 657 §3), and the maximum is nine years (657 §2). Thus, a religious could make perpetual profession less than four years after becoming a novice and cannot remain in initial formation longer than eleven years and six months.

122 1983 *CIC*, c. 646.

123 *CO* 262, 264, 265, 266.

124 *CO* 262.

125 *CO* 268.

and is gradually introduced to the way of life.[126] The next stage, the novitiate, has a duration of two years.[127] Temporary profession is made initially for three years and then renewed annually so that at least five years and no more than nine years are completed before perpetual profession.[128]

Nuns in the United States and Europe have commented that the required duration of initial formation is excessive. There is, of course, the possibility of requesting a dispensation for individual candidates. Meanwhile, some monastic leaders have written to the Holy See asking for greater flexibility regarding the length of formation, especially the requirement of five years in temporary profession. The abbot primate of the Benedictine Confederation, in a letter to the CICLSAL prefect, pointed out the diversity of candidates as a reason for flexibility. He noted that women in Europe and the Americas usually enter at a more mature age and many of them have had positions of responsibility, whereas in Africa and Asia, women enter very young.[129] The abbots and priors of the Salzburg Abbots Conference sent a letter to Pope Francis, noting that the nine-year period of formation "is a great hardship for candidates who have often already reached the age of 30 in our countries, as the final decision is only made at an advanced age."[130]

Concluding Thoughts

Pope Francis' apostolic constitution *Vultum Dei quaerere* and its implementing instruction, *Cor orans*, require significant changes on the part of monasteries of nuns. The obligation to be federated, the broadened scope of the role of a federal president in relation to member monasteries, and the lengthened duration of initial formation have garnered the most attention. The final provision of *Vultum Dei quaerere* is that monasteries revise their constitutions once they have adapted to the new papal legislation.[131] Our sisters in contemplative religious life will be engaged in implementing the new papal legislation for some years ahead.

It should also be noted that, with the provisions of *Cor orans*, the Congregation for Institutes of Consecrated Life and Societies of Apostolic Life commits itself to greater engagement with monasteries of nuns, including by establishing *ad hoc* commissions when the real autonomy of life of monasteries becomes fragile

---

126 *CO* 275-276.

127 *CO* 279.

128 *CO* 287.

129 Right Rev. Gregory J. Polan, O.S.B., letter to His Eminence Cardinal João Braz de Aviz, October 16, 2018 (unpublished).

130 Salzburger Äbtekonferenz, letter to "Heiliger Vater," undated (unpublished). The letter notes that the abbots and priors of the conference unanimously approved the letter on April 26, 2019. It is signed by more than thirty abbots and priors.

131 *VDq* 14 §2.

or non-existent and by appointing religious assistants to federations. According to the "Final Dispositions" of *Cor orans*, CICLSAL will assign monasteries to existing structures of communion if they have not become federated within one year of publication of the instruction. That deadline has passed and there are still unfederated monasteries. Pope Francis' new legislation for nuns will be effective only if CICLSAL is able to do its part in the implementation.

A final thought: canonists who are called upon to assist monasteries of nuns as they implement *Cor orans* will want to be mindful of the purpose of the new norms, which is to help "contemplative women to attain the goal of their specific vocation," which is to seek the face of God.[132]

132 *VDq* 12; *CO* Introduction.

Seminar

Canonical Norms Regarding Place of Marriage: Both a Challenge and an Opportunity

The Reverend Sean P. Bransfield, JCL

I remember well the moment I was first asked to write an article and give a seminar presentation at the 2019 General Convention of the Canon Law Society of America. It was during the late winter/early spring of 2018, and Father Jim Conn called me on my cell phone as I was driving in the car. He was calling me to ask me if I would be willing to undertake this task. I was quite surprised when he did ask me, feeling myself unworthy to be the one to lead such a discussion. At a certain point during our conversation, I asked him why he thought I'd be a good person to give this seminar. He immediately responded by saying that, in his opinion, he thought that, working in the chancery for a number of years now, I had a good amount of practical knowledge in this area. He then went on to remind me of a story I once told him, about ten years ago, involving a request from a couple to allow their marriage to take place in a grounded hot air balloon (the request was denied). I do actually remember that request, it was one of the more unusual permissions that has been asked of me. Father Conn thought that helped qualify me to lead this presentation at a convention seminar. I guess, upon further thought, that his reasoning is good as any!

Like everyone else working in canon law these days, requests such as the grounded hot air balloon marriage venue are not altogether shocking. While that specific venue request may be new to some, we are all familiar with the changing landscape of marriage both within and outside the Catholic Church. Not only is the definition and meaning of marriage a much-discussed topic of conversation in our broader society today, but how marriage is celebrated continues to evolve, and we all have heard many stories about the various ways in which marriage ceremonies are taking place. As local churches, we are all trying to balance how to protect, promote and defend the Church's understanding of marriage. At the same time, local churches are continually asking questions and exploring ways to evangelize more effectively, especially to younger Catholics. More and more, local churches are being asked to allow marriages to take place in non-traditional venues, and as these requests are considered, finding the balance between protecting and safeguarding the Catholic understanding of marriage while effectively evangelizing to people, who are often in need of deeper catechesis,

comes into play. How do we remain faithful to the Church's understanding of marriage, and how can this fidelity on our part serve as an invitation to greater faith for those who wish to have their marriages take place with the blessing of the Church? In short, how can we better accompany as many people as possible on their faith journeys, especially as these journeys relate to the celebration of their marriages? No one article or seminar, of course, will be able to answer these questions, but hopefully this presentation can further advance the discussion and perhaps offer some insights and enlightenment on these important and relevant topics in our Church's life today.

Regarding the scope of this paper, my intent is first to review canons 1115 and 1118, as they most specifically address the current norms regarding place of marriage for marriages involving at least one Latin Catholic. It is to be noted that this paper will limit itself to marriages involving Latin Catholics. Secondly, some statistical information will be offered to show what some recent and longer-term trends have been as far as Catholics and their sacramental practices in the Church are concerned. Next, the results of an unscientific survey conducted by me regarding (arch)diocesan marriage policies, specifically as they relate to place of marriage questions, will be discussed so as to show in an unscientific way what is being done currently by local churches throughout the United States. Finally, some concluding observations and suggestions for possible future pastoral practice will be made based upon all that has been presented. These observations and suggestions will not be made in order to propose any definitive answers, but rather to further the discussion as local churches continually work at balancing the need to protect, promote and defend the Church's understanding of marriage while at the same time doing whatever is possible to accompany people in their faith and life journeys.

Canons 1115 and 1118 of the 1983 Code of Canon Law

> Canon 1115: Matrimonia celebrentur in paroecia ubi alterutra pars contrahentium habet domicilium vel quasi-domicilium vel menstruam commorationem, aut, si de vagis agitur, in paroecia ubi actu commorantur; cum licentia proprii Ordinarii aut parochi proprii, alibi celebrari possunt.[1]
>
> Marriages are to be celebrated in a parish where either of the contracting parties has a domicile, quasi-domicile, or month-long residence or, if it concerns transients, in the parish where they actually reside. With the permission of the proper ordinary or proper pastor, marriages can be

1 *Codex Iuris Canonici auctoritate Ioannis Pauli PP. II promulgatus* (Vatican City: Libreria Editrice Vaticana, 1983) c. 1115.

celebrated elsewhere.[2]

Canon 1118: § 1. Matrimonium inter catholicos vel inter partem catholicam et partem non catholicam baptizatam celebretur in ecclesia paroeciali; in alia ecclesia aut oratorio celebrari poterit de licentia Ordinarii loci vel parochi.

§ 2. Matrimonium in alio convenienti loco celebrari Ordinarius loci permittere potest.

§ 3. Matrimonium inter partem catholicam et partem non baptizatam in ecclesia vel in alio convenienti loco celebrari poterit.[3]

§ 1. A marriage between Catholics or between a Catholic party and a non-Catholic baptized party is to be celebrated in a parish church. It can be celebrated in another church or oratory with the permission of the local ordinary or pastor.

§ 2. The local ordinary can permit a marriage to be celebrated in another suitable place.

§ 3. A marriage between a Catholic party and a non-baptized party can be celebrated in a church or in another suitable place.

Let us begin by turning our attention to canons 1115 and 1118 of the 1983 Code of Canon Law, as they provide the foundation for our canonical study of the question regarding place of marriage. Beginning with canon 1115, it is important to begin by noting that this canon determines in principle the place, or more specifically the territory, where any particular marriage may be celebrated.[4] As canon 1115 states, for a marriage involving two Catholics, the normal place for marriage is where one of the contracting parties has a domicile, quasi-domicile or month-long residence, and if only one of the parties is Catholic, then it is to be where the Catholic has domicile, quasi-domicile or month-long residence.[5] Furthermore, marriages of those who have no domicile or quasi-domicile are normally celebrated where those persons actually reside.[6] As the canon states, the

2 *Code of Canon Law, Latin-English Edition: New English Translation* (Washington, DC: CLSA, 1998) c. 1115. All subsequent English translations of canons from the 1983 code will be taken from this source unless otherwise indicated.

3 C. 1118,

4 See Donal Kelly, "Marriage," in *The Canon Law: Letter and Spirit*, ed. Gerard Sheehy et al. (London: Wellington House, 1999) 627.

5 See John P. Beal, "The Form of the Celebration of Marriage," in *New Commentary on the Code of Canon Law*, ed. John P. Beal et al (New York/Mahwah, NJ: Paulist Press, 2000) [hereafter *New Commentary*] 1333.

6 Ibid.

permission of a contracting party's proper ordinary or pastor is required to licitly celebrate a marriage elsewhere.[7] Noting that the present 1983 Code of Canon Law has no longer retained the preference contained in the 1917 Code of Canon Law that the marriage be celebrated in the parish of the bride, one can see that in the present code, more freedom has been given to the spouses when choosing a place for marriage.[8]

Even this seemingly elementary norm gives rise to questions on a regular basis to priests, deacons and other pastoral ministers who prepare couples for the celebration of their marriages. Many times, couples will approach a parish and ask to have their marriage celebrated there, and it is quickly found out that neither the man nor the woman lives within the parish. Another common yet similar situation is encountered when one or both parties to the marriage grew up in the parish where they wish to be married, but now they don't live in the territorial confines of the parish, and thus are not, canonically speaking, parishioners. Furthermore, when one or both of the parties in this latter situation are asked, "What is your parish?" they immediately respond with something like, "This is my parish." Most priests, deacons and other pastoral ministers know this not to be accurate, and canonists certainly know this to be the case, but how does one respond?

According to the norm of canon 1115, permission for a couple to be married where neither person has a domicile, quasi-domicile or month-long residence needs to be granted by the proper ordinary or proper pastor of one of the contracting parties. In theory, this seems like an easy enough permission to have granted. However, many times it is the case that neither the man nor the woman are registered in the parish where one or both of them actually lives, and sometimes the reality is that neither party is practicing their faith regularly. What is one to do then? This again is one of those moments when pastors try to balance what the law mandates and what is needed, in that particular moment, to help accompany that particular couple in their journey of faith, in the hopes of leading one or both of them into a deeper participation in the life of the Church. I use the term *mandates* in the previous sentence while remembering that, at least in this instance, this norm in canon 1115 asking for the permission of one's proper ordinary or pastor to marry elsewhere is for liceity and not for validity.

Nevertheless, the requirements of this norm can serve as a pastoral aide to the one assisting a couple finding themselves in this situation who are preparing for the celebration of their marriage. Perhaps the Catholic(s) to this upcoming marriage are not attending Mass regularly (if at all) and are not registered at their canonically defined (in virtue of territory) parish. Perhaps it is also the case that a particular pastor is unwilling to provide this letter of permission to a person or

7 Ibid.

8 Ibid.

persons who have just registered in their parish but are unknown to the pastor or pastoral staff. As the pastoral minister preparing this couple for marriage, making the couple aware of this norm, even if not requiring its fulfillment in each and every case, can provide the opportunity of creating a teaching moment wherein the couple is introduced to the fact that their actual canonical parish is the one whose boundaries encompass where they actually live, and it is there, in that parish, where the Church is providing for a local community to grow in the practice of its faith, and it is through that parish that the local parishioners can be mutually supported in the ways of faith by their fellow parishioners who are also, in a very real and physical sense, their neighbors. While the norm of obtaining this letter of permission from one's proper ordinary or pastor may vary in its actual implementation, this norm can always serve as the foundation for introducing a teaching moment so that Catholics can come to better learn and understand that they are, by virtue of where they physically live, part of a "certain community of the Christian faithful stably constituted in a particular church."[9]

Having defined in canon 1115 where the proper territory is for a particular marriage to take place, canon 1118 specifies the actual location for where a marriage is to take place.[10] Canon 1118 §1 in fact is a further specification of canon 1115,[11] in that canon 1118 states that a marriage between Catholics or between a Catholic and a baptized non-Catholic party is normally to be celebrated in the parish church of one or both of the Catholic parties, but that with the permission of the local ordinary or pastor of one of the parties to the marriage, it can be celebrated in another church or oratory. What is "another church?" According to canon 1214, "By the term church is understood a sacred building designated for divine worship to which the faithful have the right of entry for the exercise, especially the public exercise, of divine worship."[12] Certainly, this is found in a parish church, but in addition to other churches that have rectors,[13] another example of a church could be a distinct church for worship that is different than a parish church. These, for example, are often found where parishes have merged, wherein two (or more) parishes have merged into one new parish but one or more of the former parish churches remain, and those churches not designated as the parish church of the newly formed parish are employed as churches for worship by the newly constituted parish. Oftentimes, norms regarding the use of these churches for worship are outlined by diocesan policies regarding place for marriage, and these policies should always be consulted when a pastor is

9 C. 515 §1: "Paroecia est certa communitas christifidelium in Ecclesia particulari stabiliter constituta, cuius cura pastoralis, sub auctoritate Episcopi dioecesani, committitur parocho, qua proprio eiusdem pastori."

10 See Kelly, 629.

11 Ibid.

12 C. 1214: "Ecclesiae nomine intellegitur aedes sacra divino cultui destinata, ad quam fidelibus ius est adeundi ad divinum cultum praesertim publice exercendum."

13 See Beal, 1337.

deciding whether or not to allow for another church to be used for the celebration of a marriage when that church is not a parish church but rather a non-parish church which is located within a parish's territorial boundaries.

What, specifically speaking, is an oratory? It is, after all, another word that gets used often in ways that are not canonically correct. According to canon 1223, an oratory is understood as "a place for divine worship designated by permission of the ordinary for the benefit of some community or group of the faithful who gather in it and to which other members of the faithful can also come with the consent of the competent superior."[14] As noted by John Huels, an oratory "is different from a church principally in virtue of who has a right to make use of it. All the faithful have the right to go to a church, but only that community or group of people for whom an oratory was established has the right to make use of it."[15] As also noted by Huels, an oratory can be established for specified groups of the faithful such as religious communities, seminary communities, other school communities, nursing home communities, etc.[16] Specifically regarding marriage, canon 1109 §2 of the 1917 code specifically prohibited the celebration of marriages in the oratories of seminaries and religious houses, but this prohibition was lifted with the issuance of the 1983 code.[17] Nevertheless, "the consent of the rector of the church or the superior responsible for the oratory is required in addition to the permission of the local ordinary or pastor."[18]

Canon 1118 §2 also allows for the celebration of a marriage between two Catholics or between a Catholic and a baptized non-Catholic to occur in another suitable place, and one immediately notes that this permission can only be given by the local ordinary and not by the pastor whose territory includes some potential "other suitable place."[19] Likewise, canon 1118 §3 allows for a non-sacramental marriage between a Catholic and an unbaptized person to occur "in a church or in another suitable place" (and here, it is noted that the norm contained in canon 1118 §3 does not require the permission of the local ordinary). So then, of course, the next question immediately comes to mind: what is "another suitable place?" This question admits no easy answer! Nevertheless, we canonists, along with others in the Church, are continually trying to determine the answer to that question, and that answer will continue to evolve for all of us.

---

14 C. 1223: "Oratorii nomine intellegitur locus divino cultui, in commodum alicuius communitatis vel coetus fidelium eo convenientium de licentia Ordinarii destinatus, ad quem etiam alii fideles de consensu Superioris competentis accedere possunt."

15 John M. Huels, "Oratories and Private Chapels," in *New Commentary*, 1433.

16 Ibid.

17 See Beal, 1337.

18 Ibid.

19 Ibid., 1338.

As noted by John Beal, a suitable place "might include the non-Catholic church or place of worship of one of the parties to a mixed marriage, a non-denominational chapel attached to a college, university, or other institution, or even a private home."[20] Furthermore, Beal notes that, "When judging the suitability of a place for the celebration of a marriage, care should be taken to ensure that the nature of the place is consistent with a religious celebration."[21] He further states that, "A suitable place for the celebration should enhance rather than distract from the religious dimension of the marriage."[22] Whether a proposed marriage employing canonical form is being planned between two Catholics, between a Catholic and a baptized non-Catholic or between a Catholic and an unbaptized person, Beal's understanding of what constitutes a suitable place is well-reasoned and balanced, as far as a general description of the term suitable place is concerned.

But more specifically, what is understood by the term suitable place? As a canonist who works daily with the granting of dispensations and permissions for marriage, as well as being someone who routinely deals with the granting of *visums* and *nihil obstats*, I certainly have come to wonder more and more, over the years, what is considered a suitable place. Furthermore, as Beal notes, one "should consult local guidelines on suitable places for marriage and use common sense."[23] But for those of us who advise our diocesan bishops and local ordinaries concerning marriage policies, we all know that there are no magic answers concerning what are suitable places for marriage. If one were to ask ten canonists to describe what is a suitable place, one could receive ten different answers, at least as far as specifics are concerned. The same would be true if you asked the same of ten bishops, ten priests, ten members of a religious congregation or ten members of any given parish council or parish liturgical committee.

Over the course of the last year to two years, when I have been spending time with various priest friends, I have asked them, in casual and informal ways, their thoughts on the possibility of outdoor weddings being allowed. Almost everyone I asked had answers that were nuanced, and all of the answers were sound and well thought out. What constitutes another suitable place? In the end, what experience is teaching us is that these answers are becoming more and more a matter of interpretation.

Sacramental Trends in the U.S. Catholic Church

While canonists and other church officials continue to grapple with the question of what constitutes sound marriage policies regarding place of marriage,

---

20 Beal, 1338.

21 Ibid.

22 Ibid.

23 Ibid.

and while many are wondering what is being done in other local churches, it seems important to try and understand better what is happening in terms of the celebration of the sacraments in general in the Church today. To what extent are Catholics still getting married today in the Church? Is the observance of canonical form still considered as important today by the average Catholic as it was in the past? If these numbers are changing, what can local churches do to help address these changing practices? Is it best to double down on catechizing the faithful as to why more traditional marriage policies are still the best way of proceeding, or is it better to accommodate and modify more traditional policies so as to perhaps more effectively meet the people where they are? There are no simple answers to these questions, and the varied answers are almost always thought out and well-reasoned. Oftentimes, it seems that understanding the best way to catechize can become a matter of interpretation. Canonists will all agree on the fact that "a fruitful liturgical celebration of marriage . . . is to show that the spouses signify and share in the mystery of the unity and fruitful love between Christ and the Church."[24] But what constitutes a fruitful liturgical celebration, and in what types of physical environments can this take place? These are questions we all are trying to continually answer as best as we possibly can.

As experience has taught us and as our own local churches have discovered, the number of people actively participating in the Church's sacramental life over the years has, by and large, continued to decrease. While it is true that the number of clergy available to minister to the faithful has continued to decline (as seen from the average number of active diocesan priests per parish having dropped from 1.8 in 1970 to 1.0 as of 2018),[25] the percentage of Catholics attending weekly Mass has also continued to drop. While survey-based estimates state that 54.9% of Catholics attended weekly Mass as of 1970, by 1990 that percentage had dropped to 32.5%. Even more noticeable, by 2015 the percentage of weekly Mass-goers was 23.4%, and by 2018, that number had dropped to a mere 21.1%.[26] Similarly, the number of infant baptisms in the Church has declined overall as well, with 1.089 million infant baptisms having occurred in 1970 but only 615,119 having occurred in 2018. However, even more noticeable is that while that same number dropped from 1.089 million in 1970 to 996,199 in 2000, a drop of slightly less than 100,000, the number had dropped from 996,199 in 2000 to 615,119 as of 2018, a drop of almost 400,000.[27]

---

24 C. 1063, 3°: "fructuosa liturgica matrimonii celebratione, qua eluceat coniuges mysterium unitatis et fecundi amoris inter Christum et Ecclesiam significare atque participare."

25 See "U.S. Data Over Time," Frequently Requested Church Statistics, Center for Applied Research in the Apostolate (CARA), https://cara.georgetown.edu/frequently-requested-church-statistics/ (accessed on 19 Jan. 2020).

26 Ibid.

27 Ibid.

More specifically, marriages and annulments have declined in the life of the Church during that same time period. Regarding the celebration of marriages, whereas in 1970 there were 426,309 marriages celebrated in the Church, by 1995 this number had dropped to 294,144, and in 2018 only 143,082 marriages had been celebrated.[28] Likewise, while 60,691 annulment cases were initiated in 1985, that number had dropped to 33,727 in 2005, and by 2018 that number was 21,661.[29] Furthermore, the percentage of U.S. Catholics marrying in the Church has continued to decline over time. In 1970, approximately 75% of all Catholics marrying in that year were married in the Church. This percentage fell below 50% in 1982, but as recently as 1996, this percentage was still as high as 50%. Beginning in 1996, however, this percentage began to experience a steady decline, and by 2016 only 29% of Catholics were marrying in the Church.[30]

The drop in the number of Catholic marriages in the Church over time taking place in the United States is startling, as seen in the fact that from 1969 through 2013, there was a 64% decline in these marriages.[31] This decline reflects a larger societal trend that shows fewer people (Catholic or non-Catholic) marrying. While in 1960, 72% of U.S. adults were married, as of 2011, only 51% of this same group were married.[32] Likewise, the median age for first marriages for U.S. adults has risen over the years. Whereas in the 1960s the median age was in the early 20s for both men and women, as of 2011, the median age for first marriages in the U.S. was 29 for men and 27 for women.[33]

While these national statistics are sobering, they are of course reflective of the situations being experienced in our local churches. For example, the statistics being seen in the Archdiocese of Philadelphia, my own local church, are no less concerning. In the Archdiocese of Philadelphia, there exists what is commonly referred to as an October Count, whereby the number of people attending Sunday Masses throughout the Archdiocese is counted for all the weekends of October. In 1990, the first year this October Mass census was taken, 416,137 people attended Mass throughout the Archdiocese in October. By 2018, that number

---

28 Ibid.

29 Ibid.

30 See "A Dip in the Adult Catholic Population," 1964 (blog), Center for Applied Research in the Apostolate (CARA), ed. Mark Gray, March 12, 2018, http://nineteensixty-four.blogspot.com/2018/03/a-dip-in-adult-catholic-population.html (accessed on 19 Jan. 2020).

31 See Thomas Baker, "The Decline of Catholic Marriages," *Commonweal*, July 15, 2015, https://www.commonwealmagazine.org/decline-catholic-marriages (accessed on 19 Jan. 2020).

32 Ibid.

33 Ibid.

had dropped to 199,101, which represents a 52% decline.[34] In addition, other archdiocesan statistical numbers, more long-range in perspective, show a steep decline in Catholic infant baptisms and marriages. In 1961, there were 37,855 infant baptisms and there were 9,017 Catholic marriages in the Archdiocese of Philadelphia. In 2018, there were 7,937 infant baptisms and 2,814 Catholic marriages celebrated in the same Archdiocese, representing a 79% decline and a 69% decline, respectively.[35]

Why have these numbers continued to decline? There are no magic answers of course, but it is without doubt that our society in general has become much more secular over the years, and the practice of organized religion continues to be in decline. Nevertheless, what are some of the possible causes for the decline in Catholic marriages? A few factors can be considered. First, there is a generally lower level of institutional allegiance among younger Catholics, as measured by Mass attendance and other traditional means of staying connected with the Church.[36] No doubt, the sexual abuse scandals that have afflicted the Church for the better part of twenty years have hurt the Church's institutional credibility. Furthermore, widespread cohabitation before marriage[37] is an indication that many people, and notably younger Catholics, are not accepting (and oftentimes are not even aware) of the Church's teaching that sexual relations are properly reserved to those who are married. Furthermore in this regard, to the extent that Catholic couples are aware of the Church's disapproval of premarital cohabitation, this may discourage couples from approaching the Church to have their weddings take place under the Church's auspices.[38]

Another factor that may be a disincentive to marrying in the Church could be pre-Cana programs, conferences, etc. As valuable and as important as the Church understands these evangelizing tools to be, especially in such an unchurched society, to what extent do these program requirements make Catholics less willing and therefore more unlikely to approach the Church for marriage?[39] Questions like these should not make us willing to abandon what we believe to be so important to the work of evangelization, but these considerations cannot be ignored either. Another factor that can be negatively impacting the number of

34 See Matthew Gambino, "Half of Catholics Attending Mass 28 Years Ago No Longer Do, Figures Show," *CatholicPhilly.com*, September 5, 2019, http://www.catholicphilly.com/2019/09/our-changing-church/half-of-catholics-attending-mass-28-years-ago-no-longer-do-figures-show-2/ (accessed on 19 Jan. 2020).

35 See Matthew Gambino, "Decline in Baptisms, Marriage Seen as Harbinger, Call to Community," *CatholicPhilly.com*, September 24, 2019, http://www.catholicphilly.com/2019/09/our-changing-church/decline-in-baptisms-marriages-seen-as-harbinger-call-to-community-2/ (accessed on 19 Jan. 2020).

36 See Baker, "The Decline of Catholic Marriages."

37 Ibid.

38 Ibid.

39 Ibid.

weddings in the Church is a general decline in the family and parental pressure being exerted on younger Catholics to marry in the Church.[40] While in certain ways this is a good thing (for example, being married in the Church simply because of parental/familial pressure and not for reasons rooted in the practice of one's faith), this decline in familial pressure can also be understood as another consequence of people practicing their faith less, which then naturally leads to less importance being placed on handing on the faith to others.

Finally, this leads to one final consideration as to why fewer Catholic marriages are taking place today (though the reasons cited above are certainly not an exhaustive list): a desire on the part of couples to have marriages take place in non-traditional settings.[41] Social media and the internet have educated people on all the different ways that weddings can take place. The venues and circumstances that present themselves as options for people to marry are seemingly endless. How is the Church to respond when people with good intentions, if not fully informed of the Church's reasons for preferring marriage to take place in the Church, approach the Church to have these non-traditional marriages take place and have them sanctioned by the Church? There are, of course, no easy answers to these questions, and yet the fact remains that we have to continually strive to evangelize more fruitfully to the Faithful that we are called to serve.

The Present State of the Question

Having now worked for the past three and a half years in chancery work, and spending part of almost every day at the office working on the processing of various marriage permissions and dispensations, I have, like so many other canonists, fielded phone calls from bishops, priests, deacons and future spouses regarding what is allowed and what is not allowed. When a permission is sought that is generally not granted, it can sometimes be very difficult to explain the *why* of the decision to say no, especially when the person asking is not a cleric or someone well-schooled in the pastoral and theological rationale that informs certain decisions. People oftentimes present their questions in good faith, and they don't understand why their requests are being denied. It is not that the ones making these decisions and then trying to explain the reasons why are incapable of explaining the rationale backing these decisions, it is oftentimes rather a question of "How do I explain this to someone in 30 to 60 seconds, oftentimes when the person is upset and emotional about the negative decision?" We do not have the luxury of having an unlimited amount of time to help lay the foundation, in general, of how the Church is looking to protect, preserve and defend the sanctity of marriage. Rather, we have one to two minutes to explain to someone on the phone (people we've usually never met) why, for example, their marriage can't take place in a catering hall with their uncle who is a permanent

---

40 See Baker, "The Decline of Catholic Marriages."

41 Ibid.

deacon presiding. These are difficult and oftentimes no-win situations, especially when one is concerned about keeping well-intentioned (if not especially well-catechized) people like this in the Church.

Having now attended over the last ten to twelve years a number of national, regional and local canon law workshops, conventions and seminars, I am well aware that these predicaments are not unique to me and to my Archdiocese. We all face the same dilemmas, and we are all wondering how best to respond. We, the Church's canonists and ministers, want to do all we can to promote, protect and defend the sanctity of marriage as the Church understands it, but how is this best done?

Having attended these same workshops, conventions and seminars, I also realized that we are all wondering what other local churches are doing to address these issues. Place of marriage policies are almost always a discussion topic at these gatherings, especially the more regional and local ones. The more it is talked about and learned what is being done on the local and regional levels, the more it has been sensed that, overall, we do not know well enough what is being done more generally across our U.S. dioceses in terms of place of marriage policies. Having been asked to give this presentation, the thought came to mind that perhaps the most practical contribution that could be made would be to help us understand a little better what is being done, at the present time, in our various local churches.

To that end, I created an online survey in the spring of 2019 regarding place of marriage policies currently being employed in (arch)dioceses across the United States, in the hopes that many responses would be made, so that we could learn, at least in the present moment, what is going on in our local churches.

While this unscientific survey was limited to Latin (arch)dioceses in the United States, 76 (arch)dioceses responded to the questionnaire, which gives an overall good sampling of place of marriage policies and practices currently being employed. The questions were grouped into three general categories. The first set of questions concerned marriages taking place between two Catholics. The second set of questions regarded marriages taking place between a Catholic and a baptized non-Catholic, and the third set of questions concerned marriages taking place between a Catholic and an unbaptized person. Within the latter two categories, each had questions concerning policies regarding marriages taking place according to canonical form as well as marriages taking place when a dispensation from canonical form is being sought. Responders to the questions were also given the opportunity to respond with additional or clarifying comments to each of the questions if they chose to do so. Finally, a couple of summary types of questions were asked as a way of rounding out the survey.

Marriages Taking Place between Two Catholics

This category was limited to three questions, as questions were only asked regarding the use of canonical form. The first question asked whether marriages involving two Catholics are allowed to take place in non-Catholic churches or houses of worship. Seventy-six answers were provided. Fifty-seven respondents (respondents being, of course, archdioceses or dioceses that responded to the survey) responded No, but 18 responded Yes. Clarifications/further comments were able to be offered with each question if any responder wished to do so. Among the 23 clarifications offered for this question, a number of responders noted that when this permission is given, it is done so when weddings take place at college or university non-Catholic chapels, oftentimes when one or both parties to a marriage is an alumnus of that institution. Some of the other reasons cited for allowing this permission (beginning with reasons most cited to reasons less cited, and this will be the order in which clarifying reasons are listed for all of the subsequent questions as well) included the following: the existence of particularly extenuating circumstances; when a good pastoral reason exists for allowing the permission; when the size of a parish church where the wedding would otherwise have been held is deemed too small; if a parish church is undergoing construction or renovation; if the wedding is taking place at a non-denominational chapel on a military base. One clarification of note for this question stated that one diocese's former bishop allowed this permission, but the current bishop does not.

The next question in this category asked whether dioceses allow marriages between two Catholics to take place in neutral, indoor settings. Seventy-six answers were provided. Sixty-three respondents answered No, while 13 respondents answered Yes. Twelve clarifications were offered. The most common clarification stated that when this permission is granted, it is usually because of particularly extenuating or pastorally based reasons (for example, the health of a bride or groom's parent making it difficult to travel to different locations during the wedding day). One respondent clarified that while their diocese's current answer to this question is No, a possible policy change is being discussed. One clarification also noted that when this permission is granted for extenuating circumstances, the wedding ceremony must take place in a permanent structure, and it cannot be the same place as the wedding reception.

The final question in this category asked whether marriages involving two Catholics are allowed to take place in neutral, outdoor settings. Seventy-six answers were provided. Sixty-four respondents answered No, while 11 respondents responded Yes. Twelve clarifications were offered. The most common clarification essentially stated that when specific permissions of this type are granted, it is because there exist compelling pastoral reasons to do so. Other clarifications noted (with most of these reasons only being offered by one or two respondents) the following reasons why this permission has been

granted in the past: this exception was made just one time; these permissions are only granted where diocesan shrines with outdoor altars exist; if the wedding is taking place on a military base and if the specific location on the base is a venue where other Catholic liturgical services are ordinarily offered. Another clarification noted that if the permission is granted, the wedding must take place on a permanent structure (such as a gazebo, a pergola or a porch, etc.), and the venue of the ceremony cannot be at the same place as the wedding reception. One responder noted that while their diocese's current answer to this question is no, possible policy changes are currently being discussed. Another response noted that when this permission is granted, it is given with the stipulation that the ceremony cannot take place within Mass (regardless of whether the permission is granted for a neutral location that is either indoors or outdoors).

Marriages Taking Place between a Catholic and a Baptized Non-Catholic

With this category, the questions were divided into two sub-categories (each sub-category inquiring about three different situations/scenarios). The first subcategory involved marriages between a Catholic and a baptized non-Catholic that take place with the use of canonical form, and the second subcategory involved marriages between a Catholic and a baptized non-Catholic where a dispensation from canonical form is being sought.

Concerning marriages involving the use of canonical form, the first of the three questions asked whether permissions for these types of marriages are allowed to take place in non-Catholic churches/houses of worship. Seventy-six answers were provided. Fifty responders answered Yes, while 24 responders answered No. Twenty-seven clarifications were offered. Among the clarifications offered, it was noted that when this permission is granted, it is generally for the following reasons: very limited permissions in this regard have been made; when it is allowed, it is allowed when the specific church is the church of the baptized non-Catholic; only for particularly compelling reasons; only when the church venue being asked is an actively used Protestant church; if the church or chapel is an alma mater chapel; if a preferred Catholic church is deemed too small for the anticipated number of attendees; only if a preferred Catholic church is being remodeled or is under renovation. It was further noted in some of the clarifications that when this permission is granted, it is only done after the non-Catholic pastor/minister of the church has been consulted and has given his/her approval.

The second question in this sub-category asked whether marriages between a Catholic and a baptized non-Catholic, employing canonical form, are allowed to take place in neutral, indoor settings. Seventy-six answers were provided. Twenty-six responders answered Yes, while 49 responded No. Twenty-one clarifications were offered. By far the most common clarification cited was that when a permission in this type of situation is granted, it is only allowed

because of the existence of particularly compelling reasons. One response noted that while that diocese's current policy is to answer no to this request, possible policy changes are being discussed. One response noted that with these types of requests, the granting or denying of the permission will depend on the specific venue being proposed for the place of marriage.

The final question in this sub-category asked whether marriages between a Catholic and a baptized non-Catholic, employing canonical form, are allowed to take place in neutral, outdoor settings. Seventy-six answers were provided. Sixteen responders answered Yes, while 59 responded No. Twelve clarifications were offered. The most commonly noted clarification stated that when a permission in this instance is granted, it is only done for particularly compelling and pastoral reasons. One responder noted that this permission is only granted if the preferred worship space is deemed too small for the anticipated number of guests. Finally, one responder noted that while the answer to this question is currently no, possible policy changes are being discussed.

The second sub-category in this larger category of Catholics marrying baptized non-Catholics involved requests for dispensation from canonical form. Again, three questions were asked in this sub-category of questions. The first question asked the following: when a Catholic is marrying a baptized non-Catholic and a dispensation from canonical form is being sought, are these dispensations granted when the venue being proposed is a non-Catholic church or house of worship? Seventy-six answers were provided. Seventy-four responded Yes, and two responded No. Eight clarifications were offered. A few clarifications essentially noted that when a dispensation in this case is granted, it is only done so for compelling pastoral reasons. One clarification noted that the dispensation is only granted when the church venue being sought is the specific church of the non-Catholic. One respondent noted that if the non-Catholic church is outside the diocese, the dispensation is only granted after first consulting the diocese whose territory includes the specific non-Catholic church where the wedding celebration is being sought (as per the norm of canon 1127 §2).[42] Finally, one clarification noted that when a dispensation in this type of instance is granted, it is done with the proviso that the couple must first complete a diocesan marriage preparation program before the dispensation is granted.

The second question is this sub-category asked the following: for marriages involving a Catholic and a baptized non-Catholic, will a dispensation from canonical form be granted when a couple wishes to marry in a neutral, indoor setting? Seventy-six answers were provided. Forty-one responded Yes, while 32

42 See C. 1127 §2: "Si graves difficultates formae canonicae servandae obstent, Ordinario loci partis catholicae ius est ab eadem in singulis casibus dispensandi, consulto tamen Ordinario loci in quo matrimonium celebrator; et salva ad validitatem aliqua publica forma celebrationis; Episcoporum conferentiae est normas statuere, quibus praedicta dispensation concordi ratione concedatur."

responded No. Twelve clarifications were offered. The most common clarification noted that when dispensations in this specific instance are granted, it is only because there exists a particularly compelling pastoral reason. A small number of clarifications noted that when this dispensation is granted, it is only done after the specific wedding venue has been deemed public as well as *suitable* (there's that word again!).

The third and final question in this sub-category asked the following: for marriages involving a Catholic and a baptized non-Catholic, will a dispensation from canonical form be granted when a couple wishes to marry in a neutral, outdoor setting? Seventy-six answers were provided. Twenty-eight responded Yes, while 47 responded No. Seven clarifications were offered. A few clarifications noted that when a dispensation in this instance is granted, it is only done so because a particularly compelling pastoral reason exists. Some clarifications noted that when a dispensation is granted under these circumstances, it is only done when the location is asked by way of a special and specific request and the location is subsequently deemed both public and suitable. Finally, one clarification noted that when a dispensation is granted for this type of situation, it is only granted for a compelling reason and with the proviso that the place where the vows are exchanged is separate and distinct from the place where the reception will take place.

Marriages Taking Place between a Catholic and an Unbaptized Person

As in the previous section, the questions regarding marriages between a Catholic and an unbaptized person were divided into two subcategories, with each subcategory containing three questions. The first subcategory involved marriages taking place according to canonical form, and the second category involved marriages where a dispensation from canonical form is being sought.

The first question in the first subcategory asked whether marriages between a Catholic and an unbaptized person, when using canonical form, are permitted to take place in non-Catholic churches/houses of worship. Seventy-six answers were provided. Forty-four responded Yes, 28 responded No, and 18 clarifications were offered. Regarding the clarifications, the most common was that when these permissions are granted, it is only because of the existence of compelling pastoral reasons. Other clarifications were the following: the permission is only granted if the unbaptized person is active in the practice of their faith; only if the church/house of worship is at other times used for the celebration of Mass (for example, at a college chapel); and only when the unbaptized person is a member of a recognized world religion (meaning the non-baptized person is not an atheist).

The second question in this subcategory asked whether marriages involving the use of canonical form between a Catholic and an unbaptized person are permitted to take place in neutral, indoor settings. Seventy-six answers were

provided. Forty-three responded Yes, 30 responded No, and 20 clarifications were offered. The clarification most cited was that when this permission is granted, it is only given due to the existence of compelling pastoral reasons. A few clarifications noted that the permission is only granted if the proposed venue is deemed suitable. The following once mentioned clarifications were also noted: the permission is granted only if the unbaptized person is active in the practice of their faith; the permission is only granted if the venue is a non-denominational chapel and not some other neutral setting; a permission in this instance is only granted if the marriage is between a Catholic and an unbaptized person; finally, one last clarification noted that this permission is only granted when the unbaptized person is a member of a recognized world religion (again, meaning the non-baptized person is not an atheist) and there is a specific, compelling reason to grant the permission.

The third and final question in this subcategory asked whether marriages involving the use of canonical form between a Catholic and an unbaptized person are permitted when the proposed wedding venue is a neutral, outdoor setting. Seventy-six answers were provided. Twenty-four responded Yes, 51 responded No, and 11 clarifications were offered. The most common clarification offered was that when this permission is granted, it is only done because of the existence of a compelling pastoral reason. A couple of clarifications noted that this permission is only granted if the venue is deemed suitable or appropriate. One clarification noted that the responding diocese's current answer to this permission is no but that potential policy changes are being discussed.

The second subcategory in this larger category of marriages involving Catholics and unbaptized persons involved marriages where a dispensation from canonical form was being sought. The first question in this subcategory asked whether marriages between a Catholic and an unbaptized person would be dispensed from canonical form if the venue for the marriage is a non-Catholic church/house of worship. Seventy-six answers were provided. Sixty-seven responded Yes, while 9 responded No. Twelve clarifications were offered. As with so many other questions in the survey, the most common clarification noted that when this dispensation is granted, it is due to the existence of some compelling pastoral reason. A few other once-mentioned clarifications included the following: a dispensation in this instance is only granted when the church/house of worship is deemed suitable; the dispensation is only granted if the church/house of worship has special significance for the unbaptized party; and the dispensation is not granted if the church/house of worship is not the same faith tradition of the unbaptized person. Finally, one clarification noted that while the diocese's former bishop allowed this dispensation in these instances, the new bishop may not continue with that policy of his predecessor.

The second question in this subcategory asked whether dispensation from canonical form requests are granted when a Catholic and an unbaptized person

wish to marry in a neutral, indoor setting. Seventy-six answers were provided. Sixty-one responded Yes, while 14 responded No. Sixteen clarifications were provided. The most common clarification noted that when this dispensation is granted, it is because of the existence of a compelling pastoral reason to do so. A couple of clarifications noted that this dispensation is only granted if the proposed wedding venue is deemed suitable. A few once-mentioned clarifications noted the following: the dispensation is only granted if the proposed officiant is a religious leader; the dispensation is only granted if the setting is a non-denominational chapel; the dispensation is only granted if the proposed venue has some special significance for the non-Catholic party.

The third and final question in this subcategory asked whether dispensation from canonical form requests are granted when a Catholic and an unbaptized person wish to marry in a neutral, outdoor setting. Seventy-six answers were provided. Thirty-seven responded Yes, 38 responded No, and 9 clarifications were provided. The most common clarification noted was again the fact that this dispensation request is granted when a compelling pastoral reason exists for doing so, and some clarifications noted that this dispensation request is granted only if the proposed place or venue of the marriage is deemed suitable.

Final Summarizing Questions Asked at the Conclusion of the Survey

Following these questions, there were two final, summarizing types of questions. The answers provided to these questions were extremely enlightening and, I believe, help serve as a springboard for further discussion. The first of these two final questions asked if a diocese's place of marriage policy had been altered in the last ten years, and if so, how. About two-thirds of the respondents answered No to this question, though many noted that exceptions to their policies are sometimes/oftentimes granted on a case-by-case basis due to the existence of compelling pastoral reasons. There were, in addition, a number of interesting responses, a few of which will now be noted. One diocese noted that their bishop is considering changing the diocesan policy so as to allow two Catholics to marry in a neutral indoor or outdoor setting, but no decision has yet been made. One respondent noted that there have been some rumblings about that diocese's episcopal province agreeing to allow outdoor weddings but no concrete discussions have yet taken place. One respondent noted that the primary reason the diocese has relaxed its place of marriage policies is because there is a pastoral concern that if these requests are denied, the disaffected couples will, in response, leave the church. One diocese noted that consideration is being given to making a possible policy change a topic of discussion at a future presbyteral council meeting. One diocese noted that while its official policy has not changed in the past few years, its praxis has. Because a number of surrounding dioceses have relaxed their policies, requests that were previously denied are now being considered (and oftentimes granted) on a case-by-case basis by the bishop.

There were further noteworthy responses to this same question. One diocese noted that it is considering modifying its policy in the near future. Another diocese noted that its policy was changed so that marriages between a Catholic and an unbaptized person taking place according to canonical form must now take place only in a church, an oratory or in some other authorized chapel. One diocese noted that even though possible changes to its policies have been discussed for over a year, no decisions have yet been made. One diocese noted that in the past year its policy has been relaxed concerning dispensations from canonical form. In a similar response, another diocese stated that policies regarding dispensations from canonical form have been modified to allow for much greater latitude in the granting of these. One diocese noted that its policy was changed in regard to marriages involving Catholics and baptized non-Catholics in that they now must marry in a Christian church, but preferably in a Catholic church. One diocese noted that its territory is in a destination wedding locale, and so its policy has been very careful to make it clear what it will allow or not allow, so as to protect the sanctity of marriage. One diocese noted that its previous bishop was much more permissive in his place of marriage policies, seeing a greater allowance for weddings in non-traditional venues as being a tool for greater evangelization, but the new/current bishop does not share that same philosophy and so the diocesan policies have been made more strict. One diocese noted that since implementing a more expansive/permissive policy for marriages involving its own subjects, one particularly challenging aspect of implementation has been obtaining the *nihil obstat* of another diocese when the wedding is to take place in that other diocese. Another diocese noted that while its previous policy did not allow for outdoor weddings, the new policy provides a pathway for these to take place. Finally, one respondent noted that the diocesan policy has added a list of prohibited places for marriage. This list of prohibited places includes secular or commercial wedding chapels as well as places well known for their policies that are inconsistent with Church teaching regarding marriage.

The final question of the survey simply asked respondents if they wished to offer any further comments. More interesting answers were provided. One respondent simply answered that the diocese follows what the bishop does, which ultimately is true for every diocese! One respondent answered that the diocese prohibits weddings from taking place in a neutral setting so as to give witness to the sacred nature of marriage and to the communal dimension of the sacramental commitment. Others expressed the opinion that weddings need to take place in a sacred space and that churches are specifically sacred spaces, while neutral settings are not, whether they be indoor or outdoor. The observation was also made by some that dioceses which allow for the use of canonical form in venues other than church buildings make it difficult for dioceses which do not allow such permissions. As has been noted at various times in this presentation, a number of dioceses are considering the possibility of making changes to their current policies, even if these changes have not yet been made. Another responder, making an observation that was shared by others, astutely noted that dioceses

that are more destination wedding locales, if they allow more expansive place of marriage policies, will make the workload more burdensome for pastors whose territories include popular wedding venues. Not only would the processing of wedding paperwork be more burdensome to these pastors, but these pastors would presumably also have to officiate at so many more weddings.

There were further interesting observations/responses. One responder noted that while the diocese generally has a "no neutral place, indoors or outdoors" policy, when exceptions to the policy are made, it is usually because antipathy exists as far as entering into sacred spaces foreign to one's own faith tradition are concerned. One responder spoke at length about the bishop's decision to allowing newer, more permissive policies in the past few years. Recognizing that making this decision creates positive and negative consequences, the responder nevertheless focused on the positive reasons that motivated the bishop's decision to change his diocese's policy. It was first noted that allowing Catholics to marry in non-traditional venues allows their marriages to be valid from the very beginning of their marital unions. Secondly, it allows for more couples to be evangelized through diocesan pre-Cana programs. Thirdly, these more permissive policies allow for a Catholic cleric (priest or deacon) to be personally involved in the wedding liturgy, as opposed to rent-a-clerics being hired to officiate. Having clergy in good standing involved in the liturgy helps ensure that the Catholic Rite of Marriage is celebrated with Scripture and a homily, along with Catholic prayers. When all of these elements are present, it helps to reinforce to all attending the wedding the realities of the presence of God, the sacramentality of marriage and the goods of marriage. All of this makes good catechesis possible, with the liturgy itself being a powerful teaching tool.

One responder noted that his bishop has clearly stated that the diocese's wedding policy will not change if that change will go contrary to the episcopal province's shared policy. Another responder noted that the United States bishops' general insistence on marriage taking place in a sacred space deprives the U.S. Church of the opportunity to catechize for the sacrament. Expanding on this idea, the responder noted that for many couples, the wedding venue is one of their most important considerations in planning their wedding. When the Church says No to their proposed venue, the Church loses the opportunity to catechize, and, most likely, that couple's (and their future family's) future relationship with the Church will be adversely affected.

Finally, as a way of summarizing these comments in a way that looks ahead to what other dioceses may or will likely do, if they have not done so already, one responder noted that the current diocesan policy is under review, and the diocese is open to more substantial changes in the future, especially considering the fact that other (arch)dioceses are also open to making policy changes and/or have begun making changes to their policies. Another responder, one from a wedding destination locale, stated that because of its location, the diocese deals

with a large number of wedding requests from couples who live outside of their dioceses. This responder looks forward in the future to considering the wedding locale as a possible evangelization tool.

Where Do We Go from Here?

As the latter months of 2017 became the early months of 2018, I found myself in a predicament. A family from my first priestly assignment in the Archdiocese of Philadelphia with whom I have become very close friends told me that their son was getting married in the summer of 2018. Having also become friends with the groom-to-be and his fiancée, I was becoming increasingly worried that I would not be able to attend their wedding because they were planning on marrying in a non-Catholic wedding. The groom-to-be, being Catholic, and his bride, being Jewish, were planning on marrying in an outdoor ceremony. The more I talked with the couple, I learned that while they were firm in their resolve to marry outdoors, they would like to have their marriage be considered valid by the Church, if possible. Fortunately, they were planning to marry in the bride's hometown, which is in a diocese that grants dispensations from canonical form for outdoor weddings if one of the parties is an unbaptized person. Not only was I able to help facilitate the wedding paperwork, but the couple also attended a pre-Cana program and were able to enter into a valid and licit marital union. I attended the wedding, and to be honest, it was a beautiful weekend in so many ways. Not only was I able to spend the weekend with great friends and share in a moment of unique importance in their lives, but by my being present and offering some Catholic prayers at the ceremony, I was able to witness to the Church's accompaniment of this newly married couple as they took a momentous step in their lives. I was personally grateful that the marriage was taking place in a diocese that allowed a marriage of this type to take place.

We are all well aware of what the law allows in terms of place of marriage policies, but we all continue to discern the best way of proceeding in our local churches. As the results of the informal and unscientific survey taken for this presentation/paper have shown, we as local churches are widely varied in our policies. Personally speaking (and this is only one person's opinion), I am not sure that this is good pastoral practice, particularly as seen from the vantage point of couples who show interest in marrying according to the norms and laws of the Church. Perhaps others may have better answers than I have, but if, for example, a Catholic couple were to ask me why they can't get married outdoors with a Catholic ceremony while a similar couple in a neighboring diocese can be allowed to do so, I would be hard-pressed to give them what I would consider an adequate answer. I would do my best to explain that the bishop of a local church, as that Church's proper pastor, has determined that his diocese's place of marriage policies are deemed the best way to promote, protect and defend the sanctity of marriage. And, to be honest, I could make that argument with a real level of conviction. But if that same well-informed couple explained to me

the reasons why the neighboring diocese allowed that same type of wedding in an outdoor setting and if the couple concluded that a place of marriage policy ultimately seemed to them merely a set of arbitrary rules, I believe I would be at a loss for a good response. Like everyone else, I do not have the perfect answers to pastoral challenges such as these, and it is not my place to say what every bishop/ local church should do. That said, perhaps I can offer just a few suggestions for further thought and consideration as local churches continue to discern what is the best place of marriage policies for their own (arch)dioceses.

First, and perhaps this doesn't even need to be said, we must follow the will of our own bishops. They are, after all, the pastors of our local churches, and so we owe them our respect and obedience. In (arch)dioceses that have bishops that have firm convictions regarding place of marriage policies, we are called to respect and obey these policies and implement them to the best of our abilities, even if we would like to see policies that are different than the ones that actually exist.

However, as was made clear by the results of the survey used in this presentation, many (arch)dioceses, and therefore bishops, are open to at least discussing anew, and perhaps making concrete changes, to their place of marriage policies. This willingness to re-evaluate these policies is especially being considered in light of the fact that this is being seen as a way of possibly encouraging more couples to marry in the Church, which will oftentimes help them stay better connected with the Church as they begin their marriage and family lives. If these further conversations and/or possible policy changes are being considered, allow me to offer a few practical suggestions.

First, make this discussion a broad-based one. Starting with the local level, allow parish councils to discuss the question so as to allow people to offer their opinions, with the proviso being that people are clearly told in advance that any decisions or changes being considered will be done on a diocesan level, and not merely on a parish or deanery level. With this information in hand, pastors can then meet with each other at their deanery or regional levels so that the deans/presbyteral council members can learn what the thoughts are in their local regions. The deans/presbyteral council members can then meet with the bishop and (arch)diocesan curial officials so as to have as full and informed a discussion as possible. On a side or connected note, continue also to speak about this issue at canonical conventions and meetings. Perhaps regional meetings of the CLSA would be a good place to continue these discussions. Keep talking about the issue and keep evaluating what the best policies can possibly be.

Another suggestion would be to encourage, as much as possible, a common policy for episcopal provinces and regions. It is a bishop's prerogative, of course, to establish his own policies in his (arch)diocese, but it would also be helpful to pastors and others working with couples preparing to marry if they can at least

know that many, if not most, of their neighboring (arch)dioceses share the same policies as their own. Avoiding having to provide responses to the arbitrary rules argument is to be encouraged as much as possible, because it really does seem a difficult argument to win.

If changes from stricter to more permissive policies are being considered, perhaps various middle ground approaches can first be made. For example, without making changes to marriages involving the use of canonical form, can a relaxing of policies concerning dispensations from canonical form first be made? Or, as another alternative, whether employing canonical form or not, can changes to policies be considered for marriages between Catholics and unbaptized persons, given our theological understanding that these marriages are not sacramental in nature? Admittedly, changes with this latter type of marriage may upset people who do not fall into this category (marriages between two Catholics or marriages between a Catholic and a baptized non-Catholic), so every possible policy change should be evaluated from all angles. But again, is some middle ground change to policy possible? This is something to be considered.

As another practical suggestion, if changes to policy are considered, perhaps these can be done on an *ad experimentum* basis, and this *ad experimentum* status should be publicly made known when changes are first implemented. This would allow local churches to have time to review the impacts (both positive and negative) these policy changes have made. Admittedly, it may be difficult to revert to former policies, but the implementation of newer policies on an *ad experimentum* basis (perhaps for a one or two year period) will at least make it known both at the beginning and end of these probationary periods that further policy changes, or returns to previous policies, are indeed possible.

Regardless of what policies exist in one's own (arch)diocese, it is important to make our pastoral ministers aware of the fact that policies are in fact diocesan and that those same policies are not necessarily the same in other dioceses. When priests, deacons or other pastoral ministers are asked to prepare couples for weddings that will take place in other (arch)dioceses, these same ministers would be well-advised to let the couples know that place of marriage policies can and oftentimes do differ from one diocese to another, and so couples need to be well-informed about what is or is not allowed in the territory where they wish to marry before concrete plans for their marriage begin to be made.

Furthermore, in deliberating whether or not to make place of marriage policy changes, it is important to remember, at least in terms of marriages employing canonical form, that what is being talked about here is a permission and not a dispensation. Have we made permissions more difficult to obtain than dispensations? If we as local churches routinely grant disparity of worship dispensations, for example, which bear on validity, but are much stricter in the granting of permissions, which oftentimes bear on liceity, is this not something

that should be a significant point of reflection as we continue to evaluate what our place of marriage policies should be?

Finally, respect the policies of other local churches, especially when these policies are different from those of our own. Canon 1118 does indeed provide latitude for determining these questions on a local level, and we are called to always respect the mind of the lawmaker, even if we don't personally agree with what has been decided and/or implemented. When it comes to place of marriage policies, in light of canon 1118, it is important to remember that there is no right or wrong answer. How does one define suitable? This is a question that will never admit of a definitive answer. So, as long as canon 1118 remains in effect, we need to acknowledge and respect the differences of theological and pastoral opinion that lead to the establishment and implementation of place of marriage policies, no matter how varied they may be.

Finally, continue to evaluate the question. The current state of the question is exactly that, current. What is best for our local churches in our current times and places will continue to change and evolve, just like life itself. So, let us all continue to be open to questions that the law allows us to discuss. In conclusion, let us remember that the *salus animarum* is always to be our primary goal as we continue to serve as ministers of the Church. What are the best place-of-marriage policies for the life of the Church? Let us pray for the ongoing guidance of the Holy Spirit, so that He can help us all further know how best to proceed and in turn be drawn closer to Christ, in and through His Church.

Seminar

Ten Years Later: The Special Faculties Granted to the Congregation for the Clergy, 2009-2019

The Very Reverend Georges de Laire, JCL

Introduction

The document before us is the circular letter from the Congregation for the Clergy to bishops at their sees dated 18 April 2009 with protocol number 2009 0556.[1] The document is supplemented with the "Procedural Guidelines" issued by the same congregation on 17 March 2010.[2] The letter presents to the bishops three special faculties granted to the Congregation for the Clergy to assist them with procedures to address clergy in irregular situations. Two faculties facilitating dismissal from the clerical state for priests who find themselves in particular scandalous situations, and one faculty for the dispensation from the obligations subsequent to sacred ordination, including that of celibacy, for priests who have voluntarily abandoned ministry for a period longer than five consecutive years.

To be clear, I am not presenting from the perspective of the Congregation for the Clergy, as I am not, have not been, and do not plan to be, an official of the congregation. I am presenting from the perspective of one who has processed over 45 cases of clergy who have met the criteria set forth by the special faculties. Over the years, I have benefited from the suggestions and corrections offered by officials of the congregation. Most were very helpful, while some remain unclear; but what is important to remember is that the congregation decides the cases and thus it is for us to prepare the cases accordingly. It is also helpful to note that, over the years, the changing of the officials has led to some changes in what was expected from the *acta* of the cases. Therefore, I encourage all of us to entertain helpful communications with the officials of the congregations. Such relationships will reduce the length of the processes by making sure that cases

---

1 See "Canons 1317; 1319; 1342, §2; 1349; 1399 Special Faculties for Congregaton for Clergy: Administrative Procedures for the Laicization of Priests," *Roman Replies and CLSA Advisory Opinions 2009*, ed. Sharon A. Euart et al. (Washington, DC: Canon Law Society of America, 2009) 37-47.

2 See "Canons 1317; 1319; 1342, §2; 1349; 1399 Special Faculties for the Congregaton for Clergy: Procedural Guidelines," *Roman Replies and CLSA Advisory Opinions 2010*, ed. Sharon A. Euart et al. (Washington, DC: Canon Law Society of America, 2010) 43-51.

are filed appropriately.

Therefore, this presentation is meant to be a practical and not academic perspective.

Understanding the intent for the granting of the special faculties to the Congregation for the Clergy will help in preparing cases. There are 4 elements to understanding the reasons for the faculties.

1. To protect the dignity of the priesthood, especially the "sacred power" of the one acting in the person of Christ, head and shepherd; to protect those priests who continue to do what they can to honor their priesthood.[3]

2. To provide a better theological understanding behind priestly celibacy, and the duty to observe "perfect and perpetual continence."[4]

3. Obligation for bishops to promote and protect common discipline; bishops must be attentive that their priests are faithful to their proper ministerial duties.[5]

4. The bishop is judicially responsible for making sure priests are faithful to their obligations. This establishes the faculties as a judicial tool.

   a. Peaceful resolution to a condition that may have arisen (cf. c. 1446);

   b. Observance of procedural norms in processing cases of "unfaithful" clergy (cf. cc. 1717ff, 1339-1341);

   c. Upon receipt of information, follow canons 1717-1719 (the preliminary investigation) and following. Then comes the admonition—to repair scandal, restore justice, and reform the cleric (c. 1341)—leading either to a penal process or an extra-judicial administrative process.

---

3 Cf. John Paul II, apostolic exhortation *Pastores dabo vobis* 15, March 25, 1992: *AAS* 84 (1992) 679-681; English translation at http://www.vatican.va/content/john-paul-ii/en/apost_exhortations/documents/hf_jp-ii_exh_25031992_pastores-dabo-vobis.html (accessed on 2 Mar. 2020).

4 Cf. *Codex Iuris Canonici auctoritate Ioannis Pauli PP. II promulgatus* (Libreria Editrice Vaticana, 1989) c. 277; English translation of canons of this code are from *Code of Canon Law, Latin-English Edition: New English Translation* (Washington, DC: Canon Law Society of America, 2012).

5 Cf. c. 384, 392; Second Vatican Council, dogmatic constitution *Lumen gentium* 27, November 21, 1964: *AAS* 57 (1965) 32-33.

The 2009 letter was followed with a brief letter introducing procedural guidelines. The letter is of 17 March 2010 with protocol 2010 0823. The letter states emphatically, "[I]t is essential to note the *indispensable initial requirement*, namely that the *impossibility* or the *extreme difficulty* in following the ordinary canonical means already available, be that the *via gratiosa* (dispensation) or the penal judicial route, has been clearly established beforehand."[6]

Three elements are identified as required before considering the special faculties:

1. *Objective* or *subjective* impossibility for the *via gratiosa*, for the priest in question to petition himself for dispensation.

2. Documented pastoral efforts were not successful in reforming the cleric and his return to priestly ministry.

3. Grave difficulties preventing a canonical penal trial.

I recommend making sure that the four elements of the first letter be included (or at least referenced) in the bishop's *votum*.

All three conditions found in the 2010 letter MUST be referenced in the instructor's *votum* and in the bishop's *votum*, substantiated by proper documentation in the acts. Therefore:

1. To address a grave lack of discipline by some priests and to protect those who do what they can; to promote the *salus animarum*; to respond to the needs of bishops in their duties to affirm proper continence.

2. In 2012 when I shared with a local ordinary the content of my case load, he exclaimed, "Make sure your bishop understands that the application of the faculties is not guaranteed."

The content of Faculties I and II follows.

> Special Faculty I:
>
> The Special Faculty to treat and present to the Holy Father, for His approval in *forma specifica* and His decision, cases of dismissal from the clerical state *in poenam* with dispensation from the obligations consequent to ordination, including that of celibacy, of clerics who have attempted marriage, even if only civilly, and who, having been admonished, have not withdrawn from this state, therefore persisting in an irregular and scandalous life (cf. c. 1394 §1); and of clerics

6 *Roman Replies and CLSA Advisory Opinions 2010*, 43.

guilty of grave sins against the 6th Commandment (cf. c. 1395 §§1-2).

Special Faculty II:

The Special Faculty to intervene in accord with c. 1399 *CIC*, either by taking direct action in a case or by confirming the decisions of Ordinaries, were the competent Ordinary so to request, due to the special gravity of the violation of law and the need or urgency to avoid an objective scandal.

This is granted along with the derogation from the prescriptions of canons 1317, 1319, 1342 §2 and 1349 *CIC*, with respect to the application of perpetual penalties, to be applied to deacons only for grave reasons and to priests for the gravest reasons, always requiring that such cases are presented to the Holy Father for His approval *in forma specifica* and for His decision.[7]

In short, Faculty I deals with:

- Attempted marriage, even if only civilly (Does this include homosexual nuptials?); or
- Grave sin against the Sixth Commandment.

Faculty II deals with:

- Deacons for a "grave reason" and
- Priests for the "gravest reason," such as:
    1. Special gravity of violation of law AND urgency to avoid objective scandal (i.e., the recent case of two priests who abandoned their respective ministries to civilly marry each other);
    2. Drug dealing (i.e., "Monsignor Meth" in Connecticut)[8]; or
    3. Embezzlement.

Both workshop presentations in Atlantic City showed a need to remind ourselves that *Sacramentorum Sanctitatis Tutela* (*SST*)[9] addresses delicts reserved to the Congregation for the Doctrine of the Faith (CDF) and that the current practice of the Roman Curia is to favor *SST* over the special faculties. That is to say, all gravest reasons related to the sacrament of confession would not fall under Faculty II, but *SST*. Same for delicts committed against the Eucharist

7 *Roman Replies and CLSA Advisory Opinions 2010,* 45.

8 See, e.g., "Suspended priest, 'Monsignor Meth,' gets 5-year sentence," CBS News, May 7, 2015, https://www.cbsnews.com/news/suspended-connecticut-priest-dubbed-monsignor-meth-gets-5-year-sentence/ (accessed on 11 Mar. 2020).

9 John Paul II, *motu proprio Sacramentorum sanctitatis tutela*, April 30, 2001: *AAS* 93 (2001) 737-739.

or against the faith.

Until more recently, Roman Catholic priests who abandoned ministry to join another ecclesial community were subjects to the application of Faculty II (or III if they had abandoned for more than five years). In the past couple of years, it has been my experience that, the cases presented to the Congregation for the Clergy of priests who had joined the Episcopal Church were transferred to the CDF under its jurisdiction with reference to Article 1 §1 and Article 2. It also happens that the *taxa* for CDF is greater than the *taxa* for the Congregation for the Clergy!

For both faculties, it is necessary to start the process with what the law already requires, namely the proper application of canons 1717-1719 and the preliminary investigation.

After the preliminary investigation (cc. 1717-1719) of the actions of a priest

- Make sure all documents are there. A preliminary investigation is necessary, or there must be evidence that there is no need for it, but after closure, move to canon 1720.
- You must have at least one admonition, as per canon 1347. It must be documented. Have proof of delivery for any letter; provide meeting notes and witness accounts.

  Proof of marriage

  - If the cleric does not respond to the invitation by the bishop to initiate the petition himself, he could be asked to provide a statement to that end and swear to the fact that he is now married with no intention to stop his contumacy.
  - Some states provide marriage certificates to third parties.
  - Obtain affidavits from witnesses stating their factual knowledge that the marriage has taken place. It has been known that other clerics have attended a brother's nuptials, and even former parishioners!
  - Newspaper announcements and photos are helpful documentation.
  - Internet social media posts are also very helpful as proof.

Post investigation steps to be taken by the instructor

- Announce the close of instruction. Documentation is key, as I have received letters from the congregation asking me to provide it when I failed to include it in the *acta*.

The accused has the right of defense after being presented the proofs. It is important to wait until the instruction is completed before meeting with the cleric, as he must be provided with the ability to review all the proofs presented against him. Only presenting some of the proofs would infringe upon his right of defense. This is also a good time to remind the cleric that he has the right to choose a canonist to assist him at that point. There should be documentation that the cleric was informed of this right. The norms of law regarding the advocate apply in this instance, too, such as a provision that the choice of a canonist can be restricted to those approved by the bishop (cf. cc. 1483ff.)

Review of the case with the supporting proofs with two assessors

- Include mandates of appointment of the assessors, who should be priests.
- The assessors could be stably appointed or specific to the case; either way the mandates of appointment are to be included in the *acta*.
- Document the transfer of the *acta* to the bishop and to the assessors.
- Document the meeting between bishop, assessors, notary, and instructor who are called to review the case.
- Minutes of the meeting are to be taken by an appointed notary. The minutes should be topic specific, meaning that there should be explicit reference to some of the proofs under review.
- Opinions of the assessors must be provided individually, not one opinion with two signatures.

The *votum* of the bishop

With regard to the *votum* from the bishop to apply Faculty I or II:

- It should include reference to the fact that the ordinary means of a penal trial is not possible or would be very difficult (e.g., impossibility to staff a process);
- The petition should be specific to which faculty is being applied. For Faculty II, the bishop asks for his decision to be confirmed as requested because of the gravity, urgency and objective scandal. In this instance there should be an explanation as to the objective scandal or urgency.
- Practically speaking, the *votum* can be written by someone other than the bishop (i.e., the instructor), but the bishop must sign it.

Reminder

The decisions reached after the application of the faculties are in *forma specifica*. It means that there is no possibility of appeal and no possibility of

recourse. These applications are penal processes adjudicated by a decision of the Holy Father. The rescript for Faculties I and II will indicate "*in poenam.*"

Faculty III

> The Special Faculty to handle cases of clerics, who having freely abandoned the ministry for a period of more than five consecutive years and who, after careful verification of the facts, insofar as this is possible, persist in such freely chosen and illicit absence from the ministry, taking this situation into account, to declare then their dismissal from the clerical state, with dispensation from the obligations consequent to ordination, including that of celibacy.[10]

In short, regarding Faculty III:

- It applies to priests who have abandoned ministry for a period of at least five consecutive years and who persist after being instructed to return to ministry.
- It is unclear whether this faculty applies to the cases of priests who abandon ministry and who are under the age of 40. (See the norms that apply for such cases.)

The phrase "insofar as this is possible" in Faculty III means that reasonable efforts must be made to try to locate the priest. A basic internet search is not sufficient. In one instance, after I sent the *acta* explaining my inability to locate the cleric to inform him of the bishop's intent to petition for him, the congregation located him for me and returned the case!

In keeping with the reasons behind the granting of the special faculties, the bishop of the cleric's diocese of incardination (or the superior general of the institute of consecrated life or society of apostolic life) must invite the cleric to petition himself for dispensation. The invitation becomes also an opportunity to engage the cleric on the topic of the possibility of a return to active ministry in the Church. The *via gratiosa* is always favored in these cases. Should the cleric not respond to the invitation, I recommend that a second invitation be mailed to the cleric. This might help in establishing the fact that the cleric has no intention to return and that he is content in perpetuating his contumacy.

Another tool that can be mailed to the cleric, as a follow-up, is what has been referred to as a waiver of notice and a deadline to respond. The waiver provides the cleric with a document that states in the first person singular (I), that he received the invitation to petition himself for dismissal, but he refuses to

10 *Roman Replies and CLSA Advisory Opinions 2010*, 48.

proceed and acknowledges that the bishop (superior general) will proceed with the petition. It also states:

> I have been informed of my right to have a canonical advocate of my own choosing; I consent to have this matter proceed without any objection on my part; I hereby waive notice of any of the further proceedings; I request and understand that I will be provided with a copy of the final decision on this matter by the Holy See.

I recommend sending a self-addressed stamped return envelope with the waiver as an extra enticement for the cleric signing it.

In compiling the documents of the case and conducting the instruction, other than the list of required documents provided by the Congregation for the Clergy, I recommend including:

- Sacramental history: Baptism, Eucharist, Confirmation, Holy Orders, with certificates if they are available.
- Education history: Where and what schools were attended and degrees obtained.
- Application process: Seminary application documents.
- *Do not* include the psychological testing results. (Cf. c. 220.)
- Yearly scrutinies from seminary faculty.
- Reception of Lector and Acolyte and dimissorial letters if any were issued.
- Letter requesting ordination to diaconate.
- Decree of ordination and dimissorial letters if any were issued.
- Letter requesting priestly ordination.
- Decree of ordination and dimissorial letters if any were issued.
- History of diocesan or extra-diocesan assignments with notes, if applicable.
- If the priest has gone through rehabilitation or similar program, notation to that effect; *do not* share treatment results. (Cf. c. 220.)
- Any documents leading to departure from active ministry, letter of resignation of pastorate, acceptance of resignation, abandonment, etc.
- Letter of admonition, if there is one. There was a period in the Church when bishops encouraged the priest for his abandonment, wished him well and so on.
- All subsequent communications.

- Documents that may support the lack of suitability to return to ministry.
- Communications regarding laicization process.

During the presentations of this seminar in Atlantic City in October of 2020, one participant pointed out that, as is common with most of these processes, the disposition of the congregation may vary, and thus the congregation has also been known to have the approach of "less is more" when it comes to documents in the *acta*. Remember that the minimum is what is on the provided list of required documents that can be found at the end of the 2010 letter to the bishops.

In the instructor's *votum*, if there is documentation, I would reference it somehow. The *votum* should include page numbers of the documents after the file has been paginated.

Make sure there is a document closing the instruction.

Make sure there is a *votum* from the promoter of justice. The *votum* does not have to be elaborate, it can be simple, but it should always be specific to the case in question. Here is an example of the *votum* of the promoter of justice in the cases I instructed:

> I, the Reverend Patrick Cleric, J.C.L., the undersigned Promoter of Justice for the above referenced case, having reviewed the acts, with particular attention to the unique facts relative to the Reverend John Ontherun, his right of defense, and believing the public good will be best served by the cleric being returned to the lay state, have no objection to the proposed action.

Make sure there is a written statement transferring all documents to the bishop for his review and *votum*, including *vota* of the instructor and the promoter of justice.

Make sure all the acts are notarized.

Include a cover letter introducing the case to the Congregation for the Clergy.

Send three copies, never the originals.

I always recommend using the Nunciature for transmittal to Rome.

Independent of whether there was a "waiver of notice" as part of the *acta*, the congregation will respond to the petitioning hierarch acknowledging receipt of the case, with the proper attribution of the protocol number. With the letter to the hierarch, the congregation provides a letter to the cleric informing him that the hierarch has filed the petition and that the cleric can provide documentation

challenging the petition. Because there is a deadline to be observed by the cleric, I recommend sending the letter from the congregation to the cleric with proof of delivery.

The letter from the congregation to the hierarch will also be the first vehicle for the corrections the congregation "suggests" to the instructor. It will include whether documents are missing, whether it is not clear that the cleric must be given an opportunity to have canonical representation, and so on.

As with any communications with the Roman Curia, when providing added documents or anything else, remember to include the proper protocol number, as well as the cleric's name.

Re: Prot. N° 2019 0001
Reverend John Ontherun

Once the case has reached conclusion, the congregation will send the petitioning hierarch a cover letter giving notice of the decision, guidelines on notifying the (no-longer) cleric, and the inevitable *taxa*. More recently, the decisions I have received also included an "unofficial" translation of the decree, the original being in Latin.

Again, note that the decisions are reached by the Congregation for the Clergy and presented to the Holy Father for the final decision. The decisions of the Holy Father are *in forma specifica* and therefore not open to appeal or recourse. Special Faculties I and II result in a dismissal from the clerical state while Special Faculty III results in a dispensation from the obligations subsequent to sacred ordination, including that of celibacy. The decisions are effective by the approval of the Holy Father, whether the cleric accepts notification or not. Should the cleric refuse to come to receive notification, the congregation asks that the decrees be returned to Rome. I recommend that you make a copy of the decree before sending the originals back, whether signed or not. When returning the decrees to Rome, the congregation asks for a summary of how the notification took place and if there is anything in particular to note.

And then there is the *taxa*!

Seminar

Qui propter nos homines et propter nostram salutem: Justice and Mercy in the Distribution of the Salvific Goods of the Church

The Very Reverend Peter A. Faulk, JCL

1. Introduction

Virtually no other topic has had as much ink spilled over the last 40 years in the field of canonistics as the tension between justice and mercy in the administration of justice in the Church.[1] Whether it is a question of theory, a question of *praxis*, a question of orthodoxy and protecting the deposit of faith or a question of the application of the principles of justice on a practical, case by case basis, the justice-mercy question fundamentally concerns a correct understanding the *ius* and its correct application, especially in a modern hyper-kinetic, rapidly transforming techno-globalized societal context. Justice and mercy concern the dialogue between natural law and positive law, vindicating the rights of the subject of law while simultaneously upholding the common ecclesial good, as well as the relationship between that which is the object of justice and the formalized norm.[2]

In the context of the practical reality of credibly realized missionary discipleship, a correct understanding of the classical conception of the *ius* concerns a thoroughly updated and enlightened pastoral approach to ecclesiastical discipline, governance and administration. Primary among these tasks is the just and equitable distribution of the spiritual goods of the

---

1 This study does not seek to be a taxative cross-referencing of the canons pertinent to the distribution of the sacraments, but more of a systematic *ius*-philosophical analysis of the theoretical underpinnings of the specific principles inherent in the documents of the Second Vatican Council and their import upon the entire *forma mentis* by which the Church's ministers should approach the subject of a just and equitable distribution of the Church's spiritual goods. For a taxative analysis of the canons correlative to this subject see D. Le Tourneau, "Le canon 213 sur le droit aux biens spirituels et ses conséquences sur les droits et les devoirs fondamentaux dans l'Église," *Studia Canonica* 47 (2013) 407-466.

2 See Javier Hervada, *Cos'è il Diritto? La moderna risposta del realismo giuridico* (Roma: EDUSC, 2015).

Word of God, the Sacraments and pastoral charity. However, this becomes a question of the classical conception of the *ius* as the object of justice and as that which is concretely required *in hoc saeculo*.[3] Jurgen Habermas in his book *Between Facts and Norms* highlights the Post-Enlightenment legal and political transformation from historically traditional civilizations in which credibility and validity were given to norms which emanated from sacred authority by virtue of habit and custom. Secular modernity has replaced sources of sacred authority with mechanisms such as representative consent of the governed, fundamental equality before the law and mutually furnished consensus to concede validity to formalized norms emanated from a legitimately constituted state.[4] The Church's response to this is witnessed in reflecting upon the depths of inter-Trinitarian life as the perfect *communio* society as an updating of our understanding of both the lived vertical and horizontal aspects of missionary discipleship as an externalization of the interior mystery of perfected brotherhood, equality and peace in a pluralistic-globalized modern context. The sacramental nature of the Church, where *communio* properly understood, signifies that the fundamental rights of the hierarchy and Christ's faithful are enucleated, structured, and revolve around the mystery of the Word and the Sacraments.[5] This constitutional totality challenges us to always be developing an inter-ecclesial consensus and culture where rigorous scientific accuracy is a minimal criteria for both theoretical and practical pastoral application. The canonical professional must rely on the role of the Thomistic distinction and apply this distinction by a methodology of spiritual discernment of the intricacies of each case as he calibrates the law to the facts in order to render what is truly just. As Ulpian tells us, the jurist is the expert of both what is just and what is unjust.

In the United States, as well as everywhere else in the world, we have a specific national as well as ecclesial-national culture in which the faith is received, formed and nourished. As a Church rooted in a nation which is a child of the Enlightenment, we embrace its paradigms while simultaneously cultivating the riches of our Greco-Roman intellectual and civilizational heritage. Pope Benedict observed in this regard in the Regensburg address that the Post-Enlightenment, Post-Scientific Revolution reality—which for our purposes we will refer to as the techno-globalized modern world—increasingly is forming people in an ever

---

3 See Javier Hervada, *Critical Introduction to Natural Law* (Montreal: Wilson & Lafleur, 2006).

4 See Michele Dillon, *The Authority of the Holy Revisited: Habermas, Religion, and Emancipatory Possibilities*, Sociological Theory, vol. 17, no. 3 (Madison: SAGE Publications, 1999) 290-306.

5 See Javier Hervada, *Las raíces sacramentales del derecho canónico. Sacramentalidad de la Iglesia y Sacramentos: IV Simposio Internacional de Teología de la Universidad de Navarra* / edición dirigida por Pedro Rodríguez . . . [et al.] (Navarra: Servicio de Publicaciones de la Universidad de Navarra, 1983) 359-385.

more de-Hellenized intellectual paradigm.[6] The nature of a more positivistically-scientistically stratified *ausbildung* and worldview is rendering people such that they are unable to recognize the entire universe of Hellenic symbology of which the Church is the great custodian. Hence, mercy becomes a matter of realizing that the great majority of faithful do not have the luxury of a formal liberal arts or seminary education and need assistance and encouragement as they seek greater integration and belonging into the family of God which is the Church. This component of the much referenced "evangelization of culture" calls for identifying where the best impulses of modernity, as a *Logos* tradition, synergize with the truth of reason and the Gospel and to create new avenues of edification and development of the life of faith of the People of God who live and are formed in this new de-Hellenized milieu.

In a word, justice and mercy are about us as canonists in our role of engaging in a renewal and pastoral conversion of structures, which is always rooted in personal conversion and renewal.[7] Furthermore, it is about strengthening the Church's kerygmatic witness, which is our fundamental mission. The totality of these realities and dynamics form a task for us as canonical professionals. A just and merciful application of law and rights in a Church of missionary disciples requires that we engage the *ius* always as an art and a science with ever greater theoretical and practical precision. If one sifts through the scores of discourses and reflections upon the theme of justice and mercy in the last 40 years, I would posit that it is really a question of our present and urgent task of understanding and assimilating the principles of the Second Vatican Council. This is still a task which awaits completion.

2. A Catholic Renaissance

One of the most important thinkers in the life of the Church since the Second Vatican Council is Henri De Lubac. As a key theologian at the Council, John Paul II, Benedict XVI as well as Pope Francis have all recognized the centrality

6 See Benedict XVI, speech Glaube, Vernunft und Universität. Erinnerungen und Reflexionen, September 12, 2006, https://w2.vatican.va/content/benedict-xvi/de/speeches/2006/september/documents/hf_ben-xvi_spe_20060912_university-regensburg.html (accessed on 20 Jan. 2020).

7 See Francis, apostolic exhortation *Evangelii Gaudium* 27, November 24, 2013: *AAS* 105 (2013) 1019-1137.

> The renewal of structures demanded by pastoral conversion can only be understood in this light: as part of an effort to make them more mission-oriented, to make ordinary pastoral activity on every level more inclusive and open, to inspire in pastoral workers a constant desire to go forth and in this way to elicit a positive response from all those whom Jesus summons to friendship with himself. As John Paul II once said to the Bishops of Oceania: "All renewal in the Church must have mission as its goal if it is not to fall prey to a kind of ecclesial introversion."

English translation at http://www.vatican.va/evangelii-gaudium/en/files/assets/basic-html/page25.html (accessed on 20 Jan. 2020).

of his influence on the Council as well as the importance of his thought for its correct implementation. Henri De Lubac wrote extensively after the close of the Council that what he observed in the life of the Church was merely a slow trickle of renewal envisioned by the Council Fathers. Finally, at the end of his life, he lamented that what was happening on a worldwide scale was simply what took place at the end of the Council of Trent in France. Due to *ad intra* and *ad extra* political, social, as well as ideological pressures, the robust reform and renewal of Trent was stalled for a century in France. De Lubac assessed that after the close of the Second Vatican Council, a similar dynamic was occurring, but in this case, on a worldwide scale. Hence, he assessed that the New Pentecost envisioned by Pope John XXIII would effectively be stalled for about a 100-year period.[8] Hence, the slow trickle moves toward being a much-anticipated torrent of dynamic and revitalized inter-ecclesial life.

De Lubac also wrote that the *aggiornamento* and revitalization which was envisioned by the Council Fathers would manifest itself in the form of, in his words, a "Catholic Renaissance" which would be in harmony with the advancements of science and culture of the emerging techno-globalized modern society. We see elements of this in the emphasis of John Paul II's Christian humanism: man in Christ as the measure of all things, as well as in Benedict XVI's horizontal focus of the community and social bonds of the Christian life as the completion of the baptismal call to live out the vertical mystery of the soul's spiritual and mystical union with the Triune God.

It was in one of his last speeches before his resignation from office that Pope Benedict tackled this specific topic of an appropriate understanding of the truth of the Council for its correct implementation. This text contained some of the autobiographical anecdotes and catch phrases which had been repeated from time to time throughout his pontificate. Nevertheless, this discourse is of immense importance and merits careful study, especially in the context of the original intention of the Council Fathers.

> There was an incredible sense of expectation. We were hoping that all would be renewed, that there would truly be a new Pentecost, a new era of the Church, because the Church was still fairly robust at that time – Sunday Mass attendance was still good, vocations to the priesthood and to religious life were already slightly reduced, but still sufficient. However, there was a feeling that the Church was not moving forward, that it was declining, that it seemed more a thing of the past and not the herald of the future. And at that moment, we were hoping that this relation would be renewed, that it would change; that the Church might once again be a force for tomorrow and a force for today. And we knew

8 See Christopher J. Walsh, "De Lubac's Critique of the Postconciliar Church," *Communio: International Catholic Review*, 19.3 (1992) 404-433.

> that the relationship between the Church and the modern period, right from the outset, had been slightly fraught, beginning with the Church's error in the case of Galileo Galilei; we were looking to correct this mistaken start and to rediscover the union between the Church and the best forces of the world, so as to open up humanity's future, to open up true progress.[9]

The Holy Father's highlighting of the Galileo Crisis as a starting point for the Council touches upon an acute neuralgic point. Essentially, what has evolved in Western Culture since the Galileo incident is a growing disenchantment and mistrust of the Church as an ally in the great project of humanizing culture and civil society. It was a mistake and fumbling of the issue on the Church's part, as hierarchical leadership condemned heliocentricism as heretical. No doubt, Church leaders were attempting to uphold a correct and authoritative interpretation of the principles of Scripture and Tradition. Nevertheless, the Fathers of the Council acutely delineated this controversy as a pivot point in the consciousness of the West which began the process of a tragic separation of faith and culture, so lamented by Paul VI.[10] Hence, the Second Vatican Council was envisioned as a new watershed moment from which the phoenix of the Gospel could arise from the ruins and ashes of a dysfunctional relationship that the Church has developed with modernity.

The reforms of the Council were flattering in many ways to the Church in the United States in regard to the concepts of religious liberty and a global Church situating itself in open dialogue within the Post-World War II international pluralistic context. However, in a post *Humanae Vitae* and post 2002 Dallas Charter reality, the Church in the United States finds itself in the midst of a crisis of explanation, a crisis of internal governance and a crisis of exteriorized identity. We also find ourselves quite humbled, if not to say paralyzed. The 2004 John Jay Report pinpointed the central issue concerning the handling of the sexual abuse crisis as incompetence on the part of leadership in regard to governance and implementation of our own policies and protocols.[11] A more in depth study of this analysis reveals that Church leaders had policies and procedures in place and either did not know of their existence or if they did, they did not follow the letter

---

9 Benedict XVI, speech Discorso del Santo Padre Benedetto XVI: Incontro con i parroci e il clero di Roma, Giovedì, February 14, 2013, http://www.vatican.va/content/benedict-xvi/it/speeches/2013/february/documents/hf_ben-xvi_spe_20130214_clero-roma.html (accessed on 20 Jan. 2020).

10 See Paul VI, apostolic exhortation *Evangelii Nuntiandi* 20, December 8, 1975: *AAS* 68 (1976) 18-19, http://www.vatican.va/content/paul-vi/en/apost_exhortations/documents/hf_p-vi_exh_19751208_evangelii-nuntiandi.html (accessed on 20 Jan. 2020).

11 See John Jay College of Criminal Justice, "The Nature and Scope of Sexual Abuse of Minors by Catholic Priests and Deacons in the United States 1950–2002" (Washington DC, United States Conference of Catholic Bishops, 2004).

of the law. Improvisation took place and disaster followed in its train.[12]

However, we should not be afraid. We should have confidence. Christ did not call us and send us the Holy Spirit to protect a mere fallen and imperfect human institution. He called us and chose us to be witnesses to the Resurrection. And it is in this context that the reality of a Church of mercy is properly understood. It is not some cloy catch phrase for a banner or bumper sticker. It is a serious call for the Church to once again surprise everyone and emerge on the stage of history as Herself again; as a loving mother. A Church of Mercy is one that understands authority as Codeero understood *auctoritas*—not so much as the power to command, but validity which has been conceded through an ability to render a correct interpretation.[13] This is brought about by the Church forming its ministers to render ever more scientifically acute distinctions as well as creating masters of the art of spiritual discernment. Under the aegis of this highest, most penetrating, and most subtle form of legitimacy, will the Church be once again bestowed with the respect and permission to assist modern man in interpreting the nature of his origin, purpose and ultimate destiny?

3. A Church of Divine Mercy

The concept of a Church of Divine Mercy was indicated in the officially recognized visions of Saint Faustina Kowalska in Poland in the 1920's. The centrality of mercy was, later that century, indicated by Pope John XXIII at the solemn opening of the Second Vatican Council as its constitutive and hermeneutical interpretive key. Mercy, viewed in light of divine revelation, is an intrinsically theological concept. The mission of theology is always faith seeking *intellectus*. Once again Pope Benedict in his final discourse to the Roman clergy stated that "[T]he Council of the Fathers was conducted within the faith—it was a Council of faith seeking intellectus, seeking to understand itself and seeking to understand the signs of God at that time, seeking to respond to the challenge of God at that time and to find in the word of God a word for today and tomorrow. . . ."[14] In light of the Council's self-perceived mission as laying the path to healing the rift between faith and culture, a new beginning of the evangelization of culture finds a crystalline leitmotif in the theme of mercy as understanding and empathizing with the other as other, willing the good of the other as other, and utilizing the power of reason—*fides quaerens intellectum*—to propel the Church's proclamation of the Gospel of mercy, compassion, assistance

12 See John P. Beal, "The 1962 instruction *Crimen sollicitationis*: Caught red-handed or handed a red herring?" *Studia canonica* 41 (2007) 199–236.

13 See J.P. Balsdon, "*Auctoritas, Dignitas, Otium*," The Classical Quarterly 10 (May, 1960) 1: 43-50.

14 Benedict XVI, speech *Meeting with the Parish Priests and the Clergy of Rome*, February 14, 2014, http://www.vatican.va/content/benedict-xvi/en/speeches/2013/february/documents/hf_ben-xvi_spe_20130214_clero-roma.html (accessed on 20 Jan. 2020).

and mutual understanding to a world which expects, and even demands, that the Church to live up to its most high calling. Hence, we discover the intersection of justice and mercy in this concept of *intellectus*—in reason enlightened by faith and faith disciplined by reason. The minister of justice finds the perfectly calibrated methodology of application in drawing an adequate, scientifically rigorous distinction while simultaneously following a path of penetrating spiritual discernment to gaze into the heart of situations to render what is truly just.

4. The Church as *Communio*

In Pope Benedict XVI's final discourse to the Roman clergy he also shared a fundamental insight of the Council as that of understanding the Church as a *communio.* He stated in this regard that:

> [T]he relationship between People of God and Body of Christ creates a new reality—*communio.* After the Council it became clear, I would say, that the Council really discovered and pointed to this concept: *communio* as the central concept. I would say that, philologically, it is not yet fully developed in the Council, yet it is as a result of the Council that the concept of communion came more and more to be the expression of the Church's essence, communion in its different dimensions: communion with the Trinitarian God—who is himself communion between Father, Son and Holy Spirit—sacramental communion, and concrete communion in the episcopate and in the life of the Church.[15]

Lumen gentium tells us in paragraph one that "the Church is in Christ like a sacrament or as a sign and instrument both of a very closely-knit union with God and of the unity of the whole human race."[16] Throughout the history of Christianity, spiritual anti-juridicisms have arisen which have taught that the dimension of justice in the Church is an imposition on charism and divinization.[17] However, faith informed by reason tells us that law and justice are intrinsic dimensions of the sacramentality of the Church's life. From Ulpian's classic definition, *Iustitia est constans et perpetua voluntas ius suum cuique tribuendi*, we can extrapolate that the Church's obligation is to render that which is due in justice to each to provide for charisms and growth in the spiritual life of the

---

15 Benedict XVI, *Meeting with the Parish Priests and the Clergy of Rome.*

16 Second Vatican Council, dogmatic constitution *Lumen gentium* 1, November 21, 1964: *AAS* 57 (1965) 5; English translation at https://www.vatican.va/archive/hist_councils/ii_vatican_council/documents/vat-ii_const_19641121_lumen-gentium_en.html (accessed on 20 Jan. 2020).

17 See Carlos J. Errazuriz, *Justice in the Church: A Fundamental Theory of Canon Law* (Montreal: Wilson & Lafleur, 2009) 6-45.

faithful to flourish.[18] Hence, the Church is to distribute its salvific goods in such a manner that those who retain the title to these goods have an authentic and saving encounter with the person of Christ. One's notion of law and rights depends on one's own vision of man and of society. *Communio*[19] as interpreted on the juridic plane, ensures that justice in the Church is encountered in an efficacious manner, "like a sacrament" and creates ambits of liberty[20] for its members to grow in the perfection of freedom, master the art of missionary discipleship and exercise the

---

18 See *Catechism of the Catholic Church* 1897, 2nd ed. (Washington, DC: United States Catholic Conference, 2000), http://www.vatican.va/archive/ccc_css/archive/catechism/p3s1c2a2.htm (accessed on 19 Mar. 2020), which quotes Pope Leo XIII in n. 1897: "Human society can be neither well-ordered nor prosperous unless it has some people invested with legitimate authority to preserve its institutions and to devote themselves as far as is necessary to work and care for the good of all." It continues in n. 1898 stating that "every human community needs an authority to govern it. The foundation of such authority lies in human nature. It is necessary for the unity of the state. Its role is to ensure as far as possible the common good of the society." Hence, man in Christ, that is, incorporated into the mystery of the Church by virtue of baptism and created in the image of the Triune God is destined to live out and manifest this communion in the world through a life of actualized missionary discipleship. The invisible bonds of communion as externalized in the bonds of justice and charity are manifested in the order, which is regulated by the Church's law, ie., canon law or as *ius canonicum*, and can also be translated: *rights in the Church*. The idea of *communio*, a theological category which makes its way into canonical scholarship necessitates a conceptualization on the jurdic plane which is able to delimit and properly situate the concept according to the intrinsic exigencies of justice.

19 See Eugenio Corecco, *Diritto*, in *Dizionario Teologico Interdisciplinare* (Torino: Marietti, 1977) I: 147.

> The concept of "*communio*," which on the constitutional level of the relationship between the universal and the particular Church is realized as the "*communio* Ecclesiarum," seems to grasp the specific substance of ecclesial social life, through which eschatological salvation is realized and anticipated in history. This category, which includes the eschatological aspect in so far as it is immanent to the Church, seems to be capable of expressing the unmistakable contours of the constitution and the canonical institutions which regulate ecclesial life. The "*communio*" is at once the reality to be realized and the modality according to which canon law must be structured in order to realize it. It is, furthermore, the result of the convergence of the categories "People of God," "Mystical Body," and "Word and Sacrament," which form the foundation of the existence of canon law itself.

20 Pedro Lombardia, *Lezioni Di Diritto Canonico* (Milano: A. Giuffrè, 1985) 105. "La Chiesa e una società strutturata in maniera organica, ha senso attribuire rilevanza nel campo del diritto alle affermazioni del Magistero ecclesiastico che indicano come condizione del popolo di Dio la dignità e la libertà o che vedono nella recezione dei carismi personali il fondamento del diritto e del dovere di esercitarli."

apostolate according to the *mens Ecclesiae*.[21]

5. The Juridic Framework of Mercy and Justice Understood as *Intellectus*

Another important component of Pope John XXIII's call for *aggiornamento* stemmed from the idea that the Church is to redefine and update her own self-understanding in light of the Universal Declaration of Human Rights and the new world synthesis whose self-understanding was defined by it.[22] Pastorality, in this new world, now becomes a matter of transmitting the faith—in the fullness of truth, as a gift while simultaneously respecting the rights of those who understand themselves as radically free persons.[23] It was in light of these historical dynamics that *Lumen gentium* also carefully delineated the relationship with *autoritatis* and *sacra potestas* as defined and interpreted through the prism of *diakonia.* Those who serve in administration and governance are to protect and defend the rights of the faithful and eliminate every form of abuse and arbitrariness. In this same regard, Russell Hittinger points out, the victory of the Enlightenment "was a *Logos* tradition that was not only in dialogue with Christiantiy, but helped to lead Christianity to appreciate more deeply its own tradition of reason."[24] The valid technical advancements of the Enlightenment as well as valid critiques of historical religion-state alliances which propagated injustice is true progress and has assisted Christianity to purify its self-understanding and return to its true nature. The *societas perfecta* finds a more textured *approfondimento* in the notion of the Church as *communio* and *diakonia.* This development of our understanding of the *mysterium ecclesiae* in the distinction of powers proves to be of great practical consequence as it enhances our ability to achieve just solutions as well as providing for a more comprehensive and just ordering of

---

21 See Congregation for the Doctrine of the Faith, *Communionis notio* 4, May 28, 1992, http://www.vatican.va/roman_curia/congregations/cfaith/documents/rc_con_cfaith_doc_28051992_communionis-notio_en.html (accessed on 11 Apr. 2020); see also *Lumen gentium* 8. The idea of juridical relationship comes to us from Montesquieu, in his famous work *De l'esprit des lois*, who coined the term *rapport juridique*. It is also translatable in English as relationship of justice. Through Friedrich Karl von Savigny, this concept was injected into the mainstream of legal scholarship in the 19th century. This was all part of a greater movement to emphasize the horizontal, social, and cultural aspects of the juridical phenomenon. In the life of the Church, these horizontal bonds of *communio* as fundamentally constituted relationships of justice find their externalized and visible expression modeled upon and mystically originating in the inter-Trinitarian *communio divinarum personarum*.

22 See S. Valentan, "Freedom of Religion in International Law," *The Canonist* 10 (2019) 25-36.

23 See Jürgen Habermas, *Between Facts and Norms: Contributions to a Discourse Theory of Law and Democracy* (Cambridge: MIT Press, 1996) 174.

24 F. Russell Hittinger, "Natural Law and Public Discourse: The Legacies of Joseph Ratzinger," *Loyola Law Review* 60 (2014) 262.

ecclesial activity (c. 135).[25]

Following this line of thought, we see that the saving dispensation of the Church's salvific goods is an expression of the mystery of communion[26] which lies at the heart of the Church as willed by Christ himself for the salvation of all. A just distribution of Word and Sacrament on the theological, pastoral and juridic plane is one which recognizes the right of all of the faithful to receive the salvific goods of the Church while simultaneously recognizing the right of the legitimate pastors to ensure that the faithful fulfill the Church's requirements for reception of these goods.[27] Needless to say that the nature of law, constituting the norm as an ordinance of reason, always necessitates that the Church's pastors be sensitive to all the dimensions of each case, not in a spirit of laxism and exaggerated permissiveness, but through mercy and justice intersecting in *intellectus*, exercising the use of right reason to draw the truth from the complex weave of dynamics inherent in each juridical situation. Following this criterion and methodology, the nimble mind of the judge makes a calibrated and just decision so that the members of Christ's faithful encounter not a cold, outdated and unreasonable institution, but an efficacious administration of justice and good pastoral governance.

6. What Is Just in the Church's Distribution of Spiritual Goods

In his 2005 encyclical *Deus caritas est*, Pope Benedict XVI highlights that "the Church's deepest nature is expressed in her three-fold responsibility: of proclaiming the word of God (*kerygma-martyria*), celebrating the sacraments (*leitourgia*), and exercising the ministry of charity (*diakonia*). These duties

---

25 See Jorge Miras, Javier Canosa, Eduardo Baura, *Compendio di diritto amministrativo canonico* (Roma: EDUSC, 2007); Pio V. Pinto, *Diritto amministrativo canonico*: La Chiesa mistero e istituzione (Bologna: EDB, 2006) 91-112.

26 See Second Vatican Council, decree *Optatam totius* 16, October 28, 1965: *AAS* 58 (1966) 724, indicating that the *mysterium ecclesiae* is the inescapable reference point of canonical science stating that: "[T]he teaching of canon law and of Church history should take into account the mystery of the Church, according to the dogmatic constitution *De Ecclesia* promulgated by this sacred synod." English translation at http://www.vatican.va/archive/hist_councils/ii_vatican_council/documents/vat-ii_decree_19651028_optatam-totius_en.html (accessed on 11 Apr. 2020). Hence, the essence of law (and rights) in the Church as having its roots in mystery. At the center of the mystery of the Church one finds the mystery of the person and his inviolable dignity which is a prior before any ideology or system. The communitarian dimension of the Church as a mystery of charism and institution finds a full expression in the notion that the "I" of faith, which finds its origin and development in the "we" of the Church.

27 Two great canonists, Mörsdorf and Hervada, intuited first the intrinsic juridicality of the word and of the sacrament and second the sacraments as right-object of justice.

presuppose each other and are inseparable."[28] The Church's spiritual goods at the service of communion: the Word of God, the sacraments and liturgical life of the Church and the work of charity; hence, are all composed of a salvific immediacy. The faithful thus are able to base their right to receive the spiritual goods of the Church upon the dispensing will of the Lord which he has entrusted to the Church and its ministers.

The concept of the Church as a mystery of communion also points us to the reality that the law of the Church is rooted in the sacraments. The ecclesiastical society is manifest in the spatio-temporal realm as structured and organized around the sacraments. As Tomas Rincon-Perez has written that "the fundamental equality of all the baptized, both faithful and the hierarchy, are based respectively on the sacrament of baptism and the sacrament of Holy Orders, and both in the sacrament of the Eucharist, source and summit of communion and interaction between the priesthood of all the faithful and the ministerial priesthood."[29] The sacraments, as channels of grace, are shared goods which are concrete and visible signs of the invisible reality. Hence, they are *res iustae* which have as their foundation not the merits of the minister but the effectiveness *ex opere operato*, that is the merits of Christ.[30] The juridical title that belongs to every believer is based on the foundational will of Christ who instituted the sacraments a true right-object of justice *propter homines*.

The public aspect of the dispensation of the sacraments in an integral dimension of the relationship of justice between the requesting faithful and the sacred ministers. On the normative plane, those laws which make up sacramental law are not only juridical-administrative norms that regulate and delimit conduct, on a more radical plane they help define the identity of the missionary disciple insofar as they are norms that seek to guarantee the vindication and exercise of real, concrete rights. The formalized norms which govern the administration of these externalized goods should reflect the Church's faith in the sacraments and should make access to Divine Mercy not something that is onerous or traumatic, but one that empowers missionary discipleship in the world. The formalization of these fundamental rights in the 1983 Code assumed a *favor libertatis* and were thus constructed to assist the faithful in their living the Gospel.[31] Moreover, these norms regulate and stabilize the ecclesial society as they provide a clear path of access to the plan of salvation envisaged by Christ Himself, who leaves the flock to save one lost sheep. In fact, "the fundamental rights of the faithful, in their

28 Benedict XVI, encyclical *Deus caritas est* 25, December 25, 2005: *AAS* 98 (2006) 236; English translation at http://www.vatican.va/content/benedict-xvi/en/encyclicals/documents/hf_ben-xvi_enc_20051225_deus-caritas-est.html (accessed on 11 Apr. 2020).

29 Tomás Rincon-Perez, "Derecho Administrativo y relaciones de justicia en la administracion de los sacramentos," *Ius Canonicum* 28 (1988) 59, n. 55.

30 See Aquinas, *Summa Theologica* 3.62.5.

31 See Rincon-Perez, 61.

constitutionality, prevail over the volition of the public authority."[32]

Canon 682 of the Pio-Benedictine code of 1917 established that "Laity have the right of receiving from the clergy, in accordance with the norm of ecclesiastical discipline, spiritual goods and especially the aid necessary for salvation."[33] Canon 213 of the 1983 code, placing emphasis on the fundamental equality of all of the baptized and the recognition of rights, states that "The Christian faithful have the right to receive assistance from the sacred pastors out of the spiritual goods of the Church, especially the word of God and the sacraments."[34] In accord with *Lumen gentium* n. 37: "The laity have the right, as do all Christians, to receive in abundance [*abundanter accipiendi]* from their spiritual shepherds the spiritual goods of the Church, especially the assistance of the word of God and of the sacraments."[35] Canon 843 of the 1983 code further stipulates that the Church's "[s]acred ministers cannot deny the sacraments to those who seek them at appropriate times, are properly disposed and are not prohibited by law from receiving them."[36] According to justice, the administration of the sacraments must appropriately conform with the rights to receive them which the faithful enjoy. Within this juridical matrix the radical duty of the hierarchical *ordo* is of a ministerial nature, that is to say, it finds its *raison d'etre* in the spiritual goods of the Word of God and the sacraments being distributed *in abundance*. But this duty should not be viewed solely as an obligation of the office of the minister, but as a vindication of the rights of the faithful.

The Church's sacred ministers are also obliged to furnish for the faithful the proper preparation for the sacraments (c. 843 §2) as well as components of forming the laity in the logic of the Gospel, which is the axis upon which the Church is animated, lives and flourishes. Pastors should always teach and preach *in nomine Ecclesiae* and avoid any type of communication of subjective

---

32 Ibid., 67.

33 *Codex Iuris Canonici Pii X Pontificis Maximi iussu digestus Benedicti Papae XV auctoritate promulgatus* (Rome: Typis Polyglottis Vaticanis, 1917) c. 682; English translation in Edward N. Peters, *The 1917 Pio-Benedictine Code of Canon Law in English Translation with Extensive Scholarly Apparatus* (San Francisco: Ignatius Press, 2001) 258.

34 *Codex Iuris Canonici auctoritate Ioannis Pauli PP. II promulgatus* (Vatican City: Libreria Editrice Vaticana, 1983) c. 213; English translation in *Code of Canon Law. Latin-English Edition: New English Translation* (Washington, DC: Canon Law Society of America, 2012) 279. All subsequent English translations of canons from the 1983 code will be taken from this source unless otherwise indicated.

35 *Lumen gentium* 37; English translation at https://www.vatican.va/archive/hist_councils/ii_vatican_council/documents/vat-ii_const_19641121_lumen-gentium_en.html (accessed on 11 Apr. 2020).

36 1983 *CIC* 843 §1.

ideology.[37] Properly executed education, catechesis and preaching awaken a mature and adult confession of faith and a formation for the evangelical mission.

7. Forming Just and Virtuous Ministers: The *Ordo-Plebs* Binomial

The great Italian jurist Aldo Schiavone writes that with every great systematization of law, there is a danger that something would be lost of the purity and genius of ancient sources, original authors and authorities who animated such crystallizations.[38] Hence, one must always be attentive to maintain connection with the spirit and texts of the ancients, especially when synthesizing them.[39] The great systematization of Gratian in the eleventh century saw the dawn of a new canonical flourishing which was situated within the context of the illustrious reforms of Gregory IX. Nevertheless, a conception of the early Church—that of fundamental equality amongst all of the faithful—began to vanish and instead be replaced by the *duo genera christianorum*. Essentially, the idea gradually evolved that there were two classes of Christians: those who form the clerical and religious caste who are called in a unique and singular to holiness and mission and the rest of the baptized, who do not share the same call to sanctity and apostolate. As Massimo del Pozzo has written: "The ontological and chronological priority of the *communio fidelium* and of the common priesthood of the faithful is practically obscured and placed in the background. Popular cooperation, among other things, is often reduced to the serving and passive role of the recipients of pastoral action (*coetus serviens et oboediens*)."[40] The *ordo-plebs* binomial which existed in the early Church was taken directly from ancient Roman political culture, where the *ordo* was viewed as every much a part of the *plebs*, save for the fact that it consisted of those who had been merely called to a role of service within and for the *plebs*. From this we draw the famous *senatus populusque*.

Professor Del Pozzo continues by stating that:

> In the sources of the *ius antiquum*, there is no logical conceptualization of the figure. However, the Church Fathers and the ecclesiastical authors manifest a remarkable perspicacity and acuity in grasping the composite structure of ecclesiastical society. In the first centuries of Christianity popular cooperation is active and responsible. The *populus christianus*

---

37 See Carlos Errázuriz, *La parola di Dio quale bene giuridico ecclesiale: il munus docendi della Chiesa* (Roma: EDUSC, 2012).

38 Aldo Schiavone, *The Invention of Law in the West* (Cambridge: Harvard University Press, 2012) 19-31.

39 One notes this dynamic as the impetus which animated the Council Fathers at the Second Vatican Council as they sought for *intellectus* within a delicate balance and holding in creative tension the concepts of *ressourcement* and *aggiornamento*.

40 Massimo Del Pozzo, "La struttura 'ordo-plebs' cardine del sistema costituzionale canonico," *Ius Ecclesiae* 26 (2014) 32.

> or the *plebs* (the two concepts are largely equivalent) constitute the point of reference and the identifying factor of the community. The original ecclesiastical organization, albeit still very elementary and embryonic, considered the clergy more according to disciplinary and normative aspects rather than according to jurisdictional ones [...] Practically *ab origine* there has been a clear awareness of the influence of the hierarchical principle in the Christian order. The first, however, to formalize the transfusion in the ecclesiastical sphere of categories of Roman public law doctrine seems to have been Tertullian. "The authority of the Church has established a distinction between the *ordo* and the people (*plebs*)." Origin also repeatedly utilizes Roman municipal distinctions. Later, in St. Cyprian the *plebs* emerges as much in contrast with the *clerus* as the Christian people in general. St. Augustine, in a very well-known passage, explained the duality of position which he assumed (Bishop and Christian) as well as the consciousness of the advantageousness of the common condition of the faithful. Other such verifications of this concept could obviously be multiplied. Patristics ultimately delineates the terms of organic differentiation in the Mystical Body of Christ with clarity.[41]

The Second Vatican Council, hence, paved the way for a revitalization of Christian life by means of a rediscovery of fundamental equality exemplified by the ordo-plebs binomial within the People of God and of baptismal dignity. However, part of this overhaul of ecclesiological self-understanding is addressing the "problems and misunderstandings" which arise when the constitutional logic of the *ordo-plebs* passes to the personalistic logic of states (*clerus-laicatus*). "The incentive for joint cooperation (although historically the principal shortcoming concerns the role of the laity), is therefore not a sort of 'class struggle' or 'promotion of the third state' but an affirmation of the shared co-responsibility of the baptized."[42]

One specific emphasis of Pope Francis has been to challenge priests and religious to rediscover their great dignity and to embrace their duties with new zeal, new methods and new expressions. Following the writings of Henri De Lubac, Pope Francis has emphasized the reality that a kind of "ecclesiastical secularism" has crept into the inner life of the Church through the centuries.[43] It is fair to assert that one of the core dimensions of Pope Francis' challenge to the Church and the *ordo* who are its servants is to understand the intersection of justice and mercy in the search for *intellectus*: the courage to make distinctions and master the art of spiritual discernment, in relation to how we justly distribute

---

41 Ibid., 37.

42 Ibid., 43.

43 Henri de Lubac, *Entretien autor de Vatican II* (Paris: France Catholique CERF, 1985) 25.

the spiritual goods of the Church. For instance, the post-synodal apostolic exhortation *Amoris laetitia* n. 202 states that "ordained ministers often lack the training needed to deal with the complex problems currently facing families."[44]

To effectively minister in today's ever more specialized, expansive and intellectually kinetic and demanding globalized marketplace of ideas, the Church's ministers must cultivate a greater awareness of the insights and valid sophistication of the social sciences, sociology and psychology, personality and behavioral sciences, neuroscience, among other disciplines. Defending the unchanging deposit of faith does not mean falling into another Galileo moment where we publicly embarrass ourselves and weaken our kerygmatic mission. The Church's traditional patrimony of philosophical and theological ideas are composed of such an unparalleled excellence and refined legitimacy that we must give Christ's teaching its due. This is also a challenge for those charged with the formation of the Church's ministers to continue integrate valid insights from the social sciences so that the intersection of mercy and justice in a search for *intellectus* in making scientifically acute distinctions as well as mastering the art of spiritual discernment can be woven into the fabric of inter-ecclesiastical culture. We can anchor ourselves in the wisdom of the Desert Fathers, who were spoken of as great spiritual masters as well as experts in human nature.

When we talk about a just distribution of the spiritual goods of the Church, namely, the Word of God and the sacraments, we are fundamentally talking about inter-ecclesiastical culture and the ministers formed within it. It was Charles Borromeo who formed the seminary system according the latest insights and innovations of culture at the time. Are we doing the same to form the outstanding men who sacrifice fortune and family to serve the family of God in this distribution and ministerial service? When we speak of justice, we treasure and adhere to our traditional patrimony of Aristotle, Aquinas and the natural law tradition. Yet, in the face of multi-dimensional layers of De-Hellinization, the Second Vatican Council envisioned a richer biblical, patristic and Thomistic scientific engagement with new ways of exploring and articulating human reality which would buttress and defend the natural law tradition.

8. Conclusion

The notion of the inherent sacramentality and ministeriality of justice and mercy in the Church is found in the virtue of those practitioners, canonists, jurists and those who are responsible for pastoral leadership and governance. Virtue in the sense of Aristotle's understanding of *hexis*—the ability to balance and maintain a healthy tension between disparate, seemingly paradoxical and even

44 Francis, post-synodal apostolic exhortation *Amoris laetitia* 202, March 19, 2016: *AAS* 108 (2016) 391-392; English translation at https://w2.vatican.va/content/dam/francesco/pdf/apost_exhortations/documents/papa-francesco_esortazione-ap_20160319_amoris-laetitia_en.pdf (accessed on 11 Apr. 2020).

counter-intuitive dynamics. Mercy and justice fused and synergized under the banner of *intellectus* will see the Church's ministers and us as jurists utilizing the tools of right reason, both in theory as well as praxis. This provides us canonical professionals with great confidence in applying Magisterial teaching in combination with the valid developments of the sciences, law and culture. In a word, we need to deepen our internal juridical culture. To restore what is just in the Church and in society to its ancient prestige, we must become better trained and be better, more assiduous adherents to what is articulated in the classical conception of the *ius*. All that is needed for pastoral application, such as the principles of *aequitas* and *epikeia,* as well as all legitimate legal institutions, are valid means to render *iustitia dulcore misericordiae temperata.*

Justice and mercy in the realm of the dispensation of the Church's spiritual goods is fundamentally about the faithful's right to spiritual aid so that they may properly live the dynamism of the missionary vocation. The *munus docendi* and the *munus sanctificandi* are correlative to right to formation for the apostolate as well as the protection of the legitimate autonomy of the faithful in carrying out their mission in the world. The totality of this spiritual assistance is envisaged to see the Church at its best: being like a sacrament. On a vertical plane this consists of discipleship—a transformational encounter with the living and risen Christ so that those who actively, intentionally and vigorously participate in the sacramental life of the Church are formed as true disciples of the Master. On a horizontal plane—these fervent and assiduous disciples are empowered and equipped by the members of the *ordo* to take up the missionary mandate of Christ to transform the world as witnesses to the Resurrection.

Seminar

Proceed with Caution: Canon 1071 and Licit Assistance at Marriage

The Reverend David Fulton, JCD

In the juridic discipline of Catholic marriage, there are circumstances which can impede a person from validly marrying. There are other non-invalidating circumstances requiring a cleric or a delegated layperson to proceed with caution and not to assist at marriage without the permission of the local ordinary. The majority of such circumstances have been catalogued in canon 1071. This paper will consider the substance of the circumstances of canon 1071 as they were stipulated in Trent, in the pontificate of Benedict XIV and in the 1917 Code of Canon Law. It then will examine the circumstances as specified in canon 1071 and consider their significance in marriage preparation.

The so-called new natural lawyers (Germain Grisez, Joseph Boyle, John Finnis, Robert George) have proposed seven "basic human goods" which enable human flourishing and give rise to the precepts of the natural law that offer direction or directives for living a moral life. Such basic goods include self-integration, authenticity, justice and friendship, religion, human life itself, knowledge of the truth and appreciation of beauty, playful activities and skilled performances.[1] Germain Grisez and John Finnis propose an eighth stand-alone basic good: the good of marriage.[2]

One may wish to agree with Finnis and Grisez and accept marriage as a basic human good; one may disagree and consider marriage not to be a basic good but a useful good for human flourishing.[3] In either case, one can propose that, as a result of the good of marriage, whether basic or instrumental, the right to marry

---

1 See John Finnis, Germain Grisez and Joseph Boyle, "Practical Principles Moral Truth, and Ultimate Ends," *American Journal of Jurisprudence* 99 (1987) 103-113.

2 See Joshua D. Goldstein, "New Natural Law Theory and the Grounds of Marriage: Friendship and Self-Constitution," Social Theory and Practice 37, no. 3 (2011) 461-482..

3 For a comprehensive exposition of what new natural lawyers propose as basic goods, see Sabina Alkire, "The basic dimensions of human flourishing: a comparison of accounts," in *The Revival of Natural Law: Philosophical, Theological, and Ethical Responses to the Finnis-Grisez School*, ed. Nigel Biggar et al. (Burlington, VT: Ashgate, 2000) 73–100.

is a core human right.

While the right to marry is a fundamental human right, this right is not absolute. The current Code of Canon Law acknowledges both the right to marry and its non-absolute nature. Canon 1058 puts it this way: "All persons *who are not prohibited by law* can contract marriage" (emphasis added).[4]

The legal prohibitions to marry referred to in canon 1058 are principally set forth in the code's list of matrimonial impediments, by virtue of which a person is rendered unqualified to contract matrimony validly.[5] The code, in canon 1095 and following, also implicitly prohibits marriage by persons whose consent for marriage is misplaced or is somehow seriously defective.

There are two other sorts of canons that do not prohibit persons from contracting marriage validly, but rather touch on the lawful contracting of marriage or assisting at a marriage. The first of these is typified in canon 1124, which addresses the couple contracting marriage and prohibits a Catholic and a baptized non-Catholic from marrying without the express permission of competent authority.[6] The second of these canonical prohibitions is not about the couple who wish to marry; rather, it is about the minister who is to preside at the wedding. Stipulations of this type prohibit clergy or other designated ministers from assisting at marriage until certain conditions have been met. Canonical stipulations of this type are, at heart, warnings to the assisting minister in his or her pastoral preparation of a couple planning marriage; they require the assisting minister to proceed with particular caution. Disregarding the warnings encased in these stipulations would not result in a marriage's invalidity; it would not render the consent to marriage illicit. Rather, disregard of these warnings would render assisting at such a marriage illicit.

Canon 1106 is one example of this sort of prohibiting canon. It lays down the following stipulation:

---

4 *Codex Iuris Canonici auctoritate Ioannis Pauli PP. II promulgatus* (Vatican City: Libreria Editrice Vaticana, 1983) [hereafter 1983 *CIC*] c. 1058: "Omnes possunt matrimonium contrahere qui iure not prohibentur." English translation from *Code of Canon Law, Latin-English Edition: New English Translation* (Washington, DC: Canon Law Society of America, 2012). All subsequent English translations of canons from this code will be taken from this source unless otherwise indicated.

5 See 1983 *CIC* c. 1073: "Impedimentum dirimens personam inhabilem reddit ad matrimonium valide contrahendum." See canons 1073-1094 for the code's list of diriment impediments.

6 See 1983 *CIC* c. 1124: "Matrimonium inter duas personas baptizatas, quarum altera sit in Ecclesia catholica baptizata vel in eandem post baptismum recepta, altera vero Ecclesiae vel communitati ecclesiali plenam communionem cum Ecclesia catholica non habenti adscripta, sine expressa auctoritatis competentis licentia prohibitum est."

> Marriage can be contracted through an interpreter; the pastor, however, *is not to assist* at it unless he is certain of the trustworthiness of the interpreter.[7]

A second example of a law prohibiting assistance at a marriage is canon 1071. This canon not only requires caution on the part of the assisting minister; it requires the minister to seek a second set of eyes to examine the matter and to receive permission of a local ordinary before proceeding with the wedding. This canon's imposing caution, requiring a second set of eyes and stipulating permission of a local ordinary is what we will be considering today. Here is the text of the canon:

> §1. Except in a case of necessity, a person is not to assist without the permission of the local ordinary at:
>
> 1° a marriage of transients;
>
> 2° a marriage which cannot be recognized or celebrated according to the norm of civil law;
>
> 3° a marriage of a person who is bound by natural obligations toward another party or children arising from a previous union;
>
> 4° a marriage of a person who has notoriously rejected the Catholic faith;
>
> 5° a marriage of a person who is under a censure;
>
> 6° a marriage of a minor child when the parents are unaware or reasonably opposed;
>
> 7° a marriage to be entered into through a proxy as mentioned in can. 1105.
>
> §2. The local ordinary is not to grant permission to assist at the marriage of a person who has notoriously rejected the Catholic faith unless the norms mentioned in can. 1125 have been observed with necessary

7 1983 *CIC* c. 1106: "Matrimonium per interpretem contrahi potest; cui tamen parochus ne assistat, nisi de interpretis fide sibi constet."

adaptation.[8]

In considering canon 1071, I will first consider historical roots of the canon's list of persons and circumstances that require special caution. Next, I will offer observations on the construction of the canon as it has been presently formulated in the code. Finally, I will offer comments on some of the details of the canon and how these details touch on the way that priests and designated ministers need to engage in marriage preparation.

I. Some historical underpinnings of elements of the canon

The classes of persons and the circumstances of the proposed marriages requiring caution and permission by canon 1071 §1 are not entirely new to the 1983 code. Some of them can be found in the Council of Trent; another has been included in the jurisprudence of Benedict XIV; others are stipulated in the 1917 Code of Canon Law. Moreover, some items in the list of canon 1071 are quite ancient and are included in the *Corpus Iuris Canonici*. The following exploration of the canon's historical roots is not exhaustive, nor does it propose to illuminate the entire range of such historical roots. It offers instead an examination of the major underpinnings and juridic directions of the elements of the canon.

A. Canon 1071 §1, 1° Marriage of *vagi*

The *Tametsi* decree of Trent, in chapter 7, addresses the caution that is needed in the marriage of *vagi,* as well as the stipulation prohibiting priests from assisting at such marriages without the permission of an Ordinary. Here is the English text:

> *Vagi* are to be married with caution. There are many persons who are *vagi*, having no settled homes; and, being of a profligate character, they, after abandoning their first wife, marry another, and very often several in different places, during the lifetime of the first. The Holy Synod, being desirous to obviate this disorder, gives this fatherly admonition to all

---

8 1983 *CIC* c. 1071:

§ 1. Excepto casu necessitatis, sine licentia Ordinarii loci ne quis assistat:
1° matrimonio vagorum;
2° matrimonio quod ad normam legis civilis agnosci vel celebrari nequeat;
3° matrimonio eius qui obligationibus teneatur naturalibus erga aliam partem filiosve ex praecedenti unione ortis;
4° matrimonio eius qui notorie catholicam fidem abiecerit;
5° matrimonio eius qui censura innodatus sit;
6° matrimonio filii familias minoris, insciis aut rationabiliter invitis parentibus;
7° matrimonio per procuratorem ineundo, de quo in can. 1105.

§ 2. Ordinarius loci licentiam assistendi matrimonio eius qui notorie catholicam fidem abiecerit ne concedat, nisi servatis normis de quibus in can. 1125, congrua congruis referendo.

> whom it may concern, not easily to admit this class of *vagi* to marriage; and It also exhorts the civil magistrates to punish such persons severely. *But it commands parish priests not to be present at the marriages of such persons, unless they have first made a careful inquiry, and, having reported the circumstance to the Ordinary, they shall have obtained permission from him for so doing.*[9]

The stipulation of *Tametsi* is incorporated into *Ne temere,* the 1907 decree of the Sacred Congregation of the Council, which, in part V §4, makes the following provision about *vagi*:

> With respect to *vagi*, except in cases of necessity, it is not permitted for the pastor to assist at their marriages, unless, having referred the matter to the Ordinary or a priest delegated by him, he obtains permission to do so.[10]

Canon 1032 of the 1917 code incorporates the stipulations of *Tametsi* and *Ne temere* and legislates as follows:

> For the marriage of a *vagus* (refer to Can. 91) the pastor is never to assist, except in the case of necessity, unless, after the matter has been given to the Ordinary of the Place or to a priest delegated by him, [the pastor] shall have received the permission for assisting. [11]

In the above-cited treatment of *vagi* there are two notable elements. First, *Tametsi, Ne temere* and the 1917 code detail the caution to be exercised by pastors in examining items that must precede the celebration of marriage as part of their establishing no prior existing bond of marriage and thus the freedom of a couple to marry. Second, both *Ne temere* and canon 1032 carve out an exception to the prohibition to assist: the circumstance of *a case of necessity.*

B. Canon 1071 §1, 4° Marriage of a person who has notoriously rejected the Catholic faith

---

9 Council of Trent, decree *Tametsi*, November 11, 1563; English translation from *The Canons and Decrees of the Sacred and Oecumenical Council of Trent*, transl. J. Waterworth (London: C Dolman, 1848) 202.

10 Pius X, decree *Ne temere*, 19 April 1908, V §4, *ASS* 40 (1907) 528: "Quoad *vagos,* extra casum necessitates parocho ne liceat eorum matrimoniis adsistere, nisi re ad Ordinarium vel ad sacerdotem ab eo delegatum delata, licentiam adsistendi impetraverit." English translation by the author.

11 1917 *CIC* c. 1032: "Matrimonio vagorum de quibus in can 91, parochus, excepto causu necessitatis, nunquam assistat, nisi, re ad loci Ordinarium vel ad sacerdotem ab eo delegatum delata, licentiam assistendi obtinuerit." Hereafter, English translations from the 1917 code are those of the author, unless otherwise noted.

Although some local synods addressed the problem of the rejection of the Catholic faith as early as 1626 in the Synod of Sion in Switzerland,[12] the situation of the rejection of the Catholic faith seems to have gotten the particular attention of the Holy See in the second half of the nineteenth century. This was a result not only of the secularization of France but also of the growing anti-Church sentiment in Italy. The 1917 code addressed the matter in canon 1065 §2:

> A pastor is not to assist at the weddings [of those who have notoriously rejected the Catholic faith, even if they have not gone over to a non-Catholic sect, or those who are enrolled in a society condemned by the Church] without consulting the Ordinary who, after having inspected all the circumstances of the matter can permit him to be present for the marriage, provided there is a grave cause urging this decision, and provided that the Ordinary, in his own prudent judgment determines there is sufficient caution in place for the Catholic education of all the children and as well as that the danger of perversion of the other spouse is removed.[13]

The term *notorious* needs a bit of parsing. Notoriety can be either notoriety of fact or of law. Notoriety *of fact* is notoriety that "would be publicly known and is committed in such circumstances that it could not be concealed by subterfuge nor excused by juridic opinion."[14] Notoriety *of law* is notoriety that "comes into existence after the sentence of a competent judge which has become a *res iudicata*, or after the confession of a delinquent in a trial, made according to the norm of [law]."[15] The notoriety of canon 1065 of the 1917 code is, in virtually every imaginable case, notoriety of fact. Additionally, this canon clearly and principally targets *Catholics* who have enrolled in a society condemned by the Church. Whether the pastor who is preparing a non-Catholic who has joined condemned societies requires permission of the ordinary, in addition to a dispensation from mixed religion or disparity of worship, was a matter of some

---

12 "Inter baptizatum Catholicum et Haereticam, aposticam, et excommunicatum. Validum quidem est Matrimonium, set non licitum. *Hartzheim,* IX, 388." Quoted in John Joseph Heneghan, *The Marriages of Unworthy Catholics* (Washington DC: The Catholic University of America Press, 1944) 20-21.

13 1917 *CIC* c. 1065 §2: "Parochus praedictis nuptiis ne assistat, nisi consulto Ordinario, qui, inspectis omnibus rei adjunctis, ei permittere poterit ut matrimonio intersit, dummodo urgeat gravis causa et pro suo prudenti arbitrio Ordinarius iudicet satis cautum esse catholicae educationi universae prolis et remotioni periculi perversionis alterius coniugis."

14 1917 *CIC* c. 2197, 3°: "*Notorium notoritate facti* si publice notum sit et in talibus adjunctis commissum, ut nulla tergiversatione celari nulloque iuris suffragio excusari possit."

15 1917 *CIC* c. 2197, 2°: "*Notorium notorietate iuris*, post sententiam iudicis competntis quae in rem iudicatam transierit aut post confessionem delinquentis in iudicio factam ad normam can. 1750."

dispute for the interpreters of the 1917 code.[16]

Issues of notorious rejection of the Catholic faith and membership in forbidden societies resulted in specific questions about membership in the Masons, in the Communist party and in an atheist sect. The Holy Office, responding to questions about this canon, stated that a priest could, with the permission of his ordinary, assist at the weddings of members of the Communist party.[17] It further stipulated that those who were members of an atheist sect were to be treated as members of a non-Catholic sect, and thus needed to fulfill the *cautiones,* promising to raise as Catholic the children of either sex who were born of the marriage.[18]

C. Canon 1071 §1, 5° Marriage of a person under censure

As a result of the excommunications connected with membership in anti-Catholic organizations such as the Freemasons in Europe, the marriage of persons under censure became something of a common question in the nineteenth century. The issue of the marriage of public sinners and persons under censure, however, dates well before the 1800s, indeed to the earliest days of the Church.

I Corinthians 13:1-5 considers the exclusion from the community of a man guilty of serious sexual immorality. Early practices of ecclesiastical penance included excluding a sinner who had confessed from full participation in the *communio* of the Church until public penances had been performed. By the eleventh century excommunication had gained the status of juridic institution. In the thirteenth century all excommunications, by decree of Gregory IX, were to be understood as "major excommunications." A part of such major excommunications was the Church's declaration of a person's unworthiness to contract marriage. By the fifteenth century, the draconian institution of solely major excommunication was softened. In his constitution *Ad vitanda* in 1418, Pope Martin V re-established the distinction between excommunicated persons *tolerati* and those *vitandi*. As a result, a system developed in which two distinct sorts of excommunications were in place: mild excommunication, by virtue of which the person excommunicated was tolerated in and by community, and severe excommunication, by which that person was to be avoided, even expelled from church community and church services.

Excommunication, in its mild forms, whether notorious or not, did not mean exclusion from the community of the Church; it meant denial of the goods of the Church, particularly the goods of the sacraments. It was in the middle of the nineteenth century when exclusion from matrimony as a result of

---

16 See, e.g., Heneghan, 102-103.

17 See Supreme Sacred Congregation of the Holy Office, *Dubium: De Celebratione Matrimonii Inter Acatholicos*, June 30, 1949: *AAS* 41 (1949) 427-428.

18 Ibid.

excommunication came under scrutiny.

On December 10, 1860, the Sacred Penitentiary responded to a query on the procedure to be employed by pastors when a person planning marriage had incurred ecclesiastical censure. The Penitentiary recommended that every effort should be made to reconcile the censured person to the Church. If the person refused reconciliation, and *if grave evil seemed imminent unless marriage was allowed*, the pastor was prohibited from assisting at the marriage unless he had consulted with the ordinary. The Penitentiary noted that the ordinary was not only to consider the relevant circumstances of the case, but was also to refer to approved authors, especially St. Alphonsus, in making his decision on permitting the pastor to assist. In any event, even if the pastor received permission to assist at the wedding, no celebration of Mass at the wedding was to be included in the permission.[19]

The Penitentiary's reference to St. Alphonsus concerned his teaching on a pastor's assisting at marriages of public sinners and publicly unworthy persons. St. Alphonsus held that assistance at such marriages or serving as a witness at such marriages might very possibly involve cooperation in the sin of another. However, he noted, the pastor would be excused from wrongdoing if he assisted in order to avoid death or in order to prevent some even greater evil coming upon the community or upon the bride and groom. An example of avoiding a greater evil, Alphonsus proposed, would be to keep the bride and groom from living for a long time without marriage and thus in the state of sin.[20]

Building on this history, canon 1066 of the 1917 code considered this situation:

> If a public sinner or a person who is notoriously under censure refuses to approach confession or refuses to be reconciled with the Church, the pastor is not to assist at his or her marriage, unless grave cause urges it, about which, if possible, he should consult with the Ordinary.[21]

D. Canon 1071 §1, 6º Marriage of a minor child when the parents are unaware or reasonably opposed

The issue of status as a result of age has been convoluted in the Church's history. Juridic communities have, from time immemorial, understood that capacity to marry requires a minimal level of mental and emotional capacity

19 See *Codici Iuris Canonici Fontes,* ed. Pietro Gaspari (Typis Polyglottis Vaticanis, 1923-1939) 6426.

20 See Alphonsus de Ligouri, *Theologia Moralis,* ed. Gaude (Rome: 1912) IV, n. 54.

21 1917 *CIC* c. 1066: "Si publicus peccator aut censura notorie innodatus prius ad sacramentalem confessionem accedere aut cum Ecclesia recnciliari recusaverit, parochus eius matrimonio ne assistat, nisi gravis urgeat causa, de qua, si fieri possit, consulat Ordinarium."

to intellectually understand, evaluatively appreciate and personally embrace the reality of marriage. Additionally, capacity to marry involves sexual maturity on the part of both of the partners that would enable them to engage in coitus and thus to consummate the marriage. As a result of their considering matters of psychological and sexual maturity, juridic communities have set in law a minimum age for marriage.

In Roman law, the age of fourteen was the legally stipulated age at which a boy was released from guardianship and began to enjoy the full rights of citizenship. Fourteen was also the age which Roman law established as the minimum for a male to marry. Roman law stipulated that for females, the minimum age was twelve. There was a presumption embedded in the ages of fourteen and twelve, viz, that, at these statutory ages, puberty had occurred and sexual coitus was possible. The law also presumed that, by the age of fourteen and twelve, the partners had achieved the minimal mental and emotional maturity needed to marry. The Church of the Western Empire adopted Roman law on the issue of the minimum age for marriage.

Justinian's Codex employed the same minimum age for marriage in the Empire of the East as it was in the West. But there was one significant difference: in the East, the ages of fourteen and sixteen were statutory, and not statutory but presumptive, as in the West. As a result, "legal puberty rather than actual puberty became the minimum age for marriage in the Eastern churches."[22] Thomas Aquinas weighed in on the issue of teenage marriage. In the Summa theologiae he stated, "Upon reaching puberty, a free person may dispose of his own person in matters such as making a commitment to enter religion or marriage."[23] In the West, actual puberty rather than merely statutory puberty remained the norm until the 1917 code.[24]

Despite the minimum ages established in East and West, customary law in the West during the early middle ages seems to have afforded parents the liberty of arranging childhood marriages, for their children between the ages of seven and statutory puberty. However, upon reaching statutory puberty the children of childhood marriages could escape them and their binding force. Moreover, the parents who had arranged these childhood marriages could not insist that such marriages should bind their children to conjugal vinculum.[25]

---

22 John P. Beal, "Title VII: Marriage," in *New Commentary on the Code of Canon Law,* ed. John P. Beal et al. (New York: Paulist Press, 2000) 1283.

23 Aquinas, *Summa Theologiae* [hereafter *S.T.*] II-II.88.8, ad 2.

24 See Beal, 1283.

25 See R.H. Helmholz, *The Spirit of Classical Canon Law* (Athens, GA: The University of Georgia Press, 2010) 237-238.

Building on this history, the Corpus iuris canonici is clear in its stipulation that marriage of a female who has not completed her twelfth year and a male who has not completed his fourteenth is invalid. The 1917 code changed the minimum age, however, raising the minimum age for both the male and the female by two years. This is how canon 1067 §1 put it: "A man before the sixteenth year of age having been completed and a woman prior to having completed fourteen years are unable (non possunt) to enter a valid marriage."[26]

Raising the minimum age for marriage is consistent with the 1917 code's stipulations about status in the church as a result of age. Canon 88 declared anyone under the age of seven to be an infant; it declared anyone under twenty one to be a minor; and it also declared minor males who had completed their sixteenth year and minor females who had completed their fourteenth year to be termed *pubes.*

More than merely stipulating minimum age for a valid marriage, and more than simply considering the right to marry as an unobstructed right, some theologians have noted that the exercise of sexuality and its proper marital context need to be considered in the context of a minor's position within a family. Thomas Aquinas is worth noting in this regard, particularly in his treatment of the species of lust he terms seduction. For Aquinas, seduction describes a situation in which a man convinces a woman who is still under the care and protection of her father to engage in sex. Although the woman may be a willing participant, this sexual act damages, even destroys, the good of a proper marriage. Extending Aquinas' rationale, it may be argued that, since a father has special responsibility of care and protection for minor children until they reach adulthood or are emancipated, marriage of a *pubes* whose father is unaware or reasonably unwilling would undermine the social good of family security as it potentially undermines the social good of marriages having a place within the family from which the minor child has come.[27]

The second paragraph of canon 1067 of the 1917 code acknowledged the validity of the marriage of a *pubes;* but it proposed a caution for pastors of souls in such marriages. It stated:

> Although contracting matrimony past the above stated age may be valid, nonetheless pastors of souls need to take care to dissuade young people from marrying before an age at which, according to the accepted

26 1917 *CIC* c. 1067 §1: "Vir ante decimum sextum aetatis annum completum, mulier ante decimum quartum item completum, matrimonium validum inire non possunt."

27 See *S.T.* II-II.154.2.

mores of the region, marriage is wont to be entered into.[28]

A further caution is offered by the code, as it considered the obligations of pastors dealing with a marriage of *pubes* whose parents were unwilling that the proposed marriage proceed or unaware that the marriage had been proposed. Here is how canon 1034 of the 1917 code put it:

> The pastor is to seriously exhort minors who are still children in a family not to enter marriage if the parents are either unaware or reasonably opposed to it. If they refuse [not to marry] then the pastor is not to assist at the marriage unless the Ordinary of the place has been consulted.[29]

E. Canon 1071 §1, 7º Marriage to be entered into through a proxy

Proxy weddings have been part of the western legal tradition since the time of late Roman law.[30] Marriage is a contract in Roman law, whose only requirement for validity is consent that is mutually expressed. The expression of this consent could be in person; but it could also be by letter, or through the use of an agent, a messenger, or a proxy. By the middle of the sixth century the corpus iuris civilis required Christian parties to "bring the fact of marriage to the notice of the church."[31] Despite the requirement for presence of the parties at church, ecclesiastical law, interestingly, did not dismiss marriage by proxy as invalid.[32]

By the thirteenth century, during the papacy of Innocent III, proxy marriages were declared valid, with the possibility of either husband or wife employing a proxy at the wedding ceremony.[33] A century later, during the papacy of Boniface VIII, a number of canonists began to object to proxy weddings; but, despite these objections, the Church continued to view proxy weddings as valid. This view of the validity of proxy marriage was not overturned by the Council of Trent. The tradition of the validity of a proxy marriage was incorporated into the 1917 code in canon 1088 §1: "For matrimony to be contracted validly, it is necessary that

---

28 1917 *CIC* c. 1067 §2: "Licet matrimonium post praedictam aetatem contractum validum sit, current tamen animarum pastores ab eo avertere iuenes ante aetatem qua, secundum regionis receptos mores, matrimonium inire solet."

29 1917 *CIC* c. 1034: "Parochus graviter filiosfamilias minores hortetur ne nuptias ineant, insciis aut rationabiliter invitis parentibus; quod si abnuerint, eorum matrimonio ne assistat, nisi consulto prius loci Ordinarius."

30 For more on the classic treatment of proxy marriage and its history, see Ernest G. Lorenzen, "Marriage by Proxy and the Conflict of Laws," Harv. L. Rev. 32 (1919) 473-488, https://digitalcommons.law.yale.edu/fss_papers/4561 (accessed on 21 Jan. 2020).

31 Ibid., 476, note 35.

32 See Andrea B. Carroll, "Reviewing Proxy Marriage," LSU Journal Articles 166 (2011) 8-9, https://digitalcommons.law.lsu.edu/faculty_scholarship/166 (accessed on 21 Jan. 2020).

33 See Lorenzen, 474.

the contracting parties be present, either per se or through proxies."[34]

Citing precedents in the *Corpus Iuris Canonici,* canon 1089 of the 1917 code required particular caution for weddings that used a proxy. It stipulated that there needed to be a special mandate for contracting marriage with a particular person which was signed by the mandating party and also by the pastor, or by the ordinary of the place where the mandate was made, or by a priest delegated by either of them, or by at least two witnesses.[35]

Canon 1091 enlarged upon canon 1089, specifying an even further caution to be observed by pastors when not only a proxy but also an interpreter is to be involved in a marriage ceremony. The caution enjoined by the canon also required the permission of the ordinary if at all possible. Here is how canon 1091 put it:

> Pastors shall not assist at marriages contracted through proxies or interpreters unless there is a just cause and there can be no doubt about the authenticity of the mandate or the trustworthiness of the interpreter, and unless the permission of the Ordinary is obtained, if time allows for this.[36]

Of the seven circumstances listed in the first paragraph of canon 1071 of the 1983 code, five of them can be found in the 1917 code and have their origin in rules of law that far predate the early twentieth century. Moreover, it is notable that the five circumstances of the 1917 code that restricted a pastor's assistance at a wedding or required the prior consent of the ordinary of the place were not located in a single context in the 1917 code, but were situated in three distinct contexts:

- The weddings of *vagi* (c. 1032) and of a minor whose parents were unaware or unwilling (c. 1034) were located in the chapter dealing with the items that need to be in place prior to the wedding and were concerned with discovering the existence of canonical freedom and social propriety.

- The weddings of those who had notoriously abandoned the Catholic faith (c. 1065) and of public sinners and those under censure (c. 1066) were

34 1917 *CIC* c. 1088 §1: "Ad matrimonium valide contrahendum necesse est ut contrahentes sint presents sive per se ipsi sive per procurators."

35 See 1917 *CIC* c. 1089: ". . . ut matrimonium per procuratorem valide ineature, requirit mandatum speciale and contrahendum cum certa persona, subscriptum a mandante veet vel a parocho, aut Ordinario lovi in quo mandatum fit, vel a sacerdote ab alterutro delegato, vel a doubus saltem testibus."

36 1917 *CIC* c. 1091: "Matrimonio per procuratorem ve per interpretem contrahendo parochus ne assistat, nisi adsit iusta causa et de authenticitate mandate vel vide interpretis dubitari nullo modo liceat, habita, si tempus suppetat, Ordinarii licentia."

treated in the chapter on impedient impediments.

- The weddings employing a proxy (c. 1091) were treated in the chapter on matrimonial consent.

II. The construction of canon 1071 as it is formulated in the 1983 code

Prior to discussing the text of canon 1071 it is important to rehearse some details of the work of revising the code of 1983. The following pages will, first, offer an overview of the work of the revision of the Code of Canon Law. Next, they will comment on the first set of changes that were made in what would become canon 1071 between the years 1977 and 1980. Finally, they will note the changes made prior to the canon's final form, made between 1980 and 1982.

A. An overview of the revision of the Code of Canon Law

In the revision of the Code of Canon Law, a commission for the work was appointed by the pope, from which a number of committees were formed. Each committee of the Commission for Revision was to work generally as an independent group under the Commission's general supervision, discussing and re-working the sectors of the code assigned to them. When sectors of work were completed a schema would be constructed, and the president of the Commission sent each schema to the so-called organs of consultation: the Holy Father himself, the cardinal-members of the central commission, the dicasteries of the Roman Curia, ecclesiastical universities and faculties, the Union of Superiors General and the episcopal conferences of the world. Every schema for the new code was sent out by 1977. The organs of consultation were asked to respond to each section and were given no less than six months within which to offer their responses. Largely for purposes of organization, the ten individual schematic sectors were joined together into an over-all collection, called the Schema of 1977.

From 1977 until 1980 the committees and the central commission synthesized the responses from the organs of consultation and discussed them. Committees and the commission met to incorporate some of the received suggestions, and to introduce some of their own recommendations. After the individual schemata had been revised, they were given to the Secretary of the Commission, who produced a second schema, published on June 29, 1980. This schema was discussed and criticized by the cardinal-members of the commission and also by other experts on canon law, who were selected by episcopal conferences throughout the world and made members of the commission. The result of their work was sent to the Commission Secretary, who prepared a synthesis of observations which was sent to members of the Commission in August of 1981. Following this, a plenary session of the Commission for Revision met in October of 1981. The work of the Commission and its committees was performed in planned stages.

The basic strategy was to consist of: (1) preparation of revisions to the law by the working committees; (2) organization of revisions into schemata by the working committees and the Commission; (3) world-wide transmission of schemata for comment; (4) re-working the schemata and preparing an over-all schema taking into account the comments received; (5) discussion of the second schema; (6) preparation of another schema, and repetition of the process of consultation, as required.

The Roman pontiff convoked a plenary session of the commission, which met from October 20 until October 28, 1981. At this session the material under consideration was the Schema of 1980. The result of the plenary session was the Schema of 1982. This schema, which polished the Latin text of the Schema of 1980, emended some of the 1980 schema and added canons from the Schema on the Fundamental Law of the Church, was presented to John Paul II on April 22, 1982. He made some changes to the schema, and, on January 25, 1983, he promulgated the revised Code of Canon Law.

B. Changes between the 1977 schema and the 1980 schema

The discussion of the Commission began by bringing together and organizing under the single rubric of pastoral preparation circumstances that were scattered in the text of the 1917 code and which were presented in four distinct places in the *Schema de Sacramentis*.[37] When the text of the 1977 schema was presented to the committee's consultors for consideration, the Relator had brought into one paragraph elements that were scattered in the original 1977 schema, mirroring the scattering of the 1917 code. In this single paragraph constructed by the Relator, there were six circumstances where the permission of the local ordinary would be required for licit assistance at a wedding. Moreover, the Relator's single paragraph set down an exception to the requirement of the permission of the local ordinary for all six circumstances. The exception: *cases of necessity*.[38]

At the very beginning of their discussion of the text proposed by the Relator the consultors unanimously decided to eliminate one of the six circumstances proposed in the text.[39] The deleted circumstance proposed the case of a marriage between those who, while a prior marriage perdured, had committed adultery with each other and had attempted a civil marriage.[40] The reason for deleting the

37 See Pontifica Commissio Codici Iuris Canonici Recognoscendo, *Schema documenti pontifici quo disciplina canonica de sacramentis recognoscitur (*Typis Polyglottis Vaticanis, 1975*)* 255, 281, 258, 307 [hereafter *Sacramentis*].

38 In the original sectors of the 1977 schema, the exception of cases of necessity was offered only in the case of the marriage of *vagi.*

39 See *Communicationes* 9 (1977) 143.

40 See *Communicationes* 9 (1977) 143: "De matrimonio eorum qui perdurante priore matrimonio adulterium inter se consummaverunt et matrimonium per civilem actum attentaverunt."

circumstance was the difficulty of proving adultery.

The other five circumstances proposed for discussion were: (a) the marriage of *vagi*; (b) a marriage that, for any reason whatsoever, could not be civilly acknowledged or celebrated; (c) the marriage of a person who had notoriously rejected the Catholic faith even if she or he had not gone over to a non-Catholic community or had enrolled in a forbidden society; (d) the marriage of minor children which parents opposed; and (e) a marriage contracted through a proxy.

During the discussion, two circumstances were added to the five: (1) marriage of someone who is bound by natural obligations toward another party or to children who had been born in a previous union; (2) marriage of one who is under censure. The first of these changes was altogether new; the second, although present in the 1917 code, had simply been omitted in the *schemata de sacramentis*.

When the case of the person under censure was reintroduced into the commission's discussion, the text agreed upon by the consultors changed the circumstance as stated in the 1917 code. There, canon 1066 required oversight and permission for a person who was "*a public sinner* or a person who is *notoriously* under censure and refuses to approach confession or refuses to be reconciled with the Church." In its construction by the consultors and its inclusion in the text of the Schema of 1980, the person is described simply as *one who is under censure*. The text of the 1980 schema does not mention public sinners and does not require either that the censure be notorious or that the person under censure refuses to go to confession or to be reconciled with the Church.

The discussion that resulted in the text of the 1980 schema made two more slight changes in its considering a person who had notoriously abandoned the Catholic faith: (1) it adjusted the mood of the verb *abiecere,* altering it from the perfect indicative to the perfect subjunctive; (2) it altered the 1977 schema's term *acatholicam* (which is also the terminology of the 1917 code) to *non catholicam.*

As a result of their discussion, the consultors added a second full paragraph to the text of the 1977 schema that was to be included in the text of the Schema of 1980.[41] The added paragraph states:

> The Ordinary of the place is not to grant permission to assist at the marriage of a person who has notoriously rejected the Catholic faith unless the norms mentioned in can 1079 have been observed with

---

41 Originally the substance of the added paragraph had been included in the text of the circumstance concerning one who had notoriously abandoned the Catholic faith. The consultors considered the requirement of the *cautiones* to be important enough to warrant a separate paragraph in the proposed canon. See *Communicationes* 9 (1977) 145, 146.

necessary adaptation.[42]

C. Changes between the 1980 schema and the 1982 schema

With the two additional circumstances requiring the permission of the local ordinary, the deletion of public sinners and notoriety of censure from the circumstance's description, and the inclusion of an entire second paragraph to the proposed canon, the received text of the 1980 schema was taken into the Schema of 1982, but with one significant change: modifying the term used to denote the person who would be assisting at a marriage ceremony in which the permission of the ordinary of the place would be required. Reflecting the language of the 1917 code, the assisting minister in the schemata of 1977 and 1980 was designated as *parochus*—the pastor. Moreover, the designation *parochus* was used in the Schema of 1977 for each of the circumstances enumerated.

For example, norm 225 of the Schema of 1977 puts it this way:

> Except for a case of necessity a *parochus* is not to assist at the marriage of *vagi* unless, after the matter has been given to the Ordinary of the place, he has obtained permission for assisting.[43]

And norm 258 of the same schema puts it this way:

> The *parochus* is to admonish minor children of a family not to enter into marriage if the parents are unaware or are reasonably opposed. If a minor refuses [not to marry] he is not to assist unless the Ordinary of the place has first been consulted.[44]

Even in the 1980 schema, the term *parochus* was still employed to designate the one who was to assist at the marriage; but naming the *parochus* in each of the circumstances requiring permission was moved to the introductory stipulation that applied to all of the circumstances that would follow. Thus, the Schema of 1980 began by stipulating "*Parochus sine licentia Ordinarii loci ne assitat,*" and then described seven circumstances in which such permission would be needed.

In the Code Commission's discussion of the 1980 schema, however, the subject of the negative jussive subjunctive verb *ne assistat* was left indefinite. Moreover,

42 *Communicationes* 15 (1983) 226: "Ordinarius licentiam assistendi matrimonio eius qui notorie catholicam fidem abiecerit ne concedat, nisi servatis normis de quibus in can. 1079, congrua congruis referendo."

43 *Sacramentis*, 255: "Matrimonio vagorum parochus, excepto casu necessitatis, ne assistat, nisi, re ad loci Ordinarium delata, licentiam assistendi obtinuerit."

44 *Sacramentis*, 258: "Parochus filiosfamilias minores admoneat ne nuptias ineant, insciis aut rationabiliter invitis parentibus; quod si abnuerit, eorum matrimonio ne assistat, nisi consulto prius loci Ordinarius."

reflecting the construction of the 1980 schema, the name of the assisting person is not *parochus.* Further, the person assisting is offered only once, in the canon's first paragraph, which opens by stipulating, "One is not to assist . . . ," after which the seven circumstances requiring permission are listed. This change in the name of the assisting person is a result of the Code Commission's recognition that, since it was not only a pastor who could legitimately assist at a marriage, the language of the canon needed to reflect the fact that persons other than the pastor are obliged to consult and obtain permission of the ordinary of the place.[45]

III. Details of canon 1071 and the task of ecclesial ministers in marriage preparation

Having set the historical backdrop for the circumstances contained in canon 1071 and having discussed the construction of the canon in its present form, this study shall now examine the elements of the canon's two paragraphs. It will detail the first paragraph's seven circumstances and comment on the caution needed by those who are to assist at marriage, and note the prudence demanded of the ordinary who must give permission for the marriage.

"Except in a case of necessity"

The very first words of canon 1071 posit an exception to its rules stipulating caution: the exception that arises in the case of necessity. The inclusion of necessity by the law itself as a cause exempting from the stipulated requirements of the canon not only offers some prudential flexibility to the person preparing a couple for marriage; it also suggests that the Code of Canon Law is not draconian or absolutist, and leaves open the possibility of applying canonical equity to a case.

This is not to say that, under the claim of necessity or equity one may simply avoid the requirements of the canon. These canonical requirements result from the presumption that the circumstances specified by the canon very possibly pose a threat to a socially stable conjugal community within a community of faith, fellowship and worship. Thus, the gravity of necessity needed to trump the requirement of obtaining permission must clearly outweigh the possible dangers that may arise in each of the enumerated circumstances.[46]

---

45 See *Communicatones* 15 (1983) 226: "Cum alli praeter parochum matrimonio legitime assistere possint. . . non patet cur hic solo de parocho sermo sit . . . *Responsum: Admittitur admadversio et canon ita modificatur: 'Excepto casu necessitatis, sine Ordinarii loci ne quis assistat.'*"

46 See Thomas P. Doyle, "Title VII: Marriage," *The Code of Canon Law: A Text and Commentary,* ed. James A. Coriden et al. (New York: Paulist Press, 1985) 756.

A. Canon 1071 §1, 1° The marriage of *vagi*

The language of the canon is clear and concise: Except in the case of necessity—which can apply to all the circumstances listed in the paragraph—one is not to assist at the wedding of vagrants without the permission of the ordinary of the place.

As noted above, the caution needed for the marriage of vagi has been contained in the rule of law since Trent; it has been the rule of law as stipulated in canon 1032 of the 1917 code. The ecclesial minister's caution and the local ordinary's required permission extend to the homeless, to gypsies (Romani), to those who are unsettled by culture, by circumstances, or by choice. On July 4, 1921 the Sacred Congregation for the Discipline of the Sacraments stipulated that permission was required to assist at the wedding of immigrants or emigrants.[47] On June 29, 1941 this stipulation was repeated in another instruction by the same congregation.[48] This would seem to mean that caution by the ecclesial minister and permission of the local ordinary extend to include refugees, to those who are on the move to another country, and to migrant workers.

The first-level rationale for such required caution and permission, as Trent has stated, is to guarantee that the freedom to marry and the absence of ligamen have been sufficiently established. There is another reason that may well be operative here: persons who are unsettled in terms of domicile or quasi domicile are sometimes unsettled in terms of practical judgment, of prudence, of phronesis. Ecclesial ministers who are preparing vagi and local ordinaries giving permission need to be clear that the unsettledness does not extend to practical or emotional intelligence.

B. Canon 1071 §1, 2° A marriage that cannot be recognized or celebrated under the norm of civil law

This circumstance is one that was not included in the 1917 code. Many reasons can be offered for its inclusion. Perhaps the impossibility of recognition or celebration of a given marriage is because a person who wishes to marry wants no civil recognition of the marriage because he or she is radically antinomian and is totally opposed to the authority of a particular governmental system. In such a case the impossibility rests entirely within the will of the person wishing to marry on his or her terms. Perhaps the impossibility has to do with differences between canon law and civil law about the minimum age for marriage. Perhaps

47 See Sacred Congregation for the Discipline of the Sacraments, *Instructio Ad Rev.mos Ordinarios Locorum Super Probatione Status Liberi Ac Denuntiatione Initi Matrimoni*, July 4, 1921: *AAS* 13 (1921) 348-49.

48 See Sacred Congregation for the Discipline of the Sacraments, *Instructio De Normis A Parocho Servandis In Peragendis Canonicis Investigationibus Antequam Nupturientes Ad Matrimonium Ineundum Admittat (Can. 1020)* 6, June 29, 1941: *AAS* 33 (1941) 303.

it is because a couple whose marriage is invalid because of lack of form want to validate the marriage but are unwilling to obtain the re-marriage license that some states require. Perhaps it is because one of the parties to the marriage is an undocumented alien and there is a practice of a particular local government to establish this fact. The more common situation in which the non-recognition of a wedding might come into play is the case of a widow and widower who could not manage economically if the widow's pension were to disappear as a result of a second marriage.

The rationale for the requirements of this circumstance is the Church's general desire to ensure that a canonically valid marriage is also one that has full recognition by civil society. It is when such civil recognition or civil celebration is impossible that the caution of the assisting minister and prudence of the local ordinary come into play.

C. Canon 1071 §1, 3° A marriage of a person who is bound by natural obligations toward another party or children arising from a previous union

As noted above, this circumstance is new in the 1983 code. This circumstance is very possibly the most vexing of the seven circumstances listed in the canon's first paragraph. Moreover, considering natural obligations that may have arisen from former intimate relationships requires considering the nature of such intimate relationships, whether marital or non-marital.

When intimate relationships are genuinely marital but non-sacramental, when such are regarded as juridically valid, and when such marriages are dissolved by pauline privilege or privilege of the faith, there are moral-ethical obligations that continue, which arise from charity and justice. When, on the other hand, a putative marriage, sacramental or non-sacramental, has been declared null by judicial sentence, moral-ethical obligations of the parties toward each other and toward their children continue to exist. In view of the notion of justice and its relationship to the common good and to juridic structures,[49] the Church's rule of law notes how the obligations of justice, charity and equity arising from a former

---

49 Cf. *S.T.* II-II.58.5:

> It follows therefore that the good of any virtue, whether such virtue direct man in relation to himself, or in relation to certain other individual persons, is referable to the common good, to which justice directs: so that all acts of virtue can pertain to justice, in so far as it directs man to the common good. It is in this sense that justice is called a general virtue. And since it belongs to the law to direct to the common good, as stated above (I-II.90.2), it follows that the justice which is in this way styled general, is called " legal justice," because thereby man is in harmony with the law which directs the acts of all the virtues to the common good.

S.T. II-II.58.6: "Accordingly, just as charity which regards the Divine good as its proper object, is a special virtue in respect of its essence, so too legal justice is a special virtue in respect of its essence, in so far as it regards the common good as its proper object."

marriage should have an impact on an upcoming marriage. But because of the specific differences that can exist from case to case, the code's stipulations of the impact of these obligations are generic, not specific.

There are two loci in the code that consider the matter:

(1) Canon 1148 §3 actuates the sixteenth-century papal constitutions dealing with obligations of a former non-baptized polygamist toward a first wife and dismissed wives. The canon imposes an obligation on the local ordinary to see that the requirements of justice, Christian charity and natural equity are observed. Here is how 1148 §3 puts it:

> Keeping in mind the moral, social, and economic conditions of places and of persons, the local ordinary is to take care that the needs of the first wife and the others dismissed are sufficiently provided for according to the norms of justice, Christian charity, and natural equity.[50]

(2) Canon 1691 §1 stipulates elements to be included in a judicial sentence of marital nullity. It requires the judge-ponens to address ethical obligations that have arisen between the parties and their children. In the words of the canon:

> In the sentence the parties are to be reminded of the moral and even civil obligations which may bind them both toward one another and toward their children to furnish support and education.[51]

In constructing the 1983 code there was some discussion of such obligations that would arise when a marriage was invalid because of lack of form. One member of the Code Commission recommended that, in view of justice and the common good, prior civil bond should be included in the new code as a matrimonial impediment. The commission determined, however, that the caution established in what would become canon 1171 should be sufficient.[52] As this is the case, then it would appear that natural obligations from an intimate relationship that was either authentically marital or non-marital would be the object of the

---

50 1983 *CIC* c. 1148 §3: "Ordinarius loci, prae oculis habita condicione morali, sociali, oeconomica locorum et personarum, curet ut primae uxoris ceterarumque dimissarum necessitatibus satis provisum sit, iuxta normas iustitiae, christianae caritatis et naturalis aequitatis."

51 1983 *CIC* c. 1691 §1: "In sententia partes moneantur de obligationibus moralibus vel etiam civilibus, quibus forte teneantur, altera erga alteram et erga prolem, ad sustentationem et educationem praestandam."

52 See *Communications* 9 (1977) 362.

caution of §1, 3°.[53]

First and foremost, and expressly mentioned in the text of the canon, are the obligations toward children born of the prior relationship. Such obligations are certainly financial ones, which are typically established by judicial determination or mutual agreement; but there are other obligations as well, which not only include physical security and nourishment, but which touch upon emotional intelligence, education, and moral guidance. Thomas Aquinas, in his discussion of the wrongness of fornication, addresses the obligations toward children born of intimate relationships.

> It is evident that the upbringing of a human child requires not only the mother's care for his nourishment but much more the care of his father as guide and guardian, and under whom he progresses in goods both internal and external.[54]

Besides the obligations to children there are obligations toward former partners in intimate relationships, whether from a canonically valid marriage, a putative marriage, an invalid marriage, or a non-marital relationship. These obligations are not only financial but also moral-ethical ones, touching upon the very nature of fidelity and friendship that probably existed at some point and for some time in a former relationship and cannot, morally and ethically, simply be dismissed.

The rationale for employing caution and prudence in assessing obligations toward children and former partners is to honor and secure the common good, which "takes account of all those social conditions which favor the full development of human personality."[55] Moreover, securing the common good is a core objective of the virtue of justice, in both its legal and domestic forms.[56]

D. Canon 1071 §1, 4° A marriage of a person who has notoriously rejected the Catholic faith

This cautionary provision, as we have noted, was found in the 1917 code, in the chapter on impediments; its traditional rationale was to assure the non-perversion of the Catholic party and to guarantee the Catholic education of the couple's children. During the Code Commission's discussion of the Schema

---

53 See *Familiaris consortio* §§80-82 lists non-marital relationships as trial marriages, de-facto free unions, and Catholics in solely civil marriages. See John Paul II, apostolic exhortation *Familiaris consortio*, November 22, 1981: *AAS* 74 (1981): 81–191.

54 *S.T.* II-II.154.2.

55 John XXIII, encyclical *Mater et magistra* 65, May 15, 1961: *AAS* 53 (1961) 401-464; alternative English translation available at *The Pope Speaks* 7 (April 1962) 295-343.

56 See *S.T.* II-II.58.5-7.

of 1977 there was a proposal to make the circumstance in which a person had notoriously rejected the Catholic faith a diriment impediment. This proposal was rejected by a plurality of consultors, who preferred the circumstance to require caution on the part of the minister and prudence on the part of the local ordinary rather than to establish an impediment to the *ius ad matrimonium.*

The cautionary provision assumes a situation in which one of the parties to marriage has notoriously rejected the Catholic faith. Notoriety, as noted above, means notoriety of fact. This factual notoriety, the Commission consultors noted, can be explicit or implicit. It is explicit if the baptized person's rejection of the faith is positive and public and explicitly clear; it is implicit if a person has become a member of a manifestly atheistic or anti-Christian association.[57]

The provision allows for the possibility of the local ordinary granting permission for assisting at the wedding of a Catholic and a non-believing baptized former Catholic. It does not explicitly consider three specific situations: (a) a situation in which a validly baptized person who has notoriously rejected the Catholic faith marries a practicing Catholic; (b) the situation of a validly baptized former Catholic marrying a baptized or non-baptized non-Catholic; (c) the situation in which both validly baptized Catholics have notoriously rejected the Catholic faith. The third of these situations is extremely problematic. It proposes a scenario in which two persons, validly baptized as Catholics, have notoriously rejected the Catholic faith but wish to marry in the Catholic Church for social or aesthetic reasons rather than for religious ones.

Since all sacraments are sacraments of faith, some theologians have wondered whether a marriage contracted by two validly baptized Catholics who have explicitly rejected the Catholic faith would be valid. Here is how the International Theological Commission presented the issue:

> Where there is no trace of faith (in the sense of "belief"—being disposed to believe), and no desire for grace and salvation is found, then a real doubt arises as to whether there is . . . truly sacramental intention and whether the contracted marriage is validly contracted or not.[58]

St. John Paul weighed in on the question in *Familiaris consortio*, where he offers more a cautious observation than a theological statement. Here is how he put it:

> [I]t is true that in some places engaged couples ask to be married in church for motives which are social rather than genuinely religious.

57 See *Communicationes* 9 (1977) 145.

58 International Theological Commission, "Propositions on the Doctrine of Christian Marriage," 2.3, *Origins* 8 (1978-79) 237. Cf. S.T. II-II.58-59.

> This is not surprising. Marriage, in fact, is not an event that concerns only the persons actually getting married. By its very nature it is also a social matter, committing the couple being married in the eyes of society. And its celebration has always been an occasion of rejoicing that brings together families and friends. It therefore goes without saying that social as well as personal motives enter into the request to be married in church.
>
> Nevertheless, it must not be forgotten that these engaged couples, by virtue of their Baptism, are already really sharers in Christ's marriage Covenant with the Church, and that, by their right intention, they have accepted God's plan regarding marriage and therefore at least implicitly consent to what the Church intends to do when she celebrates marriage. Thus, the fact that motives of a social nature also enter into the request is not enough to justify refusal on the part of pastors. Moreover, as the Second Vatican Council teaches, the sacraments by words and ritual elements nourish and strengthen faith: that faith towards which the married couple are already journeying by reason of the uprightness of their intention, which Christ's grace certainly does not fail to favor and support.
>
> As for wishing to lay down further criteria for admission to the ecclesial celebration of marriage, criteria that would concern the level of faith of those to be married, this would above all involve grave risks. In the first place, the risk of making unfounded and discriminatory judgments; secondly, the risk of causing doubts about the validity of marriages already celebrated, with grave harm to Christian communities, and new and unjustified anxieties to the consciences of married couples; one would also fall into the danger of calling into question the sacramental nature of many marriages of brethren separated from full communion with the Catholic Church, thus contradicting ecclesial tradition.[59]

The question is not a new one and has been discussed as early as the fourteenth century. The frame of reference for the question is itself an unsettled question, which may be stated as follows: It is clear that marriage as a contract and marriage as a sacrament are distinct. But are marriage-as-contract and marriage-as-sacrament separable?

Carlo Caffarra claims that theologians such as Duns Scotus and Alphonsus Ligouri would argue for the separability of contract and sacrament. Robert Bellarmine argued that contract and sacrament are not only inseparable but are identical. Bellarmine's position would be taken up and somewhat adapted by his

59 *Familiaris consortio* 68. English translations at http://www.vatican.va/content/john-paul-ii/en/apost_exhortations/documents/hf_jp-ii_exh_19811122_familiaris-consortio.html (accessed on 13 Apr. 2020).

contemporary fellow Jesuits Francisco Suarez and Tomas Sanchez.[60]

What was something of an open theological question in the seventeenth century became less open in the nineteenth century, when European political theory argued that the marriage contract was a matter of secularity and should be under the control of the state, whereas marriage as a sacrament was a religious matter, and under the control of the Church. Leo XIII, considering this to be an invalid intrusion of the state upon the Church, issued the encyclical letter *Arcanum divinae sapientiae,* in which he held for the inseparability of sacrament and contract. Here is how he put it:

> Let no one, then, be deceived by the distinction which some civil jurists have so strongly insisted upon - the distinction, namely, by virtue of which they sever the matrimonial contract from the sacrament, with intent to hand over the contract to the power and will of the rulers of the State, while reserving questions concerning the sacrament of the Church. A distinction, or rather severance, of this kind cannot be approved; for certain it is that in Christian marriage the contract is inseparable from the sacrament, and that, for this reason, the contract cannot be true and legitimate without being a sacrament as well. For Christ our Lord added to marriage the dignity of a sacrament; but marriage is the contract itself, whenever that contract is lawfully concluded.[61]

The inseparability of contract and sacrament of *Arcanum* found its way into the 1917 code. Canon 1012 stated the following:

> §1 Christ the Lord elevated the marriage contract itself to the dignity of a sacrament among the baptized.
>
> §2 Therefore, among the baptized, there can be no valid contract of marriage without, *eo ipso,* its being a sacrament.[62]

In the 1983 code the words of the second paragraph of canon 1012 of the 1917

---

60 See Carlo Caffarra, "Marriage as a Reality in the Order of Creation and Marriage as a Sacrament," in *Contemporary Perspectives on Christian Marriage,* ed. Richard Malone and John R. Connery (Chicago: Loyola University Press, 1984) 127-130. Caffarra's moral theology was a major influence in the moral theology of St. John Paul II. This is evident in *Familiaris consortio;* it is evident especially in *Veritatis splendor*. See John Paul II, encyclical *Veritatis Splendor*, August 6, 1993: *AAS* 85 (1993) 1133-1228.

61 Leo XIII, encyclical *Arcanum divinae sapientiae* 23, February 10, 1880: *ASS* 12 (1880) 385-402.

62 1917 *CIC* c. 1012: "§1 Christus Dominus ad sacramenti dignitatem evexit ipsum contractum matrimonialem inter baptizatos.

§2 Quare inter baptizatos nequit matrimonialis contractus validus consistere, quin sit eo ipso sacramentum."

code are repeated *verbatim.*

As a result of the canonical position of the inseparability of contract and sacrament, St John Paul II asserted that in cases in which the Catholic faith is entirely lacking in both parties, and when a marriage in the Church is planned principally for social motives, "the pastor of souls [who well may be the ordinary of the place who has been asked for permission to assist at the wedding] cannot admit them to the celebration of marriage."[63] The International Theological Commission addresses the issue more theologically than John Paul, and questions whether baptized persons who have rejected the Catholic faith can marry validly since they cannot validly celebrate a sacrament of faith.

The issue as presented by the International Theological Commission opens once again the possibility of invalidity of a church marriage contracted by two unbelieving but baptized Catholics. The Commission declines to resolve the difficulty or to answer its own question. It states, "This gives rise to new problems for which a satisfactory answer has yet to be found."[64]

However, until the theological issue of the validity of a marriage by non-believing baptized Catholics is to be finally resolved, the practical situation as presented by John Paul II is clear, workable, and should be followed: whenever a marriage is requested by two persons both of whom have renounced Catholic faith and for whom no semblance of belief can be awakened, whether or not this renunciation of faith is notorious or not, the ecclesial minister needs to inform them that she or he cannot assist at their wedding. Moreover, the ordinary of the place, if he becomes involved, should refuse to grant permission for the wedding.

E. Canon 1071 §1, 5° A marriage of a person who is under a censure

The censures of excommunication and interdict in this canon apply to Catholics planning to marry who are over the age of sixteen (over the age of eighteen for *latae sententiae* censures).[65] Since both of these censures prohibit Catholics from celebrating or receiving sacraments, it might be concluded that persons under censure are in all cases prohibited from marrying another baptized person in the Church. This circumstance as presented in canon 1071, however, suggests that the exclusion of a person under censure from marrying and the prohibition of an ecclesial minister from assisting at the wedding are not exactly absolute. Moreover, the non-absolute nature of such an exclusion and prohibition is not new to the 1983 code; it can be found in canon 1066 of the 1917 code.

---

63 *Familiaris consortio* 68.

64 International Theological Commission, "Propositions on the Doctrine of Christian Marriage" 2.4 (1977) 237, http://www.vatican.va/roman_curia/congregations/cfaith/cti_documents/rc_cti_1977_sacramento-matrimonio_en.html (accessed on 23 Jan. 2020).

65 Cf. c. 1324 §2.

The 1983 code simplifies the norm of canon 1066 of the 1917 code:

- The present norm no longer requires the permission of the local ordinary in the case of public sinners who are not under censure.
- The present norm does not require notoriety of censure as a condition for the needed permission of the ordinary.
- The present norm does not specify that the person under censure has refused to approach confession or to reconcile with the Church.

This simplification, however, does not imply that a person who is under censure and who refuses to be reconciled with the Church should be considered eligible to marry without specific permission of the local ordinary. It is to suggest, as does pastoral practice as old as St. Alphonsus, that a local ordinary can give permission for assisting at marriage if such permission sets aside greater evils for the couple.

There is a final point that is relevant in an ecclesial minister assisting at the wedding of a person under censure. If the person under censure is to marry a non-baptized person, the proposed marriage is not sacramental and, thus, is not forbidden to the person under censure by virtue of canons 18 and 1331, 2°. Even if such non-sacramental marriage is not prohibited by canon 1331, the prescription of canon 1071 §1, 5° requires the permission of the local ordinary for assisting at the wedding—*any* wedding—of a person under censure. And it appears that only a grave cause and the exercise of extreme prudence should result in a local ordinary giving permission to assist at such a marriage.

F. Canon 1071 §1, 6° A marriage of a minor child whose parents are unaware or reasonably opposed

The 1983 code has simplified the descriptions of persons by age. Rather than repeating the division of the age of minority into infant, *inpubes* and *pubes* as did the 1917 code, the present code divides age into minority and majority. Prior to seven years of age the minor is called infant; after seven, he or she is simply called minor. Moreover, the 1983 code has reduced the age of achieving one's majority from twenty-one to eighteen.

While making some changes in describing persons by age, the 1983 code has maintained the minimum age for valid marriage set in 1917 code at fourteen for females and sixteen for males. Although canon 1083 §2 of the 1983 code enables an episcopal conference to decree a higher age for marriage, that higher

age is not for the marriage's validity, but only for its liceity.[66] It is notable that the USCCB has not acted on this, and has not raised the minimum age for a licit marriage beyond the fourteen/sixteen.

Lack of age can, in most states in our nation, be a detriment to marriage. In most states, the legal minimum for marriage is sixteen, and if a partner to a proposed marriage is below the age of eighteen, most states require parental permission and/or a court decree.[67]

Canon 1071 requires consultation with the local ordinary and his permission to assist at the marriages of all minors—even those who have received a dispensation from the impediment of age—if their parents or one of their parents does not know of the proposed marriage or is reasonably opposed.

Canonists in the United States, aware of the perils of teenage marriages that so often wind up in the diocesan tribunal, are concerned about the advisability of easily allowing the weddings of young people below the age of twenty-one. Even though canon 1071 requires caution, and canon 1072 requires pastors of souls to exercise special care in dissuading young people from marrying, Professor Edward Peters has admirably summed up potential weaknesses in applying these canonical cautions by parish ministers and their requesting permission to assist.

> First, canonical training for pastoral ministers is not what it used to be, and canon 1071 is sometimes simply overlooked by priests and deacons ignorant of its existence. Second, a surprisingly long list of diocesan personnel qualify as "local ordinaries" for purposes of consultation (canon 134), a fact that can facilitate inconsistent approaches toward teenage marriages within the same local church, approaches that might not even be those of the diocesan bishop.
>
> Third, beyond the dubious implication that parents' opposition to their children's teenage wedding plans could be deemed by ministers as unreasonable, hence exempting those ministers from any consultation requirement, there is still no parental consultation requirement even in cases where parental opposition is considered reasonable. Fourth, 18- and 19-year-olds, still teenagers and still prone to failed marriages, are not covered by the terms of canon 1071 because they are not canonically considered " minors" (canon 97). For all of these reasons, canon 1071 is

---

66 See 1983 *CIC* c. 1083 §2: "Integrum est Episcoporum conferentiae aetatem superiorem ad licitam matrimonii celebrationem statuere."

67 Cf. Sheri Stritof, "State-By-State Legal Age Marriage Laws," updated October 15, 2019, https://www.thespruce.com/legal-age-marriage-laws-by-state-2300971 for a state-by-state listing of minimum age and parental consent requirements for teenage marriages (accessed on 30 Mar. 2020).

not much of a deterrent to teenage weddings.[68]

Stanley Hauerwas maintains that it is a "peculiar sensibility of modernity to think that if our marriages have gone bad, it is because we did not know what we were doing when we 'chose' the person we married."[69] Hauerwas continues:

> The anomaly behind this set of presumptions is that one could ever know what one was doing when one got married. I take it that the wisdom of the Christian tradition has been that the church witnesses a couple's marriage, not because we think they know what they are doing, but because they do not. That is why we as Christians (should) insist that we can only have marriage witnessed in the church among people who will hold us to our promises.[70]

Whether or not Hauerwas' assessment is accurate is a matter of some dispute. What seems indisputable, however, is that the marriages of teenagers are especially precarious; and the marriages of teenagers that take place without their parents' knowledge or against their parents' reasonable objections hover near the disastrous. The well-taken cautionary comments of Professor Peters notwithstanding, the stipulation of canon 1071 §1, 6° is particularly prudent in requiring a second review of the matter as well as the permission of the local ordinary.

G. Canon 1071 §1, 7° A marriage to be entered into by proxy

As has been noted above, proxy marriages were established in Roman Law, were confirmed as valid in the Law of Justinian, were not revoked by Trent, and were held to be a valid exercise of the canonical form of marriage in the 1917 code.[71] Repeating the norm of the 1917 code, the 1983 code stipulates that proxy weddings are a valid expression of canonical form. Canon 1104 §1 states the following: "To contract a marriage validly the contracting parties must be present together, either in person or by proxy."[72]

Canon 1105 has laid down a number of requirements for valid proxy weddings in the Church. These regulations largely guarantee that a proxy does not function

68 Edward Peters, "Too young to marry," *America* (June 22-29, 1996) 14-16.

69 Stanley Hauerwas, "Killing Compassion," *Dispatches from the Front: Theological Engagements with the Secular* (Durham, NC: Duke University Press, 1994) 168.

70 Ibid.

71 A number of significant figures married in proxy weddings. Among them are Lorenzo de Medici, who married Clarice Orsini in 1469, Marie de Medici, who married King Henry IV of France in 1600, and Napoleon I, who married Archduchess Marie Louise in 1810.

72 1983 *CIC* c. 1104 §1: "Ad matrimonium valide contrahendum necesse est ut contrahentes sint praesentes una simul sive per se ipsi, sive per procuratorem."

fraudulently and that the proxy is actuating the intent of the contracting party at the time of the wedding. Here is the text of the canon:

> §1. To enter into a marriage validly by proxy it is required that:
>
> 1° there is a special mandate to contract with a specific person;
>
> 2° the proxy is designated by the one mandating and fulfills this function personally.
>
> §2. To be valid the mandate must be signed by the one mandating and by the pastor or ordinary of the place where the mandate is given, or by a priest delegated by either of them, or at least by two witnesses, or it must be made by means of a document which is authentic according to the norm of civil law.
>
> §3. If the one mandating cannot write, this is to be noted in the mandate itself and another witness is to be added who also signs the document; otherwise, the mandate is invalid.
>
> §4. If the one mandating revokes the mandate or develops amentia before the proxy contracts in his or her name, the marriage is invalid even if the proxy or the other contracting party does not know this.[73]

Although proxy weddings are possible in canon law, in the United States, there are only four states in which proxy weddings are allowed: Montana, California, Colorado and Texas.[74] Thus, in these four states the cautionary review and permission by the local ordinary is required for anyone assisting at a proxy wedding; in all other states, cautionary review and permission by the local ordinary would be required not only by virtue of canon 1071 §1, 7°, but also by virtue of §1, 2°, requiring oversight and permission for weddings that cannot be celebrated according to the norms of civil law.

In all cases of proxy weddings, oversight and permission by the local ordinary is stipulated principally in order to assure that the elements of canon 1105 that are necessary for the validity of a proxy wedding are in place. A secondary

73 1983 *CIC* c. 1105.

74 In all of these states proxy marriages are allowed for members of the armed forces. In Montana, simply being a member of the armed forces qualifies a person for a proxy wedding. In California a person has to be deployed overseas and has to be serving in a war or conflict. Colorado permits proxy weddings additionally for military contractors who are working in another country and are supporting a combat or military operation. Texas does not require a situation of armed conflict to qualify a person in the military who is serving abroad. Moreover, Texas also allows persons incarcerated in Texas prisons to have proxy weddings. Montana, in some of its jurisdictions, allows double-proxy weddings, where, if one party is deployed in the armed services, neither bride nor groom needs to be a Montana resident, and where neither bride nor groom needs to be personally present as the ceremony takes place.

but not unimportant reason for oversight and permission by the local ordinary is the caution that should be in place prior to a wedding that is hasty, or may be being performed for the wrong reasons (e.g., to get medical benefits, post exchange privileges, or admission into the United States for the spouse who is not deployed).

Canon 1071 §2: The local ordinary is not to grant permission to assist at the marriage of a person who has notoriously rejected the Catholic faith unless the norms mentioned in canon 1125 have been observed with necessary adaptation.

The "norms mentioned in canon 1125" to which the second paragraph of canon 1071 refers are the *cautiones*, which set down a level of caution to be exercised prior to the local ordinary giving permission for assisting at mixed marriage. Whereas the second paragraph of canon 1071 is clear in its reference to the employment of the *cautiones*, what remains unclear is this: what are the "necessary adaptations" that are to be employed in the *cautiones* for the wedding of a person who has notoriously rejected the Catholic faith? In an effort to provide a good answer for this, it would be helpful to look at the path taken by the *cautiones* over the past sixty years, and then to estimate which version of the *cautiones* might best be employed by the local ordinary if he is to permit a person to assist at the marriage of a Catholic who has notoriously rejected the faith.

The *cautiones* have had an interesting history over the last half century. The 1917 code was specific in its requiring both parties in a mixed marriage to engage in promises about their future life together. Canon 1061 therein stipulated that the Church did not dispense from the impediment of mixed religion unless the non-Catholic spouse promised to remove the danger of perversion from the Catholic spouse, and that *both spouses* promised that all children would be baptized and educated only as Catholics.[75] The canon of the 1917 code includes the same requirement for the *cautiones* in dispensing from disparity of worship.

In 1966 the *cautiones* of the 1917 code were modified. In the Instruction of the Congregation for the Doctrine of the Faith titled *Matrimonii sacramentum*[76] the non-Catholic party no longer has to make a promise about the Catholic baptism and education of the children. In this Instruction, the non-Catholic is invited to promise, openly and sincerely, that she or he will not create any obstacle to the Catholic party's obligation to have children baptized and raised as Catholics. It is noteworthy that, if the non-Catholic party cannot make this promise without

---

75 See 1917 *CIC* c. 1061: "Ecclesia super impedimento mixtae religionis non dispensat, nisi: . . . 2° Cautionem praestiterit coniux acatholicus de amovendo a coniuge catholico perversionis periculo, et uterque coniux de universa prole catholice tantum baptizanda et educanda."

76 See Sacred Congregation for the Doctrine of the Faith, instruction *Matrimonii sacramentum,* March 18, 1966: *AAS* 58 (1966) 235-239; see also *CLD* 6 (1963-1967), 592-596.

harming his or her conscience, "the Ordinary should refer the case with all its elements to the Holy See."[77]

In 1970 the *cautiones* were modified again. In the motu proprio *Matrimonia mixta*[78] Pope Paul VI stipulated that the Catholic party to a mixed marriage would make a declaration and a promise, whereas the non-Catholic party would have to promise nothing, but simply be informed of the declaration and promise made by the Catholic party. To quote from the English translation of the *motu proprio* provided by the Holy See:

> 4. To obtain from the local Ordinary dispensation from an impediment, the Catholic party shall declare that he is ready to remove dangers of falling from the faith. He is also gravely bound to make a sincere promise to do all in his power to have all the children baptized and brought up in the Catholic Church.
>
> 5. At an opportune time the non-Catholic party must be informed of these promises which the Catholic party has to make, so that it is clear that he is cognizant of the promise and obligation on the part of the Catholic.[79]

It is notable that the change of the *cautiones* in *Matrimonia mixta* is not the last word for all cases of mixed marriages. On April 30, 2001 the Congregation for the Doctrine of the Faith issued an instruction setting forth norms on the preparation of the process for the dissolution of the marriage bond in favor of the faith.[80]

In Article 5, the Instruction stipulates the following:

> § 1. A Catholic party who intends to contract or to convalidate a new marriage with a person who is not baptized or with a baptized non-Catholic is to declare that he or she is prepared to remove dangers of defecting from

---

77 *Matrimonia sacramentum,* I, 3.

78 See Paul VI, apostolic letter *Matrimonia mixta,* October 1, 1970: *AAS* 59 (1970) 257-263; see also *CLD* 7 (1968-1972) 711-717.

79 *Matrimonia mixta,* 4-5; English translation at http://www.vatican.va/content/paul-vi/en/motu_proprio/documents/hf_p-vi_motu-proprio_19700331_matrimonia-mixta.html (accessed on 23 Jan. 2020).

80 See Congregation for the Doctrine of the Faith, instruction *De conficiendo processu pro solutione vinculi matrimonialis in favorem fidei*, April 30, 2001 (Vatican City: Editrice Libreria Vaticana, 2001), http://www.vatican.va/roman_curia/congregations/cfaith/documents/rc_con_cfaith_doc_20010430_favor-fidei_en.html (accessed on 20 Mar. 2020). See Frederick C. Easton, "Favor of the Faith Cases and the 2001 Norms of the Congregation for the Doctrine of the Faith," *CLSA Proceedings* 64 (Washington, DC: Canon Law Society of America, 2002) 97-119.

> the faith and *the non-Catholic party is to declare that he or she is prepared to allow the Catholic party the freedom to profess his or her own religion and to baptize and educate their children as Catholics.*
>
> § 2. The favor of the dissolution is not conceded unless this declaration in writing has been signed by both parties.[81]

In considering what adaptations are possible and which adaptations should be employed, a local ordinary needs to examine each specific case. He need not develop a one-size-fits-all template; he need not restrict himself to the *cautiones* as they have been modified and have found their way into the 1983 code. If he deems it necessary, the local ordinary can require a person who has notoriously rejected the faith to sign a declaration prior to granting permission for a juridically competent person to assist at that lapsed Catholic's marriage to a practicing Catholic, who would also have to make a declaration and promise, either in writing or orally.

This completes our exploration of canon 1071.

Stanley Hauerwas has, in scattered utterances, proposed three truisms for contemporary marriages: (1) You always marry the wrong person; (2) Your children always disappoint you; (3) There's no good time to have a baby. Whether or not Hauerwas is on the money, marriages can be easily shattered. Canon 1071, with its stipulation for a second set of prudential eyes to review the matter, and a required permission to assist at certain marriages may not make these marriage less intrinsically fragile; but it can enable particularly fragile marriages to be addressed, *ab initio*, with caution and with care.

---

81 CDF, *De conficiendo processu pro solutione vinculi matrimonialis in favorem fidei*, 5 (emphasis added): "§1. Si pars catholica novum matrimonium intendit contrahere vel convalidare cum persona non baptizata vel baptizata non catholica, declaret se paratam esse pericula a fide deficiendi removere atque pars acatholica declaret se paratam esse relinquere parti catholicae libertatem propriam religionem profitendi atque filios catholice baptizandi et educandi. §2. Gratia solutionis non conceditur nisi haec declaratio in scriptis ab utraque parte subsignata fuerit."

Seminar

The Separation of the Spouses: Old Law, New Questions

Mr. Vincent Gardiner, JCL

Introduction

I suspect that a seminar on this subject would not have been scheduled five or ten years ago, and, if it had, it would have attracted much less interest. While it would be inaccurate to state that this topic has attracted no scholarly interest since the promulgation of the 1983 Code of Canon Law, it has certainly not attracted widespread interest among scholars of the law. Yet even the little academic attention it has attracted has in fact been greater than the attention given it by practitioners of the law—that is, those of us laboring at the canonical coalface, primarily in tribunals considering the nullity of marriage, and also from time to time, considering other questions passing across the episcopal desk. It would be little exaggeration to say that the first thirty years following the promulgation of the revised code was a period in which the canon law regarding the separation of the spouses never had reason to be considered in the majority of tribunals and chanceries in this country.[1]

So why are we here? In the past few years many dioceses have begun to receive queries regarding the canon law applicable to the separation of the spouses and civil divorce. Increasingly, dioceses are receiving not only general inquiries and complaints, but true petitions related to specific marriages, submitted according to a template petition form distributed online. The petitions request, among

1 In contrast to the United States and the great majority of other countries, dioceses in (the former) Czechoslovakia and a handful of other countries appear to have made relatively prolific use of judicial procedures regarding the separation of the spouses. For example, in 1988, 278 judicial cases of the separation of the spouses were introduced throughout the world. Of these, 21 (the entire African total) came from the Central African Republic, and 151—a majority of all the cases in the Catholic Church—came from Czechslovakia. See Juraj Kamas, *The Separation of the Spouses with the Bond Remaining: Historical and Canonical Study with Pastoral Applications*, Tesie Gregoriana, Serie Diritto Canonico 20 (Rome: Editrice Pontificia Università Gregoriana, 1997) 304. Kamas provides a fascinating snapshot of the unique canonical treatment of separation, together with permission to receive the sacraments in Czech and Slovak dioceses in the 1980s and 1990s. Ibid., 305-309. The author concluded, "[I]t seems that this method of pastoral care does not attain the desired purpose of the better maintenance of discipline." Ibid., 308.

other things, an ecclesiastical declaration of the separation of the spouses due to "malicious abandonment;" for the bishop or tribunal to impose a punishment on the departed spouse; and that the departed spouse be denied Holy Communion if he or she should "persevere in the grave manifest sin of marital abandonment," and damages to be paid to the petitioning spouse. In this context, then, my purpose in this talk and paper is not to give a complete history of the canonical institute of the separation of spouses, but to provide some of the information which may be most applicable when addressing these situations as they arise in your dioceses.

1. Separation and Departure

1.1 Departure

According to canon 1151, "Spouses have the duty and right to preserve conjugal living unless a legitimate cause excuses them."[2] For those subject to canon law, it is not permitted to suspend the conjugal life except for causes which may be defined by the law. But let us not miss the fact that the canon says, "unless a legitimate cause excuses them;" it does *not* say "unless permitted by the local Ordinary" or "only with ecclesiastical permission." Again, to repeat: it does not say that the only manner in which spouses can be dispensed from the obligation of preserving conjugal living is via the active intervention of ecclesiastical authority. It states that they are to preserve conjugal living "unless a legitimate cause excuses them."

It is not permitted to suspend the common conjugal life for reasons entirely of one's own devising; for example, for reasons that are frivolous, light, or immoral. However, it is permitted to suspend the common life for reasons and in a manner provided by law. Canon 1153 §1 names some of these reasons.[3] Here, I have to comment on the current CLSA English language translation. The translation renders *seu animi seu corporis* as "mental or physical."[4] *Anima* has many meanings, both literal and figurative, among which is certainly included cognates of "mental." However, the tradition stretching back to the 1917 code,

---

2 *Codex Iuris Canonici auctoritate Ioannis Pauli PP. II promulgatus* (Vatican City: Libreria Editrice Vaticana, 1983) [hereafter 1983 *CIC*] c. 1151: "Coniuges habent officium et ius servandi convictum coniugalem, nisi legitima causa eos excuset." English translations from the canons in this code will be taken from *Code of Canon Law, Latin-English Edition: New English Translation* (Washington, DC: Canon Law Society of America, 2012), unless otherwise indicated.

3 See 1983 *CIC* c. 1153 §1: "Si alteruter coniugum grave seu animi seu corporis periculum alteri aut proli facessat, vel aliter vitam communem nimis duram reddat, alteri legitimam praebet causam discedendi, decreto Ordinarii loci et, si periculum sit in mora, etiam propria auctoritate."

4 Ibid.

which had a very similar Latin phrase,[5] and prior, clearly shows that this should to be understood as a moral danger; as a threat to the eternal salvation of the spouse or the children: "Canonical doctrine has tended to interpret this cause for separation as protection of the religious life of a person when either his or her salvation or the peaceful practice of his or her faith could be in danger. In short, it has come to be identified with inducement to sin."[6]

Regarding danger to the soul, commentaries and Rotal sentences from the first half of the twentieth century were forthright in their opposition to separation because it would threaten the moral development of the children regarding the indissolubility of marriage; I think we must respect and accept that as a foundation, and also be willing to apply those same principles more broadly. We must recognize that serious and persistent mistreatment of a spouse, or any other manner of giving the children an example severely contrary to the essential rights and obligations of marriage, could well constitute a grave danger to the souls of the children within the meaning of canon 1153 and therefore be a legitimate reason for departure.

The dangers must be likely to be recurrent;[7] a single past event which is not going to occur again cannot justify a departure under this part of the canon (though of course, the recurrent nature of domestic abuse must be taken into account). A spouse can also depart if the common life becomes "too difficult" or "too hard" (*nimis duram*). This effectively opens up the reasons for departure beyond any specific categorization. Still, the reason for departure must be serious enough to be proportionate to the dignity of the matrimonial covenant; marriage is for sinners, and the spouses accept each other "in good times and in bad" or "for better, for worse."[8]

---

5 See *Codex Iuris Canonici Pii X Pontificis Maximi iussu digestus Benedicti Papae XV auctoritate promulgatus* (Rome: Typis Polyglottis Vaticanis, 1917) [hereafter 1917 *CIC*], c. 1131, §1: "Si alter coniux sectae acatholicae nomen dederit; si prolem acatholice educaverit; si vitam criminosam et ignominiosam ducat; si grave seu animae seu corporis periculum alteri facessat; si saevitiis vitam communem nimis difficilem reddat, haec aliaque id genus, sunt pro altero coniuge totidem legitimae causae discedendi, auctoritate Ordmarii loci, et etiam propria auctoritate, si de eis certo constet, et periculum sit in mora" [emphasis added]. Summarized (in part) as "is causing grave spiritual or corporal danger" in *Canon Law: A Text and Commentary*, 4th ed., ed. Lincoln Bouscaren et al. (Milwaukee: Bruce, 1963) 635; translated (in part) as "grave danger to the soul or body" in Edward N. Peters, *The 1917 Pio-Benedictine Code of Canon Law in English Translation with Extensive Scholarly Apparatus* (San Francisco: Ignatius Press, 2001) 388.

6 Escrivá Ivars, "Separation While the Bond Remains," *Exegetical Commentary on the Code of Canon Law, English language edition,* ed. Ernest Caparros et al. (Chicago and Montreal: Midwest Theological Forum and Wilson & Lafleur, 2004) 3: 2.

7 Ibid., 1585.

8 International Commission on English in the Liturgy, *The Order of Celebrating Matrimony*, 2nd ed. (Collegeville: Liturgical Press, 2016) para. 62.

The reason for the departure does not need to be imputable to the moral fault of one or both spouses; "These threats or dangers may come from the malice of the other spouse, as well as from causes for which neither spouse is directly responsible."[9] Classic examples would be a contagious disease or a mental illness. Commenting on licit reasons for departure, the *New Commentary* states that canon law has a "fault-based system for separation," even while acknowledging that "a psychological disorder may diminish or, at times, extinguish the spouse's moral culpability."[10] Unfortunately, the former quotation has been taken up by some recently, apparently to argue in favor of an unreasonably high or inflammatory standard of proof to justify a departure or separation. Rather than "fault-based," perhaps "for cause" would be a better way of describing the Church's understanding of reasons for departure and separation, distinguished from various civil legal systems which require no particular reason.

If there is danger in delay, departure is legitimate even on one's own authority. Perhaps we ought to consider that if there is truly grave danger to soul or body, or the common life is truly too difficult—if that threshold has truly been reached—then very likely there would also be a danger in delaying any longer. I would suggest, therefore, that the number of situations where departure is permissible only with the prior intervention of the local ordinary may be relatively few.

Canon 1153 §1 is not principally describing canonical separation in the narrow sense: it is enumerating the legitimate reasons for departure. Nowhere in this paragraph, in Latin or any known English translation, do we see *separationis*, "separation." This paragraph is speaking of legitimate reasons for departure: *discendi, discessio*; the practical severance of the common conjugal life. Although these same reasons could be used to justify a separation properly understood,[11] this paragraph is not referring directly to the separation of the spouses. This distinction is missed in much of the post-1983 commentary, including both CLSA commentaries.[12] However, the distinction is recognized by, among others, Hervada in *Canons and Commentaries on Marriage*, where he explains that "*de facto* separation should not be confused with . . . legal separation. [*D*]*e facto separation* . . . requires no formal declaration . . . although the right to live

---

9 Escrivá Ivars, "Separation While the Bond Remains," 1584.

10 John P. Beal, "Separation with the Bond Remaining," in *New Commentary on the Code of Canon Law,* ed. John P. Beal et al. (New York/Mahwah, NJ: Paulist Press, 2000) 1377.

11 For example, the sentence *coram* Caberletti (Tribunal of the Roman Rota, definitive sentence c. Caberletti, *Separationis*, January 20, 2011: *RRDec* 103: 1-21) at 7 and 12 clearly relies upon CCEO c. 864 §1, the Eastern counterpart to 1983 *CIC* c. 1153 §1, as it makes a decision regarding separation.

12 See Thomas P. Doyle, "Marriage," in *The Code of Canon Law: A Text and Commentary*, ed. James A. Coriden et al. (New York/Mahwah, NJ: Paulist Press, 1985) 821; and Beal, "Separation with the Bond Remaining," 1377.

together may be suspended."[13]

Another argument in favor of the difference between departure and canonical separation is to be found by comparing canon 1153 §1 to canon 1692 §1. Canon 1153 §1 says that the local ordinary can decide; canon 1692 §1 says that the diocesan bishop or a judicial sentence can decide. If these canons were both referring to true canonical separation, they would be contradicting each other regarding who is competent to decide it. No: the first is regarding departure from the common life, while the second is regarding the establishment of the canonical status of separation. Even if a local ordinary gave a decree recognizing the cause for departure as canon 1153 §1 says is possible, this would not establish the separation of the spouses per canons 1692-1696 unless those procedures were also followed and explicitly stated in the decree. There are two different canonical objects of decision: whether there is a legitimate cause for departure and whether canonical separation is to be established.

There is no process in the external forum by which a departure on one's own authority can be reviewed by ecclesiastical authority. Even if a spouse were to request a decree recognizing legitimate cause for departure from the local ordinary and the local ordinary decided, after considering the circumstances, not to issue such a decree, this would not constitute a prohibition against departure nor necessarily be a judgment on the private decision to depart in the belief that there was a danger in delay.

What is the status of spouses after the departure of one of them; that is, living apart and suspending the practical exercise of some marital rights and duties but without established separated status? A spouse who departed for an insufficient or spurious reason is undoubtedly morally obliged to return and to make amends. However, the legislator has not seen fit to establish penal law to address the violation of the obligation of marital cohabitation; this ought to be borne in mind upon receipt of one of the more wide-ranging petition templates demanding, for example, that the departed spouse be given some punishment by the diocesan bishop. Just as nobody is obliged to petition for the declaration of the nullity of his marriage unless he wishes to regain his freedom, so also spouses *de facto* separated are not obliged to seek permission for a departure effected with danger of delay, nor the establishment of canonical separation unless they actually want or need the status of a separated person in law. The law does not oblige the departed spouse to establish separated status through ecclesiastical authority. Nor does it oblige the spouse left behind to attempt to do the same by claiming "malicious abandonment;" this fact alone is sufficient to reassure many would-be petitioners that they are free to concentrate on saving their marriages rather than being distracted by an ecclesiastical process they had not previously heard

13 Javier Hervada, "Matrimonial Law," in *Canons and Commentaries on Marriage*, ed. Ignatius Gramunt (Collegeville: Liturgical Press, 1987) 98.

of but now apparently are being told is their obligation to pursue. In short, while *de facto* separation is provided for by law, in its concrete situations it needs to be addressed largely as a moral and pastoral matter; it does not create canonical questions requiring juridic resolution.

1.2 Canonical separation

True canonical separation effects a change in the juridic status of the parties, while mere departure from the home—even if declared to be a legitimate reason by the local ordinary—does not. Canonical separation removes the matter from the consideration of the spouses alone and redefines their rights and obligations towards each other. Given that the departure was already potentially legitimate, there are few practical uses to separated status in the United States. There may be occasions when separated status provides some pastoral benefit, especially if a person is troubled in conscience regarding the obligations remaining towards a *de facto* separated spouse. Those who receive negative decisions regarding the nullity of marriage but who have no interest in attempting marriage again, may benefit from this suggestion, especially since the evidence may have been gathered already and the separation could be instituted by an administrative process. I would suggest, however, that these are relatively rare exceptions, and really ought to be utilized only when the potential petitioner is the one whose conscience seriously is burdened regarding the obligations remaining towards the divorced spouse despite explanation of the law regarding legitimate departure.

Separation would be necessary for one who wished to enter into religious life while bound by the bond of marriage. It may also be suitable to consider regarding a married cleric—for example, a permanent deacon—whose marriage appears to have been shipwrecked.[14]

1.3 Adultery

Adultery as a reason for separation or departure is classified separately in the law. Historically speaking, it was the classic—and sometimes the only—reason for separation. It is now codified in canon 1152. Since it is not especially relevant to the petitions and complaints now being received, I will not dwell on it except

14 The *National Directory for The Formation, Ministry, and Life of Permanent Deacons in the United States* (Washington, DC: United States Conference of Catholic Bishops, 2005) has a paragraph (n. 76) addressing "A Deacon and Family Confronting Divorce." The lack of mention of formal ecclesiastical involvement in the departure or separation may be taken as an indication of how these institutes are either unknown or deprecated, even when they may be relevant. The universal norms on which the U.S. document is based has no equivalent paragraph. See Congregation for Catholic Education and Congregation for the Clergy, *Basic Norms for the Formation of Permanent Deacons: Directory for the Ministry and Life of Permanent Deacons* (Vatican City: Libreria Editrice Vaticana, 1998).

insofar as it can illuminate departure and separation as a whole.

There is argument that separation on one's own authority for adultery, in contrast to the reasons mentioned in canon 1153, is not only licit as a reason for departure but also effects the true canonical status of the separation of the spouses.[15] However, I would like to mention one relevant part of the canon regarding separation for adultery. Canon 1152 §3 states, "If the innocent spouse has severed conjugal living voluntarily, the spouse is to introduce a cause for separation within six months to the competent ecclesiastical authority . . . ." The mention of introduction of a cause for separation within six months was significantly weakened between the 1972 and 1978 *schemata*, for reasons that are not entirely clear in the published notes. The draft originally stated that the non-adulterous spouse ". . . *debet intra sex menses causam separationis . . . deferre*."[16] This was changed to ". . . *intra sex mensem causam separationis deferat* . . . ."[17] Huels notes that *debet* (as in 1972) indicates a "strong positive command," such as "must;" while the present subjunctive (as in 1978) indicates a "mild command [or] exhortation . . . best translated as 'should.'"[18]

> Therefore, it is reasonable to conclude that the change from '*debet . . . deferre*' to '*deferat*' indicates that the *coetus* wanted to give a greater degree of autonomy in the exercise of the right of the innocent party to separate by his or her own authority, since recourse to the ecclesiastical authority is merely an exhortation rather than a strong obligation.[19]

Since ecclesiastical separation effects a change in the obligations the spouses have towards each other, including financial matters and the care of the children, approaching the competent authority provides the opportunity for these matters to be decided, since they would not have been addressed by a separation *propria auctoritate*. Whatever the strength of the obligation or exhortation to approach ecclesiastical authority within six months, failure to do so would not affect the liceity of the departure already effected or the separation *propria auctoritate* already established.

15 See Anthony St. Louis-Sanchez, "Separation of Spouses Propria Auctoritate and the Nature of Ecclesiastical Intervention," *Studia Canonica* 48 (2014) 2: 493–530.

16 "Coetus Studiorum «De Matrimonio» Session XVI," *Communicationes* 34 (2002) 243.

17 "Opera Consultorum in Apparandis Canonum Schematibus: Coetus Studiorum de Iure Matrimoniali," *Communicationes* 10 (1978) 119.

18 John M. Huels, *Liturgy and Law: Liturgical Law in the System of the Roman Catholic Church* (Montréal: Wilson & Lafleur, 2006) 234–35.

19 St. Louis-Sanchez, "Separation of Spouses Propria Auctoritate," 519.

1.4 Malicious abandonment

The canonical core of the petition templates circulating is the request for a declaration of the separation of the spouses due to "malicious abandonment" or "malicious desertion" (*malitiosam desertionem*). Although this concept does not appear in text of the Code of Canon Law, it is not fictional; it is a part of the canonical tradition and is recognized in jurisprudence. The basic concept is this: if a spouse has some reason to be defined as a separated spouse in canon law, most likely for its civil effects or possibly to enter into religious life, but cannot factually claim to have suffered another recognized reason for separation (e.g., adultery, or grave danger to soul or body, or an unduly hard common life, etc.), but instead the other spouse has simply left—possibly without even claiming that the departure was legitimate—then the abandoned spouse would need some reasoning or argument by which to claim the status of a separated spouse. The concept of "malicious abandonment" is that reasoning. A more thorough explanation of the concept of malicious abandonment is given in the *Exegetical Commentary*.[20] Briefly, malicious abandonment can be declared where there is, in fact, a suspension of the common conjugal life by one party; where this is done with the deliberate intent to abandon conjugal rights and obligations at least for a time; and where there was no legitimate reason to do so.

The petitions received mostly focus on the cessation of cohabitation, with some supplementary reference to the education of the children. Of course, more rights and obligations than these are tied up in marriage. But there is, I think, one very notable omission from the claims in these petitions: they do not mention incontinence. Commentaries from the first half of the twentieth century seem to consider as one of the primary ills of separation the possibility that a spouse would be tempted to unchastity as a result of no longer receiving the owed marital debt. A typical example quotes a sixteenth century moralist and canonist thus: "[Tomas] Sanchez held that by no means must an ecclesiastical judge permit young married persons to be separated because of the danger of incontinence."[21] The Roman Rota reasoned similarly in 1910: "Separation . . . exposes the consorts to the danger of incontinence. . . . For matrimony also exists as a remedy for concupiscence and, if common life is dissolved by separation, immediately it opens the door to adulterous amours and illicit associations."[22] And again in 1930, "separation from bed, board and cohabitation, even temporary, is a *res*

---

20 See Escrivá Ivars, "Separation While the Bond Remains," 1585–1586.

21 "Quare judex Ecclesiast. nullo modo permittere debet conjuges illvenes separatos esse ob incontinentiæ periculum." Tomás Sánchez, *Disputationum de Sacramento Matrimonii*, lib. IX, disp. 4, n. 5, p. 178, quoted in Eugene A. Forbes, "The Canonical Separation of Consorts," Dissertationes Ad Gradum Laurea in Facultatibus Ecclesiasticis Consequendum Conscriptae, Series Canonica 15 (Ottawa: University of Ottawa Press, 1948) 141.

22 Tribunal of the Roman Rota, definitive sentence c. Lega, *Separationis*, July 5, 1910: *RRDec* 2: n. 11; translated in Forbes, "The Canonical Separation of Consorts," 142.

gravis inasmuch as it . . . is fraught with dangers to the consorts, especially the danger of incontinence."[23] When the object of matrimonial consent was the *ius in corpus*,[24] and when the remedy for concupiscence was one of the secondary ends of marriage given in the law,[25] then it is logical that the first casualty of the severance of the common life would be that the spouses would be tempted into sexual sin. If one were truly trying to enter into the mindset of the pre-personalism commentators and Rotal judges, the headline complaint about a departed spouse would be that the abandoned spouse could consequently be tempted to unchastity. The complete absence of mention of this issue cannot be a coincidence or an oversight.

The supporting source collations which are often mailed together with the petitions quote liberally from the same sources mentioned herein by the present author; there must have been, on some level, a choice not to advance claims based on the *ius in corpus* and the danger of incontinence. Perhaps it reflects a certain superiority on behalf of those who would submit these petitions; the assumption that the one petitioning would never be tempted to unchastity, no matter how long the absence of the spouse. Or perhaps it is because even those who are attempting to return to a prior era of marriage law by trying to force the return of a departed spouse, are unwilling to return completely to that mentality in all its aspects. All of this is an aside to illustrate a theme to which I will be returning: that it is not always possible to import parts of the prior law and commentary regarding separation into our present law and anthropology of marriage as a whole.

1.5 Forcing a spouse to return

One of the key themes underlying these petitions, sometimes implicit and sometimes explicit in the cited sources, is the idea that a departed spouse can be *ordered* or *forced* to return—to return, it is claimed, not merely to residence in a common home but to the resumption of married life in every way. As I explained earlier, the decision to depart is fundamentally not justiciable according to a close reading of the current canon on departure. Nevertheless, the question of whether or not a spouse can be forced to return needs addressing since it does have some pedigree.

Many commentaries on the prior law take for granted that the resumption

23 Tribunal of the Roman Rota, definitive sentence c. Julienn, *Separationis*, August 6, 1930: *RRDec* 22: 523-534, n. 11; translated in Forbes, "The Canonical Separation of Consorts," 142.

24 See Charles J. Scicluna, *The Essential Definition of Marriage According to the 1917 and 1983 Codes of Canon Law: An Exegetical and Comparative Study* (Lanham, Maryland: University Press of America, 1995) 84.

25 See 1917 *CIC* c. 1013 §1: "Matrimonii finis primarius est procreatio atque educatio prolis: secundarius mutuum adiutorium et remedium concupiscentiae."

of the common conjugal life can be ordered by ecclesiastical authority, at least in theory. One from 1948 states, "The injured spouse has the right to petition the public ecclesiastical authority to force the return of his partner who has departed for an unjust reason."[26] "If the guilty [spouse] refuses to return, he can be forced to do so by ecclesiastical sentence and sanction."[27] Several post-1983 commentaries essentially agree, even if they avoid the term *force*. Woestman states, for example, that "both canon law and civil law grant the right to an action to enjoin one's spouse to maintain or restore common living," though he immediately follows this with "most frequently this is not the most expedient or propitious means to achieve marital harmony."[28] While respecting those later commentators, I wonder whether they may have been incorporating unchanged some assumptions from the prior law regarding separation, without taking into account the more fundamental changes to the canon law of marriage. One of these most important changes is surely the changed object of matrimonial consent.

Gaudium et spes described marriage as an "intimate communion of . . . life and love,"[29] and a "mutual gift of two persons."[30] Marriage comes into being with a "human act whereby spouses mutually bestow and accept each other."[31] Known as "personalism," this new understanding saw the object of matrimonial consent as the spouse him- or herself, in contrast to the 1917 code which defined the object of matrimonial consent as the perpetual and exclusive right to the body.[32] Borrowing from *Gaudium et spes*, canon 1057 §2 of the 1983 code redefined matrimonial consent as the act "by which a man and a woman mutually give and accept *each other*" [emphasis added]. If something as important as the definition of the object of matrimonial consent can be changed, we need to be ready for this to have far-reaching consequences. While there may not be a straight line to be drawn from a personalist object of matrimonial consent to the *ipso iure* abrogation of a previously understood ability to order the return of a departed spouse, the change should force us to reconsider with a critical eye commentary on the prior law insofar as it seems to rely on the abrogated definition of the object of matrimonial consent.

---

26 Forbes, "The Canonical Separation of Consorts," 137.

27 Ibid., 227.

28 William H. Woestman, *Special Marriage Cases*, rev. ed. (Ottawa: Saint Paul University, 1992) 64. See also Ladislas Örsy, *Marriage in Canon Law: Text and Comments, Reflections and Questions* (Dublin: Dominican Publications, 1986) 234.

29 Second Vatican Council, pastoral constitution *Gaudium et Spes* 48, December 7, 1965: *AAS* 58 (1966): "*Intima communitas vitae et amoris* . . . ." All translations of the texts of the Second Vatican Council are taken from Walter M. Abbott, *Documents of Vatican II* (New York: America Press, 1966).

30 *Gaudium et Spes* 48: "*. . . mutua duarum personarum donatio* . . . ."

31 Ibid.: "*Ita actu humano, quo coniuges sese mutuo tradunt atque accipiunt* . . . ."

32 See 1917 *CIC* c. 1081 §2: "Consensus matrimonialis est actus voluntatis quo utraque pars tradit et acceptat ius in corpus, perpetuum et exclusivum, in ordine ad actus per se aptos ad prolis generationem."

Many of the commentaries cited by the new proponents of judicial solutions to marital distress come from the first half of the twentieth century and must have sounded outdated even then. For example, one considered the questions "whether the husband is bound to provide food for his wife, and, more particularly, whether he is bound to take his meals at the same table with her."[33] We are told that the husband is obliged to provide food if he received a dowry with his wife, but he is not obliged to provide sustenance if she came with no dowry—except "when the wife performs domestic work in place of a servant, then he is bound to provide sustenance for her, at least as he would do for a servant."[34] On the other hand, it does say that the husband is obliged to eat at the same table as the wife unless a just cause excuses.[35] These are the same books which are selectively cited today in favor of enforcing the alleged law regarding the separation of spouses and civil divorce.

Many of these commentaries were produced in a time of rapid secularization and growth in divorce; a time of challenges to the Church's legal and cultural predominant dominion over marriage. I would suggest that these commentaries should not be viewed as the best summary of the Church's authentic law and teaching regarding marriage; as a zenith reached before being corrupted by a perceived "wider post-Conciliar malaise regarding the defense of marriage."[36] Instead they ought to be seen as products of their era and of their authors: unsuccessful attempts to stem the tide of divorce by any means possible, produced by men who even as they wrote complained that the law was seldom known and never enforced, and who recognized that their brother priests and bishops, and the Church in general, were moving in a different direction.[37]

If those who are promoting these petitions wish to be consistent in their very literal understanding of the vindicability of ecclesial rights at the competent ecclesiastical forum[38] combined with an unquestioning regurgitation of selectively chosen commentary on the prior law, why stop at malicious abandonment? Why not be prepared to bring a petition from the wife claiming that the food she receives is lesser than would be given to a servant, and then to hear the husband's defense that the wife does not provide servant-quality work to earn such food?

33 Forbes, "The Canonical Separation of Consorts," 131.

34 Ibid., 132.

35 See ibid.

36 Edward N. Peters, "Do Catholics Need Ecclesiastical Permission to Divorce?" *Fellowshop of Catholic Scholars Quarterly* 40 (2017) 1: 62.

37 For example, a general commentary more representative of the era states, "A party seeking separation should normally be referred to the Ordinary. However, ... it will usually be well not to insist on this obligation if the parties are unaware of it, especially if the separation is already in effect and there is no great scandal connected with it." *Canon Law: A Text and Commentary*, 4th ed., ed. Lincoln Bouscaren et al. (Milwaukee: Bruce, 1946) 572.

38 Cf. 1983 *CIC* c. 221 §1.

The answer, I suspect, is that everyone now instinctively understands that marriage is no longer to be understood as the simultaneous fulfilment of defined rights while physically located under the same roof. It is an "intimate communion of life and love,"[39] a "partnership of the whole of life."[40] These aspects of the prior law regarding the separation of spouses, considered in light of the present law of marriage as a whole, appear now to be so foreign that they cannot be applied without damage to both the institution of marriage and the rule of law in the Church.[41]

2. The bishop's permission to approach the civil forum

Canon 1692 §2 states: "Where an ecclesiastical decision has no civil effects or if a civil sentence is not contrary to divine law, the bishop of the diocese of the residence of the spouses, after having weighed the special circumstances, can grant permission [*licentiam*] to approach the civil forum."[42] Taking this paragraph, and some traditions stretching back prior to 1983, some currently claim that there is an obligation to receive the permission of the diocesan bishop prior to seeking civil separation or divorce. While this inference is not entirely unreasonable when considering this translation of the paragraph outside of its context, closer examination demonstrates that this interpretation misunderstands completely the purpose of the canon.

2.1 Universal law prior to 1983

Dating back to the mid-nineteenth century, there are records of various responses from different dicasteries of the Apostolic See regarding approaching the civil authorities for civil separation or divorce.[43] However, it should be noted that these are not requests for permission in the canonical sense; they are requests for moral advice. The usual situation is that a person in some kind of combined marital-financial distress would ask her confessor whether she could divorce her husband in the civil court without sinning. The confessor, the diocesan bishop

---

39 *Gaudium et Spes* 48: "*Intima communitas vitae et amoris . . . .*"

40 1983 *CIC* c. 1055: "Matrimoniale foedus, quo vir et mulier inter se totius vitae consortium constituunt, indole sua naturali ad bonum coniugum atque ad prolis generationem et educationem ordinatum, a Christo Domino ad sacramenti dignitatem inter baptizatos evectum est."

41 Cf. Mark 2:22.

42 1983 *CIC* c. 1692 §2: "Ubi decisio ecclesiastica effectus civiles non sortitur, vel si sententia civilis praevidetur non contraria iuri divino, Episcopus dioecesis commorationis coniugum poterit, perpensis peculiaribus adiunctis, licentiam concedere adeundi forum civile."

43 See Forbes, "The Canonical Separation of Consorts," 206–215.

or even groups of bishops if there were many similar cases, would approach the Sacred Penitentiary or the Holy Office for an opinion on the morality of the request, whether specific or general. Answers were usually negative to the request, with the exception of one oracular "*[o]rator consulat probatos auctores*:"[44] "the requester is to consult approved authors." This makes even more clear that what was being requested was not permission in any canonical sense; advice was being given about the morality of what were, in the mid-nineteenth century, relatively new situations in many countries. Not until 1906 was an answer given clearly in the affirmative, when the Holy Office gave a number of steps to ensure that the civil divorce would not be confused with a breaking of the bond of marriage. An identical reply was given consistently through at least the mid-1940s.[45] Still, what was actually being given was moral advice, not permission; there was no requirement for permission to approach the civil forum in the universal law either before or after 1917.

2.2 The Third Plenary Council of Baltimore

There was, however, particular law in the United States relevant to this matter. Canon 126 of the Third Plenary Council of Baltimore ("Baltimore III") promulgated in 1886 states, in part: "To all those who are joined in marriage, we give the precept that they are not to approach the civil courts to obtain separation from bed and table without consulting (*ne inconsulta*) ecclesiastical authority. But whoever has attempted this is to know that he has incurred grave guilt to be punished by judgment of the bishop."[46] Notice what it says: *ne inconsulta*, without consulting. Yet barely was the ink dry before this canon was being used to claim an obligation to receive permission—which is very different from consultation.

There is an argument that this canon is referring only to separation, not divorce, by the phrase "separation from bed and table," *a thoro et mensa*. This is the common law tradition phrase for separation; the canonical historical term would be *tori, mensae et habitationis*[47] (bed, table and dwelling).[48] I wonder

44 Response of the Sacred Penitentiary, June 30, 1892, cited by Forbes, "The Canonical Separation of Consorts," 209–10, and apparently not published elsewhere.

45 Forbes, "The Canonical Separation of Consorts," p. 210, cites James P. Kelly, "Separation and Civil Divorce," *The Jurist* 6 (1948) 2: 221, as having seen one from 1945.

46 *Acta et Decreta Concilii Plenarii Baltimorensis Tertii. A.D. MDCCCLXXXIV* (Baltimore: Joannis Murphy, 1886) 64–65: ". . . iis omnibus, qui matrimonio conjuncti sunt, praecipimus, ne inconsulta auctoritate ecclesiastica, tribunalia civilia adeant ad obtinendam separationem a thoro et mensa. Quod si quis attentaverit, sciat se gravem reatum incurrere et pro Episcopi judicio puniendum esse." English translation by the author.

47 See Forbes, "The Canonical Separation of Consorts," 130.

48 Note that the canonical and civil traditions use different spellings of the word for "bed."

if this argument may well be taking the Baltimore canon too literally; a more plausible explanation may be that the bishops at Baltimore did not even want to recognize divorce in calling it by its name, but were instead intending to be clear that such a civil sentence could not sever the bond of marriage as it pretends to. Still, this canon establishes a penalty and therefore needs to be interpreted strictly.[49]

Many twentieth century American commentators appear to conflate the two different practices—consultation of the Apostolic See for difficult moral issues, and Baltimore III's specific canonical requirement to consult the local ecclesiastical authorities—into sweeping claims that have little basis in the texts themselves. For example, an article in *The Jurist* from 1946 claims that canon 126 explicitly states that spouses are bound and "that they may not seek a civil divorce without the explicit permission of the Holy See, or at least of the local Ordinary."[50] As we noted previously, the canon requires consultation not permission. Furthermore, the Holy See is not mentioned at all in the canon cited, and in practice gave not permission but only guidance. Similarly, a *vademecum* for priests from 1948[51] uses "consultation" and "permission" apparently interchangeably; the author translates the canon itself as meaning "permission," notes a lack of episcopal consultation in his first case study, yet in the third case study mentions the lack of consultation in the proposition of the scenario but the lack of permission in the resolution to the same situation. I suggest, then, that many of the mid-twentieth century commentaries on this matter are not only irrelevant to the present law; they were often also irrelevant to the law of their own era.

It is commonly argued that neither the 1917 nor 1983 codes abrogated canon 126 of the Third Plenary Council of Baltimore. This claim is correct inasmuch as neither code abrogated particular penal law issued in a plenary council. Yet this ignores the fact that laws can also cease to be laws by the very fact of their widespread non-observance: "the law initially might be accepted, but could become obsolete or harmful over time and fall into desuetude, the phenomenon known as the intrinsic cessation of law."[52] This description appears to correspond exactly to what has occurred regarding Baltimore III's provisions regarding approaching the civil authorities in matrimonial matters.

It is not completely clear whether the norm of canon 126 of the Third Plenary Council of Baltimore—obliging consultation of ecclesiastical authorities before recourse to the civil court—still has the force of law; it may have been abrogated

49 See 1983 *CIC* c. 18.

50 Kelly, "Separation and Civil Divorce," 233–34.

51 See Alford, "Cohabitation and Separation of Married Persons."

52 John M. Huels, "General Norms," in Beal, *New Commentary on the Code of Canon Law*, 59.

either by subsequent legislation or by desuetude. Even if it did still nominally exist as law, I would suggest that it could not be applied today without raising troubling questions about the role of law in the life of the Church.

2.3 The 1983 Code of Canon Law

Canons 1692-1696 of the 1983 Code of Canon Law are entirely new; "The 1917 Code contained no such chapter; it contained no canons regulating procedures for separation cases; these canons were first introduced in the 1976 schema."[53] This canon appears in Book VII (*De processibus*), Part III (*De quibusdam processibus specialibus*), Title I (*De processibus matrimonialibus*), Chapter II (*De causis separationis coniugum*); it addresses the special procedural norms for cases of the separation of the spouses. It is not in the portion of the code devoted to the rights and obligations of marriage. If the code were to establish a general obligation to seek permission prior to approaching the civil authorities regarding a marriage, we might expect to find it in the title regarding marriage (cc. 1055-1165), perhaps especially in the article *de separatione manente vinculo* (cc. 1151-1155).

In response to the increasing publicity outside of specialist canonical discussion regarding the claim that canon 1692 §2 obliges a spouse to receive ecclesiastical permission before initiating a civil divorce, a bishop wrote to the Pontifical Council for Legislative Texts for clarification. The President of the Council responded with a letter dated November 4, 2015, which was subsequently published on the website of the Council.[54] Part of the letter is worth considering at length:

> Canon 1692 §1 *CIC* establishes that "unless other provision is legitimately made in particular places, a decree of the diocesan bishop or a judicial sentence can decide the personal separation of baptized spouses." Since distinct positions are possible, depending on each conference of bishops' particular legislation as well as any concordat with the civil government, the diocesan bishop's permission for a Catholic spouse to initiate civil divorce may or may not be a requirement in a given place. In practice, this means that where there is no particular legislation or concordat to direct otherwise, and where the ecclesiastical decision has no civil effects (cf. c. 1692 §2 *CIC*), the local bishop's permission would not be an obligation—whether juridical or moral.

53 Lawrence G. Wrenn, "Certain Special Procedures," in *The Code of Canon Law: A Text and Commentary*, 1016.

54 Pontifical Council for Legislative Texts, letter "Prot. N. 15181/2015: Your Excellency," November 4, 2015, http://www.delegumtextibus.va/content/dam/testilegislativi/risposte-particolari/cic/On%20whether%20a%20bishop's%20permission%20is%20needed%20for%20a%20civil%20divorce%20(can.%201692%20CIC).pdf (accessed on 17 Dec. 2019).

> However, the faithful may request advice from their bishop for reasons of prudence, pastoral clarification, or avoidance of scandals.[55]

In the PCLT's letter, then, the code's provisions regarding ecclesiastical permission to approach the civil authorities do not begin with the second paragraph of canon 1692, but with the first—which paragraph does not explicitly mention either the civil forum or permission. The first emphasized portion notes the applicability of this provision primarily to those places which do not have other provision made.[56] For example in Italy, where a Concordat provides that separation cases are to be handled by the civil authorities, they would receive recognition from the Church.[57]

The second emphasized part—the word "can"—takes a literal interpretation of *potest*; the bishop is able to decide, but is not obliged to decide, and nor is it stated that anyone is obliged to request his decision. The same interpretative approach then is applied to the second paragraph of the canon, which states that the diocesan bishop "can grant permission to approach the civil forum" (*poterit . . . licentiam concedere adeundi forum civile*). The diocesan bishop is able to grant permission, but he is not obliged to, and again it is not stated that anyone in particular is obliged to seek or to receive permission; hence the conclusion that "the local bishop's permission would not be an obligation—whether juridical or moral."

The letter seems to understand the whole of canon 1692 as referring to the canonical separation of the spouses: the first paragraph of the canon states that the diocesan bishop or the judge can decide the canonical separation of the spouses.[58] The second paragraph of the canon then states that the diocesan bishop can grant permission to approach the civil forum—which should be read in the context of the whole canon, that is, regarding canonical separation. The second paragraph does not directly address civil divorce or civil separation, though these would likely be involved in practice; it addresses the ability of the diocesan bishop to

---

55 Ibid. (emphasis in original).

56 If 1983 *CIC* c. 1692 §2 truly established an obligation to obtain episcopal permission before approaching the civil authorities for divorce or civil separation, then it would be illogical to restrict this to places where the ecclesiastical decision would have no civil effects. Indeed, places where an ecclesiastical decision *could* have civil effects would seem to be precisely the places where it would be most appropriate to receive special permission prior to circumventing the Church's own established and effective procedures.

57 "Quanto alle cause di separazione personale, la Santa Sede consente che siano giudicate dall'autorità giudiziaria civile." Pietro Cardinale Gaspari and Benito Mussolini, "Concordato Tra La Santa Sede e l'Italia," art. 34, February 11, 1929: *AAS* 21 (1929) 290.

58 See 1983 *CIC* c. 1692 §1.

attribute ecclesiastical effects to the eventual civil decision.[59]

It is sometimes argued that canon 1692 §2 must implicitly establish a requirement to receive permission before seeking civil divorce, because it would make no sense for receipt of permission to be optional—why obtain permission for something already permitted? This objection is addressed by understanding the second paragraph as referring to an alternative means to establish canonical separation. Without the authorization of the bishop, the civil authorities would have no competence regarding the canonical separation of the spouses; therefore, authorization is required only inasmuch as one wants the civil authorities to be able to create a status of canonical separation. Note the final sentence in the quoted paragraph from the letter of the Pontifical Council for Legislative Texts: "the faithful may request advice from their bishop" regarding approaching the civil forum. This is consistent with the prior practice of approaching the Apostolic See regarding civil divorce: what was given was advice, not permission or authorization.

Further clarity is achieved by considering the exact nature of the *licentia* which the bishop can give according to this paragraph. "A *licentia*—which can be translated as permission, authorization, and the like—is variously defined in doctrine. . . . Its concession makes it possible for a person to exercise some faculty or right as a prior guarantee of the validity or liceity of the permitted act."[60] Among the various categories of *licentiæ* in the law, Daniel finds that the *licentia* can be "a favor granted by rescript"[61] in which category is found "authorizing spouses to approach the civil forum for a cause of separation (*CIC* c. 1692 §2; *CCEO* c. 1378 §2)."[62] Regarding canon 1692 §2, then, less confusion might be caused if *licentiam* were translated not as "permission" but as "authorization," since "authorization" makes clearer that the purpose of the concession is to "make it possible for a person to exercise [the] faculty"[63] "to approach the civil forum for a cause of separation"[64] properly understood—that is, to obtain the status of separated spouses in the society of the Church.

All of this could certainly be made more explicit in the text of each paragraph, but I believe it does make sense in the context of the canon as a whole, and the place in the code where it is located. Still, one commentator has written, "A

59 See 1983 *CIC* c. 1692 §2. An analogy might be the "canonization" of civil contracts regarding temporal goods established by canon 1290, enabling civil law provisions to be enforceable within and by the society of the Church.

60 William L. Daniel, "The Singular Administrative Act in Canon Law," *Studia Canonica* 50 (2016) 1: 243.

61 Ibid., 244.

62 Ibid., 245.

63 Ibid., 243.

64 Ibid., 245.

casual reading of the Canons of the Code on Separation will convince one that they are not too well written."[65] Although he said this regarding the 1917 code, perhaps this is one piece of commentary on the prior law that still applies.

2.4 The *mens legislatoris*

If the meaning of a law is unclear, one of the sources to which we can turn is the *mens legislatoris*.[66] So let us consider the recent pontifical magisterium regarding separation and divorce, especially as expressed in the two Apostolic Exhortations regarding marriage and the family of the last forty years: *Familiaris consortio*[67] and *Amoris laetitia*.[68]

Familiaris consortio was published in 1981, in the last days of the 1917 code, and as the revision process was in the final stages of drafting the new Code of Canon Law. In a section dedicated to both separated and divorced persons, John Paul II writes: "Various reasons can unfortunately lead to the often irreparable breakdown of valid marriages. These include mutual lack of understanding and the inability to enter into interpersonal relationships. Obviously, separation must be considered as a last resort, after all other reasonable attempts at reconciliation have proved vain."[69]

There are a number of points in that text that apparently are not accepted by some today: that the breakdown can happen for a variety of reasons; that it can be irreparable; and that mutual lack of understanding or interpersonal problems can be the cause, rather than the clearer categorization and higher standard implied by some of the jurisprudence from the earlier twentieth century. It is clear that John Paul II is using "separation" in its everyday context, meaning a rupture in the common life; this would include situations of departure or *de facto* separation as mentioned earlier; there is no indication that he is referring only to spouses who have the canonical status of separation in the Church. There is no mention whatsoever, in the entire document, of any requirement to approach the Church regarding separation or civil divorce. One would think that if the legislator had thought that such requirements existed at the time, or if he were intending to include such requirements soon in the new code, he would have mentioned it. As Anthony St. Louis-Sanchez summarized the 1980 Synod of Bishops, which

---

65 Kelly, "Separation and Civil Divorce," 203.

66 Cf. 1983 *CIC* c. 17.

67 See John Paul II, apostolic exhortation *Familiaris consortio*, November 22, 1981: *AAS* 74 (1981) 81–191.

68 See Francis, apostolic exhortation "*Amoris laetitia*," March 19, 2016: *AAS* 108 (2016) 311–446.

69 *Familiaris consortio* 83; English translation at http://www.vatican.va/content/john-paul-ii/en/apost_exhortations/documents/hf_jp-ii_exh_19811122_familiaris-consortio.html (accessed on 13 Apr. 2020).

led to *Familaris consortio*, "Civil divorce was no longer seen as the enemy but rather as a problem in need of a solution."[70]

Amoris laetitia follows *Familiaris consortio* in recognizing that separation is something which must often be recognized as a factual reality, stating that it becomes "inevitable" in situations of "grave injustice, violence or chronic ill-treatment."[71] Again, separation is used in its everyday meaning. *Amoris laetita* in many places urges the faithful to support those in troubled marriages; nowhere does it mention canonical separation, or a requirement to receive permission to approach the civil authorities, as part of that support. *Amoris laetitia* describes situations analogous to the canonical reasons for separation or departure, reflecting both canon 1153, §1 and *Familiaris consortio*, but also develops these further as it says that these situations provide not only a right to separate, but even a moral obligation: "At times it even becomes morally necessary, precisely when it is a matter of removing the more vulnerable spouse or young children from serious injury due to abuse and violence, from humiliation and exploitation, and from disregard and indifference."[72] To my knowledge, this is the first magisterial statement that departure from the conjugal life might be not only permissible but even sometimes obligatory.

The subject is also not promoted or encouraged, as far as I can tell, in any other document emanating from any organ of the Roman Curia. Ongoing problems such as, say, theological dissent, liturgical abuses, and irregular practices in matrimonial nullity trials, have instigated a steady stream of letters, allocutions and instructions intended to address the issues. Yet there is nothing regarding the separation of the spouses or an obligation to receive permission to divorce, which would be an astonishing *lacuna* if what is being claimed as the law were actually the law. Every tribunal submits each year a statistical report to the Apostolic Signatura regarding the year's activity in the tribunal, and frequently a reply is received making some comments which the bishop moderator may be expected to address; I have never heard of a letter from the Apostolic Signatura criticizing a tribunal for hearing no cases regarding the separation of the spouses for decades in a row. I was informed by a recent graduate of the *Studium Rotale* that the three-year program to train advocates of the Roman Rota mentioned the separation of the spouses not once. In short, these present petitioners and their backers are claiming something to be the law, but their opinion does not appear to be shared by any of those responsible for the law.

---

70 St. Louis-Sanchez, "Separation of Spouses Propria Auctoritate," 515. Or, summarizing the same synod, "Divorce is simply considered a painful reality in the modern world." Kamas, "Separation of the Spouses with the Bond Remaining," 194.

71 *Amoris laetitia* 241; English ransaltion at http://w2.vatican.va/content/dam/francesco/pdf/apost_exhortations/documents/papa-francesco_esortazione-ap_20160319_amoris-laetitia_en.pdf (accessed on 13 Apr. 2020).

72 Ibid.

3. Selected Cases at the Roman Rota

There are not many cases heard or published at the Roman Rota concerning the separation of the spouses, especially from the second half of the twentieth century onwards. I summarize here a few which seem especially relevant to the present questions.

3.1 Sentence *coram* Lega, April 20, 1912[73]

This case was decided obviously prior to the 1917 code, though like the 1917 code it focuses on the question of whether the hardship in the marriage was caused by cruelty (*saevitate*). It perhaps is notable that the case was decided by the Dean of the Rota together with ten auditors; even then, it was more common to have only three auditors assigned to the case. The woman-respondent appears to be mentally ill. The judges conclude, "[I]mplacable hatred between the spouses is a just cause for the separation to be conceded."[74] The case is later summarized in its conclusions by Jarawan in a sentence of May 15, 1989, thusly: "Therefore, even if there are not cruelties, separation can be granted temporarily if there is a subjective intolerability for cohabitation, namely, if physical or psychological harm comes to the spouse due to the grave divergence of wills."[75]

Regarding temporary separation, especially in older jurisprudence, it would be a mistake to minimize the significance of temporary separation: it should not be dismissed as inconsequential as though it were not a 'real separation.' Firstly, if it is sufficient for temporary separated status, it was likely sufficient reason to depart. Secondly, given the lifelong nature of marriage itself, permanent separations should in principle be the exception and not the rule; historically the Church has been very reluctant to grant permanent separated status for any reason other than adultery. But even at the expiry of the time period established for temporary separation, while the status in canon law as separated spouses would expire, there would not be a moral obligation to return unless the reasons that originally justified the departure no longer applied.

---

73 Tribunal of the Roman Rota, definitive sentence c. Lega, *Separationis*, April 20, 1912: *RRDec* 4: 193-203.

74 Ibid., n. 12. And furthermore, "Non solum ex hoc capite (seu, saevitiis) iterum censuerunt locum esse separationi tori; sed tanto libentius inhaeserunt alteri etiam fundamento decisionis, deducto ex capitali odio et inimicitiis quae, diuturno litis processu, inter partes supervenerunt."

75 "Inde separatio, etsi saevitiae non adsint, concedi potest ad tempus si obiectiva intolerabilitas adsit conviventiae, immo si ex gravi animorum disociatione damnum physicum vel psychicum coniugi eveniat." Tribunal of the Roman Rota, definitive sentence c. Jarawan, *Separationis*, May 15, 1989: *RRDec* 81: 348-355, n. 3.

3.2 Sentence *coram* Florczak, June 30, 1928[76]

This case is not especially relevant in the history of the jurisprudence regarding separation. I raise it here because it is currently being cited by some to claim that frequent quarrels are not a cause for separation. That argument, I think, is missing the context of the decision.

The parties were in their late sixties and had been married for over twenty-five years. The petitioner's claims that his wife held a longstanding and implacable hatred for him were demonstrated to be factually false by the witnesses. The petitioner seems to want to be rid of his wife either because she argued too much with the servant, or because he wanted not to have to feed her. The respondent, who appears to be a forgiving sort, though not without a temper of her own, still desires the resumption of the common life as had endured happily for over two decades. The petitioner himself does not deny that his wife is now behaving in such a manner as to make the common life possible again. So even if the petitioner's subjective feelings about his arguments with his wife may have justified his departure in the forum of conscience, it is evident from the facts of the case that he could not be granted canonical separation in this judicial forum since his testimony which could have supported this was refuted by multiple witnesses.

This case reminds me of situations one occasionally encounters in marriage nullity trials: the court gives a negative decision because the petitioner's testimony is demonstrably false and there are few relevant facts to be had, even though it is quite possible that if one were able to get at the truth, the marriage well might be demonstrated to be invalid. It appears to me that this petitioner brought the decision on himself, perhaps with the application of some equity by the judges; it does not mean that frequent quarrels could never be a legitimate reason to separate or depart.

3.3 Sentence *coram* Jullien, August 6, 1930[77]

This sentence is quoted and translated in a 1948 doctoral dissertation, and that translation is sometimes now cited in support of the idea that separation or departure is likely unjustifiable. The oft-quoted portion reads, "It is not right that separation take place for light inconveniences, even though these are repeated, for example, incompatibility of temperament; for even more serious quarrels, arising from unusual anger and unexpected perturbation, do not exclude hope of early reconciliation; nor, *a fortiori*, for just censure and correction . . . : all these

76 Tribunal of the Roman Rota, definitive sentence c. Florczak, *Separationis*, June 30, 1928: *RRDec* 20: 267–272.

77 Tribunal of the Roman Rota, definitive sentence c. Jullien, *Separationis*, August 6, 1930: *RRDec* 22: 523-534.

do not bring with them serious injury or grave fear to a steadfast soul."[78] We need to read between the lines here. If the inconveniences are light, then obviously they cannot justify departure or separation. But if the anger and perturbation are not unusual and unexpected but frequent; if there is no hope of early reconciliation; if there is no hope of correction; if the one subject to them is not a steadfast soul, then a separation may be considered

3.4 Sentence *coram* Masala, February 19, 1975[79]

This sentence is important because it is the first published separation sentence to consider significantly the personalist understanding of marriage flowing from *Gaudium et spes*, and it quotes several times from that Pastoral Constitution on the Church. Paragraph three of this sentence is therefore quoted or referenced frequently in subsequent decisions. Like many other sentences before and after, it resists considering only an objective classification of which acts do or do not justify separation, but takes into account the subjective characteristics of the parties:

> [T]he judge is to weigh carefully all the circumstances of the case, especially keeping in mind both the objective gravity of the offenses that the aggrieved party presents as cruelty, and the character, nature, morals and consistency of both spouses, that is, of the one inflicting the cruelty and of the one suffering it (cf. Sanchez, *De matrimonio*, book X, disp. 18, nn. 7-13).[80]

3.5 Sentence *coram* Pompedda, July 26, 1976[81]

This sentence is interesting mostly because Pompedda summarizes the whole definition of what would justify separation in only one hundred words of Latin, a

---

78 "Enimvero separationem fieri nefas est ob levia quaedam incommode, quamvis repetita, puta discrepantis indolis causa; neque ob graviora iurgia, sed quae, nata ex insolita quadam ira et inopinato perturbationis motu, non excludunt spem proximae reconciliationis; nec a fortiori ob iustam reprehensionem et correctionem [...]: cuncta huismodi non inferunt gravem offensionem aut metum gravem in animam constantem." Ibid., n. 4; translated in Forbes, "The Canonical Separation of Consorts," 151.

79 Tribunal of the Roman Rota, definitive sentence c. Masala, *Separationis*, February 19, 1975: *RRDec* 76: 64–74.

80 Ibid., n. 6: "[I]udex sedulo per pendet omnia casus adiuncta, prae oculis habitis praesertim, sive obiectiva gravitate illarum offensionum, quas pars gravata pro saevitiis tra ducit, sive indole, ingenio, moribus ac constantia utriusque coniugis, inferentis nempe saevitias, easque patientis (cfr. Sanchez, De Matr., lib. X, disp. 18, nn. 7-13)." My thanks to Dr. William L. Daniel for his assistance with this translation, along with those of the sentences *coram* Pompedda and Jarawan.

81 Tribunal of the Roman Rota, definitive sentence c. Pompedda, *Separationis*, July 26, 1976: *RRDec* 77: 347–357.

quotation from Coronata's treatise on marriage;[82] perhaps this is a reminder that the law regarding legitimate reasons for separation does not need to be complex. Translated, it reads in part:

> In order to issue a true judgment about what cruelty should be thought to give sufficient cause for even a temporary separation, the judge must take into account the character and upbringing of the persons. For what is light for a woman of low estate may for the most part be serious for a woman of high estate and a good upbringing.[83]

Even if this phrasing may sit uneasily with us today, the point is clear: account must be taken of the backgrounds and characters of individual spouses, avoiding any generalized rules.

3.6 Decree *coram* Caberletti, November 14, 2007[84]

This case originated in Cleveland in 2004. The woman requested from the diocesan tribunal not separated status due to malicious abandonment, but a plain-and-simple declaration that there were no legitimate grounds for the man to have left the family home. The *libellus* was rejected due to a lack of judicial object. The petitioner appealed against the rejection of the *libellus* in accord with canon 1505 §4 to the metropolitan court of second instance, which upheld the first instance rejection. The petitioner then made recourse to the Roman Rota, which ruled that there is no recourse to third instance against the rejection of a *libellus*. Although the decree is largely focused on the procedural question of the right of recourse against a second rejection of the *libellus*, nevertheless the auditors also made space to summarize the various contradictions in the petitioner's campaign for ecclesiastical intervention in her marriage, and to quote from the first instance court's reasons for the rejection of the *libellus*: "A case for the separation of spouses is presented by the spouse who is requesting permission for the separation. The petitioner, in the case presented, does not desire a separation; hence there is no basis for a case."[85]

3.7 Sentence *coram* Caberletti, January 20, 2011;[86] sentence *coram* Sable of

---

82 See Matthaeus Coronata, *Institutiones Iuris Canonici*, vol. III (Mariatti, 1948) 923–24, n. 663e. (Coronata, Inst. Iuris Can., « De Sacramentis », III, De Matrimonio, ed. 1948, pp. 923 S., Il. 663).

83 *Coram* Pompedda, n. 4.

84 Tribunal of the Roman Rota, definitive sentence c. Caberletti, *Separationis*, November 14, 2007: *RRDecr* 25: 71–77.

85 Ibid., n. 5.

86 Tribunal of the Roman Rota, definitive sentence c. Caberletti, *Separationis*, January 20, 2011: *RRDec* 103: 1–21.

October 10, 2012[87]

These sentences regard the same marriage. The case originated with the inter-eparchial Maronite tribunal of the Lebanon, in which country the civil courts have no authority over matrimonial matters, and the decisions of the various religious authorities—including the Catholic eparchial tribunals—have civil effects. There is no civil divorce or separation in the Lebanon; all is left to the religious authorities, including temporal provisions. For this reason, cases from the Lebanon make up a disproportionately large share of the separation cases heard at the Roman Rota. They are considered according to the *Code of Canons of the Eastern Churches*, which are similar—though not identical—to the Latin code.[88]

The fact that the two codes share similar canons in this matter, however, should not deceive the reader into thinking that the law sections and arguments in these Middle Eastern cases are always entirely applicable in our own tribunals. For example, bearing an oversized importance in these cases is the question of *fault*, which if identified against a party will affect his or her ongoing financial rights and obligations in civil law.

The case involves separation as a subordinate ground, dependent on a decision regarding the nullity of the marriage. In the sentence *coram* Caberletti, after two grounds of nullity of marriage, the third part of the *dubium* was formulated *utrum restaurandus sit convictus an potius separatio declarari debeat*;[89] that is, whether the common life is to be restored or whether a separation is to be declared. The section *in iure* gives only a very brief treatment of the law regarding separation due to adultery,[90] before explaining at length *in facto* the negative responses regarding the nullity of the marriage. Only at the very end did the court turn briefly to the question of separation. The respondent was found more credible, the judges did not order the resumption of the common life (which had lasted two years, with no children being born) and a separation was ordered due to the fault of the petitioner, whose violent, adulterous and otherwise offensive behavior would have made the restoration of the common life impossible due to the danger to the woman's health.[91] The respondent, who by this point had

87 Tribunal of the Roman Rota, definitive sentence c. Sable, *Separationis*, October 10, 2012: *RRDec* 104: 258–67.

88 The principal difference is that the *CCEO* uses *consortium vitae conjugalis* and (once) *vita communis* in place of the Latin code's *convictus conjugalis*. While this may indicate an interesting shift in emphasis to illustrate the distinction between the juridic status of the parties and their actual manner of carrying out their married life, it does not fundamentally change the nature of marriage or the acts which would justify a separation. See Kamas, *Separation of the Spouses with the Bond Remaining*, 210–13.

89 See *Coram* Caberletti, n. 1.

90 Ibid., n. 7.

91 Ibid., n. 12.

become the *pars diligentior*, appealed against this decision because she wished the marriage to be declared null. In fact the higher Rotal *turnus* did find the marriage to be invalid, and therefore the question of separation was *non proponi* in the decision *coram* Sable of October 10, 2012.

The reader will note that the *dubia* used in this case at both instances at the Rota did consider whether the common life was to be restored (*utrum convictus restaurandus sit*). As previously noted, it is not possible to reconcile our current understanding of marriage with a judicial "order" to return to the conjugal life against one's will. So why do the two most recent published Rotal sentences mention it in the *dubium*? The answer is to be found in the unique interrelationship of the Lebanese civil and ecclesiastical authorities. Nobody in this case—the man, the woman, the judges—wanted or expected her to return to him; he had no interest whatsoever in resuming a life with her since he was the one who first petitioned for nullity of marriage. That part of the *dubium*, however, was a necessary prerequisite to his claim that should not pay alimony; if she could be nominally ordered to return, and then she would refuse to do so, he would not be obliged to maintain her. It is clear from both sentences that the judges did not seriously consider the possibility that she could return to him at all, never mind by judicial injunction.

3.8 Decree *coram* Jaeger, July 18, 2019[92]

A very recent decree at the Rota addresses many of the same claims we are now facing. A petitioner accused his wife of malicious abandonment and requested separation for this reason. The first instance tribunal, however, found that the petitioner was a cause of physical and moral danger to the respondent, and therefore granted the separation on that basis. The petitioner appealed directly to the Roman Rota, which declared the first instance sentence invalid due to the doubt having been incorrectly formulated.

Along the way, however, the *ponens* also clarifies a number of important points of law which explain well the appropriate response to the petitions and claims which are now reaching tribunals and chanceries. Jaeger explains that the right to depart is rooted in the spouses' human dignity and the personalist nature of marriage, analogous to a correct understanding of the *ius in corpus*, contrasted with the condition of slavery ("*servitudis*") which would be implied if the spouses were absolutely obliged to live together against the will of one of them; "a judgement about the right and duty of conjugal living is first and foremost moral; it is to be brought before the forum of conscience, and no one is to be compelled in the external forum positively to provide that."[93] Also noted

---

92 Tribunal of the Roman Rota, definitive sentence c. Jaeger, Prot N. 23.481, July 18, 2019: unpublished. Translated by Dr. Tina Marshall.

93 Ibid., n. 9.

is the fact that a canonically-established separation does not need to be formally attributed to the "fault" of one or another spouse.[94]

The decree notes the "uselessness [*inultilitate*] of a judicial process of separation that gives rise to no temporal effects"[95] in places which afford no particular effect to ecclesiastical decisions of this nature. Illustrating more clearly than ever the true nature of the separation of the spouses as an institute in canon law, we read that "cases of separation of the spouses are, for the litigating parties, first and foremost *iurium* cases" [96]—that is, they are cases to decide the temporal consequences of a marital shipwreck which has already occurred. They are not intended as a way to litigate or re-litigate who was right or wrong, at fault or innocent, in the breakdown of the relationship.

Finally, the decree hints that the petition perhaps should never have been accepted by the tribunal of first instance.[97] Quoting from the same kind of template petition as dioceses are now receiving, and also from the petitioner's own words, the decree concludes that "it is clear that the petitioner does not want separation"[98] but instead an order from the Church for the respondent to return to him.

4. Practical Considerations

4.1 Discernment of situations

As a broad generalization, these petitioners seem to fall into two distinct groups. The first group of petitioners are sincere and devout Catholics who have somehow heard of this phenomenon on the internet, and are now unsettled in conscience that they may be doing something wrong. They would like to be able to save their marriages, but they understand that it can't be forced. They look to the Church in this situation, as they have looked to the Church for answers and support at other times in their lives. They have now heard about separation, either as a canonical necessity to set them right with the Church, or as a Church-recommended means of reconciliation that may be a 'magic bullet' to fix things. These people are vulnerable, but ultimately are not too difficult to work with. They need reassurance and they need reliable information.

They need to be reassured that if they left the home because they or the children were in grave danger to soul or body, or because the married life had become unduly difficult, and there was danger in delay, they acted in accordance

94 Ibid.

95 Ibid., n. 10.

96 *Coram* Jaeger, n. 10.

97 Ibid., nn. 13-18.

98 Ibid., n. 13.

with the law and the only ecclesiastical tribunal fit to judge that decision is in the confessional, not the chancery building. They need to be told that unless they have some very specific and unusual situation, they do not need their status as a separated spouse to be formally declared by the Church. They need to be reassured that the Church's opposition to divorce does not oblige them to fight a losing battle against a civil divorce petition at ruinous cost. Most relevantly, they need to understand that the Church's assistance with their marital difficulties is to be found at Catholic Charities or the diocesan Marriage and Family Life office, not at the diocesan tribunal or by the personal intervention of the diocesan bishop.

The second and more troublesome group of petitioners—usually the husbands—seem to believe that suing a wife in ecclesiastical court is an entirely reasonable way to "save the marriage." He has been bossing his wife around for years and finding these crackpot canonical theories on the internet that confirm what he already knows to be true: the ecclesiastical court has the God-given right—indeed, obligation—to order the wife to return to him immediately. He refuses to see that putting the departed spouse in the role of respondent, obliged to justify why she feels she can no longer live with the petitioner, is only going to widen the chasm between them. This probably tells us something about the marital relationship they had, and quite possibly also why the wife left. A quotation from *Familiaris consortio* springs to mind:

> Pastors must know that, for the sake of truth, they are obliged to exercise careful discernment of situations. There is in fact a difference between those who have sincerely tried to save their first marriage and have been unjustly abandoned, and those who through their own grave fault have destroyed a canonically valid marriage.[99]

Those who have been unjustly abandoned are contrasted with those who through their own fault have destroyed a marriage. Too many petitioners see themselves in the first group, but are actually in the second. These petitioners certainly deserve pastoral care,[100] but too often they do not recognize or accept it. Every attempt to dissuade them from pursuing this petition may well be met with suspicion and accusations; that priests, tribunal staff, and the Church's ministers in general, are too accepting of divorce and are even actively working to undermine marriage. The petition becomes a campaign in itself. In contrast to the first group, these people are often difficult to work with.

I suggest that you follow every means within the law to avoid accepting the

---

99 *Familiaris consortio* 84.

100 "[T]hose who perpetrate acts of violence and abuse should not be excluded from pastoral care and concern on the part of ministers of the Gospel." Phillip J. Brown, "Legal Separation: A Pastoral Alternative," *Studies in Church Law* 4 (2008) 217.

case, whether administratively or judicially. Formal ecclesiastical intervention seems unlikely to contribute to the reconciliation of the parties, the Christian upbringing of the children, or the *salus animarum* more generally. At the same time, we would want to offer every support possible that might enable the peaceful resumption of the common conjugal life, while recognizing that as canonists we are often not the best people to provide that directly. In my experience, advising people that they should concentrate on really saving their marriages rather than pursuing an adversarial canonical process is gratefully received by those who have ears to hear.

4.2 What does the petitioner want?

What the petitioner wants is almost certainly not the status of a separated spouse in canon law. Even those who may superficially claim as such do not, on further questioning, actually want to be declared to have been maliciously abandoned and thereby entitled to separated status. Rather, the petitioner wants the Church to order the departed spouse to return. If the petitioner makes clear that he in fact has no use or desire to be established as a separated spouse, then the petition should be rejected irrespective of the boilerplate language on the petition template since there is nothing the tribunal can give him that he actually wants; there would be a lack of judicial object.

Whether or not the petition can be rejected *in limine*, there are a number of steps that can be taken by diocesan staff for the pastoral assistance of the spouses. First, contact the spouses' pastor or any other ministers who may know the couple. These couples are often very well known in the parish, and frequently the minister will be able to give a different perspective than the one given by the enquirer. Then, a letter from the local ordinary or judge to the departing spouse can be written. This is a difficult letter to write because often one doesn't know very much about the marriage; what can appear very clear after hearing the complainant can change completely after hearing the other spouse. Still, I would suggest including the following points:

- an apology for intervening in a personal matter;
- a reminder of Church teaching on divorce, perhaps with reference to the *Catechism of the Catholic Church*;
- a paraphrase of canon 1153 regarding acceptable reasons to depart, including without Church intervention;
- a reminder of the indissolubility of marriage; and
- suggestions for further pastoral support.

This letter has two purposes: first, to offer guidance and support to the departing spouse, and secondly to demonstrate to the complaining spouse that we have made an effort to help the parties and to remind him or her of the

obligations. I would not have a problem with showing this letter, upon request, to the complaining spouse, to address head-on the criticism that we are an annulment mill, or that we turn a blind eye to divorce, or that we are unwilling to do anything to help marriages in crisis.[101]

One of the checkboxes on the standard petition template which is floating around notes that it is to be used as a counterclaim in reply to citation for a cause of nullity of marriage. Turning this around, I suggest that respondents who are cited in one of these separation cases may, with the advice and support of an advocate, wish to consider whether the appropriate response to a petition for separation may be a petition for nullity of marriage. Of course, a petition for nullity of marriage should not be undertaken lightly, much less as retaliation against a petitioner sincerely trying to restore conjugal life. Still, I do believe that this would only need to happen a few times before those instigating these petitions would be forced to seriously reconsider their methods and objectives.

In a situation where a respondent, accused by the petitioner of "malicious abandonment," very evidently departed for licit reasons, the local ordinary may wish to consider issuing the decree mentioned in canon 1153 §1. This could be useful if the departed spouse requires some documentary evidence against the petitioner's (often alarmingly public) claims that she has abandoned him and is therefore to be shunned in the Church. The investigation prior to issuing such a decree would not need to be more extensive than that required by canon 50, avoiding the more involved procedure for the separation of the spouses such as the involvement of the promoter of justice. It may be important to mention in the decree, however, that the issuance of the decree is not to be interpreted as a statement that a departure on the spouse's own authority *in periculo moræ* was not or would not be legitimate.

4.3 The instruction

Hopefully, there is no instruction of the case, whether judicially or administratively; preferably the petition would have been dissuaded or rejected. Nevertheless, sometimes it may be necessary to consider the petition for separation according to a procedure. I mention here some of the matters which may distinguish it from what we are used to. Principally it is given at canons 1692-1696. It is not required to have a judicial trial. Even if a judicial petition is presented, the separation can be granted administratively, unless the respondent requests a judicial trial. The promoter of justice is required to take part in the proceedings, whether judicial or administrative, per canon 1696. However, the defender of the bond is not required to take part unless the bond itself is challenged.

101 It may be wise to refer this question to civil legal counsel, in case there may be consequences if the letter finds itself as part of the civil divorce proceedings.

Both parties should have advocates. Many tribunals train non-canonists to serve as advocates in routine marriage nullity trials; I would suggest that the novelty of a separation case makes it unsuitable for these people to serve as advocates, and that a suitable advocate would have at least a licentiate degree in canon law and a willingness to research unfamiliar areas of the law. It quickly becomes evident that many petitioners are receiving advice from somewhere, submitting pages and pages of detailed responses at every turn, making up in weight what they lack in comprehension. If this becomes apparent in the case, the judge may wish to consider invoking the provision of canon 1455 §3 whereby "the judge can bind . . . the parties . . . by oath to observe secrecy."[102] In any event, petitioners should have legitimately-appointed advocates to advise them, even, if necessary, after they have claimed that they do not want an advocate.[103]

Even more so do respondents need advocates. The respondents are very often women, and I would strongly suggest appointing a woman to be the advocate in this scenario. If your tribunal does not have a suitable woman canonist, it would be worth "borrowing" one from elsewhere. Petitioners often attempt to use these cases as a way of increasing and prolonging their ability to contact the respondent; it can be useful, therefore, for the respondent to choose to appoint the advocate also as a procurator, who can then "screen" the various communications so as not to trouble the respondent unnecessarily.

The proper *dubium* in a separation case is, "*an statuenda sit coniugum separatio, in casu*," or "shall the separation of the spouses be ordered, in this case." The ground is generic inasmuch as it is not necessary to specify in the *dubium* what are the possible reasons for the separation, for example, danger to the petitioner, or abandonment of the respondent, and so on. A separation case is not an investigation into whether or not the departure, in the past, was justified, but whether or not, for the future, a canonical separation should be established.

4.4 The decision

Sometimes the petitions include the claim that the "innocent spouse" should receive primary or sole custody of the children, and even attempt to decide child custody or access issues by ecclesiastical authority. This claim appears to originate from commentaries on the 1917 code, which did express a preference for children being in the care of the innocent spouse, or the Catholic spouse if only one were Catholic.[104] Even in the 1917 code, the local ordinary could

102 1983 *CIC* c. 1455 §3.

103 Cf. Pontifical Council for Legislative Texts, instruction *Dignitas connubii* 101 §2, January 25, 2005, *Communicationes* 37 (2005) 11-92.

104 See 1917 *CIC* c. 1132: "Instituta separatione, filii educandi sunt penes coniugem innocentem, et si alter coniugum sit acatholicus, penes coniugem catholicum, nisi in utroque casu Ordinarius pro ipsorum filiorum bono, salva semper eorundem catholica educatione, aliud decreverit."

decide otherwise if it were for the benefit of the children. The preference for the innocent spouse is no longer expressed in the successor to that canon; as Franchesci rightly argues, "the decision should always have as its first aim the welfare of the children."[105]

Canon 1154 states that "After the separation of the spouses has taken place, the adequate support and education of the children must always be suitably provided." Notably it does not state that the ecclesiastical decree or sentence must determine this; only that there is an obligation to ensure that it happens. It is not stated that the ecclesiastical authorities are to ensure that it happens; presumably the obligation remains principally with the parents. If this is to be referred to at all in the sentence or decree, I would suggest that the parties be asked to follow the directives of the civil authorities, supplemented by charity.

Concluding comments

Ed Peters recently wrote in reference to these questions regarding separation and divorce, "canonists see, and have long seen, more than one appropriate way to read legal texts that amateurs might think are unequivocal."[106] Whether or not one agrees with some of the arguments I have put forward regarding some of these questions—and I acknowledge that a number of eminent canonists have certainly written differently—we need to remember one of the maxims of both canon law and of moral theology: "*lex dubia non obligat*," "a doubtful law does not bind," expressed in the current code as "*Leges . . . in dubio iuris non urgent*."[107] Even if the claims with which we are being confronted were true in a textual or historical sense, they cannot be binding law in the fullest sense of the word as long as the Church does not seem to believe that it is the law. Even if one wanted to argue that spouses *should* be obliged to seek permission before departing or before approaching the civil authorities, I think it is impossible to argue today that they *are* obliged.

One of the suggestions I received in advance of this seminar was that I should try to include the perspective of someone trying to keep a marriage together. I did ask a woman who had been abandoned by her husband and subjected to a civil divorce she did not want and does not recognize as affecting the bond of her marriage; a devout woman familiar with canon law and with this new wave of pseudo-canonical panic, though not a canonist herself. She had two principal points: First, that the Church's ministers need to do more to help marriages in distress, especially at the moment of crisis. She believes that more marriages could be saved if clergy and laypeople alike were more willing to remind spouses

105 Héctor Franceschi, "'Bonum Prolis' in the Married State of Life and the Canonical Consequences in Case of Separation or Nullity of Marriage," *Forum* (2006) 429.

106 Peters, "Do Catholics Need Ecclesiastical Permission to Divorce?" 63.

107 1983 *CIC* c. 14.

of the gravity of their responsibilities, and of the indissolubility of marriage. Second, she is quite certain that these petitions regarding the separation of the spouses are definitely not part of the solution.

Seminar

The Permanent Diaconate: A Holy Order in Search of (Canonical) Reality

Deacon Matthew A. Glover, JD, JCL

I. Introduction

One need only ask a room full of ten people, "What is a deacon?" or "What is a deacon supposed to do?" to receive ten different answers. And those answers probably get even more varied if the ten people are canonists or theologians! I certainly would not pretend to be a professional theologian or a canonical scholar. I come to this presentation not as an accomplished expert, but simply as a relatively new deacon, canonist, and civil attorney, who has struggled (and continues to struggle) to define his role in a practical, day-to-day level in my own particular diocese and parish and in my own particular way.

I recognize that my own experiences may be very different from those of more seasoned deacons or more accomplished canonists—and mine are likely to be quite different from those in more populated or heavily Catholic areas. So, I offer this presentation not so much as definitive observations on all potential canonical issues in the diaconate, but rather as an exercise in what we in the civil law world might call "issue spotting"—pointing out the gaps, or problems, or unresolved questions for which there may be no definitive answer, or at least insufficient answers, as of yet.

If such canonical questions are abundant in other areas of the Code, I believe that is all the more so true with respect to the diaconate. To the extent that canon law can be understood as applied or practical theology, and to the extent that the Church has yet to fully flesh out the theology of Vatican II, the revisions in the 1983 code may continue to be in need of further revision. But that is even more true with respect to the canons on the diaconate (and clergy vis-à-vis the diaconate), insofar as the door to the permanent diaconate has been reopened only relatively recently.

This presentation will not spend a significant amount of time on the theological or canonical foundations of the order of deacon, as it presumes the audience is already aware of those basics. And so, after making brief mention of some of

the more key foundations, we will move to a consideration of "issue spotting" some canonical issues that occur to me. I fully recognize that these will not be exhaustive, nor are they meant to be. Indeed, any one of these topics could potentially be fleshed out into a presentation of its own. I also do not pretend to have all the answers, nor do I offer potential answers to each issue that is addressed. These reflections are offered as much to spark further questions and discussions even well after this presentation is concluded.

II. Foundations for the Order of Deacon

Most everyone is familiar with the primary scriptural foundation for the establishment of the order of deacons: Acts 6:1-6.[1] Perhaps the earliest scriptural reference is in Philippians 1:1,[2] though it does not contain much substance. The earliest substantive scriptural reference to the qualities that a deacon must possess is found in 1 Timothy 3:8-13.[3] There, Paul exhorts that deacons must be "dignified, not deceitful, not addicted to drink, not greedy for sordid gain, holding fast to the mystery of the faith with a clear conscience." They must also be "tested first" (1 Tim. 3:10).

---

1 See Acts 6:1-6:

> At that time, as the number of disciples continued to grow, the Hellenists complained against the Hebrews because their widows were being neglected in the daily distribution. So the Twelve called together the community of the disciples and said, "It is not right for us to neglect the word of God to serve at table. Brothers, select from among you seven reputable men, filled with the Spirit and wisdom, whom we shall appoint to this task, whereas we shall devote ourselves to prayer and to the ministry of the word." The proposal was acceptable to the whole community, so they chose Stephen, a man filled with faith and the holy Spirit, also Philip, Prochorus, Nicanor, Timon, Parmenas, and Nicholas of Antioch, a convert to Judaism. They presented these men to the apostles who prayed and laid hands on them.

New American Bible, Revised Edition (NABRE), http://www.usccb.org/bible/acts/6 (accessed on 26 Mar. 2020).

2 See, e.g., Phil. 1:1: "Paul and Timothy, servants of Christ Jesus, to all God's holy people in Christ Jesus at Philippi, together with their presiding elders and the deacons." *New Jerusalem Bible* (NJB), https://www.catholic.org/bible/book.php?id=57 (accessed on 26 Mar. 2020).

3 See, e.g., 1 Tim. 3:8-13:

> 8 Similarly, deacons must be dignified, not deceitful, not addicted to drink, not greedy for sordid gain, 9 holding fast to the mystery of the faith with a clear conscience. 10 Moreover, they should be tested first; then, if there is nothing against them, let them serve as deacons. 11 Women, similarly, should be dignified, not slanderers, but temperate and faithful in everything. 12 Deacons may be married only once and must manage their children and their households well. 13 Thus those who serve well as deacons gain good standing and much confidence in their faith in Christ Jesus.

NABRE, http://www.usccb.org/bible/1timothy/3 (accessed on 28 Jan. 2020).

Although it is not often discussed as a scriptural basis for the diaconate, I also look to John 13:1-20 as an implicit establishment by Jesus of what it means to be a deacon. As most are aware, John's Gospel account of the Last Supper does not actually repeat Jesus' words instituting the Eucharist (perhaps because John 6 already contains a significant discourse on the Eucharist, though that is my own personal conjecture). But what *is* contained in John's Gospel that is *not* in the Synoptics is the story of Jesus washing the feet of his apostles before the last supper. John emphasizes this act of service, rather than linking the last supper with the sacrificial act that Jesus is about to perform. And so, we see in John 13 that prior to the priestly sacrificial role, the role of a servant precedes. Jesus then orders his apostles to do for others as He has done for them. We can see in this a kind of implicit institution of the order of deacon by Jesus, immediately prior to His institution of the priesthood and the Eucharist at the Last Supper.

As for theological and canonical sources for this presentation, as well as additional food for study and thought after this presentation: In 1998, the Congregation for Catholic Education and Congregation for the Clergy issued a joint declaration titled *Basic Norms for the Formation of Permanent Deacons* and the *Directory for the Ministry and Life of Permanent Deacons* ("Vatican Directory"),[4] which contains norms of universal law on the permanent diaconate. In 2004, the United States Conference of Catholic Bishops promulgated the *National Directory for the Formation, Life and Ministry of Permanent Deacons in the United States* ("USCCB National Directory"),[5] which received the *recognitio* from the Holy See and which seeks to further implement in the United States the norms contained in the Vatican Directory.[6] Both of these directories do a good job of summarizing the historical and theological foundations for the permanent diaconate, while attempting to craft norms that help deacons live out their vocations in daily life.

On an even more scholarly level is *Understanding the Diaconate*, by the

---

4 See Congregation for Catholic Education and the Congregation for the Clergy, *Basic Norms for the Formation of Permanent Deacons, Directory for the Ministry and Life of Permanent Deacons* (Vatican City: Libreria Editrice Vaticana, 1998) [hereafter "Vatican Directory"], http://www.vatican.va/roman_curia/congregations/ccatheduc/documents/rc_con_ccatheduc_doc_31031998_directorium-diaconi_en.html (accessed on 3 Mar. 2020).

5 See United States Conference of Catholic Bishops, *National Directory for the Formation, Life and Ministry of Permanent Deacons in the United States* (2005) [hereafter "USCCB National Directory"], http://www.usccb.org/_cs_upload/8304_1.pdf (accessed on 28 Jan. 2020).

6 At their general meeting in June 2019, the USCCB approved a revised second edition of the USCCB National Directory, and that second edition is currently awaiting the necessary *recognitio* from the Holy See. Thus, while the first edition is still binding particular law for dioceses in the United States, there may soon be a new second edition taking its place. There are some substantive changes that will be referenced in this text, but most changes are to the numbering of the paragraphs.

Most Reverend W. Shawn McKnight.[7] What began as his doctoral dissertation has been transformed into an eminently readable yet thorough overview of the historical foundations and development of the permanent diaconate, with insights on continued developments (including canonical) that ought to be considered in the diaconate moving forward. Bishop McKnight's book is an invaluable resource for anyone wanting to make a serious study of the issues surrounding the permanent diaconate today, especially here in the United States.

Of course, William Woestman's canonical commentary, *The Sacrament of Orders and the Clerical State*,[8] provides helpful insights as well on the particular canons that are pertinent to the diaconate.

On a more popular level, but still very helpful, are *The Deacon Reader*, edited by James Keating,[9] and *The Emerging Diaconate* by William Ditewig.[10] These two books are not necessarily canonical in focus, nor do they necessarily constitute critical theological scholarship in the area of the permanent diaconate. But they do provide a helpful overview of the diaconate and issues pertaining to it, especially useful for those who are not looking for in-depth or technical analysis.

Finally, the USCCB recently published a collection of Pope Francis' sayings and teachings on the diaconate, in a small book titled *Deacons: Servants of Charity*.[11] I was personally pleasantly surprised by this little book, in particular how it organizes Pope Francis's sometimes extemporaneous thoughts into a more systematic organization of categories dealing with various aspects of diaconal ministry. Again, these reflections are not canonical in nature per se, but they are helpful in understanding the mind of our Holy Father when it comes to the nature of the diaconate.

III. Current Canonical Issues

As previously stated, what follows is an attempt at spotting (not necessarily resolving) some (though not all) current canonical issues with the permanent diaconate. For no other reason than ease of following along, these issues are organized more or less in the order in which they appear in the 1983 code, with

7 See W. Shawn McKnight, *Understanding the Diaconate: Historical, Theological, and Sociological Foundations* (Washington, DC: The Catholic University of America Press, 2018).

8 See William H. Woestman, OMI, *The Sacrament of Orders and the Clerical State: A Commentary on the Code of Canon Law,* 3rd ed. (Ottawa: St. Paul University, 2006).

9 See James Keating, ed., *The Deacon Reader* (New York/Mahwah, NJ: Paulist Press, 2006).

10 See William T. Ditewig, *The Emerging Diaconate* (New York, Mahwah, NJ: Paulist Press, 2007).

11 See Pope Francis, *Deacons: Servants of Charity* (Washington, DC: USCCB, 2018).

some various miscellaneous issues at the very end.

A. Deacons as Clerics

While it may be surprising to many lay Catholics, deacons and the diaconate are first treated in the section on "Clerics," under Title III of Part I (on "The Christian Faithful") of Book II (on "The People of God"). I say "surprising" because many in the Church do not think of deacons as clerics, or part of the clergy.

1. Canon 266 and Consistent Wording

The first significant reference appears in canon 266 §1: "Through the reception of the diaconate, a person becomes a cleric . . . ."[12] The diaconate is thus the entrance into the clerical state or being part of the clergy. While none of this comes as a surprise to this audience, how much of our language in diocesan policies, departments, or programming is consistent with this reality that deacons are just as much a part of the "clergy" as are priests and bishops? (I want to emphasize here that I have not forgotten and will soon come to the significant ontological distinction between the order of deacon and the orders of presbyter and bishop.) I am thinking here of things such as clergy continuing education, clergy retreat days, vicars for clergy, clergy welfare or retirement funds, and the like. If we canonists can all agree on anything, at least one of those things would be that words matter. I do not think anyone in my diocese presumes that the "Clergy Welfare Fund" is intended to support deacons in their old age or infirmity—so it is really more of a "Priest Welfare Fund." Clergy continuing education in my diocese is open to all deacons who want to attend, but it is certainly geared primarily towards our priests (as I think it should be, since the camaraderie and formational needs for priests are distinctly different from those of deacons). We do not happen to have a vicar for clergy, but for those who do, does that person work with both priests and deacons? And there are other examples. If we want to respect the identity of deacons as clerics, then we would do well to word our policies and programming consistently, both with what deacons and priests have in common, as well as where they differ.

2. Canon 273 and Obedience

The next point of discussion concerns canon 273, which states that clerics "are bound by a special obligation to show reverence and obedience to the Supreme

---

12 *Codex Iuris Canonici auctoritate Ioannis Pauli PP. II promulgatus* (Vatican City: Libreria Editrice Vaticana, 1983) c. 266 §1. English translation from *Code of Canon Law, Latin-English Edition: New English Translation* (Washington, DC: Canon Law Society of America, 2012). All subsequent English translations of canons from this code will be taken from this source unless otherwise indicated.

Pontiff and their own ordinary."[13] Insofar as deacons have "a foot in both worlds," as it were, the way in which a deacon employed in the secular world maintains reverence and obedience especially to his own ordinary can at times become more problematic. I am thinking here of deacons who work in the areas of civil law, law enforcement, public service, education, health care, immigration enforcement, and other areas that may overlap with a bishop's teaching authority within his diocese. It may be easy enough for a parish priest to show reverence and obedience to a bishop's counter-cultural teaching on a particular issue facing the secular world. But it is quite another for a deacon who actually has to work in that particular area full-time to show reverence and obedience in a practical, everyday manner—by his actions and decisions even more so than by his words. What to do when a deacon's secular employment duties run counter to his bishop's public statements? At what point might a deacon's employment demands eventually run counter to his canonical obligation of showing reverence and obedience? The possibilities seem boundless for a deacon as it pertains to activity in the secular world, insofar as a deacon's place is as much or more in the realm of the secular than it is in the sacred.

3. Canon 275 and Clerical Cooperation

Canon 275 discusses clerical cooperation, noting that since clerics all have the same ultimate goal (building up the Body of Christ), "they are to be united among themselves by a bond of brotherhood and prayer and are to strive for cooperation among themselves . . . ."[14] This may be ideal, but it seems hard enough to put into practice in many presbyterates, much less in ways that really include both priests and deacons. I know this canon aims for the ideal, and the ideal is something to which the Church should encourage us all. But one also wonders how realistic it is for deacons and priests together to actualize this ideal. In many dioceses, there are Iesus Caritas groups or other informal support groups for priests. In our diocese at least, no such support groups exist for deacons. It seems perfectly reasonable that the "bond of brotherhood and prayer" idealized in canon 275 ought not apply to all clerics alike, given the significant differences between deacons and priests, both sacramentally and in lived experience. Although we often hear of the need for priests to support one another, we may have a ways to go as a Church in forming that notion of mutual support between and among groupings of deacons within dioceses. The Vatican Directory, n.6, states that "[w]ith the permission of the bishop and in the presence or that of his delegate, it would be opportune for deacons periodically to meet to discuss their ministry, exchange experiences, advance formation and encourage each other in fidelity."[15] But other than perhaps an annual gathering, how often do deacons meet together in such support and solidarity?

---

13 C. 273.

14 C. 275 §1.

15 Vatican Directory, n. 6.

4. Canon 276 and Holiness of Life

Canon 276 deals with clerics' holiness of life. Having been "consecrated to God by a new title in the reception of orders," they are "bound in a special way to pursue holiness."[16] The canon then lists various means by which clerics are to pursue their unique call to holiness. Among those means, priests "are earnestly invited" to say Mass daily, "and deacons to participate in its offering daily."[17] Note that there is no requirement for priests to celebrate Mass each day, yet a priest's celebration of Mass daily has crept into our mindset almost as a given (which is a good thing). Note also that the canon makes no legal distinction between a priest's exhortation to celebrate daily Mass and a deacon's to *participate* in daily Mass. While it seems almost normal for a priest to be asked, "Have you celebrated Mass yet today?" it might seem odd to ask of a deacon, "Have you participated in Mass yet today?" Obviously, with a foot in both worlds, it may be impossible for most deacons to participate in daily Mass; yet in canon 276 they are "earnestly invited" to do so just as much as priests are invited to say daily Mass.[18] Interestingly, the canon does not specify whether the deacon's daily participation in Mass is intended to mean serving at a Mass as a deacon.

Another means by which deacons are to pursue holiness of life is the liturgy of the hours. Interestingly, the canon distinguishes between permanent deacons on the one hand, and priests and transitional deacons on the other. The canon defers to conferences of bishops to determine how permanent deacons are to pray the hours. While this distinction is understandable, and the effort at subsidiarity is laudable, it is also regrettable that such a firm distinction is made between permanent deacons and transitional deacons on this particular point. Permanent deacons certainly live with a foot in each world (sacred and secular), and each permanent deacon's job responsibilities will vary greatly. But the same can also easily be said for transitional deacons and certainly for priests in ministry, whose ministerial and pastoral responsibilities vary greatly. It is not clear why the code considers permanent deacons exempt from praying the full liturgy of the hours; and it is even less clear why the USCCB only requires permanent deacons to pray morning and evening prayer. Although a deacon's job duties may make the other hours difficult, surely it is not terribly difficult for a deacon to carve out additional time in the morning for the Office of Readings, or to spare five minutes on lunch break to pray mid-day prayer. The issue is not about practicality; it is about drawing a canonical distinction between permanent deacons and the rest of the clergy where there need be no distinction.

---

16 C. 276 §1.

17 C. 276 §2, 2°.

18 Ibid.

5. Canon 277 and Continence

Canon 277 is perhaps the most contentious of canons impacting deacons. It states that clerics "are obliged to observe perfect and perpetual continence for the sake of the kingdom of heaven and therefore are bound to celibacy ...."[19] It would be impossible to cover all the permutations of this issue even if the entire presentation were devoted solely to it. The issue is well researched and outlined in a 2005 article by Edward Peters.[20] In that article, Peters quotes from the Vatican Directory, specifically number 61, which states that married permanent deacons are to practice "a certain continence"[21]—without definition or explanation as to what "a certain continence" means, or how "a certain continence" might differ from canon 277's requirement of "perfect and perpetual continence."[22] Peters points to other sources of confusion in the Western tradition of continence for deacons. He also notes that James Provost addressed this same topic in a presentation to the Canon Law Society of America, wherein Provost argued that since married deacons had already acquired the rights to marital intercourse before they were ordained, and because canon 277 does not explicitly revoke those acquired rights, then canon 277's imposition of continence cannot and is not imposed on married deacons in the same way as it is for non-married deacons and priests.[23] (Provost conceded the point that the drafters of the code had initially included an express exception for permanent deacons in the drafting of canon 277, but that that exception was later removed.) Peters then concludes, in part, that the deeper principle in play is the reality that "one cannot be held to have surrendered fundamental rights without an express awareness that that is being done."[24] (I would note that the same "implicit exception" presumably applies to those married Catholic priests who have been or will be ordained pursuant to the exceptions as outlined in the Pastoral Provision.)

The only seemingly recent update from the Holy See in attempting to clarify the applicability of canon 277 to permanent deacons came from the Pontifical Commission for Legislative Texts ("PCLT"), via two separate letter responses in 2011. In the first letter, dated March 4, 2011, Archbishop Francesco Coccopalmerio as president of the PCLT stated merely that married permanent deacons "do not have the obligation of celibacy (and therefore of continence) during the marriage," and thus do not need to be dispensed from the requirement

---

19 C. 277 §1.

20 See Edward N. Peters, "Canonical Considerations on Diaconal Continence," *Studia canonica* (2005) 147-180.

21 Vatican Directory, n. 61.

22 Peters, 172-173.

23 See Peters, 176-177; James Provost, "Permanent Deacons in the 1983 Code," *CLSA Proceedings* 46 (1984) 186.

24 Peters, 177.

of canon 277.[25] The second PCLT letter, dated December 17, 2011, attempted to provide further clarification and explanation, and stated that the obligation of continence as stated in canon 277 "is inseparably linked to the obligation of celibacy to which all clerics, in principle, are bound."[26] It further states that "the current canonical discipline does not require married permanent deacons, as long as their marriage lasts, to observe the obligation of perfect and perpetual continence" as established in canon 277.[27] Ed Peters also published responses critical to both of the PCLT letters, arguing that the fundament disconnect between canon 277 and the de facto lived experience of permanent deacons (not to mention married priests) still remained. While I do not necessarily agree with all of Peters' arguments on this issue, I do think that there remains a disconnect between a plain reading of the canons and the lived experiences of married deacons—and, with a fix being a relatively simple thing to do, it strikes me as odd that the Holy Father has not simply revised the code accordingly for clarification's sake.

6. Canon 279 and the Need for More Consistent Wording

Moving to more mundane topics, canon 279 exhorts continuing study and formation for clerics. Of interest, §1 states as follows: "Even after ordination to the priesthood, clerics are to pursue sacred studies . . . ."[28] Although common sense dictates that this canon is aimed towards priests, it is odd that the wording of the canon does not make this clearer. Why reference "ordination to the priesthood" and then follow with a reference to "clerics" in general? Obviously not all clerics are bound for the priesthood. Why not simply state that *priests* are to pursue sacred studies?

7. Canon 281 on Remuneration, Support, and Retirement

Canon 279 is not the only instance of seeming internal inconsistency in using the term cleric. Canon 281 deals with financial remuneration for clerics and states that clerics "deserve remuneration which is consistent with their condition."[29] Then, §2 requires that provision be made for their social assistance "if they suffer from illness, incapacity, or old age."[30] Note that there is no distinction in §§1 and 2 between priests and deacons—only the generic term "clerics" is used. Then, in §3, the canon moves to "married deacons," stating that those who

25 *Roman Replies and CLSA Advisory Opinions 2001*, ed. F. Stephen Pedone, et al. (Washington, DC: Canon Law Society of America, 2001) 18-20.

26 *Roman Replies and CLSA Advisory Opinions 2012*, ed. Sharon A. Euart, RSM, et al. (Washington, DC: Canon Law Society of America, 2012) 12-14.

27 Ibid.

28 C. 279 §1.

29 C. 281 §1.

30 Ibid, §2

devote themselves completely to ministry must be compensated to provide for themselves and their families. And those who are employed in a civil profession must provide for their needs through their civil income.

Several potential issues would seem then to arise. What if a married deacon is terminated from his civil profession or otherwise becomes unemployed or under-employed? Is a parish or diocese required to make use of deacons' ministry on a more full-time basis, and consequently to help provide for them and their families? Common sense might dictate *No*, but the canon's language is not so clear. The Vatican Directory, n. 20, states that it is up to particular law to determine such matters: "Particular law may also determine the obligations devolving on the diocese when a deacon, through no fault of his own, becomes unemployed."[31] Meanwhile, the first edition of the USCCB National Directory n. 94 states: "In an individual situation of need, the diocesan Church ought to assist the deacon and his family in charity." However, the revised second edition of the USCCB National Directory n. 100 (which, again, has yet to receive the Holy See's *recognitio*) will revise that norm to state: ". . . the diocesan Church is to see that the deacon and his family do not lack the basic necessities of life."[32] So, while the Vatican Directory leaves it up to particular law, the first edition of the USCCB National Directory is exhortative in nature (dioceses "ought to assist"). However, the second edition of the USCCB National Directory is prescriptive: the diocese "is to see that the deacon and his family do not lack the basic necessities of life."[33] Thus, once the second edition receives *recognitio*, it would appear that dioceses must be prepared to assist deacons and their families with the basic necessities of life, at least in individual situations of need.

It remains to be seen how dioceses will interpret and treat these individual situations of need—which ones trigger the apparent requirement that the diocese sees to it that the deacon and his family do not lack the basic necessities of life. Regardless, even if a diocese decided that a particular deacon's individual situation of need did not trigger the requisite support, a deacon might well have a legitimate canonical argument that a diocese has a canonical obligation to provide for him under canon 281 §§1 and 2 should he become unemployed or under-employed, especially if it is through no fault of his own. Moreover, what if a married deacon begins to suffer from illness, incapacity, or old age, such that he can no longer suitably meet his or his family's needs? A plain reading of §2 would seem to support the conclusion that because he is also a cleric, a married deacon should be entitled to the same or similar support from a diocese or parish if and when he suffers illness, incapacity, or old age. Again, common sense might seem to dictate *No* to that point, but the wording of the canon would seem to dictate *Yes*.

---

31 Vatican Directory, n. 20.

32 USCCB National Directory, 2nd Edition, n. 100.

33 Ibid.

What about a deacon who retires from ministry? A plain reading of canon 281 §2 would seem to indicate that a deacon who has insufficient retirement funds saved up from his secular employment may have a canonical right to seek provision for social assistance that provides for his needs in his old age and retirement. This, no doubt, would open up a Pandora's box of difficult possibilities. What if a deacon's retirement funds are insufficient due to his own squandering or mismanagement? What if a deacon is permitted to incardinate into a diocese late in life? And, of course, many deacons tend to be closer to retirement age than at the time of their ordination than do priests—what if a deacon has only offered a few years of service to a parish or a diocese? Is he entitled to demand assistance in his retirement years? Again, the common sense answer would seem to be *No*. And common sense would seem to dictate that §§1 and 2 are really geared more appropriately to priests, who tend to be ordained earlier in life, and who tend to not have the kind of financial reserves built up as do deacons, relying as many of them do on the pensions or retirement funds established for them at the diocesan level.

On a practical level, one wonders how many dioceses have entities named Clergy Welfare Funds or Clergy Pension Funds and the like, the purpose of which is to care for clergy in their old age or infirmity. Presumably, the statutes and articles of incorporation of these entities clarify that the funds are to be used for priests, not all clerics including deacons. And, common sense would dictate that that is how these funds should be used—to support priests (not deacons). But, if words matter, why not rename these entities Priest Welfare Funds or Priest Pension Funds, rather than use the term clergy?

8. Canon 284 and Clerical Garb

Moving from money to garb, canon 284 states that clerics "are to wear suitable ecclesiastical garb according to the norms issued by the conference of bishops and according to legitimate local customs."[34] Canon 288, however, states that the prescripts of canon 284 do not apply to permanent deacons unless particular law establishes otherwise. Nevertheless, there is a USCCB complementary norm for canon 284, which again seems to confuse the terms *priest* and *cleric*. That complementary norm states that the usual attire for priests is "a black suit and

34 C. 284.

Roman collar."[35] But it then states that the "use of the cassock is at the discretion of the cleric." Common sense would dictate that this norm is not intended to mean that a deacon (who is a cleric) is permitted to dress in a cassock but *not* in a suit and Roman collar—but the wording in the norm is internally inconsistent. I am aware that every diocese has their own particular law on garb for deacons. In my diocese, deacons do not wear the Roman collar at any point. In some dioceses, deacons wear the collar but only while in a ministerial function (say, when serving at Mass on Sundays or performing the other sacraments).

I am not sure what this says about the notion that priests ought always to wear the collar because they are really always in ministry. While I certainly agree with that notion, I would also argue that deacons should always consider themselves in ministry, insofar as they are always to be in service. But I also would *not* be of the opinion that a deacon should *always* wear a collar. Nevertheless, why priests are expected to always be in clerics whereas deacons are rarely seen in clerics (even though they are, in fact, clerics) seems somewhat odd. (And I say this as someone who would personally prefer never to wear clerics as a deacon.) Later we will arrive at the distinctions emphasized in *Omnium in mentem*. But, for purposes of canon 284, it would seem to me that *Omnium in mentem* could and perhaps ought to be applied such that canon 284 might be revised to say "Priests are to wear" rather than the more generic "clerics are to wear," insofar as priests are ontologically different from deacons in acting *in persona Christi capitis*.

9. Canon 285 Regarding Deacons and Public Office

Canon 285 §3 states that clerics "are forbidden to assume public offices which entail a participation in the exercise of civil power."[36] However, canon 288 then states that canon 285 §3 is not binding on permanent deacons unless particular law decides otherwise. The Vatican Directory states that "[a]ctive involvement in political parties . . . may be permitted in particular circumstances."[37] And the USCCB National Directory then states that prior written permission of one's bishop is required: "A permanent deacon may not present his name for election to any public office or in any other general election, or accept a nomination or an appointment to public office, without the prior written permission of the diocesan

---

35 USCCB Complementary Norm on c. 284:
The National Conference of Catholic Bishops, in accord with the prescriptions of canon 284, hereby decrees that without prejudice to the provisions of canon 288, clerics are to dress in conformity with their sacred calling. In liturgical rites, clerics shall wear the vesture prescribed in the proper liturgical books. Outside liturgical functions, a black suit and Roman collar are the usual attire for priests. The use of the cassock is at the discretion of the cleric. In the case of religious clerics, the determinations of their proper institutes or societies are to be observed with regard to wearing the religious habit.

36 C. 285 §3.

37 Vatican Directory, n. 13.

bishop."[38] Moreover, a deacon may not even "actively and publicly participate in another's political campaign" without first obtaining written permission from the diocesan bishop.[39] Even if a permanent deacon were permitted to participate directly or even to run for public office himself, numerous conflicts could arise between the deacon's canonical obligations and his civic duties or platforms (see above discussion on c. 273, as but one example).

10. Canon 290 and Loss of Clerical State

Finally, canon 290 deals with how a cleric loses the clerical state (or, colloquially, how a cleric is "laicized"). Interestingly, a deacon may be laicized merely for "grave causes," but a presbyter only for "most grave causes."[40] This canonical distinction makes sense in light of the re-emphasis of the ontological differences in *Omnium in mentem*. However, there does not seem to be any consistent jurisprudential standard on what constitutes a grave cause versus a most grave cause. If that wording creates a standard without any real difference, why create a different standard in canon 290? As with other issues presented, I am certainly not advocating for a change in the differences of gradation—in fact, I agree that a presbyter's bar for laicization ought to be higher than that of a deacon. But if those differing standards are not actually applied in practice, how are those differing standards of any real use or meaning?

B. Hierarchical Constitution—Particular Churches and Parishes

There is scant reference to deacons in the code's discussion on the internal organization of dioceses and parishes, under the hierarchical constitution of the Church. Which seems appropriate, given that deacons are ordained in service to those hierarchical structures and to the people of God as a whole. But what role do the canons envision a deacon playing in the structural aspects of a diocese or parish?

At the diocesan level, not much of any reference is made to deacons. In fact, the canons on diocesan organization are more interesting for what they do *not* say about deacons than for what they do. Perhaps the most glaring example of an omission of the diaconate comes in the canons on diocesan synods. Specifically, canon 463 lists numerous different persons who "must be called

---

38 USCCB National Directory, n. 91. The revised second edition of the USCCB National Directory changes the numbering of this paragraph to n. 96, but makes no substantive changes to this norm.

39 Ibid.

40 C. 290: "Once validly received, sacred ordination never becomes invalid. A cleric, nevertheless, loses the clerical state: . . . 3° by rescript of the Apostolic See which grants it to deacons only for grave causes and to presbyters only for most grave causes."

to a diocesan synod as members of the synod."[41] The canon obviously calls for priests in different positions or offices to be synod members, as well as laity, members of religious institutes, seminary rectors, vicars forane and priests from each vicariate, and religious superiors. Yet, for some reason, deacons are never mentioned—meaning that hypothetically a bishop could convoke a synod without ever having to include a member of the permanent diaconate. True, §2 states that the bishop "can also call others" to the synod, which would open the door to inviting a deacon. But the role of deacons at the diocesan level seems to have been entirely forgotten or overlooked in the code's vision of diocesan consultation.

At the parish level, canon 517 permits a bishop (if there is a lack of priests) to entrust the participation in pastoral care of a parish to someone other than a priest. The canon then lists those to whom a parish's pastoral care can be entrusted: "to a deacon, to another person who is not a priest, or to a community of persons."[42] Interestingly, the canon itself does not seem to state that these are listed in any particular order of priority. However, the Vatican Directory does state that in such circumstances, permanent deacons "always have precedence over the non-ordained faithful."[43] This raises an odd dynamic for a deacon. A deacon is ordained first and foremost to *serve*, not necessarily to *lead*. Some might say that the notion of diaconal leadership is somewhat of an oxymoron. While it is understandable in part that a deacon would be an understandable choice to lead a parish insofar as he is a cleric, such a model also might seem to run counter to the very *kind* of cleric that a deacon is: a servant.

According to canon 519 the pastor of a parish is to exercise pastoral care and carry out the functions of teaching, sanctifying, and governing, "also with the cooperation of other presbyters or deacons and with the assistance of lay members."[44] Note that the pastor pastors with the cooperation of clerics, but with the assistance of lay members. While the linguistic differences may have ontological or theological foundations, in practice it would seem that in many if not most parishes the lay staff members of a parish have just as much (if perhaps not even more) influence on the ministries of a parish than do the deacons. While there has been a significant push for lay parish involvement since Vatican II, and perhaps especially during the current pontificate, many parishes seem unclear whether or how to promote diaconal involvement. We often hear of and debate things like lay leadership or lay participation in governance. But even though deacons are clerics in the Church, it seems somehow contradictory to discuss diaconal leadership or diaconal governance, insofar as the very identity of a deacon is to be a servant to others. Certainly, priests and bishops and the Pope are

41 C. 463 §1.

42 C. 517.

43 Vatican Directory, n. 41.

44 C. 519.

called to be servants as well, as indeed are the entire Christian faithful as part of their baptism. But deacons are called to be servants in a unique and distinct way, different than the kind of servant leadership to which pastors may be called. And so, how can deacons be both servants (by definition) and leaders in their parishes, without losing sight of the fact that their primary identity is always to remain in service to (not in leadership of) their pastors and the people in their parishes?

Finally, per canon 564, a chaplain by definition must be a priest. While this no doubt has deep theological foundations regarding the full care of souls or the sacramental duties that a chaplain must be able to fulfill, it also is incongruous with our everyday use of the term chaplain here in the United States. Most organizations (even Catholic organizations) that seek to name someone as their chaplain do not necessarily have in mind the full spectrum of sacramental service that only a priest can offer. Since it seems unlikely the Church will (or can) change its definition of chaplain anytime soon (if ever), dioceses and deacons would do well to make sure that deacons are not assigned or appointed to chaplaincy positions for which they are not canonically eligible. Perhaps other wording could be used that achieves the same goal, such as *spiritual director* or *diocesan/parish liaison*.

C. Deacons as Teachers and Preachers

Canon 764 gives deacons the faculty to preach everywhere, with the presumed consent of the rector of the church. Significantly, the canon makes no distinction between presbyters and deacons in the exercise of that right. Canon 767 then goes on to discuss the homily as a particular form of preaching, noting simply that the homily "is reserved to a priest or a deacon."[45] Again, canon 767 makes no distinction between deacons and priests with respect to the homily, giving the impression that, per the code, deacons and priests have equal right and faculty to preach the homily. That impression may be correct as it regards the code, but canon law is not limited merely to the code.

Pursuant to the liturgical law as defined in the General Instruction of the Roman Missal (GIRM) no. 66, "[t]he homily should ordinarily be given by the Priest Celebrant himself or be entrusted by him to a concelebrating Priest, or from time to time and, if appropriate, to the Deacon . . . ."[46] This further clarification of liturgical law raises several issues. If deacons can be said to have equal rights to preach (both in general and as it pertains to the homily) per canons 764 and 767, how can the deacon's right be restricted by GIRM 66? One answer to that question would be that although presbyters and deacons may possess the equal

45 C. 767.

46 *General Instruction to the Roman Missal* (Washington, DC: United States Conference of Catholic Bishops, 2011) n. 66, available at: http://www.usccb.org/prayer-and-worship/the-mass/general-instruction-of-the-roman-missal/ (accessed on 5 Mar. 2020).

faculty of preaching, that faculty to preach is not the same as the *right* to preach. But then what to do with canon 767's nondescript language about the homily being reserved "to a priest or a deacon," without distinction between the two?

On an even more practical level: While deacons are often criticized in general for being poor homilists, how can pastors or bishops expect their deacons to improve their homilies if they are not given the opportunity to preach more regularly? Are priests immune from giving poor homilies (surely not)? The frequency with which deacons preach at Mass certainly differs from diocese to diocese, and from parish to parish. At least one diocese has interpreted and applied GIRM no. 66 more strictly than its plain language would seem to indicate. A 2011 pastoral letter by the Bishop of Marquette on the diaconate, titled "The Deacon: Icon of Jesus Christ the Servant," includes a diocesan norm on permanent deacons giving homilies, stating as follows: "The permanent deacon may be entrusted with the homily at Mass on certain occasions, in other words from time to time, as circumstances suggest. This should not occur, however, on a routine or regularly scheduled basis."[47]

The first question that comes to mind is simply, "Why not?" There is nothing in the code that envisions such a restriction on the deacon's preaching abilities. The GIRM is certainly clear that the homily should ordinarily be given by the priest celebrant or to a priest concelebrant, and that "from time to time and, if appropriate, to the Deacon."[48] But there is nothing in the code or the GIRM that could be interpreted as precluding a pastor from regularly assigning the deacon(s) at his parish to give the homily. This is the regular practice in parishes in our diocese, and I would imagine many if not most others. Why promulgate particular law precluding pastors from exercising their own judgment and discretion in setting a homily schedule that includes deacons? Certainly, a pastor ought to have the authority and is competent to decide how often his deacons ought to preach in his parish given his unique circumstances. It may well be that certain deacons should rarely if ever be given the task of preaching a homily due to their inefficacy, but could the same not also be said for some priests? (I say all of this with the disclaimer that, but for this one disagreement with the text of the pastoral letter, the Bishop of Marquette's pastoral letter on the permanent diaconate is one of the best diocesan-level documents on the permanent diaconate that I have come across in the United States.)

None of this is intended as a push for more homily time for deacons. Personally, I am thrilled that my pastor wishes to be the primary homilist in our parish—not only because it eases the burden on me having to prepare homilies, but because

47 The Most Rev. Alexander K. Sample, Bishop of Marquette, Pastoral Letter, *The Deacon: Icon of Jesus Christ the Servant* 17, June 11, 2011, https://www.dioceseofmarquette.org/UserFiles/Bishop/PastoralLetter-Diaconate2011FullText.pdf (accessed on 26 Mar. 2020).

48 GIRM, 66.

I am convicted that the pastor's voice ought to be the primary shepherding voice that the faithful hear. But it strikes me that saying a pastor cannot put deacons on a regular homily schedule runs counter to subsidiarity, unduly restricts a pastor's governance of his parish, and is not supported by the plain language of the code or even of GIRM 66.

D. Deacons and the Sanctifying Functions

As outlined in canon 835, the principal sanctifier in any diocese is the bishop.[49] Presbyters "also exercise this function," insofar as they also share in the ministerial priesthood of Jesus Christ (§2). Deacons merely "have a part in the celebration of divine worship according to the norm of the prescripts of the law" (§3), owing to their uniquely distinct and different role in the hierarchy of sacred orders. While one of the principal roles of priests is to exercise the sanctifying function, deacons do not exercise the sanctifying functions properly speaking. Rather, they have a part in those functions to the extent permitted. As such, while deacons are often visible at liturgical functions within any given parish, it does not seem that liturgical functioning is or should be the primary means by which a deacon's presence in a parish is known to parishioners. Yet, that is how many everyday parishioners tend to view their deacons—as side and dispensable participants in the Sunday liturgies.

This viewpoint could be good or bad. It could be bad to the extent that participation in liturgical functions is the only means by which a deacon functions in a parish. But, to the extent that a deacon functions as a true servant—behind the scenes, in ways known only to the pastor or those more directly involved with parish administration or ministries—perhaps it is a good thing that a deacon's service goes largely unnoticed by many everyday parishioners.

1. Baptism

Certainly, every parish and every pastor are different, but some deacons tend to do more infant baptisms than others. Some priests and deacons read canon 861, which makes deacons an ordinary minister of baptism, and interpret that to mean that a deacon has just as much a right to perform infant baptisms as does

---

49 See c. 835:
§1. The bishops in the first place exercise the sanctifying function; they are the high priests, the principal dispensers of the mysteries of God, and the directors, promoters, and guardians of the entire liturgical life in the church entrusted to them.
§2. Presbyters also exercise this function; sharing in the priesthood of Christ and as his ministers under the authority of the bishop, they are consecrated to celebrate divine worship and to sanctify the people.
§3. Deacons have a part in the celebration of divine worship according to the norm of the prescripts of the law.

a priest.[50] That may be true in comparison to a parochial vicar, but it is not true when it comes to the pastor. Canon 530, which canon 861 references, clearly lists a number of things that are "especially entrusted to a pastor"—among them, the administration of baptism; assisting at marriages and the nuptial blessing; and performing funeral rites.[51]

Accordingly, the default presumption in any parish ought to be that the *pastor* is the one who performs all infant baptisms, weddings, and funerals, because these things are especially entrusted to him. Certainly, if a pastor wants to permit a deacon to do a baptism, then that is his prerogative. But any deacon who receives a request to do a baptism (or a wedding or a funeral) ought first to defer to the pastor, not merely out of professional courtesy, but more so out of the canonical reality of the role of the pastor in a parish.

2. Eucharist

Deacons are mentioned in several places in the canons on the Eucharist. It should go without saying, but per canon 907 deacons are not permitted to offer any prayers or perform any actions that are proper to the celebrating priest.[52]

As for vesture, canon 929 does not prescribe what a deacon is to wear, but defers instead to the rubrics.[53] GIRM 338 then states that the proper vestment for a deacon is a dalmatic over an alb and stole. But, the GIRM goes on to state that the dalmatic may be omitted "out of necessity or on account of a lesser degree of solemnity."[54] Some deacons may want to wear the dalmatic all the time, even at regular daily Mass—and such would seem to be their right, as the GIRM says "may be omitted."[55] But, whereas a priest is to always wear a chasuble when he is the principal celebrant, a deacon always has an option of downgrading to a simple alb and stole due to either necessity (which is not defined) or lesser degrees of solemnity.

The more interesting canonical issues deal with a deacon's actual functioning in Mass as a deacon and his role as an ordinary minister of Holy Communion. GIRM 116 states: "If a deacon is present at any celebration of Mass, he should

---

50 See c. 861: §1. "The ordinary minister of baptism is a bishop, a presbyter, or a deacon, without prejudice to the prescript of c. 530, n. 1."

51 C. 530.

52 See c. 907: "In the eucharistic celebration deacons and lay persons are not permitted to offer prayers, especially the eucharistic prayer, or to perform actions which are proper to the celebrating priest."

53 See c. 929: "In celebrating and administering the Eucharist, priests and deacons are to wear the sacred vestments prescribed by the rubrics."

54 GIRM 338.

55 Ibid.

exercise his office."[56] Although perhaps it exists, I do not know of a parish that actually enforces and practices this norm of the GIRM. Of course, the norm is merely exhortative—a deacon who is present *should* (not *must* or *is to*) exercise his office. But still, it seems clear that the liturgical norms encourage, even expect, that a deacon who is present exercise his office. Even if this were to be practiced, several issues arise. What if there is already a deacon (or perhaps two deacons) serving at Mass? Surely a deacon who is in attendance should not be expected to vest for Mass and sit in the sanctuary with no actual diaconal responsibilities for that Mass. Furthermore, if strictly implemented, a deacon with a wife and younger children would rarely if ever have the opportunity to attend Mass sitting with his wife and children, which would no doubt be a detriment to his spiritual role with and connection to the domestic Church.

Per canon 910 §1, a deacon is an ordinary minister of Holy Communion. An extraordinary minister may distribute Holy Communion "when the need of the Church warrants it and ministers are lacking."[57] A plain reading of these canons would seem to indicate that if a deacon is present at Mass, even if he is not vested or exercising his office, he ought to distribute Holy Communion in lieu of an extraordinary minister should there not be a sufficient enough number of ordinary ministers to distribute at that particular Mass. Again, although this may be an accurate reading of the canons, I am not personally aware of any parishes that apply the canons in this manner. Rather, it seems much more common for deacons in the congregation to be permitted to receive Communion along with the lay faithful, including alongside their wives and children, rather than asking them to come up to the sanctuary to take the place of an extraordinary minister already assigned to that Mass. I am certainly not advocating for a change to this common sense practice. I do not want to vest for every Mass that I attend (even if there is not a deacon serving). Nor do I want to distribute Holy Communion at every Mass (even if that somehow makes me a less-than-fully-pious deacon). Deacons ought to be able, in my opinion, to sit in the congregation with their wives, children, families, and friends, when they are not otherwise assigned by their pastor to serve at that Mass. This is simply to point out that the canons and liturgical norms, as currently worded, do not seem to give that kind of flexibility to pastors or deacons in deciding how they might best serve their congregations.

3. Holy Orders

Given the apparent persistent confusion over the similarities and differences between the orders of bishop and presbyter and the order of deacons, Pope Benedict XVI issued his motu proprio *Omnium in mentem* in 2009, in part to make the code conform to changes already made to the Catechism by his

56 GIRM 116.

57 C. 230 §3.

predecessor, St. John Paul II.[58] Pope Benedict XVI revised canons 1008 and 1009 to read as follows:

> Canon 1008. By divine institution, some of the Christian faithful are marked with an indelible character and constituted as sacred ministers by the sacrament of holy orders. They are thus consecrated and deputed so that, each according to his own grade, they may serve the People of God by a new and specific title.[59]
>
> Canon 1009 §3. Those who are constituted in the order of the episcopate or the presbyterate receive the mission and capacity to act in the person of Christ the Head, whereas deacons are empowered to serve the People of God in the ministries of the liturgy, the word and charity.[60]

The wording in the previous version of canon 1008 implied that all grades of orders (including the diaconate) "fulfill[ed] in the person of Christ the Head the functions of teaching, sanctifying, and governing."[61] The revised canon 1008 removes this language, and then reframes it as a new §3 to canon 1009.

Although these canonical revisions make clear the ontological distinctions between priests and deacons (priests acting in the person of Christ the Head; deacons empowered to serve in ministries of liturgy, word and charity), two things remain somewhat unclear. First, the English translation of the new canon 1009 states that priests have "the mission and *capacity* to act in the person of Christ the Head," with the word "capacity" clearly implying that those who are not priests are not *capable* of functioning in the person of Christ the Head. But the Latin original states that priests have the "*missionem et facultatem agenda in persona Christi Capitis*"—i.e., priests have the "mission and faculty" But having a faculty and having the capacity (*capax*) are two distinctly different things. The former implies that it could be delegated to and exercised by others; the latter is more restrictive, because it goes to a person's identity. Is it possible for a deacon to share in the faculty of a priest's functioning in the person of Christ the Head? Surely not. If not, then why not use the more clear term of *capax*?

Second, with these new revisions it remains unclear exactly what kind of indelible character or ontological change is imprinted upon deacons. The canons are clear that there is *some* kind of indelible mark. But ontologically and theologically, the indelible mark is much easier to explain and understand vis-à-vis the sacraments of baptism and confirmation, and ordination to the priesthood

---

58 See Benedict XVI, apostolic letter motu proprio *Omnium in mentem*, October 26, 2009: *AAS* 102 (2010) 8-10.

59 C. 1008, after issuance of *Omnium in mentem*.

60 C. 1009 §3, after issuance of *Omnium in mentem*.

61 C. 1008, prior to issuance of *Omnium in mentem*.

insofar as a priest is acting in the person of Christ the Head. But what to make of the indelible character of someone who is "empowered to serve . . . in the ministries of the liturgy, the word and charity?"[62] Are not all baptized Christians empowered in some capacity to serve in liturgy, word, and charity? If, as many contend, deacons are often too closely identified with their roles in the Sunday liturgies (rather than in their roles of service), then why are they especially empowered first to the ministry of the liturgy?

Here we see again one of the recurring dilemmas of understanding the diaconate: deacons have a foot in both worlds. They are not so essential to the life of the Church as presbyters and bishops, who act in the person of Christ the Head and who alone can confect the Eucharist, give absolution, and anoint the sick. Yet, a deacon's essential mission and faculty are not anything that could not also be done, in large part, by qualified lay people with proper appointment or delegation. Perhaps the only exception to this latter statement is that a lay person cannot give a homily, whereas a deacon can—yet, there is obviously no instance in which a deacon's inability to give a homily would result in no homily at all, since a priest is always present for the Mass.

All of which leads to reflection on the diaconate that is more philosophical than canonical: deacons are, almost by definition, expendable. Other than the homily, there is not a single sacramental or liturgical action that a deacon does that cannot also be done, under certain conditions, by a lay person.

Although it is certainly not canonical, I would propose that this notion of expendability should form the basis of a deacon's identity and spirituality. We deacons are not truly needed, at least not in the same sense as the priests or laity. But far from being a cry for defeatism, this spirituality of expendability should be a means by which deacons are able to identify with and minister to those who feel most abandoned, most ostracized, most forgotten—in short, those in most need of unrecognized, unrewarded service. This kind of service can take many forms, but the spirituality of expendability ought to serve as a foundation for any deacon's relationship with God and with the People of God. The Church can certainly go on without permanent deacons (it did so for at least a millennium!)—but the Church cannot go on without priests, or religious, or laity.

4. Marriage

We see yet another example of the deacon's expendability in the canons on marriage. Yes, a deacon can be delegated the faculty to assist at a marriage. But even if a deacon is not available, a marriage can still go on, witnessed by a qualified and properly delegated religious or lay person.

62 C. 1009 §3.

But deacons still ought to know what their faculties are with respect to marriages. This obviously varies from diocese to diocese. In our diocese, deacons have faculties to witness marriages only at the parishes to which they are assigned, whereas priests have been given the faculty to assist at marriages everywhere. This is more of a practical distinction than a theological or canonical one—priests are much more likely to move around and form relationships at multiple parishes, meaning that over time they are much more likely than deacons to be asked to do weddings outside of their respective parishes. Ours is a policy aimed at reducing the number of inadvertent invalid marriages due to a priest not having the proper faculties. A deacon, however, is much more of a stable spiritual presence over the long term for his own parish—even more so than many priests, who sometimes come and go with far too much frequency.

Deacons would do well, then to understand their own faculties, but my experience suggests that this kind of thing is something deacons rarely consider. For example, besides assisting at marriages outside of their assigned parish, I would wager that few deacons know that if they are assisting at a marriage where there is an urgent danger of death and the local ordinary cannot be be reached, then a deacon can also dispense from every impediment of ecclesiastical law (not natural or divine law, of course), whether public or occult, except the impediment arising from having been ordained a priest.[63] Deacons then should also have a basic understanding of the various impediments of ecclesiastical law—or, at least, an understanding of the fact that they exist and where they can go to find them.

5. Blessings

Finally, a brief word about blessings. Harkening back to the distinctions clarified in *Omnium in mentem*, canon 1169 creates a hierarchical distinction between bishops, presbyters and deacons. Bishops can perform consecrations and dedications; presbyters can impart blessings except those reserved to the Pope or to bishops. And, finally, a deacon can impart only those blessings expressly permitted by law.[64] (It goes without saying that the truism "if you can do the greater then you can do the lesser" applies to this canon.) Thus, although a deacon can give a blessing in the name of the Church, his ability to impart blessings is restricted to those situations where the law expressly permits it.

E. Miscellaneous Canonical Issues

A few miscellaneous canonical issues may also be worth considering, though more to spark continued discussion than to provide answers.

---

63 See c. 1079.

64 See c. 1169.

1. What's in a Name?

It seems we all know how to address priests, and most every lay person and deacon alike speak the same language in addressing priests in nearly universally the same way. But not so with deacons. In my relatively short time as a deacon, I've had any number of conversations where people ask me: "Do you prefer to be called Deacon Matt? Or just Matt? Or does it matter to you?" Just plain old "Matt" is fine by me. But note that none of us really struggles with what to call a priest. Sure, a few priests may tell certain people just to call them by their first name. But the default is to start with "Father." There seems to be no ready default for how people address a deacon. (None of this is necessarily a problem, in my opinion—it is simply a further indication of the real ontological distinction between priests and deacons, and the reality that a deacon is a cleric with a foot in both worlds.)

Clarifications from the Holy See and the USCCB do not seem to have resolved the confusion. The USCCB National Directory n. 88 states that "the Congregation for the Clergy has determined that in all forms of address for permanent deacons, the appropriate title is 'Deacon.'"[65] The problem with that assertion, however, is that the source cited by the USCCB National Directory does not seem to support it. Instead, the Congregation for the Clergy's *Joint Study of the U.S. Draft Document* issued in 2002 stated as follows:

> The introduction of the title "Reverend Mr." for permanent deacons could further complicate the issue of identity for deacons. The term "Reverend" has traditionally been associated with priests and used only for transitional deacons on their way to priesthood. As there is great sensitivity surrounding the issue of a deacon being seen as a "mini-priest," it would seem that the title "Reverend Mr." would lead to continued identification of the diaconate with the priesthood, rather than contributing to the independence and integrity of the Order of Deacon in itself. The title "Deacon" would, of course, be appropriate.[66]

Although the Congregation for the Clergy does not approve of using the term *Reverend Mr.*, neither does it ban the use of the term in the portion of the text cited by the USCCB. It seems that the Congregation for the Clergy simply expresses significant reservations about the confusion that it might cause to use the term *Reverend Mr.* when applied to permanent deacons. Moreover, the actual norm that the USCCB then promulgated in the USCCB National Directory seems to

---

65 USCCB National Directory, n. 88. The 2nd edition of the USCCB National Directory renumbers this norm to be n. 93.

66 Ibid, 49, endnote 95, http://www.usccb.org/_cs_upload/8304_1.pdf, quoting Congregation for Catholic Education and the Congregation for the Clergy, *Joint Study of the U.S. Draft Document—National Directory for the Formation, Ministry and Life of Permanent Deacons in the United States*, Prot. No. 78/2000 (March 4, 2002).

be less restrictive: "In all forms of address for permanent deacons, 'Deacon' is preferred."[67]

Although there must be some etymological, historical, or theological reasoning behind restricting the use of *Reverend* only to priests, it also seems somewhat odd that permanent deacons can be considered to be in the group known as clerics, while not being included in the group with the title Reverend. This would also seem to bifurcate the Order of Deacon into two distinct Orders: one that is transitional (destined for priestly ordination), and the other that is permanent. But there are not two Orders of Deacons—there is only "the Order of Deacon." There is really no sacramental distinction (and thus no ontological distinction) between transitional and permanent deacons, so why permit different titles?

2. Female Deacons?

I could not give this presentation without saying a word about the possibility of female deacons. As we all know, Pope Francis recently created a commission to study this possibility and report to him on their findings. Very little is known about what was actually presented to the Holy Father (which seems somewhat odd, given that one of the main purposes of the commission was to create meaningful dialogue and help educate the Church on the matter). To the extent that the Code of Canon Law is a practical application of the Church's rich theological tradition (in particular, most recently, Vatican II), then the question of female deacons is really first and foremost a theological and ecclesiological one—not a canonical one. One would presume, of course, that if Pope Francis were to declare an opening to female deacons as a legitimate development in the Tradition (or, as some would assert, a recapturing of the Tradition of the early Church), then changes in the code would necessarily have to follow suit.

One distinction by comparison that strikes me, however, is the difference in tone and approach by Pope Francis with respect to the study of female deacons versus the possibility of optional celibacy for diocesan or secular priests. Pope Francis has been relatively open to discussing the former, whereas the latter (with the exception of ordaining *viri probati* under certain unique circumstances) has been met with dismissal—even though married priests are much more evident and prevalent in the Church's history and Tradition than are female deacons.

3. Practical Issues with *Graviora Delicta*

Finally, dioceses must become more acutely aware of the potential impact of allegations of *graviora delicta* on the ministry and life of their permanent deacons. While it is true that priests tend to make the headlines, deacons are

67 USCCB National Directory, n. 88 (norm 11).

certainly not immune from such allegations. In fact, in some ways deacons have become more vulnerable to such allegations in the wake of the recent scandals and the "Me Too Movement," insofar as people are now coming forward for the first time in decades.

As a practical matter, compared to priests, permanent deacons are generally ordained later in life and, accordingly, are more likely to have had more interactions with minors as an adult prior to their ordinations to the diaconate. While any abuse of a minor *prior* to ordination may not necessarily constitute a canonical delict (insofar as the offense was committed before the person was a cleric), it *would* have to be investigated and analyzed insofar as it would impact the *suitability* of an already-ordained deacon to continue in ministry. Dioceses would do well on the front end, during a deacon candidate's years in formation, to dig into all aspects of his past in a systematic and thorough manner—helping him to recall things that he may have long since forgotten, but which could resurface after his ordination and impact his ability to minister.

IV. Conclusion

The permanent diaconate is, in many ways, a holy order that continues to be in search of a canonical reality. Tracing its roots to the apostolic era, the permanent diaconate went dormant until its restoration by Pope Paul VI in 1967. Since then, there has been much study and debate about the theological foundations for and the role of the permanent diaconate in the broader life of the Church, and particularly here in the United States. And with shifting theological debates come shifting canonical challenges. This presentation has attempted to examine where some of these theological and canonical challenges intersect, while highlighting some of the current canonical issues that remain unanswered for permanent deacons.

Although this presentation may have raised more questions than it answered, hopefully the overarching message is one of continued need for further canonical study and analysis of the permanent diaconate. The reality of the permanent diaconate is not going away, and canonists in particular have an obligation to help ensure it is integrated into the life of the Church in ways that are internally consistent within the Church's theology, laws, and praxis.

Seminar

Custom as an Expression of the Canonical Creativity of a Community of the Faithful

Dr. Wojciech Kowal, OMI, JCD

At the 59th Convention of the Canon Law Society of America (La Jolla, CA, October 13-16, 1997), John Huels gave an address with an intriguing title: "Back to the Future: The Role of Custom in a World Church."[1] In 2019, it is a perfect time to look at what was said 22 years ago, and what can be said today. This presentation is not meant to be a polemic with my colleague but rather an assessment of what was foreseen to happen in the future, what has actually materialized, and what future developments might be. This indeed may be an interesting task, as Huels was speaking about his "conviction concerning the role of custom in the Church,"[2] projecting that ". . . custom is bound to play an even greater role in the future of the world Church."[3]

Although the perspective of the talk of 1997 was *a world Church*, this presentation, potentially unlimited in its scope, will nevertheless be restricted to the North American milieu. In addition, this paper is not intended to be a comprehensive exposition of the canonical doctrine on custom, but rather a response, personal, and hopefully canonically rigorous, to some perceived developments in the understanding of the Church's legal system. It is rather an attempt to look at the role of the community of the faithful in creating a legal framework for its life and mission, uniquely suited for and expressing adequately the universal Gospel values for a given local community. One has also to add a disclaimer that the canonical literature consulted for the preparation of this

1 See John M. Huels, "Back to the Future: The Role of Custom in a World Church," *CLSA Proceedings* 59 (1997) 1-25.

2 Ibid., 1.

3 Ibid.

presentation was treated rather selectively,[4] giving priority to those writings that originated in North America and related exclusively to the Latin Church.

1. Custom as a Canonical Institute

Custom as a social phenomenon can by studied from various perspectives. This presentation is limited, however, to a strictly canonical approach.[5]

What is custom? Often it is said that it is "unwritten law." Here we encounter a problem in the English language, namely its rendering of the Latin terms *ius* and *lex*.

The word *ius* can have three meanings:[6]

a. Absolute objective right (*ius*/*droit*/right) - the object of justice, what is due, what is just;

b. Causal or normative objective right (*ius/loi*/law) - the norm in view of which the object of justice, what is due, is determined, measured. It is the corpus which says what the objective right is.

---

4 As the literature on custom is rather scarce, commentaries to the code were consulted frequently. A search for most recent articles on custom revealed the following: Giuseppe Comotti, "El canon 27 y la función interpretativa de la costumbre," *Ius canonicum* 35 (1995) 585-601; Davide Salvatori, "Il ministro della esposizione e della benedizione eucaristica," *Quaderni di diritto ecclesiale* 16 (2003) 268-281; Edoardo Dieni, "La coutume dans le droit canonique de la postmodernité. Quelques idées sommaires," *Revue de droit canonique* 53 (2003) 241-266; Marcel Metzger, "La coutume, comme modèle pour le nouveau droit liturgique," *Revue de droit canonique* 55 (2005) 251-270; G. Paolo Montini, "La diocesi comunità capace di ricevere leggi, ossia il vescovo diocesano legislatore," *Quaderni di diritto ecclesiale* 20 (2007) 117-125; Giorgio Feliciani, "La consuetudine nella codificazione del 1917," *Ius Ecclesiae* 19 (2007) 333-346; Helmuth Pree, "Diritto consuetudinario – un modo per creare uffici di laici?" *Archiv für katholisches Kirchenrecht* 177 (2008) 15-27; Derek Vidler, "The Use of the Sarum and Tridentine Rites in England before and after Trent," *Canon Law Society Newsletter* 154 (2008) 65-75; Matteo Nacci, "Le consuetudini religiose," *Apollinaris* 83 (2010) 551-570; Sebastián Terráneo, "La costumbre en el derecho canónico Indiano," *Anuario Argentino de derecho canónico* 20 (2014) 271-292; Magdalena Dziewicka, "Zwyczaj w prawie kanonicznym i w prawie polskim," *Kościół i Prawo* 4/2 (2015) 9-23.

5 The notion of custom in secular law is not addressed, as this task would exceed the competence of the author.

6 Here I depart from the distinctions proposed by Huels in his presentation, following rather a classical, comprehensive and informative exposition in Amleto Giovanni Cicognani, *Canon Law: I. Introduction to the Study of Canon Law, II. History of the Sources of Canon Law, III. A Commentary on Book I of the Code*, 2nd rev. ed., trans. J.M. O'Hara and F.J. Brennan (Westminster, MD: The Newman Bookshop, [c1934]) 10-12.

3. Subjective right (*ius/droit*/right) - power or inviolable moral or legal faculty of doing, possessing, omitting or exacting something.[7]

On the other hand, *lex* (*loi*, law) is a written norm, promulgated by the legislator, which is the source of *ius*.

There is no definition of custom in the code. However, canon 23 provides certain important elements of the description of this ecclesial reality. A custom is introduced by a community of the faithful, although in order that it have the force of law, the approval of the legislator is needed. John Huels proposes the following definition of custom: "a normative practice of a community that is adopted by the community itself."[8] Being normative differentiates custom from other practices. The Huels example refers to the practice of the people in a certain parish, to offer Christmas presents to priests. It would not be considered "normative or binding upon them" but rather "wholly optional, no matter how long the practice has been observed."[9] Huels also points to another distinction, that between a legal custom and a factual custom:

> A legal custom is one that meets all the requirements of canon law to be a custom that has the *vis legis*, the force of the law itself. A custom of fact has the same effect on the community's life as a legal custom, but it lacks one or more of the canonical requirements that would give it the same force as the law itself, e.g., a custom that has not yet been observed for thirty continuous and complete years.[10]

Both kinds of custom are practices that the community intends to be normative, nevertheless: ". . . [A] custom that has the force of law is abrogated only by a contrary custom or law (canon 28), whereas a factual custom can be abolished by a merely administrative action of a competent authority."[11]

2. Custom and Ecclesiastical Authority

One distinction is helpful: the section on custom, canons 23-28, concerns

---

7 See Francisco Suárez, *Opera omnia, Tomus sextus: Tractatus de legibus ac Deo legislatore*, Paris, Apud L. Vivès, 1856, lib. I, c. 2, no. 4: "facultas queadam moralis quam unusquisque habet vel circa rem suam, vel ad rem sibi debitam."

8 Huels, "Back to the Future," 6. Cf. T.I. Jiménez Urresti, "Introduction to the Commentary on Custom," *Code de droit annoté* (Paris: Les Éditions du Cerf, Bourges, Les Éditions Tardy, 1989) 34: Custom is "all manner of action, constant and uniform, introduced and practiced by a community." This particular commentary may serve as an example of a different canonical perspective on custom than in North America, presented by a distinct school of canon law, at the University of Salamanca in Spain.

9 Huels, "Back to the Future," 7.

10 Ibid., 8.

11 Ibid.

customs established after the promulgation of the code, while canon 5 treats on the customary law existing before. The latter reads:

> Canon 5 §1. Universal or particular customs presently in force which are contrary to the prescripts of these canons and are reprobated by the canons of this Code are absolutely suppressed and are not permitted to revive in the future. Other contrary customs are also considered suppressed unless the Code expressly provides otherwise or unless they are centenary or immemorial customs which can be tolerated if, in the judgment of the ordinary, they cannot be removed due to the circumstances of places and persons.[12]

On the other hand, canon 23 determines that "only that custom introduced by a community of the faithful and approved by the legislator according to the norm of the following canons has the force of law." The norm points to the role of each of the agents: the community of the faithful introducing "sociologically and canonically" the custom (the material aspect of custom), and the legislator's consent (the formal aspect of custom).[13]

The approval of customs deserves a special consideration. A custom introduced by a community of the faithful has the force of law only if it has been approved by the legislator. This particular canon reflects the doctrine developed during the 17th century, called "the sovereignty principle," which means that the approval of the ecclesiastical authority becomes the formal cause of a legitimate customary law. Before establishment of customary law, however, there must exist actual usage or custom, sometimes referred to as "custom de facto."[14]

A question can be asked: why would the approval of the legislator be necessary for a custom to have a force of law? Would that requirement reveal a certain distrust on the part of ecclesiastical authorities[15] as to the capacity of

---

12 *Codex Iuris Canonici auctoritate Ioannis Pauli PP. II promulgatus* (Libreria Editrice Vaticana, 1989) [hereafter 1983 *CIC*] c. 5; English translation of canons of this code are from *Code of Canon Law, Latin-English Edition: New English Translation* (Washington, DC: Canon Law Society of America, 2012).

13 See Jiménez Urresti, "Introduction to the Commentary on Custom," 34.

14 See John P. McIntyre, *Sources of Law*, class notes (Ottawa: Faculty of Canon Law, Saint Paul University, 1992-1993) 52.

15 The discussion of the consultors reveals a certain tension. During the session (*Sessio* 2) held on November 13-17, 1967, an objection was raised that canon 25: "Consuetudo in Ecclesia vim legis a consensu competentis legislatoris unice obtinet," *Communicationes* 16 (1984) 157, introduces a demand that is too harsh and perhaps including a suggestion that, as a rule, the legislator opposes creation of customs. The adjunct secretary responded that the principle that in the Church there are no customs without the consent of the legislator is fundamental as required by the hierarchical structure of the Church. See *Communicationes* 17 (1985) 35-36.

the faithful to form norms of action in the community? An answer provided by one commentator, Jiménez Urresti, points to the fact that a given community of the faithful is not isolated from the broader social milieu and it is a matter of fact that "the human community does not act exactly in accordance with evangelical standards and principles. From that, there follows the need to discern whether customs of this community of believers are or are not authentically Christian.... This final judgment—recognizing the value and endorsing the practice of custom—belongs to the hierarchy alone and is conclusive."[16] At the same time, the consultors recognized the role of the people in creating customs because they removed the word *unice* (solely) from the draft of canon 25 (corresponding to the present canon 23): "A custom in the Church obtains the force of law solely through the consent of the competent legislator ("Consuetudo in Ecclesia vim legis a consensu competentis legislatoris unice obtinet"), noting that otherwise it would be difficult to see the distinction between law and custom.[17]

The law does not specify the manner of approval. It seems that it has to be an express (explicit or implicit) approval. Nevertheless, the draft of canon 28 (corresponding to the present canon 26) contained the expression: "Nisi a competenti legislatore specialiter fuerit probata, consensu nempe expresse aut tacite manifestato . . . ."[18] All consultors agreed that a custom could be approved by a special consent of the legislator, which could be granted either expressly or tacitly, but it needed to be manifested.[19] Nevertheless, the discussion continued and at the second session (November 13-17, 1967), another formula was agreed upon, namely "consensu saltem tacite manifestato"[20] (consent manifested at least tacitly). However, during the Series Altera, session 2 (October 23-27, 1979), the *coetus* reversed its position on the matter. The session was held after animadversions and suggestions from conferences of bishops, Catholic universities and Roman dicasteries had been collected. Unanimously, a proposal of a consultor was accepted to delete the expression "consensu nempe expresse aut tacite manifestato;" otherwise, if a tacit consent sufficed, the certitude of the

16 Jiménez Urresti, "Introduction to the Commentary on Custom," 34-35.

17 See *Communicationes* 17 (1985) 36. The discussion on the draft of canon 25 was extensive, with various proposals offered; finally, the drafters agreed to a formulation which essentially is that of the present canon 23: "In the Church only that custom introduced by a Christian community and approved by the legislator according to the norm of the following canons has the force of law" (In Ecclesia ea tantum consuetudo a communitate Christiana introducta vim legis habet, quae a legislatore approbata fuerit, ad normam canonum qui sequuntur.) Ibid.

18 *Communicationes* 16 (1984) 153.

19 Ibid. ". . . consuetudo potest a legislatore probari per specialem consensum, qui dari potest sive expresse sive tacite, sed qui debet esse manifestatus . . . ."

20 *Communicationes* 17 (1985) 37, 42.

law would be compromised.[21]

Indeed, if a tacit approval were sufficient, then some uncertainty could ensue. Let us suppose that the legislator knows about the existence of a custom but does not express his judgment on the matter. Is the custom approved or not? If there is a tacit approval, then when does it take effect? It is important because with the approval, the custom acquires the force of law. Besides, canon 5 refers to toleration of customs contrary to the law. Toleration seems to be related to something undesirable, allowed to exist, although reluctantly, for "the circumstances of places and persons," when approval requires a value judgment positive as to its nature.

Who is the competent legislator? A temptation exists to consider a legislator lower than the supreme legislator as competent to approve customs contrary to the universal law. The law sanctions such customs as obtaining the force of law when they have been lawfully observed for a period of thirty continuous and complete years. Here one can find certain powers accorded to the community, operative under the conditions of reasonableness and continuous observation, with the intention of introducing a norm of action (*cum animo iuris inducendi*), by a community capable at least of receiving a law. Now, could not the same powers be acknowledged for the legislator, especially the diocesan bishop who is the pastor of his particular Church? There seems to be a certain asymmetry here: would it mean that the People of God could do more in this regard? There are some arguments pointing to a similarity of approval of customs to dispensations from merely ecclesiastical laws. However, one has to notice that dispensations concern particular cases, while customs are norms with reference to the generality of situations. Customs apart from the law do not present the same dilemma.

The prerogatives of the community could be explained by an example, related to the particular law enacted by the conference of bishops. In a certain diocese in Canada, the bishop approved a modification of penitential norms for Lenten observance. It states that in that diocese "the consumption of meat is not allowed on Ash Wednesday, Good Friday, and all Fridays of Lent. The Archbishop mandates this observance for the spiritual wellbeing of the faithful."[22] A footnote in the decree states "this is in accord with canons 87 and 88 and with Decree No. 8, paragraph 4 of the Canadian Conference of Catholic Bishops' *Complementary Norms to the 1983 Code of Canon Law*." Canons 87 and 88 refer to dispensations,

---

21 See *Communicationes* 23 (1991) 169, 200. Interestingly, *CCEO* c. 1507 §4 states: ". . . a competent legislator can approve a custom as legitimate by his consent, at least tacit (*consensu suo saltem tacito*)." *Codex canonum Ecclesiarum orientalium, auctoritate Ioannis Pauli PP. II promulgatus, fontium annotatione auctus*, Libreria editrice Vaticana, 1995, English translation *Code of Canons of the Eastern Churches: Latin-English Edition, New English Translation* (Washington, DC: Canon Law Society of America, 2001).

22 "Norms for Lenten Observance," https://bit.ly/2RCDvTL (accessed on 26 Mar. 2020).

while the decree of the conference of bishops reads: "In accordance with the prescriptions of canon 1253, the Canadian Conference of Catholic Bishops hereby decrees that the days of fast and abstinence in Canada are Ash Wednesday and Good Friday. Fridays are days of abstinence but *Catholics may substitute special acts of charity or piety on this day* [emphasis added]."[23] The act of the bishop is actually a derogation from this law, as the notion of dispensation clearly points to "relaxation" (*relaxatio*) of the law. However, derogation from a law enacted by a higher legislator is not permitted. Here there is an opportunity for the community to intervene. Creating a de facto custom could introduce a new norm of observance of a stricter penitential discipline.[24] Accepting the rule that a lower legislator cannot approve a custom contrary to a law of a higher legislator, the bishop would need to remain silent on this new usage and after thirty years, the custom would have the force of law. It seems therefore that, paradoxically, the community would have more power than the diocesan bishop would over disciplinary matters by the way of introducing customs against the law.

It seems also that often customs are looked upon as the means of liberating the community from what is perceived as "oppressive laws." The above-mentioned example points to a different attitude. The community may decide to strengthen the existing discipline or to introduce new obligations which might be associated with a certain burden freely accepted for spiritual reasons. There might also be instances of customs liberating the community from a given disciplinary norm that the people consider as hardly acceptable, and in fact not accepted by the community.[25]

Approval by the ecclesiastical authority is an essential, necessary condition for a custom to have the force of law, but it is not a constitutive element of it. Consequently, the custom draws its normative force from the community itself,[26] which introduces it with the intention of creating a norm of action (causal or normative objective right [*ius*/*loi*/law]).

3. Formation of Customs

In his conference, Huels envisaged a revival of customary law in the Church. It seems that this time has not come yet. Indeed, the role of the community

23 Decree no. 8, in Canadian Conference of Catholic Bishops, *Complementary Norms to the 1983 Code of Canon Law* (Ottawa: Canadian Conference of Catholic Bishops, 1996) 101.

24 It seems, however, that a custom must include some positive determined content, a binding practice. Therefore, a decision of the community not to do any penance on Fridays could hardly be called "practice;" it would rather not differ from abuse.

25 For instance, attempts of some legislators to mandate that the whole community remain standing after the reception of Holy Communion, until the last person in the Communion line will have received it.

26 See Jiménez Urresti, "Introduction to the Commentary on Custom," 35.

of the faithful in contributing to the creation of a legal framework in which it operates seems to be forgotten, if not disregarded these days. In the past, custom as a source of canonical norms played a significant role in the life of ecclesial communities. Nothing stands against recovering the importance of customary law in the life of the Church of today.

There are, however, some rather obvious limitations on the activity of the community in this regard. First of all, canon 24 §1 stipulates that "No custom which is contrary to divine law can obtain the force of law." Paragraph 2 introduces another determining parameter: "A custom contrary to or beyond canon law [canonical corpus of norms] (*praeter ius canonicum*) cannot obtain the force of law unless it is reasonable; a custom which is expressly reprobated in the law, however, is not reasonable."

It seems that reasonableness as used in the code is a canonical notion as canon 24 §2 states that a custom which is expressly reprobated in the law, is understood as being not reasonable. It is evident that reasonableness is not solely a logical category as one could imagine reprobation of a usage that is completely logical. Additionally, a closer look at the meaning of terms "rational" (*rationalis*) and "reasonable" (*rationabilis*) reveals some notable differences. *Rationalis* means that something is in conformity with the demands of reason (*ratio*), and as a term has a rather short history (it originated in the early middle ages), while *rationabilis* has its roots in antiquity and points to something proceeding from sound judgment, based on good sense. For instance, the stipulation of canon 396 §2 that the bishop is free to choose any clerics to be his companions on the visitation of a parish, with any other contrary privilege or custom whatsoever being reprobated, cannot be seen as the only rational option; a contrary usage is also rational, though perhaps undesirable. Similarly, one can illustrate the difference between a usage which is rational, but not reasonable. One could imagine that a certain community decided to introduce the posture of kneeling during the liturgy of the Word. Although it would be difficult to maintain that it has no imaginable *ratio* (it could be, for instance, a peculiar sense of piety when listening to the proclamation of the Word during which Christ is present, nevertheless in view of the liturgical tradition it would not be considered reasonable. Then again, demonstration of approval by clapping the hands during the readings at Mass would not only be considered not reasonable, but also not rational, as severely compromising or even nullifying the expected effect.

In fact, the canonical system demands that all objective norms (*iura*) be reasonable, and it is not enough that they be moral and just, or perhaps pious; they must be useful, timely or necessary in pursuit of the goal of the canonical legal system in a certain way, i.e. they need to enjoy intrinsic reasonableness which in turn corresponds to the principle that:

> [T]he Code is in no way intended as a substitute for faith, grace and the charisms in the life of the Church and of the faithful. On the contrary, its purpose is rather to create such an order in the ecclesial society that, while assigning the primacy to faith, grace and the charisms, it at the same time renders easier their organic development in the life both of the ecclesial society and of the individual persons who belong to it.[27]

One could also infer that custom that conforms to the law is reasonable (in the sense of reasonableness as a canonical notion), since it is modelled on the postulated reasonableness of the law that it accompanies.[28] Customs expressly reprobated by law can never be introduced because they are by definition unreasonable. On the other hand, reasonableness crosses over the boundaries of the canon law system, as it needs to be informed by theological reflection. It seems, therefore, that reasonableness is a higher standard than rationality.

This particular aspect of the process of formation of legal customs, the judgment on their reasonableness, points to a delicate relationship between the legislator and the community. What should decide what is reasonable (apart from some obvious situations like a custom contradicting a precept of divine law)? Ultimately, one can pose a question if that what is deemed reasonable in the present era would meet all the criteria that the philosophical theories of knowledge or elementary formal logic used to provide in the old days.

Canon 25 addresses the three conditions that a community must fulfil in order to create a legal custom. First of all, the community must be able to at least receive a law.[29] It seems that there is some divergence of opinions among commentators as to the criteria of determination which communities are capable of that.[30] In the North American milieu, it appears that these criteria range from the size of the group[31] to some specific canonical characteristics of a community. As for the latter, the most commonly mentioned are: possessing juridical

---

27 John Paul II, apostolic constitution *Sacræ disciplinæ leges*, January 25, 1983: *AAS* 75 pars II (1983) vii-xiv, English translation in *Code of Canon Law Annotated,* 2nd ed., revised and updated, ed. Ernest Caparros et al. (Montréal: Wilson & Lafleur Limitée, 2004) 7.

28 See Jiménez Urresti, "Introduction to the Commentary on Custom," 36.

29 See *Communicationes* 16 (1984) 152.

30 The discussion during the revision process reveals that some consultors were in favor of including in the canon draft a determination which community would be capable of receiving a law; they were, however, not satisfied with the proposed formulations. The adjunct secretary of the *coetus* was to provide a new wording for the subsequent session. It does not seem that he ever did.

31 "The community . . . must be large enough to have laws made for it." Ladislas Örsy, "General Norms, cc. 1-28," in *The Code of Canon Law: A Text and Commentary*, ed. James A. Coriden, et al. (New York: Paulist Press, 1985) 39.

personality, the fact of being established by an ecclesiastical authority, or being a group composed of persons identified by a specific canonical characteristic while belonging to the entities of either of the above two categories.[32] Others disagree, proposing different methods of identifying those communities which are capable to receive a law. One of those strategies postulates the following test: if an ecclesiastical authority addresses the whole group of communities that are identical from the point of view of their canonical structure by the means of the law, while addressing the needs of one of these communities by particular administrative acts, such a community is not capable of receiving a law.[33] Hence, a parish would not be considered a community capable of receiving a law and, consequently, not capable of introducing a canonical custom with the force of law. That seems to reduce considerably the scope of applicability of the institution of custom. Besides, it looks that an individual parish can in fact receive a law. That would be especially visible in the case of a parish erected for a community of the faithful of an Eastern Catholic Church with no proper hierarchy present in a given territory, and governed by a Latin hierarch, or for personal parishes erected for the faithful of a determined nationality, language, profession, or other distinctive characteristics. It seems that Huels provides an acceptable solution: a community capable of receiving a law is one that "[…] has been lawfully established (in canon law) and which is under the supervision of competent ecclesiastical authority."[34]

The second necessary element is the intention of the community: the community must act with the intention of establishing a legal custom, either one which conforms to the law (in this case, it confirms the force of the law), or that which is beyond or against the law. Again, in order to avoid any personification of the concept of the community of the faithful, it must be said that this intention is an objective social construct (the *finis operis* of a custom) and not the sum of the particular intentions of the members of the community.[35] Some authors maintain that the intention of the community can be verified with the necessary certainty only when the ecclesiastical authority attempts to suppress a de facto custom.[36] Nevertheless, there are different scenarios possible. I know a parish in Poland in which, some thirty years ago, the diocesan bishop decided that the parish provide sustenance for the pastor in the form of food, due to the scarce availability of monetary offerings in the region. This was what is called *id quod* of a custom, an element established by the ecclesiastical authority. However, the

32 See John M. Huels, "General Norms, cc. 1-28," in *New Commentary on the Code of Canon Law*, ed. John P. Beal et al. (New York/Mahwah, NJ: Paulist Press, 2000) 90.

33 See Jiménez Urresti, "Introduction to the Commentary on Custom," 36-37.

34 Huels, "Back to the Future," 13. One could ask if a Catholic family which founded a church may have a law applicable to them as a "board of directors" of this foundation?

35 See Jiménez Urresti, "Introduction to the Commentary on Custom," 37-38.

36 See Huels, "Back to the Future," 7.

modus quo of the custom to be formed was decided by the community itself.[37] Each week a different household in succession was to provide the pastor with the food necessary for a week.[38] It is rather obvious that this was a normative practice, with a clear intention of introducing a determined duty, and enforced by the people themselves if any family was found delinquent on that obligation. One can expect that similar arrangements might be still operative in mission countries.

The notion of the intention of the community to introduce a normative practice (*cum animo iuris inducendi servata*) deserves special attention also from a theoretical point of view. There is ample canonical literature regarding the processes of the creation of the law, searching for the motives, intentions, goals of the legislator introducing a given norm. Any extensive analysis of the history of a canonical norm would normally point to the circumstances preceding the origin of the law in question, its roots in the tradition, in previous legal enactments, and also in customs. A critical student of the process of the formation of a new law will scrutinize the developments of the legislative activity of the lawgiver, including the circumstances of the preparation of the law, the evolutive process of the discussion among the drafters, the actual redaction of the law, and the following phases of the communal understanding, reception, application, and evolution of the law in the course of time.[39] The process of formation of a new custom would seem to pose an additional challenge—while the legislative history of a written norm can, in principle at least, be traced through an analysis of written resources using properly canonical and theological tools, in the case of customs the same process of re-tracing their canonical history would require the use of anthropology of law which describes legal phenomena in a given milieu within the larger social context. According to Huels, the specific fields of interest of this scientific discipline include the response of law to changes in society, the influence of customs and beliefs on individual and social behavior, the modes of enforcing law, and similar.[40]

One can also encounter a variety of attitudes in the community. Some persons may act in good faith, judging that the concrete law is harmful, untimely, inappropriate or useless, while others may be motivated by bad faith, acting out of disobedience, not necessarily related to the content of a given law, but out of contempt for the legislator. It seems, however, that even such a morally deficient

---

37 Cf. McIntyre, *Sources of Law*, 52.

38 Unfortunately, the area was well known for raising ducks, and soon the priest—actually, my brother—could not even look at them!

39 See Gommar Michiels, *Normæ generales iuris canonici: commentarius libri I Codicis iuris canonici*, editio altera penitus retractata et notabiliter aucta, vol. 1 (Paris: Desclée et Socie, 1949) 530-533.

40 See John M. Huels, "Interpreting Canon Law in Diverse Cultures," *The Jurist* 47 (1987) 279.

intention does not prevent the custom from being introduced. If perchance the legislator would find that the custom is worthy of approval due to its objective intrinsic reasonableness, this would not mean his approval of the deficient intention, but rather an acknowledgement of the importance of that custom in the life of the community.[41]

A special approval of the competent legislator is needed for customs beyond the canonical corpus of norms (*praeter ius canonicum*) or contrary to a law (*contra legem*),[42] to obtain the force of law. What about customs which are not approved by the competent authority? Canon 26 provides for a de facto approval; customs contrary to a law or beyond the canonical corpus of laws must have been observed for thirty continuous and complete years to obtain the force of law. The custom against a law (*contra legem*) which contains a prohibiting clause must, however, be observed for one hundred years. Customs which are reprobated by the law can never obtain the force of law (see canon 24 §2).[43]

It seems that canon 27, invoking an old maxim that custom is "the best interpreter of laws (*leges*)" opens an ample, albeit not yet fully recognized opportunity for exercising a kind of "canonical service" offered to the whole Church by a community introducing a custom. The principle announced in the canon "is [also] valid for legal customs which do not introduce a new norm, but amplify the force of the practical (factual) reception of the law . . . ; [and] also for customs beyond the law or those that are contrary to a law, about which it would be better to say that custom is the best interpreter of *ius* rather than *lex*."[44]

The intellectual operation of interpretation by the way of custom requires some prior understanding of the law by the community (unless one is to assume that the community acts in an irreflective manner!). Although this pre-understanding introduced by the community does not uncover, directly and *per se,* the will of the legislator, nevertheless, it may indicate, with some level of certitude, the meaning of the law intended by the legislator.[45] As Örsy remarked, through understanding, acceptance, and practice of the law, the people of God

---

41 See Jiménez Urresti, "Introduction to the Commentary on Custom," 38.

42 Unlike some commentators, like Huels, I maintain that the first of those two notions relates to the whole system of canonical norms (c. 26 has the expression *ius canonicum* for that), while the second relates necessarily to the concrete identifiable law (*contra legem* as in c. 26).

43 See Jiménez Urresti, "Introduction to the Commentary on Custom," 38-39.

44 Ibid., 39.

45 See Michiels, *Normæ generales iuris canonici*, vol. 1, 533.

become interpreters, too.[46]

Finally, canon 28 deals with the revocation of customs, both anterior and posterior to the code, by contrary law or by opposite custom. The canon introduces therefore, next to the intervention of the legislator promulgating a contrary law and thus revoking the custom which is contrary to or beyond the law (*sive contra sive praeter legem*), a kind of "self-correcting" measure available to the community. It allows for modifying the canonical discipline established by a previous intention of introducing a given custom, now considered as no longer corresponding adequately to the reality, through forming a new intention of introducing a binding norm of action.

4. The Future of Custom

In order to talk about the future, one has to have a look at the past. John McIntyre pointed to the fact that "although the Church has recognized custom (*consuetudo*) as a legitimate source of law (*ius*), nevertheless, since the time of the Council of Trent, the role of custom diminished in favor of statutory law (*lex*)."[47] The discussion of the *coetus* reveals that the intention of the drafters was to retain the discipline of the 1917 code, with necessary adjustments.[48] McIntyre later opines: "... [T]he history of this institute [custom] illustrates the shift from the reasonable custom (intellectualist [approach]) to the 'will of the competent superior' (voluntarist [approach]) indicative of fundamental misunderstanding about the nature of custom in the first place. And so, the matter rests."[49]

---

46 See Ladislas Örsy, *Theology and Canon Law: New Horizons for Legislation and Interpretation* (Collegeville, MN: Liturgical Press, 1992) 49. This conviction brings some consequences with regard to custom. If the meaning of law is fixed at its promulgation, what would be left for the custom deemed as the best interpreter of law? How could a custom explain, modify, or clarify understanding of laws? See ibid., 60. McIntyre points to three uses of custom: as interpretative, supplemental, and abrogative. See John P. McIntyre, *Customary Law in the* Corpus iuris canonici (San Francisco: Mellon Research University Press, 1990) 87-112. The traditional reflection on the search for the "mind of the legislator" observes that recourse to the mind of the legislator takes no account of a merely internal will of the legislator. See Michiels, *Normæ generales iuris canonici*, vol. I, 554. The traditional doctrine found in Suárez' thought maintains that the mind of the other human being is not accessible in any other way than through a verbal expression. See Suárez, *Tractatus de legibus ac Deo legislatore*, lib. VI, c. 1, n. 13). Consequently, the meaning of the law cannot be obtained as something proceeding directly from the mind of the legislator, but only through the mediation effected by his words. This is even more so in the case of having reference to the drafters' discussions in the revision process: the drafters are not legislators, and therefore their intentions and argumentation offered in the process of drafting the canons of the code, cannot be attributed to the legislator; the legislator's mind will, therefore, be first of all revealed in the promulgated text itself.

47 McIntyre, *Sources of Law*, 50.

48 See *Communicationes* 9 (1977) 232.

49 McIntyre, *Sources of Law*, 51.

John Huels pointed to several factors which he regarded as favoring the activity of the People of God in creating customary norms. First, he indicated that the demographics, or to be more exact, the multiplicity of cultures within the Church's society will create the space for respecting "the autonomy, the variety of situations, and the aspirations"[50] of peoples from different cultural backgrounds. Indeed, this is something that looks almost natural as a basis for development of various customs: some of them brought into a new country with the migration of a given community (like blessings of Easter food typical for several Central or Eastern European nations), or some new ones, created in the newly acquired societal setting. Is there any perceivable activity in this regard or the newly arrived people assume rather the ways of living established in North America? This may also take a form of shunning anything that would differentiate the new immigrants from the "American" or "Canadian" Church.

Another factor which was indicated as a possible incentive for increasing the role of custom in the life of the Church was a perceived peak of legislative activity in the Church in the twentieth century, "particularly in the post Vatican II years during which we have witnessed so many changes in nearly every area of ecclesiastical discipline."[51]

> This period culminated in the two new codes, the Latin code of 1983 and the Eastern code of 1990. During this period there were two significant reforms of the Roman curia, and hundreds of executory documents were issued by the dicasteries of the Holy See. I believe this period of intense lawmaking activity that we have experienced in our own generation has largely come to an end. Although further reforms in certain areas would still be welcome, it is unlikely that we will again see another such major reform of church discipline in our lifetime.[52]

That was a bold prediction, but, in my estimate, the legislative activity thrives in the Church, including plans for the revision of the Latin code in the near future.

A lot, however, will depend on the attitude of ecclesiastical superiors towards newly formed customs of fact. John Huels maintains that the interruption of the time period for a custom contrary to a law or beyond canon law to obtain the force of law (30 continuous and complete years) can occur through a decision of the community itself or of an ecclesiastical authority. He explains "a custom that does not have the force of law can be eliminated not only by the competent legislator, but also by other officials: a lower level legislator, the vicar general or

50 Huels, "Back to the Future," 1.

51 Ibid., 1-2.

52 Ibid.

episcopal vicar, the pastor of the parish, the superior of the religious community, etc."[53] In his commentary, "General Norms, cc. 1-28," Huels supports this opinion by a reference to Gommar Michiels' *Normæ generales iuris canonici.*[54] However, a closer look at the latter source points to a different conclusion. First of all, even though canon 25 of the 1917 code stipulated that the consent of the competent ecclesiastical superior (*competentis superioris ecclesiastici*) is necessary for a custom to obtain the force of law, nevertheless, the same Michiels in his commentary indicates that this superior is to be the legislator to whom belongs the power to enact the respective norm of action.[55] Yet, later in his commentary Michiels states that a custom can be interrupted by the decision of any ecclesiastical superior who, however, has the competence to protect authoritatively the legal order in the community.[56] In my opinion, that task corresponds to the notion of executive power. Therefore, parish priests would be excluded (as they do not possess executive power, unless in specific instances when delegated by the law itself or a competent ecclesiastical superior). For the decision to interrupt the time period needed for a custom to obtain the force of law requires interpretation of the norms of law (*ius*), and moreover, an authoritative interpretation as it affects the whole community in its exercise of the right to create customs. Huels remarks that "[t]heoretically, the process of forming and eradicating customs can go on endlessly if the community and the competent authority remain at odds."[57] Actually, the attitude of ecclesiastical superiors may be one of the main reasons that customs are rare today, if they quash any attempt by the community to introduce a normative practice that does not correspond to their view of liturgical or disciplinary matters or expressions of piety. However, that kind of attitude would practically nullify the purpose of the law on custom.

A telling example can be drawn from an often-contentious question of postures during the Mass. The Institutio generalis Missalis Romani, as adapted to the Church in Canada, in no. 43 states the following: "In the dioceses in Canada, the faithful should kneel at the Consecration . . . . Where it is the practice for the people to remain kneeling after the *Sanctus* (*Holy, Holy, Holy*) until the end of

---

53 Ibid., 11.

54 On page 92, Huels makes a reference to Gommar Michiels, *Normæ generales iuris canonici: commentarius libri I Codicis iuris canonici*, editio altera penitus retractata et notabiliter aucta, vol. 2 (Paris: Desclée et Socie, 1949) 85.

55 Michiels, *Normæ generales iuris canonici*, vol. 2, 45: "Theoretice illius superioris sufficit et requiritur consensus . . . cuius potestati legiferae subordinatur ius, quod per consuetudinem, de qua agitur, constituitur vel abrogatur; cum enim competentia in superiore, requisita ea sit, per quam consuetudini facti vis legis tribui possit (can. 25), is solus competens esse potest, qui normam per communitatis usum inductam vel abrogatam pro eadem communitate statuere vel abrogare potest lege personaliter lata."

56 Ibid., 85: ". . . non solummodo a legislatore a cuius approbatione pendet vis legalis consuetudinis, sed a quolibet Superiore ad cuius competentiam pertinet tutela auctoritativa ordinis juridici legalis quo communitas consuetudinem inducens regitur."

57 Huels, "Back to the Future," 11.

the Eucharistic Prayer and before Communion when the Priest says *Ecce Agnus Dei* (*This is the Lamb of God*), it is laudable for this practice to be retained." In a certain parish, not only was it not retained but the pastor waited for the people to stand up after the Consecration and would not continue the Eucharistic Prayer until they all did. This practically eradicated this custom, although the practice seems slowly reappearing in the community. It could have been argued, though, that the custom obtained the force of the law due to its long existence but that would probably worsen the relationship of the community with the pastor.[58]

Conclusion

Perhaps there is a need to return to the inspiration offered by *Gaudium et spes*, no. 53. The Constitution points to the notion of culture:

> [Culture] renders social life more human both in the family and the civic community, through improvement of customs and institutions.... Thence it follows that human culture has necessarily a historical and social aspect and the word "culture" also often assumes a sociological and ethnological sense. According to this sense we speak of a plurality of cultures. Different styles of life and multiple scales of values arise from the diverse manner of using things, of laboring, of expressing oneself, of practicing religion, of forming customs, of establishing laws and juridic institutions, of cultivating the sciences, the arts and beauty. Thus, the customs handed down to it form the patrimony proper to each human community. It is also in this way that there is formed the definite, historical milieu which enfolds the man of every nation and age and from which he draws the values which permit him to promote civilization.[59]

As I belong to a province of the Missionary Oblates of Mary Immaculate that is devoted to the work with immigrants of the Polish descent in Canada, I am rather

---

58 Another recent controversy regards the posture after the reception of Holy Communion. In some dioceses it is stipulated (or rather it is a peculiar interpretation of the existing liturgical laws) that all faithful, including the concelebrating priests, after having received Communion remain standing until the last person in the Communion procession receives it. It may be an example of a norm (interpretation) that actually introduces disorder as some are constantly turning their heads back to estimate how long the procession still is, and some who decide to sit down in desperation, while others bravely remain standing. Though this is not a question of a custom, the whole situation may serve as a reminder that in drafting laws, or interrupting customs, one should venture beyond the mere letter of the law and look also at practical consequences. Besides, there is quite a convincing argument that this particular interpretation of liturgical laws has no foundation.

59 Second Vatican Council, Pastoral Constitution on the Church in the Modern World Gaudium et spes 53, December 7, 1965: AAS 58 (1966) 1025–1115; English translation in A. Flannery (gen. ed.), Vatican Council II: The Conciliar and Post-Conciliar Documents, vol. 1, new rev. ed. (Northport, NY: Costello Pub. Co., 1996) 958.

sensitive to cultural aspects of the religious practice of immigrant communities. It seems that no one would deny the right of Eastern rite Christians to cultivate their customs, but not necessarily the same would be true in the case of the faithful of the Latin rite. *Gaudium et spes*, no. 54 mentions among the characteristics of the contemporary culture the phenomenon of "customs and usages . . . becoming more and more uniform."[60] The characteristics in this passage of the Constitution are positive as to their nature; however, including among them the "uniformization" of customs is rather puzzling, especially in the present social context in which the promotion of particular cultures is elevated to an undisputable principle, at least in Canada. A legitimate question can be asked: is this what we are aiming at in our local church communities? If this is so, I doubt that customary law has any great future.

One should end on a more optimistic note. This is going to be ultimately the community of the faithful that will decide on contributing to the legal framework for its life and mission, to express better the Gospel values lived out in a given local community. It is better not to assume the role of a prophet in this regard, as this reflection on the role of custom teaches us. In other words, the future will tell.

60 Ibid., 959.

Seminar

From Tripoli to Abu Dhabi: The Evolution of Catholic-Muslim Relations

The Reverend Elias D. Mallon, SA, STL, PhD

I. The Situation Immediately Following Vatican II

I have chosen the title *From Tripoli to Abu Dhabi* for my presentation out of qualitative rather than quantitative concerns. In fact, neither 1976, the year of the Catholic-Muslim dialogue in Tripoli, nor 2019, the year of the visit of Pope Francis to the United Arab Emirates, is a pivotal year in Christian-Muslim relations. However, qualitatively speaking, the communiqués that came out of these two meeting throw bright light on how much mutual attitudes between Catholics and Muslims have changed and improved.

Relations between Muslims and Christians antedate 1976, and we will have an opportunity to see the early days of the encounter. Likewise, Catholic-Muslim relations are evolving in new and very fruitful ways. While this evolution has been going on for several decades, it has found new energy in the way Pope Francis interacts with partners in dialogue. The years 1976 and 2019 merely provide us with a—very graphic—context to understand the breadth and increasing depth of the Catholic-Muslim dialogue.

After the close of Vatican II, the Holy See set up the Secretariat for Promoting Christian Unity under whose auspices was the Catholic-Jewish dialogue. Housed in a building on the via del' Erba, the Secretariat for Promoting Christian Unity shared a floor with the Secretariat for Non-Christians. In 1973 Pope Paul VI made Archbishop Sergio Pignedoli a cardinal and appointed him head of the Secretariat for Non-Christians.

There had been a much longer history of dialogue between Catholics and other Christians than between Catholics and Non-Christians, and Pignedoli had his work cut out for him; there were few, if any, "road plans." On 28 October 1965 *Nostra Ætate, The Declaration on the Relation of the Church to Non-Christian Religions* was promulgated. Although erroneously—if understandably—referred to as "the decree on the Jews," the first non-Christian religions mentioned in paragraph two of *Nostra Ætate* are Hinduism and Buddhism. They are, however, mentioned only in passing. It is only with paragraph three that the real discussion

is entered into, and it begins with "The Church also has a high regard for the Muslims." Thus, while not the first mentioned, Islam is the first non-Christian religion dealt with in *Nostra Ætate.*

There are several reasons why this may have been the case. Islam and Christianity (with Catholicism being the largest form of Christianity) are the two largest religions on the planet. Millions of Catholics live in what are referred to as Muslim-majority nations. Christianity and Islam have experienced 1400 years of conflict, in which now one group and later another was the aggressor and the victim. If the Catholic-Jewish dialogue was imperative for theological and historical reasons, the Catholic-Muslim dialogue was imperative at the very least for demographic reasons and, as we shall see in *A Common Word*, the peace of the planet.

When the Catholic Church committed itself to the ecumenical dialogue, the dialogue partners were known. There were church leaders like the Patriarch of Constantinople and the Archbishop of Canterbury. There were world-wide denominational organizations like the Lutheran World Federation, the World Reformed Alliance, etc., and not least, the World Council of Churches, established after World War II and comprising more than three-hundred Orthodox and Protestant Churches.

If one can speak of a structure in Islam at all, it would be very different from what we find in almost every Christian church or denomination. Islam has no official center, no official spokesperson, no official bureaucracy, and broadly speaking no clergy.[1] This has provided—and continues to provide—a challenge to the Catholic-Muslim dialogue. While the Catholic dialogue partner's status and role are clear, that is almost never the case with the Muslim interlocutor. Thus, finding (institutionally) equal dialogue partners is difficult.

In addition, while Muslims and Christians engaged in theological debates/dialogues during the Abbasid Caliphate (750-1258), by the 13th century these encounters had stopped. This was partially due to the Mongol destruction in the Middle East and partially to a change in the intellectual atmosphere in Islam. Thus in the mid-20th century Muslims not only had not had any experience of Christian-Muslim theological discussion for well over five hundred years; they had little or no desire for it. Attempts of the Holy See to initiate such a dialogue were met with indifference at best.

---

1 Muslims will often stress this, and to some extent it is true. There is no clerical class, set off by a (sacramental) ritual to perform tasks that no other Muslim may perform. Nevertheless, in Shi'ite Islam there is a clear stratification of clerical levels according to education and peer recognition, resulting in men with the title/office of ayatollah—of which there are several levels, followed by lower levels of hujjatolislam and muballiğ al-risala. Cf., however, Nabil Mouline, *The Clerics of Islam* (New Haven: Yale University Press, 2015).

However, in May 1975 the possibility of a theological dialogue with Islam seemed to open up. Muammar Gaddafi let it be known that Libya was open to a dialogue between Catholics and leading Muslim thinkers, and the topic would be limited to religious and theological topics. The Secretariat agreed.[2]

The meeting was held 1-5 February 1976 and Cardinal Pignedoli and some of the Secretariat staff were in attendance. The four points of the conference's agenda certainly met the criteria of the Holy See for a theological conversation. In addition, the Holy See insisted that there could be no political discussions since that was not in the purview of the Secretariat for Non-Christians.

From the outset there were difficulties. Many of the Muslims speakers railed against the Crusades, western imperialism, Zionism, etc. It was decided that the conference would issue a joint communiqué. A committee was set up and a communiqué was produced and signed by Cardinal Pignedoli. Rabbi Marc Tannenbaum wrote a report on the meeting for the American Jewish Committee and noted that neither Cardinal Pignedoli nor Msgr. Rossano were given the courtesy of seeing the text in advance of its introduction, nor were they aware that it contained anti-Israel paragraphs.

In point of fact, it seems that all but one of the members of the Holy See's delegation were unaware that articles 20 and 21 of the original Arabic text contained strong anti-Israel and anti-Zionist statements. The incident was a major embarrassment for the Holy See. The day after the statement, Cardinal

2 There is some rather odd material surrounding this meeting, most of which needs to be taken with a good dose of skepticism. Peter Scholl-Latour, *Adventures in the East* (New York: Bantam Books, 1988) is an often odd and poor English translation of the original German *Allah ist mit den Standhaften*. The book has a section entitled "Qadaffi and the Cardinal" (pp. 18-29) which attempts to report on this meeting. In addition to non-English phraseology, some cranky asides about the reforms of the Vatican, and some downright inaccuracies, e.g., Christians do not worship the cross (p. 21), the section reads like an exposé. Cardinal Pignedoli is presented in an unflattering light, and it seems the purpose of the section is to give an "insider's" explanation of why the cardinal was never elected pope. A similar piece by Martin Kramer can be found at Martin Kramer, "If Not for Muammar Gaddafi, This Guy Might Have Been Pope," History News Network, The George Washington University, https://hnn.us/article/151186 (accessed on 15 Apr. 2020).

The best piece on the event is a report made by Rabbi Marc Tannenbaum to the American Jewish Committee on the meeting and its outcome. Rabbi Marc H. Tannenbaum Collection, 1945-1992, American Jewish Archives, http://collections.americanjewisharchives.org/ms/ms0603/ms0603.048.002.pdf (accessed on 26 Mar. 2020). This is perhaps the best source.

What is clear is that 1) Cardinal Pignedoli and a delegation from the Holy See took part in a Muslim-Christian dialogue/encounter in Tripoli; 2) Colonel Gaddafi played a major, manipulative role in the dialogue; 3) a communiqué was issued in which, without the knowledge of the cardinal, Israel and Zionism were condemned; 4) this was a major embarrassment to the Holy See which had to do considerable damage control after the publication of the communiqué.

Pignedoli held a press conference in which he disassociated himself from the articles. On the day after Pignedoli's press conference the Deputy Secretary of the Vatican Secretariat of State noted that the Holy See could not accept these two articles because their content did not correspond in essential points to the position of the Holy See.

Thus, one of the first encounters in dialogue between Catholics and Muslims was a disaster. It embarrassed the Secretariat for Non-Christians and embarrassed the Holy See itself. We all know that the Holy See has a very long memory. Nevertheless, it is a sign of the Holy See's commitment to the dialogue that it continued.

Moving ahead forty-three years almost to the day, on 4 February 2019 Pope Francis and Sheikh Ahmad al-Tayyeb, the Grand Imam of al-Azhar University,[3] signed *A Document on Human Fraternity for World Peace and Living Together.*[4] It is a truly extraordinary document for many reasons, the first and foremost of which is its very existence. It is also a truly joint document. All of you are aware that documents issued by the Holy See have a distinct and easily recognized style, sometimes referred to as "Vaticanese." It might be less known, but should be no surprise, that Islamic documents like *fatāwin* (singular: *fatwā*) would also have a distinctive, easily recognized style. Marvelously, both styles are represented in the document. It is a document in which both a Catholic and Muslim can recognize their tradition at work.

I see Tripoli and Abu Dhabi as symbols of what has changed in a period of forty years. The dialogue has moved from distrust, disrespect and embarrassment to genuine friendship, deep mutual respect and cooperation.

The *Document on Human Fraternity,* however, is more than just of a symbol of how far Catholic-Muslim relations have come in the past sixty years. It is also a sign of what I see as a new trajectory not only in Catholic-Muslim relations but in the interreligious encounter in general.

As I mentioned above, when the Catholic Church officially committed itself to the ecumenical movement with *Unitatis redintegratio*, The Decree on Ecumenism,[5] there may have been many new things that came with it. However,

---

3 Al-Azhar in Cairo is one of the oldest universities in the world. It was founded in 970 or 972 under the Fatimid Caliphate and is arguably the premier Muslim university in the world.

4 See Pope Francis and Ahmad Al-Tayyeb, "A Document on Human Fraternity for World Peace and Living Together," February 4, 2019, http://w2.vatican.va/content/francesco/en/travels/2019/outside/documents/papa-francesco_20190204_documento-fratellanza-umana.html (accessed on 26 Mar. 2020).

5 See Second Vatican Council, decree *Unitatis redintegratio*, November 21, 1964: *AAS* 57 (1965) 90-107.

it was not an endeavor totally foreign to Christian churches or, for that matter, to the Catholic Church which joined the movement somewhat later. The goal of Christian unity, the unity of baptism, the generally shared theological history and vocabulary, the great similarity between Christians of all denominations provided something of a road map—though not without some dead ends—as how to proceed.

The interreligious dialogue, on the other hand, had no such road map. For any number of reasons, few if any of them very good, ecumenism and interreligious dialogue began to be conflated. Interreligious dialogue became a subset or even essential part of ecumenism. Having been engaged in interreligious dialogue for more than forty years, I was often asked what the difference between interreligious dialogue and ecumenism is. The official church was always very careful to see ecumenism as a project between Christians and interreligious dialogue to be a project between Christians and non-Christians. The church was very correct in highlighting this distinction. It was, however, for the most part, unsuccessful.

The goal of the ecumenical movement is Christian unity, the restoration of full communion between all the baptized. Arriving at this means dealing with differences. The differences between Christians need to be understood by all sides. It has to be decided if the differences are church-dividing. If not, they are not an obstacle. If, however, they are church-dividing, a way must be found to overcome them while violating the conscience of no one. The goal is unity.

With interreligious dialogue and, of course, with the Catholic-Muslim dialogue the initial steps are the same, *viz.,* getting to know and understand the other. After that is reasonably accomplished, however, we are immediately in unknown territory. The goal of the Catholic-Muslim dialogue is not to produce "convergence" statements, to say nothing of achieving any type of unity in the sense of communion.

Familiar as they were with ecumenical dialogue between Christians, consciously or unconsciously Catholics soon found themselves at a "where do we go from here?" crossroads. In some places the search for commonality became more and more strained—one is tempted to say desperate—and, to be honest, more and more misleading. St. John Damascene, a member of a family of civil servants in the Umayyad Caliphate, to the contrary notwithstanding, Islam is neither an odd nor heretical form of Christianity. Islam is a separate religion. While Judaism, Christianity and Islam have strong "familial" connections, not the least of which is worshipping the same God, each religion has what I call an *irreducible particularity.* Irreducible particularity is that which makes each of these religions a religion unto itself with its own internal consistency, a consistency which is not reducible to the particularity of any other religion.

The irreducible particularities of Islam and Christianity provide rich and

rewarding opportunities for dialogue. In such an exchange there is a getting to know each other. Sometimes such a dialogue provides unexpected and surprising points of contact between Christianity and Islam. Such a dialogue can be very rewarding and satisfying. It can, however, also be very misleading. Familiarity with Islam insofar as Islam is similar to Christianity is not to see or understand its irreducible particularity. Not to understand Islam's irreducible particularity is, somewhat harshly put, not to understand Islam.[6]

II. Relations between Catholic Christianity and Islam in the Centuries before Vatican II

It is precisely at this point that the familiar intra-Christian and Catholic/Christian-Muslim dialogues part ways and do so radically. Once one gets to the stage of saying, "Oh, you hold that too! That's just like what we believe," then what is the next step? It is precisely at this point that many Catholic-Muslim dialogues simply run out of steam or run the risk of becoming trivial.

While it is true to say that the Roman Catholic Church first committed itself to the Catholic Muslim dialogue at Vatican II, for centuries open minded and broad spirited Catholics were engaged in a friendly encounter with Islam.

In 1076 Pope Gregory VII (1020-1085) wrote a letter to al-Nasir, a Muslim governor in North Africa. The tone of the letter is respectful and even warm. Gregory mentions that he and al-Nasir owe each other fraternal love in a special way, "since we confess and acknowledge—in different ways it is true—one God to whom we pray . . . ."[7] The close of Gregory's letter is extraordinary: "[W]e ask with our lips and from our heart that He [i.e., God] himself may receive you after a long stay here below, into the bosom of the most holy patriarch Abraham's beatitude."[8]

Some 800 years ago, in 1219, Francis of Assisi visited Damietta, Egypt, during the Fifth Crusade. During his stay there Francis visited Malik al-Kamil,[9] the leader of the hostile Muslim forces. While there are quasi-contemporary accounts of the visit, there are no eyewitness accounts. In recent decades something of a cottage industry has arisen around Francis' visit to al-Kamil,

---

6 Of course, this is reciprocal and is something which occurs with some frequency. Muslims understand those parts of Christianity which are similar to Islam and believe that all Christians have to do is eliminate the "falsifications" in the New Testament and renounce the "exaggeration" of worshipping Jesus (and Mary) as divine, and Christianity and Islam can become one religion.

7 Jean-Marie Gaudeul, *Encounters and Clashes: II Texts* (Rome: Pontificio Istituto di Studi Arabi e Islamici, 1984) 75; Elias D. Mallon, *Islam: What Catholics Need to Know*, 2nd ed. (Arlington, VA: National Catholic Education Association, 2018) 55.

8 Ibid.

9 Al-Malik al-Kāmil Nāṣir al-Dīn Abu al-Ma'ālī Muḥammad (1177 or 1180-1238).

including the obligatory legend that the Muslim converted to Christianity (for which there is absolutely no evidence).

If we limit ourselves to the barest, most sober account of the visit, even without details, it is still extraordinary at its core. Francis, the Christian, pays a visit to Malik al-Kamil, the leader of the Muslim forces. While the motives of Francis remain unknown, we are relatively certain that he was not going as a representative of the Christian forces. In other words, he was not visiting al-Kamil to demand his surrender. Despite all the creative hagiography we have no idea what the two spoke about. We do, however, know that Francis returned safely to the Christian camp. After his conversion, Francis was never in favor of wars—Crusades or otherwise. His lack of enthusiasm for the Crusades was, if anything, apparently strengthened by his visit to al-Kamil. On his part, al-Kamil gave generous terms of surrender to the Crusaders after they had been defeated at Damietta. The Damietta encounter is very typical of Francis of Assisi: simple and without fanfare, showing respect and love for the other; striving for peace. For any century that is outstanding; for the 13th century it is amazing.

In the time before Vatican II several Catholic figures stand out for their relationship to Muslims. What is interesting in all of them is that while they strove to understand Islam intellectually, it was done in the context of befriending Muslims and appreciating their faith. Given our limitations of time and space, it is impossible to do more than briefly mention these figures.

The first of these is Charles de Foucauld (1858-1916). A French soldier who returned to his faith and who lived first as a Cistercian priest in the Middle East and later as a hermit in Algeria, de Foucauld developed his life around the "life of Jesus at Nazareth." That is to say, that period in the life of Jesus before he began his public ministry. For Foucauld this meant a life of poverty, quietly living among the native people whom one loves and appreciates, having a daily occupation and becoming as enculturated into the native situation as possible. The Little Brothers and Little Sisters of Jesus follow the way of de Foucauld living among Muslims in North Africa and other places.

Another Frenchman, Louis Massignon (1883-1962), also returned to the practice of his Catholic faith. While suffering from a serious illness in Baghdad, Massignon had a conversion experience, which cannot be separated from his life-long work of studying the Muslim mystic and martyr al-Hallaj.[10] Hallaj was a mystic of the overwhelming transforming love of God. This love created such a unity between the Beloved and the Lover that al-Hallaj was executed for claiming that that he was The Truth, i.e., God.

Cared for in his illness by a Muslim family, Massignon had a deep love

10 Abul Muġit al-Ḥusayn bin Manṣûr al-Ḥallaj

and respect for Islam, Muslims and their culture. He advocated that Christians in Muslim countries, without doing violence to their own faith or to Islam, incorporate as much of the Islamic culture and even spirituality as possible.

Lastly, Charles Levigerie (1825-1892), founder of the Missionaries of Africa, a later cardinal and archbishop of Carthage, and Henri Marchal (1875-1957), an assistant to Levigerie, developed a theology of encounter between Christians and Muslims which is rich in possibilities. Convinced that it is God who converts, they held that arguments, power, pressure—to say nothing of force—cannot truly convert the human heart. Marchal believed that arrogance—including the arrogance of religious supremacy—legalism, pressure and a sense of religious superiority render a person resistant to God's grace. Marchal developed a theology of threefold conversion: to God, to Jesus and to Christianity. Marchal sees these three as distinct and recognized that it was theoretically possible for a person to stop after the first or second conversion. This allowed Marchal to see the possibility for a Muslim to be in a salvific relationship to God and even to Jesus without formally becoming a Christian.

While the French were by no means the only Catholics to encounter Muslims, the personal experience of Foucauld and Massignon combined with the work—both pastoral and scholarly—of the Missionaries of Africa,[11] resulted in a distinct "French flavor" to the Catholic Muslim encounter by the time of Vatican II. The Pontifical Institute for the Study of Arabic and Islam (PISAI) has been a center for the study of Islam and encounter with Muslims. Founded in Tunisia in 1926 as a training center for Missionaries of Africa, the *Institut de Belles Lettres Arab* (IBLA) moved to Rome in 1964 and became the Pontifical Institute for the Study of Arabic and Islam.

From the very beginning the Catholic Muslim encounter was personal. While IBLA and PISAI are highly respected academic institutions, they were built on the foundation of interpersonal encounters between Muslims and (mostly) French Catholics.

III. Recent Muslim Outreach to Christians

There has also been significant outreach from the Muslim side. The publication of *A Common Word*[12] in 2007 is a very important milestone in the conversation between Christians and Muslims. It is very carefully addressed by name and title to Christian leaders and "leaders of Christian Churches everywhere."[13] I

---

11 Often referred to as the "White Fathers" in the past due to the color of their habit, the preferred name of the community is the Missionaries of Africa. They were founded in 1868 by Archbishop Lavigerie.

12 Cf. *A Common Word*, https://www.acommonword.com (accessed on 26 Mar. 2020).

13 Ibid.

have listed the recipients below to show the care that was taken in terms of the titles and protocols of the church leaders addressed. This is a change from a certain indifference in the past to the sometimes-embarrassing complexities of the Christian reality. It is also a sign of the seriousness with which the letter was composed.

While dealing with theological topics, the letter is not without very practical implications. In the closing paragraphs the Muslim leaders state:

> Finding common ground between Muslims and Christians is not simply a matter for polite ecumenical dialogue between selected religious leaders. Christianity and Islam are the largest and second largest religions in the world and in history. Christians and Muslims reportedly make up over a third and over a fifth of humanity respectively. Together they make up more than 55% of the world's population, making the relationship between these two religious communities the most important factor in contributing to meaningful peace around the world. If Muslims and Christians are not at peace, the world cannot be at peace. With the terrible weaponry of the modern world; with Muslims and Christians intertwined everywhere as never before, no side can unilaterally win a conflict between more than half of the world's inhabitants. Thus our common future is at stake. The very survival of the world itself is perhaps at stake.[14]

Recognizing that not all believers (on both sides) are open to and supportive of dialogue between Christians and Muslims, those who dissent—especially violently—are addressed directly:

> And to those who nevertheless relish conflict and destruction for their own sake or reckon that ultimately they stand to gain through them, we say that our very eternal souls are all also at stake if we fail to sincerely make every effort to make peace and come together in harmony.[15]

A Common Word is one of the most extraordinary and comprehensive statements to come out of the Muslim community in its attempt to deal and live with the Christian world.

The letter was originally signed by 138 Muslim scholars.[16] For someone familiar with Islam, the diversity of the signatories is nothing short of astounding.

---

14 *A Common Word*, https://www.acommonword.com/building-communities-across-faith-boundaries/ (accessed on 26 Mar. 2020).

15 Ibid., https://www.acommonword.com/the-acw-document/ (accessed on 26 Mar. 2020).

16 That number has increased considerably in the ensuing years.

If Muslims at times have shown an indifference to the historical and theological complexities of Christianity, Christians have responded with incredible ignorance to the complexity of Islam. Among the signatories are Sunnis and Shi'ites, Salafis and Sufis to name just four rather large groupings in Islam. These groups are generally not in conversation with each other and there is often (violent) hostility between them. The very fact that such an extremely divergent group of Muslims could come to get to sign this letter is alone historical.

On a personal note, I was disappointed with the Christian response. While Muslims who deeply disagree with each other on many, diverse theological topics were able to overcome—at least temporarily—those disagreements to address Christians, most Christian churches responded individually. For one magnificent moment Muslims were able to overcome their often deep divisions. We Christians were not, even though no doctrinal issues were involved.

IV. Methodologies of Theological Analysis and Religious Aesthetic

Here I get beyond my area of expertise and more into an area of feeling. Having been engaged in the ecumenical and interreligious movements for forty years and having studied at a German university, I find the roots of the Catholic-Muslim dialogue have a certain unique "flavor"—I like to use the word "aesthetic"—that is generally not found in other dialogues. I hesitate because I do not want my reflections here to be absolutized and made into mutually exclusive characteristics, to say nothing of caricatures. They are not. However, I think the differences, while extremely (overly?) subtle, are important and rich with possibilities.

If many dialogues are characterized by great respect, academic rigor and great depth of intellectual curiosity and understanding, the foundational encounters between Muslims and people like Foucauld, Massignon, Lavigerie, Marechal and Corbin[17] are characterized by a deep and obvious affection for Muslims and Islam. This is by no means to imply a lack of intellectual and academic rigor. It is, however, very much to underline that the Catholic-Muslim encounter experienced by all of these people was grounded in a deep and personal affection. In many, if not most instances, these people learned Islam not so much from books as from Muslim friends. These initial encounters may be of importance for the contemporary dialogue.

Traditionally the Catholic-Christian dialogues have been characterized by deep theological analysis. Differences are analyzed with the ultimate, if not always immediately possible, goal of overcoming them to achieve Christian unity. Much ecumenical work was done in German- and Dutch-speaking countries, and some of the leading voices for the ecumenical commitment of the Church in Vatican II

17 Henri Corbin (1903-1978) was a scholar of Islamic mysticism.

came from theologians from these countries.

While this approach proved very fruitful for the intra-Christian ecumenical dialogue, it has been less successful in the Catholic (Christian)-Muslim dialogue. There are many reasons for this, but the most important reason is that differences—especially deep differences—between Christians and Muslims simply cannot be overcome for the sake of some kind of unity. That is simply not possible. The intra-Christian and Catholic-Muslim dialogues have radically different goals and, I believe, require different methodologies and hermeneutics. At the risk of oversimplification I would describe the methodology of the intra-Christian ecumenical dialogue as "theological analysis" and the Christian-Muslim encounter of the French scholars mentioned above as "religious aesthetic." I do not intend these to be mutually exclusive but rather more as two different approaches to the different dialogues.

A milestone in the Catholic-Muslim dialogue was the publication of *Guidelines for Dialogue between Christians and Muslims.*[18] The *Guidelines* provide the theological underpinnings as well as practical advice for Catholics in dialogue with Muslims. There is a clear differentiation between ecumenical dialogue and interreligious dialogue. Ecumenical dialogue is between baptized Christians. It has for its goal Christian Unity, i.e., one church, according to the will of Christ. It is not clear in all details what that one church would be or how it would look but Christian unity—one church in full communion—is the goal of the ecumenical dialogue. The ecumenical dialogue produces convergence statements, agreements and expressions of growing unity.

None of this is the case in the dialogue with Islam or other non-Christian religions, and the *Guidelines* are very clear about this. With extraordinary honesty, the *Guidelines* recognize:

> [T]he meeting of a Muslim and a Christian . . . carries with it a certain sense of contradiction. Each of the two religions . . . considers itself to be universal in its overall plan of salvation. . . .
>
> Does one or the other party lack in honesty or sincerity if they try to carry on dialogue . . . while all the time they have such convictions in their hearts about the universality of their message? Of course not, especially if they believe that God Most High is sovereign even over the diversity of their respective communities, and that He will someday, in His good time, let them know why "they differed."[19]

---

18 See *Interreligious Documents I: Guidelines for Dialogue between Christians and Muslims*, ed. Maurice Borrmans (Mahwah, NJ: Paulist Press, 1981).

19 *Guidelines for Dialogue*, 41.

The difference between the ecumenical and interreligious encounters is clearly delineated. With the publication of the *Guidelines,* the Catholic Church clarified the purpose and methodology of the Catholic-Muslim dialogue and provided it with a possible trajectory. Whether the *Guidelines* were successful in this remains an open question.

In my experience, many Catholic-Muslim dialogues have, at least in the west, continued to follow a pattern set by the (intra-Christian) ecumenical movement. The dialogue partners spend a great deal of time studying and discussing points of contact between Christianity and Islam. In some cases, e.g., belief in one God who is self-revealing, the similarities are deep. In other cases, *e.g.* reverence for Jesus and Mary, the differences are greater than the surface similarities. However, once discussion on the similarities between Christianity and Islam are exhausted, the dialogue often withers. If the articulated or unarticulated goal of the dialogue is agreement, it ultimately hits the proverbial "wall" of irreconcilable difference.

This should surprise no one. Islam and Christianity are two different religions, each with its own irreducible particularity, which is to say, that they cannot be reconciled in such a way as to collapse one into the other. Where does a dialogue go once it reaches the point of recognizing irreconcilable differences between the partners? In the ecumenical dialogue this would present a major obstacle. This is not, however, the case in interreligious dialogue in general or the Catholic-Muslim dialogue in particular.

First, one should not be surprised by insurmountable differences. One should expect and, indeed, welcome them. The great French pioneers of the Catholic-Muslim encounter were neither surprised nor dismayed by the insurmountable differences between Islam and Christianity. In fact, they knew from the outset that these differences existed. What drove and motivated the encounter was not the need for agreement but rather a mutual affection. Awareness of the differences between the two religions allowed them to understand each other better, but the differences did not prove to be an obstacle to affection, friendship and—very importantly—cooperation.

Pope Francis has introduced a new element to dialogue at its highest level. It is does not replace or make other elements of dialogue obsolete. It is rather very personal and connected with Francis' own personality. The element that Francis adds fits very well with what I hint above is the "French or 'aesthetic' model for Catholic-Muslim dialogue." That element is friendship. This is unselfconsciously evident in many unmistakable ways. When, for example, Pope Francis meets with Bartholomew I, Patriarch of Constantinople, or with Sheikh Ahmad al-Tayyeb, Grand Imam of al-Azhar University, it is clearly a meeting of religious leaders. However, it is—once again unselfconsciously—evident that these are religious leaders who actually like each other and have trust and affection for each other.

Francis, Bartholomew and al-Tayyeb have shown that they can work together with full integrity and faithfulness to their own faith traditions in order to address problems facing humanity: climate change, religiously inspired hatred, persecution, asylum seekers and bigotry. Francis can do this as a Roman Catholic, Bartholomew as a Greek Orthodox Christian and al-Tayyeb as a Sunni Muslim. In their integrity and faithfulness each brings something unique and irreplaceable to solving the problems facing humanity.

For the Catholic-Muslim dialogue this means that after all the discussions about how we are alike, after the somewhat disappointing discovery that we may not be as alike as we thought, the dialogue has reached a new stage, not a conclusion to say nothing of a dead end. Built on respect, trust and affection for the other, the dialogue now leads us to a place where we can use our unique God-given differences to address the problems facing humanity.

I think this is of particular relevance to a convention of the Canon Law Society. Very often canon law is seen at best on the periphery of the Muslim-Catholic dialogue answering questions of whether one can or cannot do this or that. As a total outsider, I suspect that the code has very little specific to say about the Catholic-Muslim dialogue. However, that is beside the point to a great extent. Canon law, based on theology and the Word of God, is preeminently a pastoral—a practical—discipline. This very practical nature of canon law allows for an interaction with Muslims in attempting in order to deal with problems affecting society, etc. Canon law can provide flexible ways for fruitful cooperation between Muslims and Catholics in a pluralistic society and world. This does not involve the ever-popular "paradigm shift," regardless how impressive such might sound. Rather it involves a realization that both canon lawyers and Muslim *fuqahā*[20] are attempting to help the believer live in the modern world and, at the same time, be faithful to a complex and ancient tradition. The modern world has modified that a bit in that you are attempting to help believers (plural) live faithfully but *together* in a modern, pluralistic world with all its difficulties, challenges and dangers.

The joint declaration *A Document on Human Fraternity for World Peace and Living Together* issued by Pope Francis and Sheikh al-Tayyeb shows that both our communities have come a very long way since the conference in Tripoli in 1976. There is still a long way to go, but I think Francis and al-Tayyeb show us the possibility for a new—yet not so new—way forward in the Catholic-Muslim dialogue.

---

20 Plural of *faqih*, "jurisprudent" and sometimes "theologian," especially in the Sunni world.

Seminar

Conducting a Diocesan Synod in Service of Missionary Discipleship

The Most Reverend Thomas John Paprocki, JD, JCD

It is good to be with you at this 81st Annual Convention of the Canon Law Society of America to present this seminar on "Conducting a Diocesan Synod in Service of Missionary Discipleship." I speak with you not only as a fellow canon lawyer and a member of the CLSA since 1986, but also as a diocesan bishop who has recently conducted a diocesan synod. My plan in this seminar is to describe the lived pastoral experience of conducting a diocesan synod in the service of missionary discipleship in light of the pertinent canonical norms and instructions.

In 2017 I conducted a diocesan synod in the Diocese of Springfield in Illinois on the theme of promoting missionary discipleship and stewardship. We had been talking about discipleship and stewardship in our diocese for some time, and our conversations about promoting missionary discipleship and stewardship intensified in 2014 when my vicar general, then-Monsignor Carl Kemme, was named bishop of Wichita. The Diocese of Wichita is well-known for its dedication to discipleship and stewardship, so we set out to learn from them and have continued to learn much from them on these themes in the past five years.

In conversations with my presbyteral council, diocesan pastoral council and with focus groups that we established around the diocese to discuss the concepts of missionary discipleship and stewardship, we reached a point where people wanted to take the next step of committing ourselves to the discipleship and stewardship way of life. But I knew that making a corporate and communal commitment to be a discipleship and stewardship diocese would require more than a decree from me as diocesan bishop. It would require a grassroots commitment from the clergy and the people in the pews in order to take root, grow, and flourish. It seemed to me that a diocesan synod would be the best way to go about having a broad consultation on these themes across the diocese.

This would be our fourth diocesan synod for the Diocese of Springfield in Illinois. The previous diocesan synods were held in 1889 (when our diocese was based in Alton), 1953 and 1963. (Note that canon 356 of the 1917 Code of Canon Law had set ten years as the maximum interval between diocesan synods.) Since it had been more than half a century since our previous diocesan synod, you

might say that we were long overdue to have another one!

What is a diocesan synod?

The Code of Canon Law provides nine canons (cc. 460-468) on the diocesan synod (see Appendix One for the text of these canons).[1]

Canon 460 defines a diocesan synod as a group of selected priests and other Christian faithful of a particular diocese which meets to offer assistance to the diocesan bishop for the good of the entire diocesan community. The word *synod* simply means *meeting* in Greek. Of course, meetings take place all the time in a diocese, but a diocesan synod is a special type of meeting convoking a sizeable number of people who advise the diocesan bishop in setting the direction for the pastoral ministry of the parishes and other components of the diocese itself for the next several years.

Canon 461 of the 1983 Code of Canon Law provides for a diocesan synod to be held "when circumstances warrant it in the judgment of the diocesan bishop, after he has consulted the presbyteral council." When I consulted on September 10, 2016, with the diocesan pastoral council, which includes two lay representatives from each of the seven deaneries of the diocese, and on September 12, 2016, with our presbyteral council, which represents the priests of the diocese, both of these councils enthusiastically recommended that I convoke a diocesan synod.

Canon 462 provides that only the diocesan bishop convokes the diocesan synod, not however one who presides over a diocese *ad interim*. The diocesan bishop presides over the diocesan synod; he can, however, delegate the vicar general or an episcopal vicar to fulfill this office for individual sessions of the synod.

Canon 463 indicates the persons who are to be called to the diocesan synod as its members and are obliged to participate in it. Some of these are specified, while others can be called as members to the diocesan synod by the diocesan bishop. I will discuss the membership in our diocesan synod later in this presentation.

Canon 464 stipulates that a member of the synod who is hindered by a legitimate impediment cannot send a proxy to attend in his or her name; such a member is to inform the diocesan bishop of this impediment. This question did arise in our synod.

Canon 465 provides that all the proposed questions are to be subject to the free discussion of the members during the sessions of the synod.

---

1 Unless otherwise noted, all canons quoted are from the *Code of Canon Law, Latin-English Edition* (Washington, DC: Canon Law Society of America, 2012)

Canon 466 states that the diocesan bishop is the sole legislator at a diocesan synod while the remaining members of the synod possess only a consultative vote; he alone signs the synodal declarations and decrees which can be published only through his authority.

Canon 467 indicates that the diocesan bishop is to communicate the texts of the synodal declarations and decrees to the metropolitan and to the conference of bishops.

Canon 468 allows for the diocesan bishop to suspend or dissolve a diocesan synod in accord with his own prudent judgment. If the episcopal see should become vacant or impeded, a diocesan synod is interrupted by the law itself until the succeeding diocesan bishop has decreed that it is to continue or that it is terminated.

Instruction on Diocesan Synods

In 1997, the Congregation for Bishops and the Congregation for the Evangelization of Peoples issued an *Instruction on Diocesan Synods*.[2] While the canons offer a general schema for a diocesan synod, the 1997 instruction offers more concrete assistance in how a synod is held, what is to be addressed, and who is a part of it.

The *Instruction on Diocesan Synods* describes a preparatory phase and the actual conducting of the synod, which consists properly of the synodal sessions. The preparatory phase is to consist of: (1) spiritual, catechetical and formational preparation; (2) diocesan consultation of the faithful; and (3) determining the questions (see *Instruction* III.C.2). The *Instruction* also states that "an equilibrium should be maintained between the period of preparation for the Synod and its celebration. The synodal sessions should be arranged over a period of time so as to permit sufficient time to study the questions raised during the sessions, as well as to make interventions during the discussions" (*Instruction* IV.2).

Preparatory Commission

According to the *Instruction on Diocesan Synods*, the bishop is obliged to constitute a preparatory commission:

> The members of this preparatory commission are chosen by the Bishop from amongst the clergy and other faithful who are distinguished by their pastoral prudence and by their professional competence and who,

2 See Congregation for Bishops and the Congregation for the Evangelization of Peoples, instruction *Instruction on Diocesan Synods*, March 19, 1997, http://www.vatican.va/roman_curia/congregations/cbishops/documents/rc_con_cbishops_doc_20041118_diocesan-synods-1997_en.html (accessed on 27 Mar. 2020).

> in so far as possible, reflect the various charisms and ministries of the People of God. Some members should be expert in the disciplines of Canon Law and Sacred Liturgy.[3]

Its tasks are principally to assist the bishop in matters pertaining to the organization and preparation of the synod; in drawing up and publishing the synodal directory; in the designation of the synodal members and in his determining the questions to be proposed for synodal deliberation. The diocesan bishop presides over the meetings of the preparatory commission.

In the fall of 2016, I appointed the following persons as the members of the preparatory commission:

Reverend Monsignor David J. Hoefler, V.G., Moderator
Reverend Christopher A. House, Secretary of the Synod
Reverend Daren Zehnle, Master of Ceremonies
Reverend Kevin M. Laughery, Notary of Synod
Reverend R. Dean Probst, Procurator for the Clergy
Reverend Charles "Chuck" Edwards,
Director of Stewardship and Discipleship
Reverend Brian C. Alford, Director for Vocational Services
Mr. Michael Christie, Chairman, Diocesan Pastoral Council
Mr. Zach Wichmann, Member of Diocesan Pastoral Council
Mrs. Marlene Mulford,
Director for Communication and Information Services
Mrs. Christine Malmevik, Director for Catechesis
Mrs. Brandi Borries, Superintendent of Catholic Schools
Mr. John Maxwell, Director for Financial Services
Mr. Shaun Riedell, Director for Development

Directory for the Fourth Diocesan Synod

In looking at the *acta* from our previous diocesan synods, it appeared that the official gathering of the synod took place in one day within a liturgical rite held in our cathedral. Apparently, all the preparatory work was done in advance, with the actual convocation of the diocesan synod taking place as the occasion for the official ratification and approval of the diocesan statutes.

I also looked at the experience of other dioceses which had recently conducted diocesan synods, and in most cases the official meetings of their diocesan synods took place over one weekend.

Discussing this with the preparatory commission, the presbyteral council, and the diocesan pastoral council, we decided to conduct our fourth diocesan

---

3 *Instruction on Diocesan Synods*, III.B.1.

synod over the course of the calendar year of 2017. On December 29, 2016, I issued a decree in accord with canon 461 §1, convoking The Fourth Synod of the Diocese of Springfield in Illinois to take place in 2017. I also published a *Directory for the Fourth Diocesan Synod*, which described: (1) the nature and purpose of a diocesan synod; (2) the convocation and timeline of the diocesan synod; (3) the membership of the diocesan synod; (4) the officers of the synod; (5) the preparatory commission; (6) determining the questions; and (7) rules of procedure for the synod.

Timeline for the Fourth Diocesan Synod

The general timeline started with an opening ceremony on January 22. Throughout 2017 committees drafted the synodal directory, the questions for discussion and proposed synodal declarations, decrees and statutes. There were listening sessions in the deaneries and parishes, as well as opportunities for people to offer feedback online through our diocesan website. The solemn closing of the synod took place on November 26, 2017. The timeline for the various events associated with our fourth diocesan synod was as follows:

- Sunday, January 22, 2:00 PM – Prayer Service for the Opening of the Preliminary Phase of the Diocesan Synod (at the Cathedral of the Immaculate Conception in Springfield)

- Sunday, April 2, 2:00 PM – Diocesan Synod Deanery Prayer and Listening Sessions in each Deanery with the Bishop connected by video conference to hear the needs, desires and opinions of the faithful regarding the proposed synodal topics

- Tuesday April 11, 6:30 PM – Chrism Mass with Official Opening of the Diocesan Synod (at Cathedral)

- Saturday, May 20, 10:00-2:00 – First Session of the Official Members of the Diocesan Synod (at Cathedral Atrium)

- Saturday, August 12 – Gathering of Permanent Deacons for prayer and discussion regarding the Diocesan Synod (at Cathedral)

- Saturday, August 19 – Synodal Consultation with Consecrated Religious (at Chiara Center, Springfield)

- Saturday, September 9 – Second Session of the Official Members of the Diocesan Synod (at Little Flower Parish Center, Springfield)

- Monday, September 18 to Thursday, September 21 – Convocation of Priests for prayer and discussion regarding the Diocesan Synod (at Pere

Marquette Lodge, Grafton, Illinois)

- Sunday, September 24, 2:00 PM – Diocesan Synod Deanery Prayer and Listening Sessions in each Deanery with the Bishop connected by video conference to receive feedback on proposed synodal declarations and decrees

- Wednesday, October 11, 2017 – Consultation with the Diocesan Curia

- Saturday, November 18, 10:00-2:00 – Final Session of the Official Members of the Diocesan Synod to vote on synodal declarations, decrees and statutes (at St. Joseph the Worker Parish, Chatham)

- Sunday, November 26, 2:00 PM – Mass Closing the Diocesan Synod on the Solemnity of Christ the King (at Cathedral)

Prayer for the Fourth Synod of the Diocese of Springfield in Illinois

In anticipation of the synod, the preparatory commission wrote a *Prayer for the Fourth Diocesan Synod*, which we used for all of the sessions of the synod:

> O God, who never forsake your people and ever journey with them
> through the struggles and joys of daily life,
> stir up the flame of faith in the hearts of your sons and daughters
> in our Diocese of Springfield in Illinois.
> Help us to experience anew your great love for us
> and fill us with a greater desire to love and serve you and our neighbor.
>
> Throughout this time of our fourth diocesan synod,
> help us, by the light of the Holy Spirit,
> to discern the needs of our local Church
> and better follow Christ your Son as intentional disciples.
> Open our hearts and minds to know your will,
> to speak the truth with love, and to hear each other,
> that together we might plan, with the help of your grace,
> for the strengthening and growth of our diocese.
>
> May Mary, the Immaculate Conception,
> first and greatest of all disciples, lead us closer to your Son.
> May she accompany us as we follow the call
> to live as his disciples and as generous stewards of your many gifts.

Through Christ our Lord. Amen.[4]

Questions for the Preliminary Phase of the Synod

The Synod Preparatory Commission developed a series of questions inviting people to reflect on the meaning of discipleship in their lives, namely, that being a disciple is to have entered into a personal relationship with Jesus Christ. At the diocesan synod deanery prayer and listening sessions in each deanery, the following questions were presented for table discussion in each of the deaneries, with a person designated to give a summary of their discussion by video conference.

1. SPRINGFIELD DEANERY: Describe your relationship with Jesus Christ.

- What does it look like?
- How did it come about?
- How can you start/deepen your relationship?

2. LITCHFIELD DEANERY: When Jesus asks, how do you answer these questions?

- "Who do you say that I am?" Mt. 16:13-20
- "Do you love me?" Jn. 21:16-17
- "Do you love me more than these?" Jn. 21:15 What are the "these" in my life that compete with my love of Jesus Christ?
- "What do you want me to do for you? (Bartimaeus)" Mk. 10:46-52

3. ALTON DEANERY: So - "Is he the one or are you looking for someone else?" (Like the question that came from John the Baptist) Mt. 11: 1-6

4. JACKSONVILLE DEANERY: "Ignorance of the Scriptures is ignorance of Christ." (St. Jerome and as referenced in the Catechism of the Catholic Church, par. 133) What does this quote say to you?

5. EFFINGHAM DEANERY: How do/can the sacraments help you in your relationship with Jesus Christ?

6. DECATUR DEANERY: Is your heart grateful? "Ten were healed, were they not? Where are the other nine?" Lk. 17:11-19

---

4 "Prayer for the Fourth Synod of the Diocese of Springfield in Illinois," *Acts, Declarations and Statutes of the Fourth Synod of the Diocese of Springfield in Illinois* (2017) 3, https://diospringfield.cld.bz/FourthSynodCompiledActsDeclarationsandStatutes/2/ (accessed on 27 Mar. 2020).

- How can/do you show gratitude to Jesus for your relationship and all He has done? Psalm 116

7. QUINCY DEANERY: What does stewardship mean to you?

A spokesperson for each deanery presented a summary of the answers to these questions to me and to the other participants in the deanery meetings by video conference call. A written compilation of the answers was also given to me for my review and for our records.

Membership of the Diocesan Synod

Some of the members of the diocesan synod are designated by canon 463 §1 of the Code of Canon Law, such as the vicar general, the judicial vicar, the deans, the presbyteral council, the diocesan pastoral council and representatives of consecrated religious. Canon 463 §2 provides that others can be called as members to the diocesan synod by the diocesan bishop; these can be clerics, members of institutes of consecrated life, or lay members of the Christian faithful. I decided in consultation with our preparatory commission for the diocesan synod that each parish pastoral council of our 129 parishes would select one parishioner with the approval of the pastor or parochial administrator to represent the parish as an official member of the diocesan synod.

Each of the members of the diocesan synod received a decree of appointment with a cover letter from me. In my cover letter, I wrote:

> The various elements of the Diocesan Synod will take place over the next several months, culminating in the official closing of the Synod on the Solemnity of Christ the King on Sunday, November 26th. In particular, you are asked to be present for all formal sessions of the synod to be celebrated on May 20th and November 18th, 2017, at the Cathedral of the Immaculate Conception in Springfield, as well as any other sessions that may still be determined, unless legitimately impeded, in which case you are asked to inform me of the nature of the impediment preventing you from being present.
>
> The Diocesan Synod will set the direction and tone for the pastoral ministry of the parishes and other components of the diocese itself for the next several years, if not decades, to come. In order to build a vibrant community of intentional and dedicated missionary disciples of the Risen Lord and steadfast stewards of God's creation who seek to become saints, I plan to ask the Fourth Diocesan Synod of the Diocese of Springfield in Illinois to discuss how the community of Catholic faithful in this diocese can be committed to the discipleship and stewardship way of life as commanded by Christ Our Savior and as revealed by

Sacred Scripture and Tradition.

The full text of all the synodal documentation for the Fourth Diocesan Synod of the Diocese of Springfield in Illinois is available at the Diocese's website at www.dio.org/synod/.

Mandate for the Fourth Diocesan Synod

The mandate that I established for our diocesan synod was to consider how we could make a communal commitment as a diocesan community of clergy and laity regarding discipleship and stewardship as a way of life. Specifically, I said that this would include looking at the biblical concept of tithing and defining what that means for us as a diocese in terms of stewardship of our time, talent and treasure. Closely related to this was for us to look at how we could foster community-wide support of Catholic education so that more students would be able to attend Catholic schools. This involves understanding Catholic education as being the responsibility for everyone in each parish as a means to hand on the faith to the next generation of Catholics, not just the financial burden of parents to pay for their children's education.

Since one of the outcomes of a diocesan synod is particular legislation for the diocese per canon 466, we set out to update our diocesan statutes, which may be understood as a basic constitution that officially guides the policies, procedures and practices of the diocese, the parishes and other entities of the diocese, with a special focus on how to live discipleship and stewardship as a way of life for the faithful of our diocese.

My main hope for our diocesan synod was that our clergy and laity together with me would make a heartfelt commitment to stewardship and discipleship as a way of life. We would need to overcome our doubts and fears in order to succeed in this endeavor. In the end, what makes this so important is that it is all about our future as a Church: whether we will diminish or grow as a community of faith. I said it was my fervent prayer that it will be the latter, showering our diocese with abundant blessings of unprecedented growth.

Official Opening of the Fourth Diocesan Synod

Our fourth diocesan synod was officially opened in the context of our Chrism Mass at the cathedral on April 11. One of the original reasons for scheduling the official opening of the synod in conjunction with the Chrism Mass was that the Chrism Mass is an occasion when most of our priests are present along with representatives of each of the parishes of the diocese. But as I was preparing my homily for this Chrism Mass, it became clear to me in the course of my prayer that there is an important spiritual connection between the Chrism Mass and the theme of our Synod being focused on promoting discipleship and stewardship.

If we consider the symbolism of the oils that are blessed and consecrated at the Chrism Mass, we can gain a greater appreciation for their relationship to the discipleship and stewardship way of life.

At the Chrism Mass in the cathedral of every diocese around the world during Holy Week, the diocesan bishop blesses or consecrates three kinds of oils: the Oil of the Sick, used in the sacrament of the anointing of the sick; the Oil of Catechumens, used to anoint those preparing to be baptized; and the Sacred Chrism, used to consecrate altars and church buildings and to consecrate people in the sacraments of baptism, confirmation and holy orders.

The symbolism of oil is not as apparent in our modern context in Western culture as it used to be in the past, so some words of explanation may be helpful. In the countries of the Orient and in southern Europe, olive oil has always been a staple of daily life, much more than with Americans. It enters into the preparation of food; it is used as a remedy, internally and externally; in past centuries it was the chief means of furnishing light, being burned in lamps; it was employed in ancient times by the athletes of the Olympic games, to give flexibility to their muscles. Hence, we see the various symbolic meanings employed by the Church when she uses it to give us spiritual nourishment, to cure our spiritual ailments, to spread the light of grace in our souls, and to render us strong and active in the never-ending conflict with the Spirit of Evil. The use of oil to express the imparting of spiritual strength is so appropriate that the Church employs it not only for the anointing of people, but also for altars and church buildings which are to be used to assist in the sanctification of the people of God.

All of these anointings are pertinent to the themes of discipleship and stewardship of our diocesan synod, as we would be praying for God to strengthen us with His Holy Spirit to become more dedicated disciples of our Risen Lord and more steadfast stewards of His creation.

Conducting the Actual Sessions of the Fourth Diocesan Synod

The fourth diocesan synod spanned most of the calendar year of 2017. On Sunday, January 22, we held the Prayer Service for the Opening of the Preliminary Phase of the Diocesan Synod at our cathedral in Springfield. Following our listening session on April 2 in each Deanery connected by video conference to hear the needs, desires and opinions of the faithful regarding the proposed synodal topics, the official opening of the Fourth Diocesan Synod took place in the context of the Chrism Mass at the cathedral on Tuesday of Holy Week, April 11.

The first session of the members of the Diocesan Synod took place on Saturday, May 20, in the cathedral atrium. The members of the Synod included those specified by canon law, such as the members of the Presbyteral Council,

the Deans and the leaders of religious communities serving in our diocese, as well as one appointed delegate from each of our 129 parishes, for a total of over 200 Synod Members. At this first meeting we discussed a working draft of the proposed Synodal Declarations, addressing the question of how we as a diocese could be committed to discipleship and stewardship as a way of life.

During the summer and early autumn, I conducted a number of listening sessions about our synodal topics, during which I consulted with our permanent deacons and their wives, consecrated religious women and men, as well as the priests of our diocese during our convocation of priests.

The second session of the members of the synod took place on September 9, during which a first draft of synodal statutes was proposed and discussed along with the synodal declarations.

On Sunday, September 24, we held our second listening session in each deanery connected by video conference to receive feedback on the revised synodal declarations.

Following the suggestions and modifications made by the members of the Synod, as well as those offered by the priests, deacons, consecrated religious and lay Christian faithful through the various consultations over the past several months, I revised the proposed diocesan synodal declarations and statutes in light of the feedback that I received. In the end there were 12 synodal declarations and 172 statutes in the final version of the synodal statutes, reflecting the valuable input received in the process of consultation.

Synod members offered amendments to the synodal declarations and synodal statutes prior to voting on them at the final session of the fourth diocesan synod, which took place on Saturday, November 18th, at St. Joseph the Worker Parish in Chatham. All of the synodal declarations and synodal statutes were overwhelmingly approved by the synod members, who voted using electronic voting devices.

The synodal declarations state the main themes setting the direction of the diocese with regard to discipleship and stewardship for the foreseeable future, which I projected to be at least for the next ten years. The synodal statutes cover a greater breadth of the life of the Church in our diocese consistent with the synodal declarations. Policies and procedures will fill out the details later. The starting point for the 2017 fourth diocesan synodal statutes was the 1963 third diocesan synodal statutes, to provide for continuity in the ecclesial life of our diocese while updating them to reflect changes since the Second Vatican Council and the commitment of this fourth diocesan synod to the discipleship and stewardship way of life. The twelve synodal declarations should be seen as progressing organically and cohesively from our diocesan, individual and

parochial commitments to discipleship and stewardship.

Voting Regarding Synodal Declarations and Statutes

The process of drafting the Declarations and Statutes of the Fourth Diocesan Synod started with updating the Statutes of the Third Diocesan Synod (1963) and incorporated modifications proposed in various consultations with clergy and laity. At the final session of the fourth diocesan synod, on November 18, 2017, some amendments were accepted as "friendly" and others were voted upon by the synod members. Then each synodal declaration was voted on separately and the Synodal Statutes were voted upon as a whole. The vote for each of the 12 synodal declarations is given below. Following the outline of the books of the Code of Canon Law, 172 statutes were approved by a vote of 161 Yes, 17 No, and 5 abstentions.

Summary of the 12 Declarations of the Fourth Diocesan Synod (see Appendix Two)

- Declaration 1 articulates a new mission statement for our diocese, stating that "the community of Catholic faithful in this diocese is committed to the discipleship and stewardship way of life" and to implementing the four pillars of discipleship and stewardship: hospitality, prayer, formation, and service. (Vote: Yes 183, No 2, Abstained 3)
- Declaration 2 calls for all pastoral initiatives to be set in relation to holiness and for our diocese to invite people to a life of discipleship and stewardship. (Vote: Yes 181, No 5, Abstained 0)
- Declaration 3, from my Second Pastoral Letter, calls for a culture of growth in the Church that starts with inviting people to experience the love of Jesus Christ (Vote: Yes 181, No 3, Abstained 1)
- Declaration 4 defines Catholic discipleship for an individual person as a committed approach to living a Christian life within the Catholic Church, having accepted Jesus Christ as one's Lord and Savior. (Vote: Yes 173, No 8, Abstained 6)
- Declarations 5 provides that formation for discipleship and stewardship as a way of life shall be the primary focus of the catechetical programs for all ages. (Vote: Yes 178, No 5, Abstained 2)
- Declaration 6 provides that the Sacraments of Christian Initiation shall be offered in the proper sequence (Baptism, Confirmation and Eucharist) for children as well as for adults. Children are to receive the Sacraments of Confirmation and Eucharist at about the age of reason, which in this Diocese will normally be in their third grade of

elementary school, as a way to promote discipleship and stewardship as a way of life from an early age. (Yes 147, No 35, Abstained 5)

- Declaration 7 addresses the issue of scholarships as a way for the entire Christian community to fulfill its responsibility to transmit the faith to the next generations. (Vote: Yes 166, No 16, Abstained 5)
- Declaration 8, from my First Pastoral Letter, describes the art of celebrating the liturgy properly and adoring the Lord in the Eucharist devoutly as a necessary step to inviting people to the ecclesial experience of discipleship and stewardship. (Vote: Yes 180, No 6, Abstained 1)
- Declaration 9 is the theme of my Third Pastoral Letter, which is a post-synodal pastoral exhortation, addressing how living as a Christian is a step toward the goal of everlasting happiness in eternal life. (Yes 183, No 1, Abstained 2)
- Declaration 10 indicates that those committed to discipleship and stewardship pledge to share their talents, give of their time and contribute proportionately from their financial resources for the good of the Church and those in need. (Vote: Yes 177, No 9, Abstained 0)
- Declaration 11 is a call to fulfill the Biblical command to tithe by donating the suggested amount of at least 8% of their income to their parishes and 2% to other charities as an expression of their gratitude to God and of their stewardship of His manifold gifts of creation. (Vote: Yes 147, No 34, Abstained 6)
- Declaration 12 addresses parish tithing as a replacement for the Annual Catholic Services Appeal and physically taking up second collections. (Vote: Yes 147, No 36, Abstained 4)

Official Closing of the Fourth Diocesan Synod

Our fourth diocesan synod was officially closed with the celebration of the Holy Sacrifice of the Mass at our Cathedral of the Immaculate Conception in Springfield on November 26, 2017, the Solemnity of Christ the King. During the liturgy I formally accepted the synodal declarations and statutes by signing a "Decree Promulgating the Declarations and Statutes of the Fourth Diocesan Synod of the Diocese of Springfield in Illinois" as well as a "Decree to Close the Fourth Synod of the Diocese of Springfield in Illinois." After the Post-Communion Prayer, we gave praise to God for the graces received at our fourth diocesan synod by singing the *Te Deum*.

Promulgation of the *Acts, Declarations and Statutes of the Fourth Diocesan Synod*

All of the synodal documentation was compiled and promulgated as the *Acts, Declarations and Statutes of the Fourth Diocesan Synod*, published online on our diocesan website. A version in "pdf" format is posted at:

https://www.dio.org/uploads/files/2017_Synod/FourthSynodCompiled ActsDeclarationsandStatuteswebversion.pdf.

A version in "Flipping Book" format is posted at:

https://diospringfield.cld.bz/FourthSynodCompiledActsDeclarationsandStatutes.

Hardcopy commemorative editions of the *Acts, Declarations and Statutes of the Fourth Diocesan Synod* were printed in bound book format and were sent to all parishes, priests, deacons, seminarians, staff of the diocesan curia, and to each of the members of the synod. As provided by canon 467, copies of the commemorative edition of the *Acts, Declarations and Statutes of the Fourth Diocesan Synod* were mailed to the Metropolitan Archbishop of the Province of Chicago and to the President of the United States Conference of Catholic Bishops. A copy of the commemorative edition was also sent to the Apostolic Nuncio to the United States of America in Washington, D.C. The instruction also calls for a copy to be sent either to the Congregation for Bishops or to the Congregation for the Evangelization of Peoples.

Post-Synodal Pastoral Letter

To help implement our diocesan synod, I wrote a post-synodal pastoral letter entitled, *Ars vivendi et moriendi in Dei gratia* ("The Art of Living and Dying in God's Grace"), available online with my two previous pastoral letters at https://www.dio.org/bishop/pastoral-letters.html.

In January 2019, I posted a letter to all of the cardinals, archbishops and bishops of the United States on the USCCB website for bishops with links to the online versions of the *Acts, Declarations and Statutes of the Fourth Diocesan Synod* as well as my pastoral letters.

Conclusion

In conclusion, my hope is that this seminar will prove to be helpful to those of you as canonical advisors whose diocesan bishops may be considering whether to conduct a diocesan synod. The threshold question, of course, is whether to conduct a diocesan synod. If the decision is made to have a diocesan synod, you must decide the most opportune time to do so.

In my opinion, it would have been helpful for the revised Code of Canon Law to have kept at least a recommended time period for conducting a diocesan synod. The current criterion of canon 461, "when circumstances warrant it in the judgment of the diocesan bishop, after he has consulted the presbyteral council," unfortunately translates to the default time frame being "infrequently" due to the force of basic inertia. Of course, the previous time frame of "every ten years" as set by the 1917 code apparently was not assiduously observed, as can be seen in the fact that no diocesan synod was held in our diocese from the promulgation of the 1917 code until 1953. Only once in our diocese's history was the 10-year period observed, when Bishop William O'Connor convoked a diocesan synod in 1963, ten years after the previous synod in 1953. Despite the fact that the revised Code of Canon Law was not promulgated until twenty years later in 1983, it is understandable that diocesan synods took a back seat to the Second Vatican Council (1962-1965), as particular churches needed to comprehend and implement the changes brought about in the universal Church by an ecumenical council. Now that more than half a century has passed since the close of the Second Vatican Council, it seems that a number of diocesan bishops are finding it opportune to conduct diocesan synods for their local churches.

In my own experience, I did not call for a diocesan synod immediately after my installation as Bishop of Springfield in Illinois on June 22, 2010. I found it helpful over the first five years as diocesan bishop to visit each of the 129 parishes in my diocese, as stipulated by canon 396. While a diocesan synod may be a useful way for a diocesan bishop to begin his tenure in a diocese, in my own experience I found it more helpful to visit each parish first and form my own impressions about the needs of the diocese before embarking on a diocesan synod. Knowing something about the diocese helped me to formulate the issues and the questions that would need to be addressed at the synod.

After finishing my pastoral visitations of all our parishes in 2015, we began earnestly discussing the idea of a diocesan synod. In the summer of 2017, during the year of our Fourth Diocesan Synod, I celebrated my 65th birthday, which meant that I had ten more years before I would be expected to submit my letter of resignation, per canon 401. As such, I told people that our Fourth Synod of the Diocese of Springfield in Illinois would set the direction and tone for the remainder of my time as diocesan bishop and that it would be up to my successor to call the next diocesan synod!

In sum, I would say that the experience of conducting a diocesan synod was a highly helpful way to do a broad-based consultation with the clergy, consecrated religious and laity of the diocese in order to embark on a diocesan-wide initiative such as making a communal commitment to the discipleship and stewardship way of life. Time will tell if the seeds planted in this process will bear fruit in the years to come.

APPENDIX ONE

The Code of Canon Law provides nine canons (cc. 460-468) on the diocesan synod:

Canon 460 A diocesan synod is a group of selected priests and other Christian faithful of a particular church which offers assistance to the diocesan bishop for the good of the entire diocesan com-munity according to the norm of the following canons.

Canon 461 §1. A diocesan synod is to be celebrated in each of the particular churches when cir-cumstances warrant it in the judgment of the diocesan bishop, after he has consulted the presbyteral council.

Canon 462 §1. Only the diocesan bishop convokes the diocesan synod, not however one who presides over a diocese ad interim.

§2. The diocesan bishop presides over the diocesan synod; he can, however, delegate the vicar general or an episcopal vicar to ful¬fill this office for individual sessions of the synod.

Canon 463 §1. The following persons are to be called to the diocesan synod as its members and are obliged to participate in it:

1º the coadjutor bishop and the auxiliary bishops;

2º the vicars general, the episcopal vicars and the judicial vicar;

3º the canons of the cathedral church;

4º the members of the presbyteral council;

5º lay members of the Christian faithful and members of institutes of consecrated life, to be selected by the pastoral council in a manner and number to be determined by the diocesan bishop or, where such a council does not exist, in a manner determined by the diocesan bishop;

6º the rector of the diocesan major seminary;

7º the vicars forane (deans);

8º at least one presbyter to be selected from each vicariate forane by all who have the care of souls there; also to be selected is another presbyter who would take the place of the first one selected if he were impeded;

9º some superiors of the religious institutes and societies of apostolic life which have a house in the diocese, to be selected in a manner and num¬ber determined by the diocesan bishop.

§2. Others can be called as members to the diocesan synod by the diocesan bishop; these can be clerics, members of institutes of consecrated life, or lay members of the Christian faithful.

§3. If he should judge it opportune, the diocesan bishop can invite as observers to the diocesan synod some ministers or members of churches or ecclesial communities which are not in full communion with the Catholic Church.

Canon 464 A member of the synod who is hindered by a legitimate impediment cannot send a proxy to attend in his or her name; such a member is to inform the diocesan bishop of this impediment.

Canon 465 All the proposed questions are to be subject to the free discussion of the members during the sessions of the synod.

Canon 466 The diocesan bishop is the sole legislator at a diocesan synod while the remaining members of the synod possess only a consultative vote; he alone signs the synodal declarations and decrees which can be published only through his authority.

Canon 467 The diocesan bishop is to communicate the texts of the synodal declarations and de-crees to the metropolitan and to the conference of bishops.

Canon 468 §1. It is within the competence of the diocesan bishop to suspend or dissolve a diocesan synod in accord with his own prudent judgment.

§2. If the episcopal see should become vacant or impeded, a diocesan synod is interrupted by the law itself until the succeeding diocesan bishop has decreed that it is to continue or that it is terminated.

APPENDIX TWO

Diocese of Springfield in Illinois
2017 SYNODAL DECLARATIONS

The Synodal Declarations adopted by the Fourth Diocesan Synod of the Diocese of Springfield in Illinois are as follows:

1. Statute n. 1:

a. The mission of the Roman Catholic Diocese of Springfield in Illinois is to build a fervent community of intentional and dedicated missionary disciples of the Risen Lord and steadfast stewards of God's creation who seek to become saints. Accordingly, the community of Catholic faithful in this diocese is committed to the discipleship and stewardship way of life as commanded by Christ Our Savior and as revealed by Sacred Scripture and Tradition.

b. To further this mission, the Diocese of Springfield in Illinois is committed to implementing the Four Pillars of Discipleship and Stewardship, namely:

i. Hospitality – to invite people proactively to join us in prayer, especially Sunday Mass;

ii. Prayer – to provide well-prepared celebrations of the sacraments and other occasions for prayer as signs of hope and paths of grace to heaven;

iii. Formation – to study the Bible and learn more about Jesus and our Catholic faith; and

iv. Service – to serve each other, especially those in need, by practicing charity and justice.

2. Statute n. 2: In the Diocese of Springfield in Illinois, "all pastoral initiatives must be set in relation to holiness"[5] and will invite people to a life of discipleship and stewardship.

3. Statute n. 3: "The art of growing in God's grace is the key to growth in the Church. Building a culture of growth in the Church starts with inviting people to experience the love of Jesus Christ. . . . This growth looks not only to build up the number of followers of Jesus Christ, but also – and more importantly – for Christ's followers to grow in the depth of their relationship with Jesus Christ and

5 "Nihil dubitamus ante omnia adfirmare visionem rerum illam, in qua collocari debet totum pastorale iter, esse sanctitatem." John Paul II, apostolic letter *Novo Millennio Ineunte* 30, January 6, 2001: *AAS* 93 (2001) 287.

in their commitment to observe all that he has commanded us to do."[6]

4. Statute n. 4: To be a disciple means to accept Jesus Christ as one's Lord and Savior.[7] Disciples are those who "make a conscious, firm decision, carried out in action, to be followers of Jesus Christ no matter the cost to themselves."[8] Catholic discipleship refers to a committed approach to living a Christian life within the Catholic Church.

5. Statute n. 64: Formation for discipleship and stewardship as a way of life shall be the primary focus of the catechetical programs in our Catholic parochial schools, high schools and parish schools of religion, as well as our faith formation programs for youth, adults and those with special needs, with sacramental preparation seen as a step in this process, but not the end of the process. Being a practicing Catholic must be taught as a way of life. Thus, religious education is a personal obligation that does not end with the reception of the sacraments, but continues into adulthood.

6. Statute n. 80: The Sacraments of Christian Initiation shall be offered in the proper sequence (Baptism, Confirmation and Eucharist) for children as well as for adults. To promote discipleship and stewardship as a way of life from an early age, those who are baptized as infants are to receive the Sacraments of Confirmation and Eucharist at about the age of reason, which in this diocese will normally be in their third grade of elementary school, after they have been properly prepared and have made sacramental confession.[9]

7. Statute n. 67: As a means of fulfilling the responsibility of all the Christian faithful (not just parents) to hand on the Catholic faith to the next generation and in order that cost not be a barrier for children to receive a Catholic education, our parishes and schools through the use of scholarships (public and/or private) shall help pay tuition to make Catholic education available in Catholic grade schools, high schools and parish schools of religion (K-12) for all children of their parishes whose parents agree to the terms of the Family School Agreement.

8. Statute n. 79: "The art of celebrating the liturgy properly and adoring the Lord in the Eucharist devoutly (*ars celebrandi et adorandi*) is the key to fostering

---

6 Thomas J. Paprocki, second pastoral letter *Ars Crescendi in Dei Gratia* 1, September 14, 2015, https://www.dio.org/bishop/pastoral-letters/ars-crescendi-in-dei-gratia.html (accessed on 27 Mar. 2020).

7 Cf. John 3:16; Acts 2:38, 4:12; Romans 10:9, 13.

8 United States Conference of Catholic Bishops, *Stewardship: A Disciple's Response* (Washington, DC: United States Conference of Catholic Bishops, 1992).

9 Cf. cc. 891 and 914 and the complementary norm of the United States Conference of Catholic Bishops.

the active participation of the People of God in divine worship."[10] The clergy of the Diocese of Springfield in Illinois "must consider the celebration of the liturgy as their principal duty."[11]

9. Statute n. 134: The art of dying in God's grace is the key to everlasting happiness in eternal life. The Christian faithful die to sin through the saving waters of baptism. By dying to their selfish desires through acts of mortification and self-sacrifice, the Christian faithful grow in love of God and neighbor. The whole Christian life aims at reaching this goal of everlasting happiness in eternal life by turning from sin and growing in virtue through God's grace.

10. Statute n. 143: As a diocese committed to discipleship and stewardship, the community of Catholic faithful recognizes that everything we have comes from God and that He has given us gifts not just to use them for ourselves but also to share them with others. As faithful and generous stewards of God's abundant gifts, those committed to discipleship and stewardship as a way of life pledge to share their talents, give of their time and contribute proportionately from their financial resources for the good of the Church and those in need.

11. Statute n. 144: Trusting in God's providence and giving according to their means, the Catholic faithful of the Diocese of Springfield in Illinois are called to live as disciples of Our Lord Jesus Christ by giving of their time and talent and striving to fulfill the Biblical command to tithe by donating the suggested amount of at least 8% of their income to their parishes and 2% to other charities as an expression of their gratitude to God and of their stewardship of His manifold gifts of creation.

12. Statute n. 145:

a. Each parish is a member of the Diocese and of the universal Catholic Church. As such, each parish has an obligation to contribute to the operational expenses of the Diocese and the Apostolic See. Following the Biblical model of tithing, parishes shall tithe approximately 10% of their designated annual income to the diocese, which shall be used to fund the operations of the Diocesan Curia, payment of assessments to the Catholic Conference of Illinois and the United States Conference of Catholic Bishops, financial contributions to the Apostolic See in accord with canon 1271, and donations to national and international collections.

---

10 Thomas J. Paprocki, first pastoral letter *Ars Celebrandi et Adorandi* 1, June 22, 2014, https://www.dio.org/bishop/pastoral-letters/ars-celebrandi-et-adorandi.html (accessed on 27 Mar. 2020).

11 ". . . celebrationem considerent veluti praecipuum munus." Benedict XVI, post-synodal exhortation *Sacramentum Caritatis* 39, March 13, 2007: *AAS* 99 (2007) 136.

b. Parish tithing will replace the Annual Catholic Services Appeal and regularly-scheduled second collections. Parishioners who wish to make additional donations to the scheduled diocesan, national and international collections may still do so by placing the envelope with their designated donation in the regular collection. Special second collections will be taken in support of the Annual Missionary Plan of Cooperation and may still be taken up from time to time to assist victims of natural disasters and other extraordinary causes.

c. The Diocesan Bishop shall appoint a committee, whose purpose is, in consultation with the Diocesan Finance Council and Presbyteral Council, and subject to the approval of the Diocesan Bishop, to define what constitutes the annual parish income for the determination of a formula to calculate the amount that is subject to the approximate 10% tithe.[12] Such process should take into consideration the goals of the diocese to build up the Body of Christ, to support Catholic formation and education, and to recognize the differences in parishes (e.g., those with an abundance of material wealth and those without, those that operate parish schools and those that do not). Such formula should attempt to be fair and just to all, while at the same time provide adequate financial resources to the diocese, so that the diocese can accomplish its intended mission.

---

12 Cf. c. 1263.

Officer's Report

Report of the President

Dr. Zabrina R. Decker, JCD

What a year this has been! I am convinced that the hand of God is always supporting us in all challenges and this year has produced proof. We have had many challenges but the Board of Governors that was together this year had the perfect combination of strengths to address them all and move the Society forward. They were a true blessing! I want to recognize those members leaving the Board at the conclusion of the Atlantic City convention: Monsignor John Foster, Past President, Sr. Nancy Reynolds, Treasurer; and Father John Donovan and Ms. Susan Mulheron, Consultors.

Our challenges and blessings began immediately after last year's convention in hiring a new Executive Coordinator for the Society. We were blessed to find Donna Miller. She brings so many gifts to the position! Her skills with webinars have renewed this initiative. She also brings skills as a civil lawyer. Donna and Father Patrick Cooney, the incoming chair of the Publications Advisory Board are working together to move the publications of the Society forward. This includes a reprint of the code! She has been tireless in her research of e-publication as we look to new/multiple formats for the printing of the code and other publications.

Yes, the challenges and blessings extend to the website! There is no doubt that we have moved forward exponentially with the implementation of the new site. As with any new technological endeavor, there are going to be bumps along the road. We had some drop-offs! Having acknowledged that, Colleen Crawford and Megan Boland, our gifted General Secretary and Administrative Assistant, were able to work both with the design team and our members to smooth out the path. Our site is both working and a work in progress. It will be complete and will offer real value to our members.

The finances of the Society show a recovery this year. Sister Nancy Reynolds will present her final Treasurer report on a positive note. This has come about through the careful financial stewardship of the Board of Governors. As President, I suggested a postponement of the Presidential visit to Rome. There is no doubt regarding the importance of the relationship between the Society and the Roman dicasteries but, after consultation with the Board, it was determined that we could take a break this year. Instead, some of the money was used to provide much needed updates to the hardware at the office in Washington DC. This included

new laptop computers for the staff. These laptops with docking stations make us more mobile and provide telecommuting options while retaining the power of a desktop.

The Society sponsored two open-houses for the canon law students and faculty from the Washington DC area and The Catholic University of America. Both in February and July, over 30 students and faculty stopped by the offices for lunch, conversation and publication discounts. Over 20 became members! Monsignor Foster and I were present for both and had a great time meeting and greeting while Colleen and Megan were busily assisting with publication sales and membership.

Also in July, at the offices of the Society, there was a meeting of the minds over publications. I met with Jay Conzemius, our Vice-President, Donna Miller, our Executive Coordinator, Colleen Crawford, our General Secretary, Sr. Sharon Euart, the current Chair of the Publications

Advisory Board and Fr. Patrick Cooney, the incoming Chair to share the history of the PAB (special thanks to Sr. Sharon), coordinate information on publications and gather new ideas. This was a valuable and successful effort! My personal thanks to all who participated.

Speaking of publications, a reprint of the code is very close to completion. Monsignor Bruce Miller, a Past-President of the Society has been instrumental in forming a committee of talented canonists to steer the reprint. He has also been working with Donna Miller to bring this to fruition.

Another publication update of great import is that Father John Beal has agreed to take charge and begin the process of developing a new commentary on the code. This project is in its nascent stages but will be very exciting to follow as it develops!

I did continue the tradition of travel to the School of Canon Law at St. Paul University in Ottawa, Canada. In May, I prayed and celebrated with those who were graduating, spoke to the students about the Society, welcomed more new members and gave a Presidential address that reflected on the sex abuse crisis and the canonical ability of the laity to assist in addressing the issue. Monsignor John Renken, the Dean of the School of Canon Law and Dr. Chad Glendinning, a consultor on the Board of Governors were very welcoming and Father Frank Morrisey extended the warm hospitality for which he is well-known.

The committees of the Society are doing great work! For example, the Clergy Committee is working on a project with the USCCB Committee on Canonical Affairs and Church Governance and the Laity Committee has almost completed the outline for a new canonist mentoring program. As a Board, we reached out to

new Society members to get them involved in the work of the Society and many were able to accept our invitation. We are always looking for committee member suggestions. Please sign-up or suggest a member.

The most recent challenge of my Presidential year came on September 9, 2019. Colleen Crawford, our General Secretary, submitted her resignation. This was a sad day for the Board, the Society and for me personally. Colleen has been a font of knowledge and the epitome of professionalism for the Society. She has moved on to a position that will further extend her potential. I know that I speak for all of us when I say that we wish her all the best.

The blessing that came from this challenge is that Megan Boland, our Administrative Assistant at the offices of the Society, pursued the position, interviewed with a committee from the Board of Governors and proved to be a stellar candidate. I am happy to announce that Megan has accepted the position of General Secretary. She brings practical Society experience, a love of the Church and a lot of energy. Welcome Megan!!

As I complete my presidential year, I call to mind what Paul wrote in his first letter to the Corinthians: "I give thanks to God always for you because of the grace of God which was given you in Christ Jesus, that in every way you were enriched in him with all speech and all knowledge – even as the testimony of Christ was confirmed among you – so that you are not lacking in any spiritual gift, as you wait for the revealing of our Lord Jesus Christ; who will sustain you to the end, guiltless in the day of our Lord Jesus Christ." May we be blessed as we further the work of The Canon Law Society of America!

Officer's Report

Report of the Treasurer

Sr. Nancy Reynolds, SP, JCL

As I come to the end of my third year as Treasurer of the Canon Law Society of America, I am happy to report on the 2018-2019 budget and present to you the 2019-2020 budget of the Society.

We have experienced three very stressful years financially. We were in the red for the past two budget years, 2016-2017 and 2017-2018. In the most recent fiscal year, 2018-2019, the bottom line continues to show the Society in the red as the Board of Governors and Resource and Asset Management Committee continue to search for ways to pull the Society out of this deficit. Our total income for the year was $583,281 and our total expenses were $595,967, showing a loss of $12,686 at the completion of the budget year. At least the deficit is getting to be less and less as we work on a solution.

It is always very difficult to make the budget for any convention. That budget is dependent on many items: how many people attend, if the state gives us tax exemption, convention hotel, audiovisual expenses, etc. For the 2018 convention in Phoenix, we lost $7,860, but came in under budget on the convention hotel and on audiovisual expenses. Also, the contract commission brought in $19,342.05. That piece of income is thanks to Nix Conference and Meeting Management. Per their contract with us, Nix gives the money earned on sleeping room commission to us.

The scholarship donations this past year were $11,410 and the money given for scholarships was $23,599.93. We are most appreciative of the members of the Society for their generosity in donating to the scholarship funds. The licentiate fund balance is very close to the fund balance for operations. The scholarship funds are separate from the operating budget. They should not be reported in the operating budget for the Society. I will ask that the new treasurer will present a separate financial report for the two scholarship funds from now on. Their income, expenses and investment gains or losses should be reported in a separate financial report. We have reported those numbers in the financial report for 2018-2019, but I will ask that they be removed from the proposed budget and given their own separate report.

Also, I want to point out to you that we had $7,906.46 in miscellaneous

income, which has come as part of the first distribution of the Reverend Msgr. Thomas J. Green estate. We are told that there will be an additional gift to the CLSA at the final distribution of his estate. Msgr. Green loved the Society and was such as integral part of its conventions and its work for many years. We are most grateful to Tom. He did not restrict his gift, so the BOG will consider where the gift will best serve us in his memory.

We continue to have difficulty reaching our goal for membership dues every year. Many members have seen a change in how they are funded to attend the annual convention. There are dwindling diocesan budgets due to a number of factors and thus, many are not funded by their arch/dioceses anymore and simply cannot afford it every year. We have a number of members reaching retirement age and more and more arch/dioceses filing bankruptcy. We also have had some concerns about member retention affected by the website and I assure you that is a matter of constant concern and dialogue for the General Secretary and the Board of Governors. The Board is also focused on making membership truly worthwhile. The Resource and Asset Management Committee and the Research and Development Committee are focused on analyzing more statistics to help inform budgeting and fiscal policies for the future, in conjunction with the Board.

You will note that our publications income was up this year. We budgeted $52,000 and ended just $2,153.82 short. We had new publications this year and are eagerly anticipating the publication of the third printing of the Code of Canon Law. Our new Executive Coordinator, Donna Miller, has told us that she is close to completing the work on that printing. We have been doing short runs of the second printing and selling them for the list price for bookstores and seminaries. Our third printing will show greater disparity between unit cost and list price to help the Society's bottom line.

I have certainly enjoyed my three years as your Treasurer and I am very happy to present the report for the past fiscal year. I wish the new Treasurer blessings on the work he will do in the coming three years. As I age and fade into the sunset, I know that I have grown in my canonical self by being a member of the Canon Law Society of America and serving as your Treasurer.

CUIT Quarterly Balances, Year Ending 6/30/19

	General Operations Investment Fund Balance	Licentiate Scholarship Investment Fund Balance	Doctoral Scholarship Investment Fund Balance
6/30/2016	$773,041.48	$658,694.29	$53,329.79
9/30/2016	$809,456.81	$689,723.11	$55,841.99
12/31/2016	$843,851.76	$719,030.35	$58,214.82
3/31/2017	$870,332.69	$741,594.29	$60,041.63
6/30/2017	$883,659.21	$752,949.61	$60,960.97
9/30/2017	$910,890.23	$776,152.60	$62,839.56
12/31/2017	$954,193.96	$813,050.86	$65,826.93
3/31/2018	$945,873.03	$805,960.72	$65,252.93
6/30/2018	$930,131.57	$818,120.56	$66,237.41
9/30/2018	$962,844.17	$846,893.70	$68,566.98
12/31/2018	$906,816.48	$797,613.13	$63,222.30
3/31/2019	$940,359.18	$864,243.76	$69,971.66
6/30/2019	$907,880.84	$881,066.54	$72,470.65

CANON LAW SOCIETY OF AMERICA

Financial Statements and Independent Accountant's Review Report

For the Year Ended June 30, 2019

LSWG

CERTIFIED PUBLIC ACCOUNTANTS & BUSINESS ADVISORS

Lintin Shafer Warfield & Garrett, P.A.
1803 Research Boulevard, Suite 404 •
Rockville, Maryland 20850-6118 •
301-738-8400 • FAX 301-417-4190
ROCKVILLE FREDERICK
www.lswgc pa.com

Independent Accountant's Review Report

To the Board of Governors of
Canon Law Society of America
Washington, DC

We have reviewed the accompanying financial statements of Canon Law Society of America (a nonprofit organization), which comprise the statement of financial position as of June 30, 2019, and the related statements of activities and changes in net assets, functional expenses and cash flows for the year then ended, and the related notes to the financial statements. A review includes primarily applying analytical procedures to management's financial data and making inquiries of management. A review is substantially less in scope than an audit, the objective of which is the expression of an opinion regarding the financial statements as a whole. Accordingly, we do not express such an opinion.

Management's Responsibility for the Financial Statements

Management is responsible for the preparation and fair presentation of these financial statements in accordance with accounting principles generally accepted in the United States of America; this includes the design, implementation, and maintenance of internal control relevant to the preparation and fair presentation of financial statements that are free from material misstatement whether due to fraud or error.

Accountant's Responsibility

Our responsibility is to conduct the review engagement in accordance with Statements on Standards for Accounting and Review Services promulgated by the Accounting and Review Services Committee of the AICPA. Those standards require us to perform procedures to obtain limited assurance as a basis for reporting whether we are aware of any material modifications that should be made to the financial statements for them to be in accordance with accounting principles generally accepted in the United States of America. We believe that the results of our procedures provide a reasonable basis for our conclusion.

Accountant's Conclusion

Based on our review, we are not aware of any material modifications that should be made to the accompanying financial statements in order for them to be in accordance with accounting principles generally accepted in the United States of America.

Lintin Shafer Warfield & Garrett, P.A.

Rockville, Maryland
February 5, 2020

CANON LAW SOCIETY OF AMERICA
Statement of Financial Position
June 30, 2019

Assets

Current Assets		
Cash and cash equivalents	$	11,624
Accounts receivable		248
Inventory		40,603
Prepaid expenses		31,764
Total Current Assets		84,239
Furniture and Equipment - at cost		
Furniture and equipment		46,491
Less: accumulated depreciation	(23,999)	
Furniture and Equipment, Net	22,492	
Other Assets		
Security deposit		2,094
Investments		907,881
Investment - scholarship fund		953,538
Total Other Assets		1,863,513
Total Assets		$1,970,244

Liabilities and Net Assets

Current Liabilities		
Accounts payable	$	11,089
Accrued wages		1,459
Deferred revenue		6,167
Total Current Liabilities		18,715
Total Liabilities		18,715
Net Assets		
Without donor restrictions		
Undesignated		
1,036,868		
Board designated - publications		(29,206)
Total Unrestricted		1,007,662
With donor restrictions		943,867
Total Net Assets		1,951,529
Total Liabilities and Net Assets	$	1,970,244

CANON LAW SOCIETY OF AMERICA
Statement of Activities and Changes in Net Assets
For the Year Ended June 30, 2019

	Without Donor Restriction			With Donor	
	Undesignated	Publications	Total	Restrictions	Total
Revenue					
Membership dues	$249,498	$-	$249,498	$ -	$249,498
Convention and workshops	187,691		187,691		187,691
Sale of publications		49,846	49,846		49,846
Contributions				11,409	11,409
Interest and dividends	5,929		5,929	5,642	11,571
Royalties		4,448	4,448		4,448
Unrealized gain on investments	77,962		77,962	77,195	155,157
Other income	10,534		10,534		10,534
Net assets released from restrictions	31,177		31,177	(31,177)	
Total Revenue	562,791	54,294	617,085	63,069	680,154
Expenses					
Program Services					
Publications		98,329	98,329		98,329
Convention and workshops	262,873		262,873		262,873
Membership outreach	52,319		52,319		52,319
Scholarship fund	31,177		31,177		31,177
Total Program Services	346,369	98,329	444,698		444,698
Supporting Services	185,938		185,938		185,938
Total Expenses	532,307	98,329	630,636		630,636
Changes in Net Assets	30,484	(44,035)	(13,551)	63,069	49,518
Net Assets - Beginning of Year	1,006,384	14,829	1,021,213	880,798	1,902,011
Net Assets - End of Year	$1,036,868	$(29,206)	$1,007,662	$943,867	$1,951,529

The accompanying notes are an integral part of this statement.

CANON LAW SOCIETY OF AMERICA
Statement of Functional Expenses
For the Year Ended June 30, 2019

	Program				Supporting	
	Publications	Convention and Workshops	Member Services	Scholarship Fund	General and Administrative	Total
Cost of publications sold	$ 26,669	$ -	$ -	$ -	$ -	$ 26,669
Publication expenses	2,935	-	-	-	-	2,935
Royalty expense	1,272	-	-	-	-	1,272
BrightKey	43,796	-	-	-	-	43,796
Coordination	-	131,658	-	-	-	131,658
Honoraria	-	16,131	-	-	-	16,131
Printing	-	2,677	-	-	-	2,677
Program materials	-	5,376	-	-	-	5,376
Audio visual	-	26,800	-	-	-	26,800
Liturgy	-	3,596	-	-	-	3,596
Other	-	2,840	-	-	-	2,840
Postage	-	889	-	-	-	889
Supplies	-	5,802	-	-	-	5,802
Travel	-	1,731	-	-	-	1,731
Convention planning committee	-	4,071	-	-	-	4,071
Membership outreach	-	-	229	-	-	229
Constitutional	-	-	833	-	-	833
Standing	-	-	203	-	-	203
Other	-	-	641	-	-	641
Scholarships paid	-	-	-	22,486	-	22,486
Scholarships expenses	-	-	-	1,113	-	1,113
Lodging	-	-	-	-	22,690	22,690
Travel	-	-	-	-	9,161	9,161
Other expenses	-	-	-	-	1,454	1,454
Officer expenses	-	-	-	-	7,763	7,763
Executive Coordinator office	23,657	61,302	50,413	7,578	112,076	255,026
Depreciation expense	-	-	-	-	5,289	5,289
Rent expense	-	-	-	-	27,505	27,505
	$ 98,329	$ 262,873	$ 52,319	$ 31,177	$ 185,938	$ 630,636

The accompanying notes are an integral part of this statement.

CANON LAW SOCIETY OF AMERICA
Statement of Cash Flows
For the Year Ended June 30, 2019

Increase (Decrease) in Cash and Cash Equivalents		
Cash Flows from Operating Activities		
Changes in Net Assets	$	49,518
Adjustments to reconcile changes in net assets to net cash provided by (used in) operating activities:		
Depreciation		5,289
Unrealized (gain) on investments		(155,157)
Change in assets and liabilities:		
Accounts receivable		(248)
Inventory		5,517
Prepaid expenses		(15,175)
Accounts payable		4,582
Accrued wages		513
Deferred revenue		(21,508)
Net Cash Used in Operating Activities		
Cash Flows from Investing Activities		(126,669)
Purchase of investments		(1,827,420)
Proceeds from sale of investments		1,935,648
Net Cash Provided by Investing Activities		108,228
(Decrease) in Cash and Cash Equivalents		(18,441)
Cash Balance - Beginning of Year		30,065
Cash Balance - End of Year	$	11,624
Supplemental Disclosures:		
Income taxes paid	$	
Interest paid	$	

The accompanying notes are an integral part of this statement.

CANON LAW SOCIETY OF AMERICA
Notes to Financial Statements
For the Year Ended June 30, 2019

1. Nature of Activities

The Canon Law Society of America (CLSA) is a national, not-for-profit corporation, established in November 1939 in Washington DC to promote canonical and pastoral approaches to significant issues within the Roman Catholic Church. In addition to a publication service, CLSA conducts an annual convention and other symposia to promote a better understanding of church law and its pastoral applications. Major sources of revenue include: membership dues, sales of publications and annual convention and workshops.

2. Basis of Financial Statement Presentation

The accompanying financial statements are presented on the accrual basis of accounting, whereby revenue is recognized when earned and expenses when they are incurred.

CLSA adopted Financial Accounting Standards Board (FASB) Codification Standards. Under the Codification Standards, the Organization is required to report information regarding its financial position and activities according to two classes of net assets:

Net Assets Without Donor Restrictions - Net assets that are not subject to or are no longer subject to donor-imposed stipulations.

Net Assets with Donor Restrictions - Net assets whose use is limited by donor imposed time and/or purpose restrictions.

Revenues are reported as increases in net assets without donor restrictions unless use of the related assets is limited by donor-imposed restrictions. Expenses are reported as decreases in net assets without donor restriction. Gains and losses on investments and other asset or liabilities are reported as increases or decreases in net assets without donor restrictions unless their use is restricted by explicit donor stipulation or by law. Expirations of donor restrictions on the net assets (i.e. the donor-stipulated purpose has been fulfilled and/or the stipulated time period has elapsed) are reported as reclassifications between the applicable classes of net assets

3. Summary of Significant Accounting Policies

Cash and Cash Equivalents -For purposes of the statement of cash flows, CLSA considers all cash accounts and all highly liquid debt instruments purchased with an initial maturity of three months or less to be cash and cash equivalents.

Investments - Investments in marketable securities with readily determinable fair values are reported at their fair values in the statement of financial position. Investment income or loss (including gains and losses on investments, interest and dividends) is included in the statement of activities and changes in net assets as an increase or decrease in net assets without donor restrictions unless the income or loss is restricted by donor or law. Investments consist principally of two mutual funds. Fair value of investments in securities is based on the latest reported sales price at June 30, 2019.

Canon Law Society of America
Notes to Financial Statements
For the Year Ended June 30, 2019

3. Summary of Significant Accounting Policies (Continued)

Accounts Receivable - Accounts receivable are stated at the amount management expects to collect from outstanding balances. The provision for uncollectible accounts is based on management's evaluation of the collectability of accounts receivable. CLSA considers accounts receivable to be fully collectible; accordingly, no provision for doubtful accounts is required. Books and publication receivables are considered uncollectible if not collected within 90 days after the sale.

Inventory -The inventory of books and publications is valued at cost, on the first-in, first out method.

Property and Equipment - Purchases of furniture and equipment are recorded at cost. CLSA's policy is to capitalize expenditures for equipment purchased in the amount of $1,000 or more. Depreciation is calculated over an estimated useful life of five to ten years using the straight-line method. Depreciation and amortization for the year ended June 30, 2019 totaled $5,289.

Tax Status - CLSA is exempt from federal income tax under Section 50l(c)(3) of the Internal Revenue Code. CLSA has not been classified by the Internal Revenue Service as a private foundation. Income which is not related to the exempt purpose, less applicable deductions, is subject to Federal and state corporate income tax. CLSA is covered under a group religious exemption and is not required to file Form 990.

Estimates - In preparing financial statements in conformity with U.S. generally accepted accounting principles, management is required to make estimates and assumptions that affect the reported amounts of assets and liabilities, the disclosure of contingent assets and liabilities at the date of the financial statements, and the reported amounts of revenues and expenses during the reporting period. Actual results could differ from those estimates.

Financial Instruments - CLSA's financial instruments consist of investments, accounts receivable, accounts payable and accrued expenses. It is management's opinion the CLSA is not exposed to significant interest rate or credit risk arising from these instruments. Unless otherwise noted, the fair values of these financial instruments are market values of these financial instruments, and approximate their carrying values.

Revenue Recognition - Contributions are recognized when the donor makes a promise to give to CLSA that is, in substance, unconditional. Contributions received are recorded as with or without donor restrictions depending on the absence or existence and nature of any donor restrictions.

Revenues from membership dues are recognized pro-rata (on a straight-line basis) over the membership period which corresponds with CLSA' s fiscal year end. Convention and workshop registrations are recognized as revenue without donor restrictions at the point in time the meeting or program is held.

Canon Law Society of America
Notes to Financial Statements
For the Year Ended June 30, 2019

3. Summary of Significant Accounting Policies (Continued)

Membership dues, convention and workshop revenues received in advance are deferred and recognized as revenue in the subsequent year.

For revenue streams involving multiple performance obligations, the transaction (i.e. Selling) price is allocated based on relative standalone selling prices of the goods or services. If a standalone selling price is not directly observable, it is estimated using an expected cost plus margin approach.

Recently Issued Accounting Standards - In 2016, the Financial Accounting Standards Board (FASB) issued Accounting Standards Update (ASU) No. 2016-14, *Presentation of Financial Statements for Not-for-Profit Entities.* Canon Law Society of America adopted the provisions of this new standard during the year ended June 30, 2019. In addition to changes in terminology used to describe categories of net assets throughout the financial statements, new disclosures were added regarding liquidity and the availability of resources (Note 12), and disclosures related to functional allocation of expenses were expanded (Note 4).

4. Functional Allocation of Expenses

Directly identifiable expenses are charged to programs and supporting services. Executive Coordinator office expenses have been allocated among the programs and supporting services benefited based on estimated time and effort.

5. Fair Value Measurement and Investments

Financial Accounting Standards Board (FASB) Codification Standards defines fair value, establishes a framework for measuring fair value, and expands disclosures about fair value measurements and establishes a hierarchy for valuation inputs.

Fair value is the price that would be received to sell an asset or paid to transfer a liability in an orderly transaction between market participants at the measurement date. A fair value measurement assumes that the transaction to sell the asset or transfer the liability occurs in the principal market for the asset or liability or, in the absence of a principal market, the most advantageous market. Valuation techniques that are consistent with the market, income or cost approach are used to measure fair value.

The fair value hierarchy prioritizes the inputs to valuation techniques used to measure fair value into three broad levels:

- Level 1 - inputs are based upon unadjusted quoted prices for identical instruments traded in active markets.

5. Fair Value Measurement and Investments (continued)

- Level 2 - inputs are based upon quoted prices for similar instruments in active markets, quoted prices for identical or similar instruments in markets that are not active, and model-based valuation techniques for which all significant assumptions are observable in the market or can be corroborated by observable market data for substantially the full term of the assets or liabilities.
- Level 3 - inputs are generally unobservable and typically reflect management's estimates of assumptions that market participants would use in pricing the asset or liability. The fair values are therefore determined using model-based techniques that include option pricing models, discounted cash flow models, and similar techniques.

Investments in mutual funds at June 30, 2019, which are all considered level 1, consist of the following:

	Cost	Market
Mutual funds	$ 1,715,813	$ 1,861,419

By fund type at June 30, 2019:

	Cost	Market
Without donor restrictions	$834,816	$ 907,881
With donor restrictions	880,997	953,538
Total Investments	$ 1,715,813	$1,861,419

CLSA invests in a professionally managed portfolio that contains mutual funds. Such investments are exposed to various risks such as interest rates, market and credit. Due to the level of risk associated with such investments and the level of uncertainty related to changes in the value of such investments, it is at least reasonably possible that changes in risks in the near term would materially affect investment balances and the amounts reported in the financial statements.

Investment income, which is included in the statement of activities and changes in net assets for the year ended June 30, 2019 is comprised of the following:

	Without Donor Restrictions	With DonorRestrictions	Total
Net unrealized gain	$ 77,962	$ 77,195	$ 155,157
Interest and dividends	5,929	5,642	11,571
Net Investment Income	$ 83,891	$ 82,837	$ 166,728

Canon Law Society of America
Notes to Financial Statements
For the Year Ended June 30, 2019

6. Concentration of Credit Risk

CLSA maintains its cash and cash equivalents in bank deposit accounts, which at times, may exceed federally insured limits. CLSA has not experienced any losses in such accounts and believes it is not exposed to any significant financial risk on cash and cash equivalents.

7. Commitments

Office Lease

In December 2015, CLSA entered into a ten-year lease for office space. Monthly rent payments are $2,289 and increase 3% annually. Rent expense for the year ended June 30, 2019 is $27,505.

Minimum future rental obligations for the next five years by fiscal year are: 2020 - $27,944; 2021 - $28,782; 2022 - $29,646; 2023 - $30,535; 2024 - $31,451.

8. Board Designated Funds

The Board has designated that net income from the sale of publications and books be set aside for use only in the publication activities. As reported on the statement of activities and changes in net assets, the net assets from publications decreased in fiscal year 2019 by $44,035 to ($29,206).

9. Net Assets with Donor Restrictions

The activity in net assets with donor restrictions for fiscal year 2019 is as follows:

	Scholarship Fund	Doctorial Scholarship	Total
Balance June 30, 2018	$811,741	$69,057	$ 880,798
Income	13,033	4,018	17,051
Expenses	(28,273)	(2,904)	(31,177)
Unrealized gain on investments	71,384	5,811	77,195
Balance June 30, 2019	$867,885	$75,982	$943,867

10. Annual Meeting Site Reservation Agreements

CLSA has reserved hotel space for future annual meetings. The terms of these reservation agreements provide that a fee will be assessed to CSLA if the reservation is canceled due to site change, within a specified period prior to the meeting dates.

Canon Law Society of America
Notes to Financial Statements
For the Year Ended June 30, 2019

11. Executive Coordinator Agreement

CLSA has an agreement with the Executive Coordinator beginning August 1, 2017 and ending July 31, 2020, unless renewed or terminated. Subsequent to year-end, the Executive Coordinator resigned from the position.

During the year ended June 30, 2019, a new Executive Coordinator was hired, agreement beginning May 1, 2019 and ending April 30, 2022, unless renewed or terminated. In the event that the agreement is terminated without cause, CLSA has agreed to pay severance at the lesser of the Executive Coordinator salary for the remaining term of the agreement or four months.

12. Liquidity and Availability of Financial Assets

The following table reflects the CLSA's financial assets as of June 30, 2019, reduced by amounts not available for general expenditures within one year. Financial assets are considered unavailable, illiquid or not convertible to cash within one year, trust assets, assets held for others, perpetual endowments and accumulated earnings net of appropriations within one year, or because the governing board has set aside the funds for a specific contingency reserve or a long term investment as board designated endowments. These board designations could be drawn upon if the board approves that action.

Financial assets:		
Cash and cash equivalents	$	11,624
Accounts receivable		248
Investments		907,881
Investments - scholarship fund		953,538
Financial assets, at year-end:		1,873,291
Less those unavailable for general expenditure within one year, due to:		
Donor restrictions		943,867
Financial assets available to meet cash needs for general expenses within one year	$	929,424

The CLSA has a policy to structure its financial assets to be available as its general expenditures, liabilities and other obligations come due.

13. Subsequent Events

Management has evaluated subsequent events through February 5, 2020, the date that the financial statements were available to be issued. There were no significant events to report.

Supplementary Information

CANON SOCIETY LAW OF AMERICA
2019-2020 BUDGET

		BUDGET approved 7/1/18-6/30/19	ACTUAL 7/1/17-6/30/18	ACTUAL 7/1/18-6/30/19	BUDGET 7/1/19-6/30/20
INCOME					
4100	**STEWARDSHIP**				
4110	**Membership Dues**				
4111	Dues - New Members	8,000	3,000	2,325	3,000
4112	Annual Memberships	260,000	237,100	246,673	240,000
4120	**Donations**				
4121	Membership Contributions	0	0	0	0
4122	General Donations	0	0	0	0
4130	**Scholarship Contributions** *(Fundraising Income)*				
4131	Licentiate Scholarship	7,500	8,847	7,814	7,500
4132	Doctoral Scholarship	2,500	2,626	3,597	2,500
	Transfer: Designated Sch. Funds (BOG approved for awards)	32,200			17,200
	Transfer: 5% Quarterly Rolling Average of General Operations	41,708			43,968
4140	**Investment Income**				
4141	Interest & Dividend Income for General Ops (Ending 001)		13,486	5,929	8,000
4142	Interest & Dividend Income for Licentiate Scholarship (Ending 002)		11,322	5,215	8,000
4143	Interest & Dividend Income for Doctoral Scholarship (Ending 003)		916	422	500
4144	Interest & Dividend Income for Scholarship (TD Bank)		566	5	0
4150	Realized Gains/Loss		0	0	0
4160	Unrealized Gains/Loss for General Ops (Ending 001)		63,210	77,962	0
4161	Unrealized Gains/Loss for Licentiate Scholarship (Ending 002)		53,849	71,384	0
4162	Unrealized Gains/Loss for Doctoral Scholarship (Ending 003)		4,360	5,811	0
4300	**MEMBERSHIP DEVELOPMENT**				
4310	**Annual Conference - Membership Meeting**				
4311	Exhibit/Advertising	2,400	650	2,050	2,400
4312	Banquet Fees (Additional)	480	480	350	560
4313	Convention Registration	140,000	140,925	140,450	157,500
4314	W1. Pre-Convention Fees	11,550	9,725	8,388	12,600
4315	W2. Pre-Convention Fees	11,550	14,075	17,413	12,600
4316	1 Day Registration	500	375	200	500
4317	Sponsorship Donations	0	200		0
4318	Contract Commission	13,000	17,255	19,342	17,000

CANON SOCIETY LAW OF AMERICA
2019-2020 BUDGET

Code	Item	BUDGET approved 7/1/18-6/30/19	ACTUAL 7/1/17-6/30/18	ACTUAL 7/1/18-6/30/19	BUDGET 7/1/19-6/30/20
4400	**PRODUCT DEVELOPMENT**				
4410	**Publication and Resources**				
4411	Sales	52,000	45,253	49,846	50,000
4412	Reprint Permissions	0	0		0
4413	Product Partnership Royalties	5,500	6,712	4,448	5,500
4414	Shipping and Handling Fees (BrightKey)	10,000	0		10,000
4415	Miscellaneous Income	0	2,690	7,906	0
4416	Administrative Fees from Publications	N/A	0	0	N/A
TOTAL INCOME		598,888	566,608	583,281	580,828
EXPENSES					
5100	**STEWARDSHIP EXP**				
5110	**Annual Donation Distribution**				
5111	Donation	0	0	0	0
5120	**Scholarships**				
5121	Licentitate Scholarship Awards	30,000	22,500	20,288	25,000
5122	Doctoral Scholarship Awards	2,200	1,154	2,198	2,200
5123	Other Scholarship Expenses	800	0	1,113	800
5200	**PROFESSIONAL DEVELOPMENT**				
5220	**Partnerships**				
5223	Networking (Rome/Australia Trip)	11,000	9,988	0	11,000
5300	**MEMBERSHIP DEVELOPMENT**				
5310	Membership Outreach (Regional Meetings)	5,000	1,067	229	5,000
5320	**Annual Convention - Membership Meeting**				
5321	Exhibit/Advertising Exp.	0	0	0	0
5322	Hotel, Food Events	98,000	121,979	79,320	83,000
5323	Audio Visual	30,000	34,125	26,800	30,000
5324	Convention Supplies	5,000	7,020	5,802	4,500
5325	Convention Travel	4,500	1,352	1,731	11,500
5326	Convention Telecommunications	0	0	0	0
5327	Convention Postage/Shipping	1,500	2,019	889	1,500
5328	Convention Printing/Copying	3,000	4,418	2,677	3,000

CANON SOCIETY LAW OF AMERICA					
2019-2020 BUDGET		BUDGET	ACTUAL	ACTUAL	BUDGET
		approved			
		7/1/18-6/30/19	7/1/17-6/30/18	7/1/18-6/30/19	7/1/19-6/30/20
5329	Promotion, Program Materials/Banners	5,250	6,891	3,953	5,250
5330	Liturgy and Environment	2,000	0	3,596	3,000
5331	Speaker/Workshop/Facilitator/Panel/Honoraria Stipends	18,600	14,776	12,142	18,600
5332	Speaker/Workshop/Facilitator/Panel/Travel Expenses	5,000	1,300	3,989	5,000
5333	Convention Lodging/Meals/Entertainment	10,000	9,430	2,815	8,000
5334	Convention Planner	48,500	46,602	52,338	50,000
5340	**Board of Governors**				
5341	Telecommunications	100	385	1,456	400
5342	Postage/Shipping	50	0	52	75
5343	Printing/Copying	100	0	754	150
5344	Supplies	0	0	0	0
5345	Travel	9,000	7,584	8,565	8,000
5346	Lodging/Meals/Entertainment	16,400	22,519	22,501	18,000
5347	Officers' Expenses	5,000	3,469	7,764	4,500
5350	**Committees**				
5351	Constitutional Committees	4,000	3,618	833	4,450
5352	Standing Committees	3,000	1,756	203	9,575
5353	Convention Planning Committee	2,000	4,604	4,071	2,000
5354	Committee Work Contingency & Orientation	2,000	687	641	1,500
5400	**PRODUCT DEVELOPMENT**				
5410	**Cost of Good Sold - Publication and Resources**				
5411	Cost of Goods Sold	2,600	15,027	0	2,600
5420	**Expenses - Publication and Resources**				
5421	Administrative Expenses	N/A	0	0	N/A
5422	Publication Advisory Board Committee	3,500	4,925	28	3,500
5423	Books/Media Materials (Practicum on Penal Law, *CIC* Reprint,	9,000	(0)	27,697	15,000
5424	Subscriptions/Licensing	100	100	0	100
5425	Advertising/Public Relations	500	0	0	500
5426	Postage/Shipping	300	24	179	300
5427	Supplies	150	340	0	150
5430	**BrightKey - Outsourcing Publication and Resources**	40,000			40,000
5431	Equipment Lease/Purchase/Maintenance		5,396	5,228	
5432	Packing/Invoice Supplies		675	166	
5433	Project Management Fees		8,262	7,992	

CANON SOCIETY LAW OF AMERICA					
2019-2020 BUDGET		BUDGET	ACTUAL	ACTUAL	BUDGET
		approved			
		7/1/18-6/30/19	7/1/17-6/30/18	7/1/18-6/30/19	7/1/19-6/30/20
5434	Rent - Storage Space (Pallet/Quick Pick Processing)		7,471	4,193	
5435	Order Processing		3,235	2,407	
5436	Website, IT Services		3,266	3,402	
5437	Printing/Copying		3,801	4,477	
5438	Professional Services		4,099	4,368	
5439	Telecommunications		97	86	
5440	Postage/Shipping		4,330	11,477	
5450	**Expenses - Royalties Publication and Resources**				
5451	Royalties for Code of Canon of the Eastern Churchs (CCEO - 8% of	250	56	73	250
5452	Royalties for Code of Canon of the Canon Law, 6794 (CIC - 8% of	2,000	656	950	2,000
5453	Royalties for Dignitas Connubii: Norms and Commentary (Diginitas	250	85	145	250
5454	Royalties for Selected Issues (60% of NR)	100	63	104	100
5455	Royalties for Reception and Communion (Quantity Sold x $6)	25	0	0	50
5460	**Product Partnerships**				
5461	Product Partnerships	0	0	1,043	1,500
6100	**Canon Law Society Operating Expenses**				
6110	**Salaries and Benefits**				
6111	Salaries	157,726	132,188	161,923	164,246
6112	FICA	9,004	8,273	10,390	12,417
6113	Professional Development (CLSA Staff)	1,000	0	0	1,000
6114	Employee Benefit Plans	12,000	7,707	6,231	12,945
6115	Pension Plan	142	142	36	142
6116	403b Obligations	5,185	3,454	5,447	5,375
6117	DC Paid Family Leave 0.62% Taxes	N/A	N/A	209	
6118	Florida State Unemployment Insurance 2.7% Taxable Wages	N/A	N/A	84	
6120	**Operating Expenses**				
6121	Publications/Media Materials (Proceedings - Member Service)	10,000	7,976	612	11,000
6122	Membership Dues/Subscriptions/Licensing	3,700	1,602	1,596	3,000
6123	Advertising/Public Relations	1,000	840	0	1,000
6124	Gratuities (Awards/Gifts)	150	0	36	100
6125	Equipment lease/purchase/maintenance	1,700	2,160	1,753	1,800
6126	Business Insurance	1,100	1,116	1,176	1,150
6127	Rent	27,128	26,340	27,505	27,944
6128	Telecommunications	2,350	2,407	3,621	2,400
6129	Postage/Shipping	1,300	1,725	1,135	1,300

CANON SOCIETY LAW OF AMERICA					
2019-2020 BUDGET		BUDGET	ACTUAL	ACTUAL	BUDGET
		approved			
		7/1/18-6/30/19	7/1/17-6/30/18	7/1/18-6/30/19	7/1/19-6/30/20
6130	Printing/Copying	100	0	0	100
6131	Supplies	3,000	(777)	6,190	3,000
6132	Professional Services (Contracted Services)	6,000	2,514	720	4,500
6133	Bank/Financial Services Fees/Payroll Fees/Intuit Fees	13,000	17,965	13,233	15,000
6134	Accounting/Audit Fees	9,000	7,900	3,000	9,000
6135	Legal Fees	500	0	340	1,000
6136	Travel	5,000	1,687	1,389	5,000
6137	Lodging/Meals Enterntainment	1,500	3,148	1,798	1,500
6138	Website, IT, & Social Communication	34,433	18,118	30,408	7,500
6139	Bad Debt/Write-Offs	0	0	0	0
6140	Depreciation	0	5,382	0	0
TOTAL EXPENSES		686,793	619,367	595,967	646,719
NET INCOME		(87,905)	(52,759)	(12,686)	(65,891)

Note: Since Scholarship income by definition belongs to the Scholarship Fund, it cannot be used to balance the overall budget. Hence, the Scholarship income and expenses (in the darkened fields on page 1 and 2 of the budget) were not included in the Bottom Line number.

Canon Law Society of America Balance Sheet
Year Ending June 30, 2019

	Jun 30, 19
ASSETS	
Current Assets	
Checking/Savings	
1010 · TD Operating Account - 9622	448.76
1011 · TD Money Market Account - 9630	4,091.13
Total Checking/Savings	4,539.89
Other Current Assets	
1200 · Accounts Receivable	
1230 · Security Deposit (Ops)	2,094.40
Total 1200 · Accounts Receivable	2,094.40
1400 · Prepaid Expenses	
1420 · Other Prepaid Expenses	31,327.22
1422 · Other Prepaid Ex (Convention)	437.01
Total 1400 · Prepaid Expenses	31,764.23
1500 · Inventory Asset	
1510 · Inventory - Books & CDs (Pub)	46,120.08
Total 1500 · Inventory Asset	46,120.08
1600 · Investment	
1612 · CUIT Magnus-Ops (Ending 2001)	907,880.84
1622 · CUIT Magnus-Licentiate (..2002)	881,066.54
1623 · CUIT Magnus-Doctoral (...2003)	72,470.65
Total 1600 · Investment	1,861,418.03
Total Other Current Assets	1,941,396.74
Total Current Assets	1,945,936.63
Fixed Assets	
1700 · Fixed Assets	
1710 · Furniture and Equipment (Ops)	46,491.00
1790 · Accumulated Depreciation(contra	-18,710.00
Total 1700 · Fixed Assets	27,781.00
Total Fixed Assets	27,781.00
TOTAL ASSETS	**1,973,717.63**
LIABILITIES & EQUITY	
Liabilities	
Current Liabilities	
Other Current Liabilities	
2100 · Accounts Payable	
2110 · Accounts Payable	6,631.33
Total 2100 · Accounts Payable	6,631.33
2130 · Accrued Payroll	
2131 · Accrued Wages	946.00
Total 2130 · Accrued Payroll	946.00
2200 · Deferred Revenue	
2204 · Deferred Rev - Membership Dues	6,167.22
Total 2200 · Deferred Revenue	6,167.22
Total Other Current Liabilities	13,744.55

Canon Law Society of America Balance Sheet
Year Ending June 30, 2019

	Jun 30, 19
Total Current Liabilities	13,744.55
Total Liabilities	13,744.55
Equity	
3101 · Unrestricted	
3102 · Undesignated	1,006,039.53
3103 · Board designated - Publications	15,174.00
Total 3101 · Unrestricted	1,021,213.53
3120 · Temporarily restricted	880,798.00
3126 · Unrestricted Retained Earn-Scho	5,804.62
Net Income	52,156.93
Total Equity	1,959,973.08
TOTAL LIABILITIES & EQUITY	1,973,717.63

Report of the Executive Coordinator

Donna M. Miller, JD, JCL

Introduction

It is a humbling and privileged opportunity for me to deliver this report as the Executive Coordinator of the Canon Law Society of America. I began my duties on May 1, 2019, and I could not have asked to be surrounded and assisted by a better group of dedicated, knowledgeable and friendly individuals. The Executive Coordinator has been a part-time position for several years, and, thanks to technology, I am blessed to be able to serve the Society remotely from my home in Florida.

I first want to recognize the standard of excellence set by our former General Secretary, Colleen Crawford, who served the Society tirelessly for the last seven years. We now are blessed to have Megan Boland as our new General Secretary. Megan worked side-by-side with Colleen for nearly eighteen months, and now she has slipped seamlessly into the role of leading our Administrative Office in Washington, DC. I am without words to express the gratitude that I have for Megan for her impeccable attention to detail, her limitless skillset and her irreproachable work ethic in this new role. We are also blessed to have Mary Nguyen continuing to handle with competence the financial affairs in our office. I extend my deepest gratitude to both Megan and Mary.

Code Reprint Project

For the past five months, my attention primarily has been devoted to the ongoing project involving the Society's Latin-English translation of the Code of Canon Law. The last reprint to be completed by the Society was in 2012, after Pope Benedict made the first changes to the code (in *Omnium in mentem*, 2009) since the Society published its 1999 Latin-English translation. A few years after that reprint was produced, Pope Francis delivered to the world four additional documents that have changed various canons in the code. These changes have necessitated a reprint so that the newest norms can be incorporated into the text.

The documents that have changed or replaced existing canons since 2012 and that will be included for the first time in this upcoming reprint are:

- *Mitis Iudex Dominus Iesus* (15 August 2015)
- *De concordia inter Codices* (31 May 2016)

- *Magnum principium* (3 September 2017)
- *Communis vita* (19 March 2019)

I am extremely grateful to Msgr. Bruce Miller for being the driving force behind this project and for his gracious patience with me as I became acquainted with the vast work that had been done prior to my stepping onto the scene. In early June, I completed a meticulous review of the English text of all seven books of the code and compiled a list of editing changes. An unofficial committee (assembled by Msgr. Miller) was asked to consider and respond to the questions that I raised. The combined knowledge and expertise of the individual canonists who participated is an incredible blessing to the Society. We held a productive GoToMeeting session on August 1 to review the suggested handling of several edits that needed discussion. I am grateful to Msgr. Miller, Fr. Paul Counce, Fr. Peter Akpoghiran, Fr. Ulrich Rhode, Zabrina Decker and Msgr. John Renken for all that they have contributed and continue to contribute to this project.

In mid-August, I completed an exhaustive review of the Latin text of the code with the new integrated norms. With the help of Msgr. Renken, the revised Index for the code was completed. In addition, Chorbishop John Faris secured for us the tables of corresponding canons that the Canadian publisher, Wilson and Lafleur, used in their recent code update (*Code de droit canonique bilingue (latin/français) et annoté, 4e édition*, 2018). These resources were very helpful to me in editing the existing tables for our upcoming reprint.

The final edits that have been submitted to the formatter include the fontes and the Outline of the Code of Canon Law (noting changes in the headings of Book VII). We have been given a mid- November date by the formatter, by which time we anticipate the layout to be finished and the proof returned to us for additional review by the Publications Advisory Board (PAB). Those who are called to serve on this important board in the coming year will play a part in this tremendous undertaking. I am grateful to the current PAB members, under the leadership of the current chair—and former CLSA Executive Coordinator—Sr. Sharon Euart, RSM, for their unwavering patience and their willingness to assist with the reprint.

Naturally, it would have been ideal if the much-anticipated changes to Book VI of the code had been released prior to publication of this reprint. Similarly, we have been waiting for the release of the replacement for Pastor Bonus, which is being referred to as *Evangelium Praedicate*. However, the plan is to move on with this reprint and, when those changes come, we will proceed with a more complete revision—for which additional permissions and editing will be required.

For now, we have replenished our supply of the 2012 soft-bound edition of the code with Brightkey, which stores our inventory and processes many of our book purchases. We hope that this will satisfy the demand for those needing the code for the fall semester. We will re-evaluate the inventory as we push for the work-in-progress-reprint to be completed as quickly as possible.

Electronic and On-Demand Publishing

A related issue was addressed last year by my predecessor, Fr. Pat Cogan, with regard to electronic publishing and print-on-demand. We continue to analyze the issues surrounding the production of the Society's books—especially the code—in an electronic format. The unofficial committee that has helped with the code reprint (and eventual revision) is fully committed to an electronic version of the code. The Board of Governors has listened and considered the information that has been presented to them on the subject. We have examined Amazon as a potential partner in such an endeavor, and we note that there are pros and cons—in addition to unknowns—if we elect to go that route. But we will continue to look for answers and explore the possibilities, along with the required permissions that accompany such an endeavor, with the hope that we soon will be able to accommodate our members who desire an electronic version of our Latin-English translation of the code and other future publications.

Green Commentary Revision

Msgr. John Foster, who served this past year as Past-President on the Board of Governors, has headed up a revision project involving the "Green Commentary," which is to say the *New Commentary on the Code of Canon Law* that was published for the Society by Paulist Press in 2000. I am honored to be replacing Msgr. Foster in this undertaking so that he can attend more readily to the canonical matters of the Military Archdiocese. President Zabrina Decker has formulated a mandate to grant Msgr. John Beal, one of the original editors of the 2000 Commentary, the authority to oversee the revision. Paulist Press has agreed to publish the product again, as long as it is one volume. We are very optimistic that 2023 is a realistic target release year—to coincide with the 40th anniversary of the 1983 *Codex Iuris Canonici.*

The Anticipated Revival of Webinars

One of our newer initiatives, which is actually a resurrection of a previous service, is our plan to use our new subscription to GoToWebinar to host webinars for our members. The subscription includes storage for webinars that we record and access to GoToMeeting services. With GoToWebinar we can have up to 100 participants on a live session, while GoToMeeting has a capacity of 25 (with webcam accommodation). We can also conduct a "simulated live webinar"

where we pre-record the content but conduct it as a live event—people register and log-on at a scheduled time to listen to the playback. We do not plan to charge our members for webinars. We have at least two committees with webinars in the works, so our members soon should see an announcement for these upcoming events. Suggestions for webinar topics and presenters are always welcome. Please notify me via email if you have any questions or suggestions.

Oklahoma City Province and Interdiocesan Tribunal Workshop

Each year the Board of Governors strives to send a representative to each regional gathering of canonists. I was pleased to attend the two-day August event hosted by the Diocese of Little Rock for the Oklahoma City Province. The meeting was held at the St. John Catholic Center, which dates back to 1916, first as Little Rock College and then as St. John Home Mission Seminary. The presenter was Msgr. Alejandro Bunge, who hails from Argentina and is a member of the Roman Rota. His presentations (totaling over five hours) were excellent, and participants gave rave reviews. In particular his explanation of the "Briefer Process before the Bishop" captivated the audience. I appreciate the warm southern hospitality that was extended to me by the host diocese and nearly one hundred attendees.

CLSA Membership

As always, we welcome new members to the Society with open arms. I did discover that our Associate Membership, which is for individuals who are not degreed canonists, came as a surprise to several people who work in Tribunal offices. I encourage those of you who have non- canonist office staff to give them the link to our CLSA website so that they can explore the possibility of becoming an Associate Member. We would be happy to answer any questions that you or they may have about the benefits of membership.

Conclusion

When I joined the CLSA in 2002, I was a fledgling canon law student with very little knowledge of the impact that this ministry would have on my life. Now, as we approach 2020, I dare to invoke the adage that "hindsight is 20/20." I am privileged and blessed to be serving as Executive Coordinator for this storied and esteemed organization. If anyone has questions or comments, I encourage you to reach out to me or to our office staff. We are here to serve you and to make your respective ministries more fruitful through our work as canon lawyers in service of missionary discipleship.

Report of the General Secretary

Colleen Crawford

I begin this annual report with an expression of gratitude, and indeed, an acknowledgment of circumstances that were first announced publicly in the September 2019 CLSA eNewsletter. After seven years in the administrative office, I am bidding a fond farewell to the Canon Law Society of America and its remarkable membership, as I transition into a new professional position. Since I am not in Atlantic City to present my report at the 81st Annual Business Meeting, it is quite impossible to bury this lede, and I do wish to reiterate, briefly, my sincere appreciation for those members who have encouraged me and inspired me in my professional journey, and whose wisdom and friendship I will carry with me in new endeavors. I offer a special thank you to the Past Presidents of the CLSA, recent Board members and Committee chairpersons, Convention planning personnel and the incredible staff at Nix Conference and Meeting Management, and Sr. Sharon Euart, RSM – my first supervisor and educator in canon law, and indeed, by virtue of hiring me, the reason that I had the unique privilege of serving the CLSA membership.

Board officers will provide extensive commentary on the operations, financials, and Convention planning efforts of the Society's administrative office, so my remarks below will offer concentrated perspective on the CLSA website and a few miscellaneous items. As always, questions may be directed to the administrative office.

In the last calendar year, members who followed the quarterly eNewsletter became well-acquainted with advancements and complications related to the website project. The partnership with FreshySites, the Society's website developer, began in earnest in summer 2018, following extensive review of website proposals by the Board of Governors. Top priorities included the reestablishment of the Member Directory, improved member engagement and backend content, and—in the interest of promoting membership in the Canon Law Society of America—a firm desire to make public-facing pages more accessible and mission-minded. After rigorous vetting and revision of the Privacy Policy under the direction of a civil attorney, we were pleased to unveil the new website in mid-May 2019. Since its launch, we have provided extensive feedback to FreshySites Support to inform the website's continued refinement, and I thank members who have offered insight into their website experience. These experiences are crucial steps toward formally documenting errors and improving the overall website experience.

The WordPress Engine remains a new vehicle for office staff, and much like members, we too have experienced a steep learning curve. This curve is most apparent with particular administrative workflow, including individual processing time for dues remittance, applications, and registrations. As the office gains more insight into billing processes and manual interventions on WordPress (and indeed, as FreshySites continues to make workflow adjustments), CLSA staffers will be able to assume more responsibility and outsource fewer questions. On the whole, this action will improve troubleshooting for members by phone and by email, and it should reduce questions. I regret that the billing process for member dues (including subscription prompts and informal scripts/auto-notices from plug-ins) caused some unease and confusion in late June and early July. I reiterate an assurance that the office is committed to reducing and closing these gaps, and we have been forthright with FreshySites personnel about our expectations for optimizing the website.

Finally, the administrative office was, and indeed, is, particularly concerned with expanding and growing member content—ensuring that downloads, electronic publications, and archived material are available and inherently "useful" for members who serve in canonical ministries. Plans are in motion to create a series of member-friendly tutorials that will guide users through important resources and content on the website. We will also begin employing brief surveys for more regular feedback, and we look forward to the full restoration of the Electronic Advisory Opinions Index. This plan is the first of several stages to improve overall website functionality, and it will be enhanced by the renewal of the CLSA webinar series under the direction of Executive Coordinator Donna Miller.

While much of the administrative year has been devoted to supplementing gaps in member services, the office continues to perform its "regular" administrative tasks, including working alongside the Publications Warehouse to maintain product inventory and fulfill orders. Recently, publication orders have required additional manual intervention on the part of the office, and indeed, the new e-commerce platform necessitated a research-driven overhaul of the Society's shipping rubric. It has been a year of change and adaptation for the BrightKey warehouse and the administrative office, but working through these growing pains will ensure long-term member and customer satisfaction.

New book production remained minimal this year, due in part to the six-month vacancy in the Executive Coordinator position, but I offer sincere thanks to Past President John J. M. Foster for his role in seeing Proceedings 2018 to completion. Monsignor Foster promptly and thoroughly edited all contributions to the volume, and his work ethic was indefatigable, even in the wake of delays and concerns with the printer. As Donna Miller assumes the Proceedings helm, and as she continues her work on the third printing of the Code of Canon Law, I look forward to the new fruits of CLSA Publications.

The office continues to receive reporting from Committees and assist with the preparation of select Committee materials and meeting hosting, and in this vein, I would strongly encourage members to read the annual Committee reports in full and learn about recent developments and on-going projects. October is an excellent time to consider renewing service to a Committee or becoming involved for the first time. Please do contact the existing Committee Chair, speak to a member of the Board of Governors, or complete a Committee Recommendation Form to seek appointment to a Committee. The work of Committees and Task Forces is paramount to the growth and prosperity of the Society as a whole!

I conclude this report by thanking the Board of Governors for their guidance, and thanking you, the members, for your patience and kindnesses throughout the year. I offer particular gratitude to Megan Boland, who has proven herself, time and again, an invaluable asset and resource for the administrative office. I have every confidence that Megan will continue to run operations smoothly, with the financial expertise of Mary Nguyen and the recommendations of the Board of Governors. I move forward with the knowledge and comfort that operations are in excellent hands.

It has been an honor to serve as General Secretary. Please know of my prayers for the Society's ongoing mission and the particular ministries of its members.

Constitutional Committees

Committee: Nominations
Constituted: Constitutional Committee
Mandate: Articles IX and X of Constitution

To submit to the active members, at least one month prior to the date of election, the names of nominees as provided for in Article IX of the Constitution.

To formulate and recommend to the Board of Governors plans for maintaining and increasing membership in the Society. Revise all proposals so that the meaning of each is clear (Article X).

Members: Rev. Msgr. John Foster, *ex-officio*, Past President(2019)
Rev. Garry Giroux (2021)
Rev. Deacon Gerald Jorgensen, *chair* (2020)
Sr. Victoria Vondenberger, RSM (2019)

REPORT

The Committee met on January 14 and 15, 2019, at the CLSA office in Washington, D.C. The objective of the meeting was to secure at least 4 Nominees for 2 Consultor positions, 2 Nominees for Treasurer, and 2 Nominees for Vice-President/ President-Elect. The goal is to present to the Board of Governors the nominees for the three offices before the conclusion of January 2019. Committee members initially discussed the general criteria it would use to identify nominees for the three offices that will be elected at the October 2019 General Convention and Annual Meeting.

Members concurred that having served as a member of the Board of Governors was crucial for the nominees it would put forward for Vice-President/President-Elect. In regard to Treasurer, members thought it was crucial for nominees to have some financial management or budget management experience of multiple areas and accounts. Finally, in regard to nominees that the Committee put forward for Consultors, it was crucial that nominees have several years of membership in the Society and experience as a member of an active committee of the Society. Nonetheless, Committee members recognized that its criteria had to be flexible when it came to securing nominees for the offices open for election. Furthermore, committee members reminded themselves that the Board of Governors explicitly had instructed the committee that no speakers at the 2019 General Convention could be nominees for any of the positions open for election at the 2019 General Convention and Annual Meeting.

Next, committee members reviewed the lists of general convention attendees for the past three conventions, the members of committees of the Society for the current year and for the past three years, the nominations submitted by members of the Society attending the 2017 and 2018 General Conventions, and the Canon Law Society of America Slate of Nominees for the past 15 years.

Then, once the committee members had identified offices that would be open for election, discussed general criteria, and reviewed the various lists, they began to generate potential nominees, also keeping in mind gender diversity and geographic representation. Once potential nominees were identified and agreed upon by the Committee, the Chair and the Past-President divided the names between them and began making calls to secure nominees. When persons are asked if they are willing to be a nominee for a specific position, there are no guarantees that the person will say "yes;" often times some other person or persons has/have to be consulted.

During the time Committee members were waiting for return calls from the nominee, with his or her decision, they discussed whether to continue the Candidates' Forum at the General Convention. It is the Committee's recommendation to the Board of Governors that the Candidates' Forum be discontinued. Committee members based their recommendation on the following: 1) it has been Committee members' experience that since its inception the Candidates' Forum has had minimal attendance; 2) that most of the persons in attendance at the Candidates' Forum were friends and supporters of one or more candidates and already had decided how they would vote; 3) that there were few, if any, questions from the audience in attendance at the Forum; and 4) that the Convention Planning Committee and the Board of Governors could find a better, more productive use of that time for the Society at large. In place of the Candidates' Forum, the Committee recommends that all candidates be instructed to create a video presentation of a specified length in which each candidate responds to the same set of questions and then the video presentation of each candidate is posted to the Society's website for access by all members.

Moreover, the Committee recommends that the Board of Governors pursue electronic voting by qualified voters in attendance at the Society's Annual Meeting to vote for Offices, Resolutions, and any other motions requiring action at the Annual Meeting.

In conclusion, the Committee presents the following Nominees for the Offices open for election at the 2019 Annual Meeting of the Canon Law Society of America:

Consultors

1. Ms. Barbara Bettwy
2. The Reverend Jamin David
3. The Reverend Monsignor Victor Finelli
4. Mr. Michael Forbes

Treasurer

1. The Reverend Steven Callahan
2. The Reverend Kevin Niehoff, O.P.

Vice-President/President-Elect

1. The Reverend Monsignor C. Michael Padazinski
2. Mrs. Meg Romano-Hogan

Submitted by: Deacon Gerald Jorgensen, *chair*
8 July 2019

Committee: Resolutions
Constituted: Constitution, Article X 2009
Mandate: The Committee on Resolutions is established in art. X of the CLSA Constitution, with the following functions:

1. To solicit, develop and draft proposed resolutions which will express the concerns of the Canon Law Society of America;

2. To consult with the membership at large and, in particular with the Board of Governors, the standing and *ad hoc* committees of the Society, and the organizers of the annual convention;

3. To formulate proposed resolutions on given points in response to requests of the members of the Society;

4. To compose differences in the formulation of similar proposals and to revise all proposals so that the meaning of each is clear; (and)

5. To encourage resolutions which authentically express in a positive way the activities and concerns of the Society.

Members: Ms. Bertha Nwazi Nyirenda, *chair* (2019)
The Reverend David C. Gross (2020)
The Reverend Andrew Szymakowski (2021)
BOG Liaison: Mr. Jay Conzemius, Vice-President

REPORT

Our Committee receives and processes resolutions prior to and at the annual Convention, and accordingly, the bulk of the Committee's work will occur between August and October. The committee members proposed using email conference but did not have any matters arising to discuss. On July 17, 2019, we reached out to the CLSA membership, using Fr. Paul Hartmann's canon law list serve, for any topics/questions for consideration at the 2019 Canon Law Convention. At the time of this report none had been brought forward.

Submitted by: Ms. Nwazi Bertha Nyirenda, *chair*
24 July 2019

Committee: Resource and Asset Management
Constituted: *Constitution*, Article X, as last amended in 2008, 2013
Old Committee Structure: Committees on Budget, Investment and Scholarship Fund.
Mandate: The mandate of the Committee is as follows:

1. To develop a comprehensive budge for all the activities of the Society and report on the funding available for projects;
2. To submit the proposed budget for the coming fiscal year to the Board of governors for approval at its springs meeting; To conserve, invest and disburse the monies of the Scholarship Fund in accord with the criteria established by the Society; (and)
3. To advise the Treasurer on all matters pertaining to the Society's investments. (Article X, 7)
4. Membership: The Committee of Resource and Asset Management shall consist of the Vice-President, the Treasurer, and a senior consultor and two additional members appointed by the President. The Treasurer shall act as Chair of this committee. (Article X, 2)

Members: Sr. Nancy Reynolds, SP, *chair*
The Reverend Monsignor Bill King (2019)
Sr. Margaret A. Stallmeyer, CDP (2019)
The Reverend John P. Donovan, *ex officio* (2019)
Mr. Jay Conzemius, *ex officio* (2019)
Former Treasurer Mentor: The Reverend Thomas E. Cronkleton, Jr.

The Committee's report will be presented in conjunction with general remarks on the financials. The finalized budget, as modified in April 2019, will be reviewed by Nancy Reynolds, SP.

Committee: Professional Responsibility

Constituted: *Constitution*, Article X (as last amended in 1995), and the Code of Professional Responsibilities, which was adopted in 1983 (for an experimental period of three years), revised in 1987, with a Statement Concerning Professional Courtesies adopted for an experimental period of three years in October 1993, which was revised and adopted in 1996; the current version of the CLSA Revised Code of Professional Responsibility was adopted in October 2016 (Introduction).

Mandate: The mandate of the Committee is as follows:

1. Regarding complaints
2. To receive complaints of any party aggrieved with respect to provisions of the Code of Professional Responsibility of the CLSA;
3. To make an initial finding that the complaint is not frivolous but is serious in character.
4. By majority vote, to refer the matter to one of the Hearing Officers;
5. To issue advisory opinions and decisions on the application of the Code of Professional Responsibility; (and)
6. To advise on all other questions concerning the professional responsibility of canonists.

Members: The Reverend John P. Donovan, *chair* (2019)
Ms. Susan Mulheron, *ex officio* (2019)
Dr. Chad Glendinning, *ex officio* (2020)
Sr. Marie Breitenbeck, OP, *hearing officer* (2019)
The Reverend J. Michael Clark, *hearing officer* (2020)
Dr. Benedict Nguyen, *hearing officer* (2021)

Subcommittee: Mr. Jesus Cabrera
Ms. Patricia Dugan
Mr. Christopher Siuzdak

REPORT

The committee has not met since January 2019, but have had regular communications, and discussions through e-mail. We have discussed procedures, recent inquiries made, and 2019 Convention Presentations. We have acted upon the following:

A subcommittee was appointed to prepare a meeting for first time convention attendees. Originally, it was planned to be a meeting before the Keynote address, but after much discussion we decided to resume the practice of the fore new

members breakfast. Thus, the Wednesday of convention there will be a breakfast for first time attendees, opting for a more informal conversation with talking points to be provided for the veterans. Areas to be covered will be the purposes of the society regarding professional standards verses the Bar of the civil law; the importance of networking as resource; the purpose and need for continuing education through the convention, webinars and regional conferences and the ministry of a canonist.

We have addressed two complaints since last October against one member. In both instances the matter was resolved with recommendations made to the canonist to be more transparent. It was noted that our Code of Professional Responsibilities approved in 2016 should be addressed for its redundancy and recommends that a *turnus* rather than a single hearing officer be appointed to review complaints.

Submitted by: The Reverend John P. Donovan, *chair*
15 August 2019

ON-GOING COMMITTEES

Committee: Church Governance
Constituted: 2009
Mandate: The mandate of the Committee is as follows:

1. To initiate as needed any projects pertinent to the study of canon law pertaining to Church structures and governance or the implementation thereof, including but not limited to the following:
   a. diocesan and parish temporalities;
   b. consultative bodies;
   c. diocesan and parish structures;
   d. power of governance;
   e. comparative law issues;
2. To oversee projects referred to the committee by the BOG;
3. To oversee its subcommittees working on projects concerning Church governance; (and)
4. To collaborate with national organizations and other groups dealing with issues of Church governance.

Members: The Reverend Joseph L. Newton, *chair and BOG Liaison* (2020)
Ms. Mary C. Edlund (2019)
Mr. Christopher J. Fusco, Esq. (2020)
The Reverend Monsignor Charles Antonicelli (2020)
Ms. Sofia Seguel (2021)
Ms. Jeannine Marino (2021)
The Reverend Anthony Omenihu (2021)
The Reverend Gregory Luyet (2021)

Note: The committee did not submit a final report in advance of the printing of the Annual Reports Booklet.

Committee: Clergy
Constituted: 2009
Mandate: The mandate of the Committee is as follows:

1. To initiate as needed any projects pertinent to the study of canon law pertaining to the life and ministry of bishops, priests and deacons or the implementation thereof, including, but not limited to, the following: (a) canonical issues related to the sexual abuse of minors, (b) clergy personnel issues and resources, (c) advocacy for clergy in penal cases;

2. To oversee projects referred to the committee by the BOG;
3. To oversee its subcommittees working on projects concerning clergy; and
4. To collaborate with national organizations and other groups dealing with clergy issues.

Members: The Reverend William Elder (2019)
Deacon Daniel Welter (2019)
Dr. Margaret Chalmers (2020)
The Reverend Monsignor Stephen Doktorczyk (2020)
The Reverend Monsognor Edward Lohse (2020)
The Reverend Georges de Laire (2021)
Deacon Daniel Laurita (2021)
The Reverend Luke Millette, *chair* (2021)
Ms. Mary Santi, *BOG Liaison*
The Reverend Monsignor Fred Easton, *Past President Mentor*

REPORT

Since the last report, the Committee on Clergy has been working on the development of a webinar on Penal Processes. Speakers have been chosen and final content needs to be developed. The Committee for Clergy has also been in dialogue with the USCCB Committee on Canonical Affairs and Church Governance who has asked for assistance with a project. Finally, the Committee for Clergy is collaborating with the Committee for Eastern Affairs on a project addressing issues specific to MarriedClergy.

Submitted by: The Reverend Luke Millette, *chair*
5 August 2019

Committee: Convention Planning
Constituted: 1971
Mandate: The mandate of the Committee is as follows:Previous Committee Structure – Committees on Convention Planning (Constitutional) and Convention Liturgies

Members: The Reverend Jamin Scott David, Baton Rouge, *chair* (2019)
The Reverend James Conn, SJ, Boston (2019)
Mrs. Rita Ferko Joyce, Pittsburgh (2020)
The Reverend Robert Sinatra, Camden (2021)
The Reverend Monsignor John Foster, AMS; Stockton, *ex officio – Past President*

REPORT

Since the last "in person" meeting of the Committee on Convention Planning in January 2019 in Washington, the Board of Governors gave suggestions and approval of the slate of speakers for the 2020 conference in St. Louis, Missouri. Committee members have nearly completed their assignments by contacting the proposed speakers to ascertain from them their willingness and availability to engage the membership as presenters for the upcoming convention in 2020. The working theme as presented by the Committee on Convention Planning is *20/20: Evolving Laws and Practices.* Most presenters have been secured for the 2020 Convention (the current slate of speakers for the 2020 convention is attached to this report)!

The committee also has been addressing some "loose ends" regarding seminars and major addresses to be presented at the 2019 Convention in Atlantic City, New Jersey.

Aside from continued communications with prospective speakers and attendance at the annual Convention in Atlantic City in October, the Committee plans to meet again "in person" in Washington, DC on 06-08 January 2020 to begin planning the 2021 convention.

On behalf of the Board of Governors, Father David thanks Father Conn for his past three years of service to the Convention Planning Committee as his term expires in October. Father David, whose term is expiring also in October, has been honored to have served the Society as Chairperson of the Committee on Convention Planning the past three years and looks forward to further collaboration with the BOG and other members of the Society in different capacities in the coming years.

Submitted by: The Reverend Jamin Scott David, JCL, *chair*
10 July 2019

20/20 EVOLVING LAWS AND PRACTICES
12–15 October 2020
The Chase Park Plaza, St. Louis, Missouri

Keynote Address
Pope Francis: Teacher, Legislator & Pastor
The Reverend Monsignor Paul McPartlan (Catholic University of America)

Major Address
Historical Look of Where We're Going with Francis as Legislator
The Reverend Monsignor Ronny Jenkins (Catholic University of America)

Major Address
The Discipline of Bishops
Archbishop Bernard Hebda (Archdiocese of Minneapolis/St. Paul)

Seminar Topics and Presenters

Challenges to the Seal of Confession
The Reverend Monsignor Stephen Doktorczyk (Diocese of Orange)

Professional Responsibilities: Cooperation and Civility Among the Roles in a Penal Trial
Dr. J. Michael Ritty and The Reverend Alex Laschuk

Consecrated Virgins & CICLSALS's New Instruction
Dr. Christina Hip-Flores

Professional Development of Lay Canonists: A Panel
Ms. Mary Santi and Ms. Anne Bryant (Third Panelist TBD)

Tips for Collecting Proofs for Auditors, Judges & Other Investigators
The Honorable Susan Malone (AMS)

Marriage Issues and the RCIA
Ms. Barb Bettwy

Personality Disorders and the Impact on Martial Consent (Potential Repeat Seminar)
Deacon Jerry Jorgensen

Canon 1099 with Special Considerations for Marriages Involving Parties from Non-Western Cultures
TBD

Cor orans
Sister Nancy Bauer, OSB

Canon 1389
TBD

Boundary Issues: Morality vs. Criminality
Ms. Susan Mulheron

Parishes Entrusted to a Religious Institute: Canonical Considerations
The Reverend John Chrysostom Kozlowski, OP

When Eastern Catholics Marry
Chorbishop John Faris

Data Driven Canon Law: Trend Since the Promulgation of the Code
Ms. Diane Barr

The Board of Governors' Choice
TBD

The Board of Governors' Choice
TBD

Committee: National Convention Chair
Chair: The Reverend Monsignor Victor F. Finelli, JCL

2019: Atlantic City, New Jersey

Welcome to Atlantic City, the world-famous Atlantic City Boardwalk, and most importantly the 81st Annual Convention of the Canon Law Society of America! Although getting to Bally's was more challenging than some other destinations, now that you're here I hope your enjoying your stay. When we visited the location we found that this particular hotel was very equipped to serve our needs and would lend itself to having a wonderful convention. I hope that you are experiencing the same thing. Don't be scared to venture out onto the Boardwalk. There you will find many fine eateries, most especially within the various casinos, both here along the boardwalk and over in the marina. The "Jitney" is an inexpensive way to travel but so is Uber. I hope you have a great convention and find this time worthwhile, but in educational development but also in renewing friendships and developing new ones.

2020: St. Louis, Missouri

The 82nd National Convention is planned for October 12-15, 2020 at the beautiful Chase Park Plaza right in the heart of St. Louis. Planning for this convention has already begun and I have no doubt that our visit to St. Louis will be another great convention. If you recall we were there a few years ago at another beautiful venue, and for those who remember St. Louis is filled with many exciting things to do and see before and after our convention.

2021: Albuquerque, New Mexico

The 83rd National Convention is planned for October 11-14, 2021 at the Hyatt Park Place in beautiful downtown, Albuquerque. We arrive right on the tails of the famous "Balloon Fiesta" which is held every year in Albuquerque. It's a magnificent sight with dozens and dozens of beautiful hot air balloons filling the

morning sky. Come early to make sure you see this spectacular event! We will be taking over nearly the entire hotel which will afford us literally a "space of our own." The staff of the hotel, as well as the Albuquerque Visitors Bureau, seemed genuinely excited to have our group present for the week. This will be a great location for sure.

2022: We have begun planning the 84th Annual Convention with the dates being October 10-13, 2022. Seems like a long way off, but before you know it'll be here, so be sure to place it on your long-range calendars.

I am thankful to Colleen Crawford, General Secretary to the CLSA, and to Megan Boland, both of whom work diligently for our Society. It's a real corporate work with everyone sharing in the tasks. In the end, it's our goal to make these days truly a benefit to your canonical ministry, in whatever capacity that may be. It's an absolute pleasure for me to assist and serve in this capacity and to work with these fine, dedicated people. Thank you for allowing me to do so.

Submitted by: The Reverend Monsignor Victor F. Finelli, *chair*
13 August 2019

Committee: Eastern Churches
Constituted: January 2018
Mandate: The mandate of the Committee is as follows:

1. To foster the study of the law of the Eastern Catholic and Eastern non-Catholic Churches through seminars at CLSA conventions and symposia and in publications and translations.
2. To serve as a resource to respond to inquiries regarding pastoral questions involving Eastern Christians.
3. To serve as a resource to other CLSA Committees when initiatives call for consideration of Eastern Catholic issues.
4. To promote the involvement of canonists proficient in Eastern canon law in the Society.
5. To promote the unity of Churches in all publications and discussions.

Members: Chorbishop John D. Faris, *chair* (2020)
Mr. Sean Doyle (2019)
The Reverend Alexander Laschuk (2020)
Dr. Margaret Chalmers (2019)
BOG Liaison: Mr. Timothy Olson

REPORT

The major work of the Committee was to propose and, after BOG approval, prepare for a pre-Convention Workshop at the 2020 CLSA convention in St. Louis, that will be held 2-6 pm on Sunday and 8:30 am – 2 pm on Monday.

The "working plan" will be a series of six 45 presentations (with 45 minutes for discussions): 1) Theology of married clergy and the ordained ministry; 2) Formation of married men for the ordained ministry; 3) Appointments/transfers of married men and pertinent financial issues; 4) Family life and protection of child policies; 5) Married deacons; 6) Annulments, irregularities, and married clerics. We will also compile current eparchial and diocesan policies regarding married clergy.

The Chair was informed that the revised edition of the English translation of Lorenzo Lorusso's *Eastern Catholics and Latin Pastors* had been sent to the printer.

Submitted by: Chorbishop John D. Faris, *chair*
7 August 2019

Committee: Institutes of Consecrated Life and Societies of Apostolic Life
Constituted: 2009 (Revised Mandate 2019)
Mandate: The mandate of the Committee is as follows:

1. To initiate as needed any projects pertinent to the study of canon law pertaining to the life and ministry of Institutes of Consecrated Life and Societies of Apostolic Life or the implementation thereof, including, but not limited to, the following:
   a. sponsorship;
   b. mergers and restructuring of institutes;
   c. governance;
   d. membership;
   e. new forms of consecrated life;
   f. the process for private and public associations to be established as Institutes of Consecrated Life or Societies of Apostolic Life.
2. To initiate as needed any projects pertinent to the study of canon law pertaining to the life and ministry of solitary forms of consecrated life, including but not limited to, the following:
   a. eremitic or anchoritic life;
   b. hermits;

c. consecrated virgins;

d. widows.

3. To oversee projects referred to the committee by the BOG.

4. To oversee its subcommittees working on projects concerning any form of religious life listed in 1 or 2 above.

5. To collaborate with national organizations and other groups dealing with issues of any form of religious life listed in 1 or 2 above.

Member: Dr. Eileen Jaramillo, DMin, JCL, *chair* (2020)
The Reverend Joseph M. Arsenault, SSA, JCL (2020)
The Reverend Brian T. Austin, FSSP, JCD Candidate (2020)
Sr. Eloise Rosenblatt, RSM, PhD, JD (2021)
Sr. Tracey Sharp, SCRH, JCL (2020)
Sr. Therese Guerin Sullivan, SP, JCL (2021)

BOG Liaison: Dr. Christina Hip-Flores, JCD

REPORT

The committee was able to discuss and implement the mandate in various ways throughout this past year. At the 2018 CLSA Convention there was a committee meeting. It was the first time the members had the chance to meet one another face to face. Since his term of office was ending, we also had the opportunity to thank Rev. John Chrysostom Kozlowski, OP, JCD for his work on the committee. Throughout the year there were conference calls and email exchanges. One of them included welcoming our newest member, Sister Therese Guerin Sullivan, SP, JCL.

The committee dialogued about various people who might be interested in giving a seminar at the annual convention on such timely topics as: *Cor Orans,* Implementing Instruction on the Apostolic Constitution *Vultum Dei Quaerere* on Women's Contemplative Life and the Instruction *Ecclesiae Sponsa Imago* on the *Ordo Virginum*. The chair of the committee then submitted the topics and names to Rev. Jamin David, chair of the convention planning committee. Rev. David acknowledged that he discussed the suggestions with his committee. They decided to provide one seminar.

This committee also dialogued about submitting opinions for possible publication in *Roman Replies and CLSA Advisory Opinions.* Three members decided to author opinions: Rev. Brian Austin, FSSP, Sr. Therese Sullivan, SP and Dr. Eileen Jaramillo. The opinions were then circulated among the committee

members for comments and suggestions. Due to dynamics transpiring in one of the opinions, the member asked that the committee discuss the issues during one of the conference calls. Once the opinions were ready, they were forwarded to either Colleen Crawford or Sister Sharon Euart, RSM, JCD, chair of the publication advisory board.

The third item that involved committee work was the mandate. The current chair recognized that the mandate needed revision and began discussing this matter with Dr. Zabrina Decker, JCD, the then Vice-President. This conversation continued with Jay Conzemius, JCL when he was elected. The BOG indicated to the committee that a draft could be worked on and submitted to them. Since this committee is not a constitutional committee, Jay indicated that the BOG had the authority to approve changes to the mandate. Sr. Tracy Sharp, SCRH and Dr. Eileen Jaramillo worked on the initial revision. Then it was submitted to the entire committee for suggestions and approval. The chair sent the proposed new mandate to the BOG. Some modifications were made. Jay indicated to the chair that the above mandate should be inserted into this report.

At the time this report was written, the BOG was moving toward leaving out widowers in this revised mandate. While the term widows cannot be found in the 1983 Latin code, it is contained in canon 570 of the 1990 Eastern code. At best, this can be viewed as suppletory law for the Latin Church. In Number 7 of the Apostolic Exhortation *Vita consecrata* (1996) both widows and widowers are named. While VC did not establish new law, it clearly moved away from a merely feminine understanding. This inclusion is more consistent with various canons in the Latin code. The BOG was also moving toward using the term religious life in numbers 4 and 5 rather than consecrated life. Such a term is more restrictive. It is only used in the Latin code in regard to religious institutes (cc. 607 and 610). The Eastern code only uses it in canon 607.

Additionally, CLSA members may be interested in knowing that on March 19, 2019 the Apostolic Letter *Communis Vita* was issued Motu Proprio by Pope Francis. It provides for the modification of norms in the Latin code of Canon Law. These norms are related to illegitimate absences from a religious house during which religious distance themselves from the jurisdiction of the legitimate Superior. At times the religious cannot be located. The changes mean that canons 694 and 729 have been entirely replaced. These new norms would be an excellent topic for a future CLSA seminar.

As chair of this committee, I want to compliment the committee members for their hard work this past year. In the midst of all the demands that are made on their time, they remained focused on the service that is being given to the members of this society.

Submitted by: Dr. Eileen Jaramillo, *chair*
31 July 2019

Committee: Laity
Constituted: 2009
Mandate: The mandate of the Committee is as follows:

1. To initiate as needed any projects pertinent to the study of canon law pertaining to the life and ministry of lay persons or the implementation thereof, including, but not limited to, the following:
   a. Lay ecclesial ministry;
   b. Collaboration with clergy;
   c. Rights of the lay faithful;
2. To oversee projects referred to the committee by the BOG;
3. To oversee its subcommittees working on projects concerning the laity, (and)
4. To collaborate with national organizations and other groups dealing with the role of the laity in the Church.

Members: Ms. Anne Bryant, *chair* (2020)
Mr. J. Michael Ritty (2019)
Mr. Stephen Garbitelli (2020)
Ms. Elizabeth Sondag (2020)
Deacon Matthew Glover (2021)
The Very Reverend Mark Payne (2021)
Mr. Daniel Quinan (2021)
Mrs. Victoria Kaczmarek (2021)
BOG Liaison: Ms. Susan Mulheron

REPORT

The Committee on the Laity completed and had approved the proposal of its CLSA Lay Canonist Mentor Program. In April the program was sent to the deans of St. Paul University and The Catholic University for their ideas and suggestions. It is our hope that we can begin setting up and implementing the program this year so new canonists can benefit from it. We believe this to be a very worthwhile project and one that will be an advantage to the CLSA and to those who become involved in the program.

Submitted by: Ms. Anne E. Bryant, *chair*
18 July 2019

Committee: Publications Advisory Board
Constituted: Board of Governors, 2007
Mandate: The mandate of the Board is as follows:

1. To advise the BOG about all aspects of current, periodic and proposed CLSA publication projects, including financial, literary, educational and marketing issues;
2. To monitor the progress of all CLSA publication projects
3. To implement the procedures for peer review of CLSA publications;
4. To make the final recommendation to the Board of Governors regarding specific publications.
5. To review the coordination and management of the CLSA's publications activity on the part of the Office of the Executive Coordinator; (and)
6. To provide a written report to the CLSA membership at the annual convention.

Members: Sr. Sharon Euart, RSM, Chair (term ends 2019)
The Reverend Patrick Cooney, OSB (2020)
Ms. Susan Mulheron (2020)
The Reverend Monsignor Michael Souckar (2022)
VACANT
Dr. Diane Barr, R&D chair, *ex officio* (2021)

REPORT

Meetings

The Publications Advisory Board met by conference call twice during the year and via email correspondence on several occasions. No in-person meeting occurred due to the lack of clarity regarding roles and relationships for board designated work groups. The chair participated in several important conversation/ meetings regarding the history of PAB, its mandate and relationship to the BOG and the Administrative Office.

Meeting of PAB Chair and CLSA President

The PAB chair had a phone conversation with Vice-President Jay Conzemius prior to the February BOG conference call meeting and an in-person meeting with President Zabrina Decker on February 8, 2019 to discuss publication matters. The discussions addressed concerns that PAB had raised in its reports to the BOG and to the membership since 2015 and about which the current CLSA leadership and BOG were not aware. PAB provided a chronology of events and recommendations that the members hoped would be helpful in addressing misperceptions of BOG members regarding PAB's role and work.

Among the items in the chronology was a recommendation for a meeting with the CLSA president, executive coordinator, general secretary, and chair of PAB to discuss mutual concerns, communication, and the relationship among the BOG, PAB and OEC.

The PAB chair and CLSA president discussed the need for better communication between the BOG and PAB as well as follow up from the BOG to PAB's recommendations, such as, for example, that the BOG retain the CLSA protocol for publishing, particularly the peer review process. Regarding the peer review, PAB noted the difference between publishing as an individual and publishing as a representative of an organization, with the latter reflecting on the scholarship and credibility of the organization as well as the individual. The members noted that peer review protocols are not uncommon for scholarly or professional journals.

Meeting of PAB Chair with Fr. John Beal, Msgr. John Foster and Paulist Press

The chair of PAB met with John Beal, John Foster and a representative of Paulist Press in late January to discuss the possibility of a revision of the *CLSA Commentary*. A report on Paulist's response and a decision by the BOG will be announced prior to the convention.

Meeting of CLSA President and Vice-President, Executive Coordinator, General Secretary, out- going and in-coming Chair of the PAB

On July 16 a meeting to address CLSA publications and the respective roles of the PAB, the Executive Coordinator Administrative Office, and the BOG was held at the CLSA Offices. It was a very fruitful meeting. The discussion helped clarify the role of PAB, the Executive Coordinator and the BOG considering the history and role of the PAB since its establishment in 2007 and developments since that time. It was particularly helpful to Donna Miller, the new executive coordinator and Rev. Patrick Cooney, OSB, new chair of PAB.

CLSA Administrative Office

Colleen Crawford, General Secretary, updated PAB throughout the year on the publication activities of the CLSA Administrative Office.

Vademecum for *Mitis Iudex*:

The status of the *vademecum* is somewhat unclear at this time pending a decision from the USCCB regarding whether the Society is competent/authorized to produce a document which generally is prepared by bishops in their role as an episcopal conference. PAB noted the importance of determining who is or will be the publisher (CLSA, CCLS, USCCB, St. Paul's, CCCB) and how the material will be made available, electronically or written material.

PAB recommended that the Sacramental Law Committee consider using the

already-prepared materials by members of the Sacramental Law Committee as advisory opinions, webinars or self- standing pastoral resources.

Third Printing of Code

During the February 8 meeting with CLSA President Zabrina Decker, the PAB chair was informed that following the October 2018 convention, Fr. Bruce Miller assumed responsibility for the Third Printing of the code. PAB has not been involved in the project since that time. The chair was consulted during the April BOG meeting for historical information on several issues related to reprinting the code including the use of the vernacular, Vatican licenses, and permissions and procedures for publishing the code. PAB recommended that the BOG clarify the nature of the next publication of the code – a third printing or a revised translation of the code and the procedures necessary for each.

Pastoral Resources

Though year-to-date numbers for sales of pastoral resources including the code were good, the financial impact continues to raise serious concerns. The cost of short runs of the Second Printing of the code is high and given the low price for purchase of the text, especially for non- members, this is and will continue to affect the Society's bottom line. PAB supported the General Secretary's recommendation for a higher differential between the price of the code for members and non-members.

Currently two publications are in process and at different stages of completion. The updated *Eastern Catholics & Latin Pastors* with English translation by Chorbishop John Faris is in print production. A second publication initiated just last Spring is in the exploratory stage.

RRAO 2019

PAB expresses deep gratitude to Msgr. Jack Alesandro for his service as editor of *Advisory Opinions* for over ten years and for his many years working with PAB, beginning with serving as chair of the Publications Task Force. PAB is grateful for the willingness of Msgr. Michael Souckar and Rev. Patrick Cooney, OSB to assume the responsibilities as editors of *Advisory Opinions* for 2019. Sr. Sharon Euart, RSM will serve as editor of *Roman Replies* for the 2019 edition.

CLSA Resource Database

With the launching of the new CLSA website, the transition of the database to the website has taken place. The General Secretary is working with consultants to ensure a smooth transition for handling the technical aspects of the database. Msgr. John Renken will continue to coordinate the content for the database and Fr. Mark Gantley will continue to oversee document ingestion.

PAB received a question regarding what permissions might be needed to ingest USCCB original materials (e.g., complementary norms, guidelines

for canonization, etc.) in the database. The PAB Chair contacted the USCCB Permissions office which responded that the USCCB would grant permission after reviewing a list of the documents that the CLSA wishes to include in the database. There is no permission needed for links (e.g. to complementary norms on the USCCB website). The director indicated that a standard fee might be worked out for the Society. Mark Gantley sought advice regarding copyrights for translations of Vatican documents by other sources. The PAB chair contacted legal counsel for an opinion.

2018-2019 Budget

At the writing of this report the June 30 actual vs. budget figures were not available. However, the May 31 financial report indicated that the CLSA Publications would show a significant deficit at the end of the fiscal year due to delays in book production. PAB noted that the delay in the publication for *Proceedings* 2018 and recommends that office procedures be modified to ensure a reasonable timeline for publication by requiring a drop-dead timeline after which the entry will be dropped, and no honorarium paid to the speaker.

In closing, I want to take this opportunity to express my gratitude to the PAB members, current and past, who have served the Society extremely well, and at times tirelessly, in carrying out PAB's mandate. Colleen Crawford's assistance has been invaluable in providing the necessary data for PAB's recommendations and decisions and we are grateful for her service, insights and numerous contributions. The Society has been well served by Colleen Crawford and all those members who have served on PAB since its establishment in 2007. I also want to wish Pat Cooney, OSB well as he assumes the chair of PAB following the 2019 convention. I have asked Pat to respond to any questions in my absence. I will continue to work together with Pat, Colleen and Donna on transition issues regarding roles and relationships.

Submitted by: Sr. Sharon Euart, RSM, *chair*
July 2019

Committee: Research & Development
Constituted: 2008
Mandate: The mandate of the Committee is as follows:

1. To initiate or cooperate in all CLSA research projects such as seminars, symposia and special studies;

2. To design and implement Think Tanks that will allow for diverse views on issues of ecclesial life having canonical implications;

3. To develop and recommend themes for the annual Conventions for submission to the Board of Governors for approval and subsequent referral to the Convention Planning Committee for implementation;

4. To maintain close communication with all the committees of the Society in order to facilitate needed research and discussion;

5. To interact with the Publications Advisory Board in order to assess the current and contemplated publications of the CLSA and offer suggestions and guidance for publication planning.

Members: Dr. Diane Barr, *chair* (2021)
The Reverend Joseph C. Scheib (2019)
Mrs. Meg Hogan (2020)
The Reverend Monsignor Ronny Jenkins (2021)
The Reverend Paul Hartmann (2021)
The Reverend Manuel Rodrigues (2021)
The Reverend Sean Bransfield (2021)

BOG Liaison: Jay Conzemius, *ex officio*, Vice President
The Reverend Msgr. John Foster, Past President

REPORT

Four members of the Research & Development Committee met person during the CLSA Convention in Phoenix in October. The purpose of the meeting was to continue to brainstorm the themes for the 2021 Convention. The following ideas were generated:

General Title: Canon Law and Civil Law: Transparency and Privacy

Future Meetings:
The Committee will meet by conference call in late to further refine the suggestions for the 2021 convention, to suggest themes for the 2022 Convention and to review other projects of interest to the committee membership. The Committee is also scheduled to meet during the upcoming CLSA meeting in Atlantic City.

Submitted by: Dr. Diane Barr, *chair*
September 2019

Committee: Sacramental Law
Constituted: 2009
Mandate: The mandate of the Committee is as follows:

1. To initiate as needed any projects pertinent to the study of canon law pertaining the sacramental life of the Church or the implementation thereof;
2. To oversee projects referred to the committee by the BOG;
3. To oversee its subcommittees working on projects concerning the sacramental life of the Church;
4. To offer suggestions to the BOG for marriage topics for pre-convention workshops; (and)
5. To collaborate with national organizations and other groups dealing with the sacramental life of the Church.

Members: Sr. Maureen McPartland, O.P., *chair* (2019)
The Reverend Peter Akpoghiran (2019)
Ms. Anna Marie Chamblee (2019)
The Reverend Arthur Mollenhauer (2019)
The Reverend Shawn Tunink (2019)
The Reverend Peter Eke (2019)
The Reverend Matthew Furgiuele (2019)
Mr. Michael Forbes (2019)
The Reverend John Boyle (2019)
The Reverend John Lessard-Thibodeau (2019)
The Reverend Michael Johnson (2020)
The Very Reverend Christopher House (2020)

BOG Liaison: Dr. Chad Glendinning

REPORT

Members surfaced topics of interest when they met during the CLSA convention in Phoenix. Those topics were: the age of confirmation; issues pertaining to the anointing of the sick; irregularities and impediments to the exercise of orders, baptism and same-sex godparents or parents; the role of the deacon at Mass; confession, the appropriate place and what falls under the seal; extraordinary form of the Roman rite: what is permitted?; and mass offerings. Older committee reports indicated that some past topics of interest were: faculties/drafting a *pagella*: experts and what to ask for; the revision of the Roman Missal; Eastern Catholics in Latin Church; and sacramental ministry to Hispanic immigrants. Members were polled regarding their interests, and

the topics of the extraordinary forms/Roman Missal, irregularities to exercise ministry and issues regarding anointing of the sick were of greatest interest. The committee then divided into two subgroups. One is surfacing issues related to the Latin Liturgy that might be of interest to CLSA members. The other is looking at issues surrounding the anointing of the sick. That only two of the committee members will remain after the 2019 convention will be an immediate difficulty, but the topics identified should be helpful for future planning.

The topic of Mass offerings was suggested to the BOG as a possible convention presentation and a presenter was suggested.

Since the *Mitis Iudex* vademecum involves an alliance with external partners (CCLS, SPU, USCCB), it was referred to a special subcommittee. Chad Glendenning, former chairperson of this committee, initially agreed to continue collaborating on this effort.

Submitted by: Sr. Maureen McPartland, OP, *chair*
5 August 2019

VARIA

CANON LAW SOCIETY OF AMERICA
EIGHTY-FIRST ANNUAL BUSINESS MEETING
Atlantic City, New Jersey
16 October 2018

MINUTES

CALL TO ORDER AND OPENING PRAYER

Dr. Zabrina Decker, President, called to order the Eighty-First Annual Business Meeting of the Canon Law Society of America (CLSA) on 16 October 2018 at Bally's Hotel in Atlantic City, New Jersey, at 11:03 a.m. She presided over the meeting as Chair.

Following the opening prayer, led by the Chair, Dr. Decker announced that Monsignor Fred Easton would serve as Parliamentarian for the Business Meeting and that *Robert's Rules of Order* would resolve matters not provided for in the CLSA's *Constitution* or *Bylaws*.

The Chair then gave instructions on the voting procedures to be observed for the elections during the Business Meeting. The procedures were adopted as presented by the Chair.

The Chair then entertained a motion that Associate Members present at the meeting would have the opportunity to address the assembly, as called for in Article 5.3 of the CLSA *Constitution*. The motion was seconded and approved by the assembly.

The Chair noted that the Minutes of the Eightieth Annual Business Meeting of the CLSA, written by Mr. Timothy Olson, Secretary, were provided in advance for review as published in *Proceedings* for the 2018 convention, on pages 435-441, as well as having been distributed electronically to the membership. The Chair entertained a motion not to read the minutes aloud. The motion was seconded and approved by the assembly. The Chair then called for any corrections to the minutes as submitted; no corrections were proposed. Therefore, the Chair announced that the minutes of the Eightieth Annual Business Meeting stood approved by the assembly.

ELECTION OF OFFICERS AND CONSULTORS

The Chair called Deacon Jerry Jorgensen, Chair of the Nominations Committee, to present the slate of nominees for officers and consultors.

Following the introduction of each set of candidates, the Chair called for nominations from the floor; there were none, and the nominations were closed.

The Chair then read the provisions of the CLSA's *Bylaws* regarding elections. The active members of the CLSA were instructed to cast their votes. The tellers collected the ballots and retired to a separate room to count them. Later in the Business Meeting, Deacon Jorgensen informed the Chair of the election results.

For the Office of Vice President/President-Elect:

192 valid ballots were cast; 97 were needed for election. There were no invalid ballots and no abstentions. The votes cast were as follows:

The Reverend Monsignor C. Michael Padazinski: 137
Ms. Meg Romano-Hogan: 55

The Chair declared an election with Reverend Monsognor C. Michael Padazinski selected as Vice President/President-Elect. The election was received with applause.

For the Office of Treasurer:

192 valid ballots were cast, 97 were needed for election. There were no invalid ballots and 1 abstention. The votes cast were as follows:

The Reverend Monsognor Steven Callahan: 91
The Reverend Kevin Niehoff, OP: 101

The Chair declared an election with Reverend Kevin Niehoff, OP selected as Treasurer. The election was received with applause.

For the Office of Consultor:

192 valid ballots were cast, 97 were needed for election. There were no invalid ballots and 1 abstention. The votes cast were as follows:

Ms. Barbara Bettwy: 117
The Reverend Jamin David: 79
The Reverend Msgr. Victor Finelli: 103
Deacon Michael Forbes: 79

The Chair declared an election with Ms. Barbara Bettwy and Reverend

Monsignor Victor Finelli elected as Consultors. The election was received with applause.

REPORTS

PRESIDENT'S REPORT

The Chair referred the assembly to pages 19-20 of the *2019 Annual Reports Booklet*, distributed at the convention registration, for the full text of the President's Report.

The Chair additionally noted that this year had unique challenges, including significant staff turn over. She acknowledged Megan Boland as our new General Secretary. Ms. Boland was received with applause.

The website is functioning, but still not ideal and complete. Work continues on this project through the diligent effort of our office staff. Dr. Decker made assurances that the website will work.

The finances of the Society show recovery this year, which will be further explicated by the Treasurer.

The open houses and campus visits this year were successful in adding new members.

Reverend John Beal has agreed to begin a revision of the *New Commentary on the Code of Canon Law* that was published in 2000.

The committees of the Society are doing excellent work. Dr. Decker summarized several of the initiatives currently underway.

No questions or observations regarding the President's Report were posed.

TREASURER'S REPORT

The Chair next invited Sister Nancy Reynolds, SP, Treasurer, to the podium to provide the Treasurer's Report. She noted that the written report is found on pages 21–30.

The Report shows that the operating budget and the JCL scholarship are nearly equal. This shows the generosity of our membership regarding the scholarships.

Regarding the 2018-2019 budget, Sr. Nancy noted that the gray areas on the budget should not be counted in the totals. When we changed our accounting system, these were erroneously included in operating expenses, but they should not be in separate funds and do not, in reality, count towards the operating

expenses. We ended up with approximately a $12,000 loss. We had previously projected a loss of $87,905. The treasurer is hopeful that next year will have a balanced budget.

Monsignor Tom Green, who passed away on 28 April 2018, has given the Society $7906 as a bequest. Another gift from his estate may be forthcoming at the final distribution. Reverend John C. Hergenrother, who passed away on 8 July 2019, has also provided a bequest to the Society's scholarship fund. He was from the Archdiocese of Chicago. The Society is grateful for the generosity of these devoted priests.

Regarding the 2019-2020 budget, we currently are projecting a $65,000 deficit for 2019-2020. However, we have reached projected income for the convention and, indeed, have received more funds than expected from preconvention workshops.

Our third printing of the *Code of Canon Law, Latin-English Translation* hopefully will be out soon and should provide substantial income.

No review from the audit company was provided before the convention. The audit company had some staff turnover, and they failed to complete the audit in a timely manner.

Reverend Tom Cronkleton requested that future balance sheets include a prior year comparison to be included in proceedings. The Treasurer indicated that it was not done this year because the changes in our accounting system would have led to inaccurate comparisons.

EXECUTIVE COORDINATOR'S REPORT

The Chair next invited Mrs. Donna Miller, Executive Coordinator, to the podium to give the Executive Coordinator's report. She noted that the written report was found on pages 31-33.

Over the last five months Mrs. Miller's focus has been on the third printing of the *Code of Canon Law*. There is some consultation that still needs to occur with the USCCB. She is hopeful that it will be ready by the end of the year. She noted that we are committed to working toward an electronic publication of the code.

She asked that members seriously consider writing an advisory opinion and/or presenting a webinar. The Executive Coordinator is happy to assist anyone who is willing to contribute. She also asked for proposed questions or topics for advisory opinions or for webinars.

Mrs. Miller noted that the major address by Sherry Weddell had led to her

wonder if part of the reason that we have lost members is a loss of trust in the Society. She noted that our personal relationship with absent and former members is important to the health of our society. She additionally noted that an issue of trust is that the database is down; it will be a primary focus to get the database up and running.

No questions or observations regarding the Executive Coordinator's report were posed.

GENERAL SECRETARY'S REPORT

The Chair invited Mrs. Megan Boland, General Secretary, to the podium to give the General Secretary's report. The written report of the former General Secretary, Ms. Colleen Crawford, can be found in these 2019 *Proceedings*, following that of the Executive Coordinator. Mrs. Boland began by noting that, having just been hired as General Secretary three weeks ago, her observations will be limited.

She expressed her gratitude to the society for their support as she took on her new role.

There were no questions or comments posed.

RESOLUTIONS

The Chair read the applicable CLSA *Bylaws* that govern the proposal of resolutions from the floor and asked if there were any such resolutions to be presented. A resolution was presented from the floor. Ms. Nwazi Nyirenda led the discussion of the resolution.

Resolution from the Floor

PROPOSED BY: Ms. Patricia Dugan, Sr. Victoria Vondenberger, RSM, Reverend Paul Golden, CM, Reverend Francis Morrisey, OMI

TITLE: Study of (the) U.S. National Tribunal for Clergy Penal Cases

STATEMENT OF RATIONALE:

WHEREAS, a national tribunal for clergy penal cases has been raised and discussed at all levels of canon law;

WHEREAS there has been a proliferation of penal cases against bishops, presbyters, and deacons;

BE IT RESOLVED THAT the CLSA commission a study regarding the desirability and feasibility of a U.S. national tribunal for penal cases, the results to be reported to the Society at the 2020 convention.

IMPLEMENTATION BY MEANS OF: The establishment of a committee.

ANTICIPATED COST: $1000

COST SUPPLIED BY: CLSA

The resolution was moved by the committee.

Patricia Dugan spoke in favor of the resolution. She noted that there are several national tribunals and that the Netherlands just erected the first national penal tribunal. She noted some issues that would need to be addressed, such as civil liability, qualifications, etc.

Reverend Phil Brown spoke in favor of the resolution. He noted a recent article in *First Things* magazine related to the backlog of penal cases. The resolution will allow us to look into the issue.

Deacon Matt Glover recommended that regional tribunals be considered as part of the proposal.

Reverend Jack Ward spoke in favor of the resolution. He noted that it is difficult to get a consistently fair trial for the accused, depending on whether the bishop is following the law, and whether the Congregation for the Roctrine of teh Faith (CDF) adequately moves things forward.

Most Reverend Thomas Paprocki asked for a clarification regarding the use of the term "bishop." It gives the impression that the bishops would also be subject to a national tribunal, when they are only subject to the Holy See. He proposed a friendly amendment regarding "clergy." The friendly amendment was accepted.

The Chair requested other interventions in favor of or against the resolution.

The Chair called the question on the resolution; the resolution was adopted by the membership with the requisite simple majority having voted in favor.

OLD BUSINESS

The Chair then opened the floor to discuss any Old Business of interest to the assembly; there was none.

NEW BUSINESS

The Chair opened the floor to discuss any New Business of interest to the assembly; there was none.

VARIA

The Chair invited visiting officials of other canon law societies to address the assembly.

The Reverend Ken Cafe, from the Canon Law Society of Australia and New Zealand (CLSANZ), noted that their society runs an institute of tribunal practice, as well as a three-year program in canon law for religious leaders. He told us about the impact of the royal commissions on the Church in Australia and New Zealand. He informed the assembly of the anticipated Plenary Council 2020 within Australia. Papua and New Guinea are now attempting to establish their own canon law society. He invited anyone in attendance to become a member of the CLSANZ and to subscribe to their publication *The Canonist*. The next conference is in Melbourne, starting on 31 August 2020. He provided a gift of a stuffed koala to the President.

The Reverend Francis Bradley, from the Canon Law Society of Great Britain and Ireland (CLSGBI) offered his appreciation to the Society for the invitation and hospitality received. He passed along the greetings of his society. The CLSGBI annual convention next year will be 4-8 May 2020 in Galway, Ireland.

The Reverend Michael Fahlman, from the Canadian Canon Law Society (CCLS) offered greetings from the president and noted his appreciation for his reception. The CCLS convention will be held in Quebec City, Quebec, next week, 21-24 October 2019. Next year's CCLS convention will be held in Calgary.

The Reverend Monsignor Pius Kii was recognized. He is the president of the Canon Law Society of Nigeria.

ADJOURNMENT

The Chair entertained a motion to adjourn. The motion was seconded and approved by the assembly. The eighty-first annual business meeting adjourned at 12:29 p.m.

Respectfully submitted,
Mr. Timothy M. Olson
Secretary

VARIA

CONVENTION MASS HOMILY WEDNESDAY OF THE TWENTY-EIGHTH WEEK IN ORDINARY TIME

The Reverend John Donovan

For those who do not know me I am Father John Donovan, a priest of the Diocese of Syracuse. I am a member of the Board of Governors, ending my term in the next 8-10 minutes. Please, if called upon to serve on committees or to run for the Board of governors, respond yes. It is a rewarding experience, enriching your knowledge of law and the many resources we are to one another. That is the end of my commercial.

I am truly honored and humbled that our soon-to-be Past President, Zabrina Decker, asked me to give this homily. This goes back to a lesson taught when I was young: "Ask questions before you agree." I was pleased to say yes to Zabrina and forgot completely the irony faced each year until I looked at the readings. And again, I am humbled.

Humility is often hard to come by in our role as canonists; we need to be confident, emphatic and at times forceful. In a discussion a few years ago with my now retired ordinary, I began a sentence with, "In my humble opinion." He stopped me from going any further and stated, "John, there is nothing humble about your opinion." We are often accused of not paying "attention to judgment and to love for God." We, like the Pharisees, are often charged with maintaining the rule, upholding the very law that is to serve as preserving freedom; possibly forgetting at times that the law is an instrument towards salvation, not salvation itself.

My niece Christine was just shy of three, it was Pentecost Sunday and she came to the parish I was serving. She said to me later that day at dinner, "Uncle John, I saw you at Church today." I said, "Yes, Christine I saw you too." She said, "You were wearing a big red thing." Now this was the late 80s, it was a chasuble from Slabbink, and it had yellows and oranges in it; it was very loud, as the fabric basically depicted flames. You also must know, my hair then was still very bright red, so red was not a color I wore. I said, "Yes, Christine, it is Pentecost and I wear red on Pentecost." She said, "You were really ugly." So, humility is not hard to come by with family or the honesty of small children.

We do not always have those honest voices around us. In fact, we are very aware that we rarely hear the truth, be it in marriage testimony or addressing a grave delict. For those involved in administration and personnel work, it is easy to assume that people are lying to us, which often leads us to become defensive, or even dogmatic. Woe to us who do not respond with a kind heart, even when we know we are being played.

We cannot truly serve without making every effort to listen with the ears and the heart of God. That is the beauty of our system of law: the ideal is stated, and we can respond pastorally within the law. We are instruments of God's mercy and compassion. As we hear today from St. Paul: "Or do you hold his priceless kindness, forbearance, and patience in low esteem, unaware that the kindness of God would lead you to repentance?" [Romans 2:5]

We are intelligent people who know that in the end the one with the most toys does not win. Yet we collect our toys; be they our gadgets, crystal, books, golf, or our travel. I suggest that we add to that collection: the time we focus on how busy we are, add another title on our CV and every time we think, "Them--those people—they just don't get it." Our role is to accompany people on their faith journey, even as contentious as our situations may become. We are the baptized, Missionary Disciples, whose role is distinct, but not removed from the responsibility of the "perseverance of good works."

Humility is not self-deprecation, but rather the use of our skills, our knowledge, our wisdom to build others up, so they, too, serve as Missionary Disciples. We are to teach and empower gently, correct justly and serve compassionately.

"Woe also to you scholars of the Law" [Luke 11: 45]. Who do you see in the mirror? Are you the "minister" you wish your mother would encounter? Is the law a hindrance to your relationships, if so, what needs to change? Do people wish to emulate your compassion, mercy and kindness? We each know the answer, and the answer we hope to give. Who are the Missionary Disciples accompanying you in this faith journey, or does pride prevent that?

My four-year-old great niece, Londyn, the daughter of my niece Christine who I spoke of, lives in Charlotte and was in town this summer; she is a pip! I was making dinner, and she was "visiting" grandma and great-grandma and turned to her mother and asked, "Why is Uncle John wearing a red apron?" Christine responded, "So his clothes don't get dirty while he is making dinner." Londyn then stated, "But Mommy it clashes with his face." Once again, I was put in my place, humbled, not because of who I am, or how I have served. It is a reminder that we need to understand and listen to the questions and needs, because we are not always on the same path or addressing the same thing. Londyn was asking about red, not an apron.

We are on a journey of faith. Our baptism calls us to be Missionary Disciples, to serve. Our role is just that, a role, not what defines who we are as individuals or as believers. How we live that role, defines our commitment as a faithful disciple. I am particularly fond of the words of St. Augustine in his sermon to pastors; I believe they apply to all of us. He states:

> I must distinguish carefully between two aspects of the role the Lord has given me, a role that demands a rigorous accountability, a role based on the Lord's greatness rather than on my own merit. The first aspect is that I am a Christian; the second, that I am a leader. I am a Christian for my own sake, whereas I am a leader for your sake; the fact that I am a Christian is to my own advantage, but I am a leader for your advantage.
>
> Many persons come to God as Christians but not as leaders. Perhaps they travel by an easier road and are less hindered since they bear a lighter burden. In addition to the fact that I am a Christian and must give God an account of my life, I as a leader must give him an account of my stewardship as well.

-St. Augustine's sermon on Pastors, Office of Readings, 24th Sunday of Ordinary Time

Let's be clear: we have very needed skills which assist us in our roles. As Missionary Disciples we cannot let our roles or our skills get in the way of the journey we share with those we serve. We are Christians and leaders who are accountable to God and one another wherever our journey takes us.

VARIA

ROLE OF LAW CITATION
Doctor Zabrina Decker

Our Role of Law recipient was born in the previous millennium and lived in the same city up until retirement. The public school system educated our recipient for elementary school and then he attended four diocesan seminaries, three of which are now closed. He did not have an outstanding academic career but managed to obtain a Bachelor of Science degree in Biology, before Mastering Divinity and being ordained a diocesan priest in 1977.

Early in his career as a parish priest, he became involved in the newly established ministry to the separated and divorced, which led him to ask the Tribunal if it needed any assistance. He did not envision that lasting 27 years. After a two year internship at the diocesan tribunal, during which time he became a member of the Canon Law Society of America, he pursued canon law studies at St. Paul University in Ottawa, Ontario, where he obtained his Doctorate of Canon Law in 1987, under the guidance of Frank Morrisey, with Dean Jean Thorn occasionally having to scrape him off the ceiling.

After the completion of his degree, he returned to the diocesan tribunal, where he served at various times as Advocate, Promoter of Justice, Defender of the Bond, Adjutant Judicial Vicar, and Judicial Vicar. He also had several terms on the Interdiocesan Court of Appeals. For the last ten years, the job of Vicar for Canonical Services was added to his duties, during which time he had to learn the ins and outs of penal law, often with the help of Bill Woestman's books. He also served in parochial ministry at two different parishes, mostly in intercultural settings, and participated in various types of canonical education throughout the diocese, as well as on the presbyteral council and college of consultors.

After leaving full-time canonical ministry, he was appointed chaplain to the Catholic students in a university setting, where he served until his retirement in 2017. From 1996 to 2009, he was an adjunct professor at the only diocesan seminary he has not closed. Since 2005, he has taught canon law at Catholic Theological Union and, since 2009, in the Catholic University of America's summer program. He has given several pre-convention workshops for the CLSA, as well as a number of seminars and major addresses. His articles have appeared in *The Jurist and Studia canonica*, among other publications.

I am honored to present this year's Role of Law Award to Monsignor Patrick Lagges.

VARIA

ROLE OF LAW RESPONSE

The Reverend Monsignor Patrick R. Lagges, J.C.D.

This is the third time that the Canon Law Society of America has presented the Role of Law Award to a priest of the Archdiocese of Chicago. Ray Goedert received the award in 1975 for his work "On Due Process," and John Dolciamore in 1981 for his work in establishing the modern-day Tribunal. Both of these priests made my job infinitely easier, since I just had to step into what they had already set up. I also had the privilege of working in Chicago with two other Role of Law Award recipients: Barbara Anne Cusack and Bill Woestman, who also enriched my understanding of the law in so many ways. And, over the years in the summer program at the Catholic University of America, I taught with three other Role of Law Award recipients: Rose McDermott, John Beal and Tom Green. I also served on the Board of Governors with another Role of Law Award Recipient, Bob Deeley.

So I wasn't born a canon lawyer. I was instead, always surrounded by what the author of the Letter to the Hebrews termed a "vast cloud of witnesses," who all pointed to the pastoral application of the law. And, along the way, I stole a lot from a lot of people. But from the first time I heard Frank Morrisey talk at the Mundelein Institute in 1982, I knew that canon law could be a useful tool in bringing God's grace to the community of God's people. And whether it was the precise analysis of Gus Mendonca, the dynamic teaching of Roch Page, or the love of the law exhibited with such creativity and with such insight by Jim Provost and Tom Green, all of these—and many more—allowed me to see the life-giving ways that the law could be used in the service of God's Spirit.

It is our privilege as canon lawyers to be able to combine the law of love with the love of law. But we need to do so with what Pope Francis most recently referred to at the opening of the Synod on Amazonia as a "daring prudence."

Most of us, at one time of another—and we heard it again in Sherry Anne Weddell's talk this morning—have used the quote of St. John Paul II in *Sacrae disciplinae legis* that "The Code is in no way intended as a substitute for faith, grace and the charisms in the life of the Church and of the faithful. On the contrary, its purpose is rather to create such an order in the ecclesial society that, while assigning the primacy to faith, grace and the charisms, it at the same time renders easier their organic development in the life both of the ecclesial society and of the individual persons who belong to it." The challenge of that quote, though, is to see, in the work that we are asked to do, the faith, grace,

and charisms behind the work that we do; to keep the law at the service of the faith, grace, and charisms that exist in the Christian community. So that, instead of asking *what is the law?* we first must ask *what is the charism? Where is the grace?* Only after recognizing the charism and the grace and the faith of the Church can we assist it with the "daring prudence" that is in the law.

One of the areas of the law that I have come to later in life, in teaching at Catholic Theological Union in Chicago, was religious law. One of the things that I found there was the call to "daring prudence" that is exemplified in canon 605 about new forms of religious life. The canon urges bishops "to strive to discern new gifts of consecrated life granted to the Church by the Holy Spirit." This canon contains a reminder that the Spirit is constantly bestowing upon the Church new gifts, and that the duty of bishops is to discern those gifts. The bishop is not to wait for the gifts to come to him. He should be actively searching them out among God's people, to understand how God might be enriching the community that has been entrusted to his care. Pope Francis, in opening the Synod last week, expanded that to include all those entrusted with pastoral care in the Church. He said, "It is the virtue of the pastor who, in order to serve with wisdom, is able to discern, to be receptive to the newness of the Spirit," with that "daring prudence" that is itself the gift of the Spirit. That, too, is the task of canonists.

When I teach, particularly when I teach sacramental law, I always tell my students that the purpose of the canons is to make God's grace more accessible to God's people. That's why the canons set the bar so low on what is required minimally for the reception of the sacraments: for baptism, an unbaptized child; for confirmation, the ability to renew one's baptismal promises; for the Eucharist, the ability to distinguish the body of Christ from regular bread, and so on. The code sets the bar low so that God's grace might be poured out on God's people in abundance. We are not the guardians of God's grace, but the dispensers of it. That's why, as Bill Woestman reminded us in accepting the Role of Law Award a few years ago, canonists were called in an earlier age *priests of justice*, those who represent and embody the righteousness of God on behalf of God's people.

That means that, before we answer a question, before we give a canonical opinion on something, we ought to re-connect ourselves with the One whose righteousness we embody. I served on the Metropolitan Tribunal for twenty-seven years. As those of you who also serve on tribunals know, people are not always at their best when they call us. (Bishops aren't, either, in my experience.) Especially in my early years, there were a number of stormy phone calls. They were never satisfying. But, as time went on, I tried doing something different before those calls—and sometimes in the middle of them. I tried praying. Before I returned a call—sometimes in the midst of a call—I asked God to allow me to say what the person needed to bring them God's peace. And I found that it worked. My angry phone calls diminished. And even when I was telling the person things that they didn't want to hear, or things that they disagreed with, the

words that I used were not hurtful; they were words that were aimed at healing, and words that in some way communicated God's grace.

I continued those prayers before the other things I did as well: in handling sexual misconduct cases, in writing decrees closing parishes or decrees establishing institutions within the Archdiocese, in dealing with the sometimes messiness of parish life or diocesan life, and even before the canon law classes that I teach. (I hope that my students don't find that discouraging – "THAT was the result of prayer?") In addition to the adage, "Think before you speak," I added "Pray before you speak." Bring Jesus into the conversation.

It is part of keeping before one's eyes the salvation of souls. I found that it was the way that I did that: looking first for the charism to which I would apply the law; looking for the ways to make God's grace more accessible to the community; praying for the wisdom to say the right thing.

I thank the Board of Governors for this honor. But most of all I thank all of those canonists with whom I was privileged to work and who have taught me so much along the way.

Varia

U.S. Tribunal Statistics

2018

Since 1975, the CLSA has published Tribunal Statistics annually in Proceedings. These statistics are provided voluntarily by participating tribunal offices in the United States. Tribunals were asked to submit a copy of the report sent annually to the Apostolic Signatura, as well as some basic financial information. Submissions came by mail to the administrative office or by online entry (via custom tribunal membership tiers) on www.clsa.org. This electronic change implemented several years ago has resulted in a more accurate comparison of statistics among U.S. tribunals.

The requested template for Tribunal Statistics for calendar year 2016 was modified by former Executive Coordinator Roger Keeler, to match more closely new information being asked by the Signatura. Collections for calendar years 2017 and 2018 were temporarily suspended due to website reconstruction. Now that the website is operational, statistics will be sought and collated for 2019 during the Spring of 2020.

While analytics were not available for reproduction in this booklet, the statistics and subsequent commentary will resume with the edition of *Proceedings of the 82nd Annual Convention.*

Varia

Board of Governors

Zabrina Decker, JCD
President

Jay Conzemius, JCL
Vice-President/President-Elect

The Reverend Monsignor John J. M. Foster, JCD
Past President

Timothy Olson, JCL
Secretary

Sr. Nancy Reynolds, SP, JCL
Treasurer

The Reverend John Donovan, JCL
Consultor

Susan Mulheron, JCL
Consultor

Chad Glendinning, JCD
Consultor

Christina Hip-Flores, JCD
Consultor

Mary Santi, JCL
Consultor

The Reverend Joseph Newton, JCL
Consultor

Administrative Staff

Mrs. Donna Miller, JD, JCL
Executive Coordinator

Ms. Colleen Crawford
General Secretary

Mrs. Megan Boland
Administrative Assistant

Varia

Convention Contributors

The Reverend Jobe Abbass, OFM Conv., JCD, Retired Professor of Canon Law

Dr. Diane L. Barr, JD, JCD, PhD, Chancellor, Archdiocese of Baltimore, Maryland (Pre-convention workshop)

Sr. Nancy Ann Bauer, OSB, JCD, Assistant Professor of Canon Law, The Catholic University of America, Washington, DC

The Reverend John P. Beal, JCD, Professor of Canon Law, The Catholic University of America, Washington, DC (Pre-convention workshop)

The Reverend Sean Bransfield, JCL, Vice Chancellor and Assistant to the Vicar for Clergy, Archdiocese of Philadelphia, Pennsylvania; Parochial Vicar, Saint Matthias Parish, Bala Cynwyd, Pennsylvania; Adjunct Professor of Canon Law, St. Charles Borromeo Seminary, Wynnewood, Pennsylvania

The Most Reverend Andrew H. Cozzens, STD, DD, Auxiliary Bishop, Archdiocese of Saint Paul & Minneapolis, Minnesota

The Very Reverend Georges de Laire, MEd, MDiv, JCL, Judicial Vicar, Vicar for Canonical Affairs, Liaison for Religious, Diocese of Manchester, New Hampshire

The Very Reverend Peter A. Faulk, JCL, Judicial Vicar, Diocese of Alexandria, Louisiana

The Reverend David Fulton, STD, JCD, Associate Professor of Moral Theology, St. Mary's Seminary and University, Baltimore, Maryland

Mr. Christopher J. Fusco, JD, JCL, Associate General Counsel, Diocese of Metuchen, New Jersey; Associate Director of Civil Law, The Resource Center for Religious Institutes, Silver Spring, Maryland (No seminar text)

Mr. Vincent Gardiner, JCL, Chancellor and Judge, Diocese of Cleveland, Ohio

Deacon Matthew Glover, JD, JCL, Chancellor for Canonical Affairs and General Counsel, Diocese of Little Rock, Arkansas

Dr. Wojciech Kowal, OMI, PhD, JCD, Vice-Dean of the Faculty of Canon Law, Saint Paul University, Ottawa, Ontario

The Reverend Elias Mallon, SA, STL, PhD, KHS, External Affairs Office, Catholic Near East Welfare Association

The Most Reverend Mark O'Connell, JCD, Auxiliary Bishop, Archdiocese of Boston, Massachusetts; Pastor, St. Theresa Parish, North Reading, Massachusetts

The Most Reverend Thomas John Paprocki, JD, JCD, Bishop of Springfield in Illinois

Ms. Siobhan Verbeek, JCD Cand., Director of Canonical Services, United States Conference of Catholic Bishops, Washington, DC (No seminar text)

Ms. Sherry Weddell, Executive Director, Catherine of Siena Institute

Varia

List of Participants

Jobe Abbass
Ottawa, ON
Joseph Abraham
Reno, NV
Anne Ameno
Buffalo, NY
John Amos
Gaylord, MI
Diana Anderson
Orlando, FL
Bruce Ansems
Kansas City, KS
William Anton
Plainview, TX
Christopher Armstrong
Washington, DC
Joseph Arsenault
Kansas City, KS
Nazario Atukunda
Portland, OR
Joseph Augustine
Wheeling, WV
Luke Austin
Middlebury, VT
Alberto Avella
Grats, NM
Paul Baillargeon
London, ON
Diane Barr
Baltimore, MD
Mark Bartchak
Altoona, PA
James Bartoloma
Camden, NJ
Nancy Bauer
Washington, DC
John Beal
Erie, PA

John Bell
Allen, TX
Joseph Bellerive
Orlando, FL
Iden Bello
Laredo, TX
William Benwell
Metuchen, NJ
Barbara Bettwy
Harrisburg, PA
Mary Gen Blittschau
Evansville, IN
Michael Boccaccio
Bridgeport, CT
Douglass Bond
Chicago, IL
James Bonke
Indianapolis, IN
Paul Bouchard
Manchester, NH
Michael Bradley
Chicago, IL
Francis Bradley
President CLSGBI
Sean Bransfield
Philadelphia, PA
Christopher Brashears
Guymon, OK
Cecilia Brennan
Monterey, CA
Ken Broussard
Lafayette, LA
Phillip Brown
Baltimore, MD
Anne Bryant
Houston, TX
Linda Budney
Bethesda, MD

Raymond Bueno
Stanwood, WA
Michael Burke
Orlando, FL
Kurt Burnette
Passaic, NJ
Jeffrey Cabral
Fall River, MA
Jesus Cabrera
Milwaukee, WI
Ken Cafe
President CLSANZ
Carl Caldwell
Euclid, OH
Steven Callahan
San Diego, CA
Gregory Caridi
Dallas, TX
Javier Castrejon
Raleigh, NC
David Castronovo
Joliet, IL
Charles
Chaffman
San Antonio, TX
Margaret Chalmers
Birmingham, AL
James Clark
Memphis, TN
John Michael Clark
Owensboro, KY
Paul Clark
Harrisburg, PA
Linda Collins
Fort Worth, TX
Jay Conzemius
Pittsburgh, PA

Patrick Cooney
Owensboro, KY
Edwin Coreas
Houston, TX
James Coriden
Washington, DC
Paul Counce
Baton Rouge, LA
Thomas Cronkleton
Cheyenne, WY
Eric Culler
Toledo, OH
Jamin David
Baton Rouge, LA
Georges de Laire
Manchester, NH
Zabrina Decker
Milwaukee, WI
Robert Deeley
Portland, ME
David Deibel
Monterey, CA
Jesus Del Angel León
Fresno, CA
Louis DeNinno
Pittsburgh, PA
John Dermond
Trenton, NJ
Lee Descoteaux
Rockville Centre, NY
James DeViese
Wheeling, WV
Jane Devlin
Boston, MA
Javier Diaz
Trenton, NJ
John Dickinson
Portland, ME
Paul DiGirolamo
Philadelphia, PA
Anthony Dill
Harrisburg, PA
Melanie DiPietro
Greensburg, PA

Francis Dolan
Chicago, IL
Carlos Donato
Memphis, TN
John Donovan
Syracuse, NY
Patricia Dugan
Philadelphia, PA
Brian Dunn
Antigonish, NS
Frederick Easton
Bloomington, IN
Juan Echavarria
Worcester, MA
Mary Edlund
Dallas, TX
Peter Eke
Gaylord, MI
Chidi Ekpendu
Los Angeles, CA
William Elder
Lake Charles, LA
Michael Fahlman
Vice President, CCLS
John Faris
Glen Allen, VA
Eric Fasano
Rockville Centre, NY
Robert Fath
Fairbanks, AK
Thomas Feeney
Corpus Christi, TX
Karla Felix-Rivera
Sacramento, CA
Christopher Ferrer
Austin, TX
Victor Finelli
Allentown, PA
Ryan Fitzgerald
Houston, TX
Michael Forbes
Austin, TX
Debbie Foreman
Lake Charles, LA

Shannon Fossett
Portland, ME
John Foster
Washington, DC
Christopher Fraser
Phoenix, AZ
Matthew Frisoni
Albany, NY
Canuto Emeritus
Fuentebella
Aruba
Matthew Furgiuele
Gaylord, MI
Christopher Fusco
Metuchen, NJ
Gerardo Galaviz
Los Angeles, CA
Mark Gantley
Honolulu, HI
Stephen Garbitelli
Portland, OR
Chris Garcia
Silver Spring, MD
Jose Garcia
Houston, TX
Vincent Gardiner
Cleveland, OH
Joseph Gehret
Indianapolis, IN
John Giel
Orlando, FL
M. Margaret Gillett
Dallas, TX
Garry Giroux
Ogdensburg, NY
Chad Glendinning
Ottawa, ON
Matthew Glover
Little Rock, AR
Jason Gries
Evansville, IN
Janice Grochowsky
Dodge City, KS
Ralph Gross
Milwaukee, WI

David Gross
Grand Rapids, MI
Kathleen Hahn
Grand Island, NE
Joseph Hannawacker
Trenton, NJ
Andrew Hart
Little Rock, AR
Robert Hayes
San Jose, CA
Christina Hip-Flores
Camden, NJ
Thuan Hoang
San Francisco, CA
Christopher House
Springfield, IL
Rina Huntwork
Grand Island, NE
Robert Hyde
Syracuse, NY
James Innocenzi
Lawrenceville, NJ
Fernanda Jaimes
Austin, TX
Eileen Jaramillo
Lansing, MI
Cesar Jaramillo
Paterson, NJ
Jolene Jasinski
Beaver Falls, PA
Ronny Jenkins
Washington, DC
Lawrence John
Amarillo, TX
Gerald Jorgensen
Dubuque, IA
Rita Joyce
Pittsburgh, PA
Michael Joyce
Saint Louis, MO
Victoria Kaczmarek
Louisville, KY
Thomas Kadera
Wheatland, WY

David Keene
Chicago, IL
Daniel Ketter
Atlanta, GA
Pius Kii
Port-Harcourt, Nigeria
Adela Maria Kim
Peoria, IL
Wayne Kirkpatrick
Toronto, ON
David Klein
Camden, NJ
Daniela Knepper
Muskego, WI
Joji Reddy
Konkala
Amarillo, TX
Thomas Koons
Allentown, PA
Patrick Lagges
Chicago, IL
Bonnie Landry
Lake Charles, LA
Daniel Laurita
Athens, AL
Raphael Lee
Newark, NJ
Rafael Leon
Raleigh, NC
John Lessard-Thibodeau
Springfield, MA
Andres Ligot
San Jose, CA
John List
Lexington, KY
Laton Lohmann
Bismarck, ND
Debra Luenser
Fort Worth, TX
Paul Luniw
Stamford, CT
Gregory Luyet
Little Rock, AR
John Lyttle
New York, NY

Paul Madrid
Austin, TX
Sandra Makowski
Charleston, SC
Edward Malesic
Greensburg, PA
W. Curtis Mallet
Lafayette, LA
Charles Mangan
Sioux Falls, SD
Salvatore Manganello
Buffalo, NY
Jeannine Marino
Washington, DC
David Masello
Providence, RI
Joseph Matt
Kansas City, MO
Reynaldo
Matunog
Los Angeles, CA
Alberto Maullon
Houston, TX
Robert McBride
Newark, NJ
Jaclyn McEachern
Washington, DC
Micheál McGavigan
Derry, Ireland
Wendy McGrath
Manchester, NH
Maureen
McPartland
Dubuque, IA
Joseph McQuaide
Wilmington, DE
Mark Mealey
Wilmington, DE
Lester Mendonsa
Vicariate of S. Arabia
Gloria Mendoza
Fort Worth, TX
Felix Menendez
Atlanta, GA

Gerard Mesure
Philadelphia, PA
Clare Millea
Hartford, CT
Pamela Miller
Cheyenne, WY
Bruce Miller
Alexandria, LA
Donna Miller
The Villages, FL
Richard Millette
Houston, TX
Edith Miranda
Oklahoma City, OK
Arthur Mollenhauer
Bridgeport, CT
Chris Moore
Baltimore, MD
Laura Morrison
Camden, NJ
Francis Morrissey
Ottawa, ON
Peter Mottola
Rochester, NY
Susan Mulheron
Saint Paul, MN
Patrick Mullins
Brisbane, Australia
Luis Navarro Hernandez
Stockton, CA
Dennis Nesser
Charleston, WV
Joseph Newton
Indianapolis, IN
Benedict Nguyen
Corpus Christi, TX
Kevin Niehoff
Grand Rapids, MI
Valere Nkouaya Mbandji
Ottawa, ON
Anthony Norcio
Annapolis, MD
Aaron Nord
St. Louis, MO

Nwazi Nyirenda
Austin, TX
Mark O'Connell
Boston, MA
Peter O'Donnell
Herington, KS
Kelly O'Donnell
Thousand Oaks, CA
Kathy Olsen
Oklahoma City, OK
Timothy Olson
Fargo, ND
Anthony Omenihu
New York, NY
George Oonnoonny
Verplanck, NY
Jose Opalda
Baltimore, MD
Michael Padazinski
San Francisco, CA
Sara Paglialunga
Fort Worth, TX
William Palladino
Boston, MA
Duaine Pamment
Lansing, MI
Thomas Paprocki
Springfield, IL
Gregory Parkes
St. Petersburg, FL
John Payne
Lake Charles, LA
Mark Payne
Milwaukee, WI
F. Stephen Pedone
Worcester, MA
Lori Peery
San Antonio, TX
Grzegorz Podwysocki
Joliet, IL
Andrea Ponzone
Boston, MA
Daniel Quinan
Saint Paul, MN

Lawrence Rasaian
Tyler, TX
Michael Ravenkamp
San Diego, CA
Amalraj Rayappan
Portland, OR
John Renken
Ottawa, ON
Nancy Reynolds
Louisville, KY
Mark Richards
Sacramento, CA
Kenneth Riley
Kansas City, MO
J. Michael Ritty
Feura Bush, NY
Carmine Rizzi
Newark, NJ
Meg Romano–Hogan
Dallas, TX
Lee Roos
Manassas, VA
Ana Romero
Oklahoma City, OK
Eloise Rosenblatt
San Jose, CA
Daniel Ross
Indianapolis, IN
Magdalen Ross
New York, NY
James Rowland
Tyler, TX
Luis Sanchez
Brownsville, TX
Michael Sanders
Louisville, KY
Mary Santi
Seattle, WA
Noel Sanvicente
San Jose, CA
Michael Scaperlanda
Oklahoma City, OK
Edward Schaefer
St. Rose, IL

Kelly Schaffer
Toledo, OH
Joseph Scheib
Pittsburgh, PA
Sofia Seguel
Washington, DC
Christopher Seibt
Syracuse, NY
Gilbert Seitz
Baltimore, MD
Julianne Shanklin
Boston, MA
Tracey Sharp
Los Angeles, CA
Donetta Shaw
Kansas City, MO
Tara Sheringer
Indianapolis, IN
Langes Silva
Salt Lake City, UT
Robert Sinatra
Camden, NJ
Michael Sinclair
Brisbane, Australia
Louis Sirianni
Rochester, NY
Christopher Siuzdak
Portland, ME
Helen Roberta Small
Seattle, WA
Daniel Smilanic
Chicago, IL
Patricia Smith
Aston, PA
Rosemary Smith
Jersey City, NJ
Janie Snead
Kansas City, KS
Anthony St. Louis-Sanchez
Denver, CO

Jeffrey Staab
Richmond, VA
Richard Stansberry
Oklahoma City, OK
Karen Sullivan-Kight
St. Augustine, FL
Margaret Sullivan
Brighton, MA
Terry Sullivan
Downington, PA
Therese Guerin Sullivan
Cuyahoga Falls, OH
David Szatkowski
Nesbit, MS
Andrew Szymakowski
Redmond, OR
Amy Tadlock
Saint Paul, MN
Michael Taylor
Manchester, NH
John Robinson Thason
Tyler, TX
William Thompson
Owensboro, KY
Rose Marie Timmer
Toledo, OH
Gregory Trawick
Cadiz, KY
Mark Tucker
Washington, DC
Jeffrey Tudgay
Scranton, PA
Ann Tully
Indianapolis, IN
Shawn Tunink
Kansas City, KS
Elisa Ugarte
Richmond, VA

Daniel Ulishney
Greensburg, PA
Benedetto Vaghetto
Pittsburgh, PA
Rodrigo Valdivia
San Diego, CA
John Vaughan
Owensboro, KY
Paul Jesus Velazquez
Los Angeles, CA
Siobhán Verbeek
Washington, DC
Ruben Villarreal
Lake Charles, LA
Ashley Voeller
South Portland, MN
Victoria Vondenberger
Cincinnati, OH
Justin Wachs
Feura Bush, NY
Richard Wahl
Houston, TX
John Ward
Baltimore, MD
Joseph Waters
St. Petersburg, FL
Daniel Welter
Chicago, IL
D. Reginald Whitt
Baltimore, MD
Thomas Wisniewski
Darby, PA
Geri Woodward
New Orleans, LA
V. Dominic Anthony Xavier
Austin, TX
Gary Yanus
Cleveland, OH

Made in United States
North Haven, CT
10 November 2026

22088271R00192